Management of Patients with Dementia

Kristian Steen Frederiksen
Gunhild Waldemar
Editors

Management of Patients with Dementia

The Role of the Physician

Springer

Editors
Kristian Steen Frederiksen
Danish Dementia Research Centre
Department of Neurology
Rigshospitalet
University of Copenhagen
Copenhagen, Denmark

Gunhild Waldemar
Danish Dementia Research Centre
Department of Neurology
Rigshospitalet
University of Copenhagen
Copenhagen, Denmark

ISBN 978-3-030-77903-0 ISBN 978-3-030-77904-7 (eBook)
https://doi.org/10.1007/978-3-030-77904-7

This Springer imprint is published by the registered company Springer Nature Switzerland AG
The registered company address is: Gewerbestrasse 11, 6330 Cham, Switzerland

Preface

This textbook may be the first to give a comprehensive and broad overview of many of the various aspects of medical management of patients with dementia. The book focuses on those aspects in which the physician has a central role in planning of care. Nevertheless, healthcare professionals with other educational backgrounds, e.g. nurses, psychologists or therapists, may also benefit from reading the book. The aim is to provide evidence-based hands-on guidance to clinicians who manage patients with dementia in daily practice, also when high-level evidence may not be available. Here, the authors, many of whom are dementia specialists, give advice based on their own clinical experience.

The first chapters of the book present an overview of the diagnostic work-up of patients suspected of dementia, and the most common causes are given. The main focus of the book is, however, the symptoms, medical comorbidities and complications of dementia which require attention from the physician whether in primary care or at the hospital.

The aspect of medical management of patients with dementia and related areas covered in this book is an ever-evolving field. Future research may change practices leading to new diagnostic tools or treatments. Although the authors have strived to describe generally accepted practices, the application of the knowledge in this book remains the professional responsibility of the practitioner. It is the responsibility of the practitioner to be up to date with all developments related to the contents of this book and to be informed of any local or national guidelines relevant.

Copenhagen, Denmark — Kristian Steen Frederiksen
Copenhagen, Denmark — Gunhild Waldemar

Contents

About the Authors

Kristian Steen Frederiksen, MD, PhD, is a consultant neurologist and director of the Clinical Trial Unit at the Danish Dementia Research Centre, Department of Neurology, Rigshospitalet, in Copenhagen, Denmark. His research focuses on the effects of physical exercise as well as development of diagnostic biomarkers and other aspects of biomarkers in dementia diagnosis. Dr Frederiksen is also the co-chair of the European Academy of Neurology's Scientific Panel on Dementia and Cognitive Disorders and is the lead author on the European guideline on medical management issues in dementia.

Gunhild Waldemar, MD, DMSc, is professor of neurology at the Faculty of Health and Medical Sciences at the University of Copenhagen and director of the Danish Dementia Research Centre at Rigshospitalet in Copenhagen, Denmark. Professor Waldemar has extensive clinical and research experience within various aspects of the dementia field. Professor Waldemar is a member of the executive committee of the European Alzheimer's Disease Consortium and was the lead author of the first European guideline on diagnostic evaluation of dementia.

Management of Patients with Dementia: An Introduction

1

Kristian Steen Frederiksen and Gunhild Waldemar

List of Abbreviations

AD	Alzheimer's disease
FTD	Frontotemporal dementia
LBD	Lewy body dementia
VaD	Vascular dementia
ADL	Activities of daily living
MCI	Mild cognitive impairment

About This Book

Continuous health and care for patients with dementia involves a multidisciplinary, multi-professional team. This book focuses specifically on the role of the physician in this multi-professional team. The types of professions involved in the care of patients with dementia will vary across a patient's disease course, but physicians often play a role in all phases of the disease. Therefore, this book addresses the role of the physician from the initial diagnosis to the end of life. In many regions of Europe and the World, physicians in certain specialties such as neurology, geriatrics, psychiatry, and general practice will play a more prominent role. However, other specialists will also have patients with dementia in their care. Patients with dementia will present in many settings such as inpatient and outpatient services and in surgical specialties and other medical specialties, requiring physicians in these settings to be knowledgeable about dementia. Thus, this book not only aims to

K. S. Frederiksen (✉) · G. Waldemar
Danish Dementia Research Centre, Department of Neurology, Rigshospitalet, University of Copenhagen, Copenhagen, Denmark
e-mail: Kristian.steen.frederiksen@regionh.dk

K. S. Frederiksen, G. Waldemar (eds.), *Management of Patients with Dementia*, https://doi.org/10.1007/978-3-030-77904-7_1

inform those physicians who are in specialties usually associated with the management of patients with dementia, but also a wider audience. The book will offer chapters devoted to those medical issues that physicians are faced with in everyday clinical practice in the management of dementia and aims to give specific recommendations for dealing with such issues. The book is not intended to give an in-depth overview of specific mechanisms of disease and pathology for which we refer to other textbooks. In this chapter, we will give a brief overview of epidemiology and causes of dementia.

There are many reasons why the management of patients with dementia requires specific knowledge on the part of the physician. (1) Patients with dementia are often reliant on other persons for the maintenance of everyday life and activities. This may include family members, and at some point, also professional caregivers, but variation will occur. Caregivers are paramount in the diagnosis, and follow-up as many patients with dementia has reduced insight or will forget symptoms they are experiencing. Patients may not volunteer these or divulge them when asked. Patients may also underestimate the need for care or be unaware of the strain their caregivers may be under. It is therefore very important to include caregivers, and at the same time, be mindful of caregiver burden. (2) Disease conditions may give rise to atypical symptoms in patients with dementia. For example, painful conditions (e.g., dental disease, chest pain due to myocardial infarction, glaucoma, arthritis) may result in altered behavior such as aggression or agitation, or apathy but may not necessarily give rise to verbal complaints of pain. (3) Knowledge of commonly occurring medical comorbidities and complications associated with dementia is also important. This may include specific cognitive symptoms such as spatial orientation difficulties, sleep disorders, an increased risk of delirium, etc. For this and other reasons already mentioned, patients with dementia often have a need for preplanned follow-up with a physician. (4) Communicative issues may also arise due to cognitive impairment. Outright speech and language impairment may be one issue, but also adjusting communication to offset the impact of other cognitive deficits may be necessary. This could include delivering only one piece of information at a time, simplifying the message, or supplementing verbal information with written or visually presented information. (5) Safety of the patient may also be cause for vigilance. For example, patients may be more prone to falls or other accidents due to motor impairment, visuocognitive deficits or poor judgment. This includes driving, which needs to be evaluated regularly. Patients with REM-sleep behavior disorder may also be at risk of falling out of bed with injuries as a result. (6) Issues with pharmacological treatment may arise and may also be a safety concern in terms of, e.g., accidental overdosing if the patient forgets that he or she has already taken the prescribed dose. Compliance issues may also result in the converse—i.e., undertreatment. Another aspect is that patients with dementia are more susceptible to the development of adverse drug reactions and side effects due to brain disorder, age, or comorbidities. Examples include anticholinergic effects, sedating effect, and increased morbidity and mortality in the case of anti-psychotics. (7) Lastly, informed consent for treatment or investigational procedures or participation in research should as always be sought, but competency may often be impaired and thus needs to be evaluated.

Overview of the Dementia Landscape

What Is Dementia?

The definition of dementia has changed over time. In recent times, dementia refers to a syndrome of acquired cognitive impairment which is associated with the decline in the ability to function independently in everyday life. This is also referred to as activities of daily living (ADL). ADL includes managing finances, cooking, shopping, making appointments, cleaning, washing clothes, dressing, personal hygiene, and other activities. This definition also implies that dementia is not a disease in and by itself, but a syndrome that may be caused by many different diseases affecting the brain. Moreover, the definition clearly differentiates dementia from intellectual disabilities present from birth. Dementia is also most often thought of as a chronic condition, but diseases that are reversible may give rise to symptoms that are indistinguishable from dementia. The most widely used diagnostic criteria for dementia are the International Classification of Disease (World Health Organization) [1] with the 11th edition to be published in 2022, and the Diagnostic and Statistical Manual (American Psychiatric Association) [2], the latter using the term major neurocognitive disorders in the latest version (Version 5). Both diagnostic criteria mandate that at least two cognitive domains are affected. See Table 1.1 for a list of the most commonly used diagnostic criteria.

Epidemiology of Dementia

In 2015 an estimated 46.8 mio people lived with dementia worldwide, a figure which is projected to increase to 131.5 mio by 2050. The corresponding figures for Europe were 10.5 in 2015 and 18.6 in 2050 [16]. The estimated worldwide socioeconomic costs associated with dementia amounts to 818 billion USD [16]. When considering the rapid increase, particularly in low and middle-income countries, the impact on human life in patients as well as in family caregivers, and the need for timely planning of care in all societies, the World Health Organization in 2012 defined dementia as a public health priority [17]. The report on dementia as a public health priority was expected to facilitate governments, policy-makers, and other stakeholders to address the impact of dementia as an increasing threat to global health [17], and in fact, many countries have developed national dementia plans.

The age-related prevalence rates have been relatively stable over the past few decades [18], so the increasing overall prevalence observed in most countries [16, 18–21] is related to higher life expectancy and demographic changes, and possibly to the fact that people with dementia may live longer time with the diagnosis. The fact that a slight decline in incidence has been observed in some high-income countries UK, the USA, and Sweden [18, 20] and Denmark [21] are encouraging, but cannot counteract the continuous increase in overall prevalence.

Mortality rates have been stable or declined during the past 2–3 decades [18, 22] with reported mortality rate ratios between 2 and 3. It is possible that the benefits of better cardiovascular health in the general population have also been of benefit for

Table 1.1 Commonly used diagnostic criteria

Condition	Criteria	References
Dementia	*ICD-10*	[1]
Mild cognitive impairment	*ICD-10*	[1]
Major neurocognitive disorder	*DSM-5*	[2]
Minor neurocognitive disorder	*DSM-5*	[2]
Mild cognitive impairment	*Petersen criteria*	[3]
Mild cognitive impairment (Including multi-domain)	*Winblad criteria*	[4]
Alzheimer's disease	*ICD-10*	[1]
Preclinical Alzheimer's disease	*National Institute of Aging-Alzheimer's Association (NIA-AA)*	[5]
Mild cognitive impairment due to Alzheimer's disease	*NIA-AA*	[6]
Dementia due to Alzheimer's disease (including non-memory variants)	*NIA-AA*	[7]
Asymptomatic at risk for Alzheimer's disease	*International Working Group (IWG)*	[8]
Presymptomatic Alzheimer's disease	*IWG*	[8]
Typical and atypical AD	*IWG*	[8]
Criteria for Alzheimer's disease based on biomarkers. Staging according to symptoms.	*NIA-AA Research framework*	[9]
Lewy body dementia	*DLB Consortium*	[10]
Prodromal dementia with Lewy bodies	*DLB Consortium*	[11]
Vascular cognitive impairment	*VASCOG*	[12]
Semantic dementia, non-fluent primary progressive aphasia, logopenic aphasia	*International primary progressive aphasia working group*	[13]
Behavioral variant frontotemporal dementia	*International behavioral variant frontotemporal dementia consortium*	[14]
Limbic-predominant age-related TDP-43 encephalopathy	*LATE Consensus working group*	[15]

people with dementia. However, it is important to note that the mortality rate ratios stay elevated for people with dementia, when compared to people without dementia (6). In fact, according to a recent large nationwide study, the mortality rate ratios gap for dementia has remained unchanged during the past two decades in contrast to the mortality rate ratios gaps for cancer and ischemic heart disease, which have narrowed considerably during the same time period, due to efficient new therapies [22]. Therefore, initiatives for improving health and decreasing mortality in dementia are still highly relevant.

Causes of Dementia

Dementia may be caused by many different neurodegenerative disorders and diseases. Moreover, a number of other medical conditions may cause a dementia-like syndrome. For example, depression may cause significant cognitive impairment and associated impairments in ADL. Vitamin deficiency, thyroid dysfunction, infections of the central nervous system, other psychiatric disorders, and substance abuse may similarly cause cognitive impairment. However, strictly speaking diagnostic criteria for dementia are rarely met in these instances, and the aforementioned conditions may have to be excluded before a specific neurodegenerative dementia disorder is diagnosed. It is important to be vigilant regarding these disorders when diagnosing patients suspected of cognitive impairment and dementia as some of the conditions are potentially reversible.

Neurodegenerative dementia disorders encompass a large number of disorders. However, only a handful are responsible for the vast majority of cases, and include Alzheimer's disease (AD), frontotemporal dementia (FTD), Lewy body dementia (LBD), Parkinson's disease dementia (PDD), and vascular dementia (VaD). Strictly speaking, VaD is not a neurodegenerative disorder, but it shares a number of clinical characteristics of neurodegenerative disorders and commonly occurs alongside neurodegenerative disorders in the same patient (e.g., AD and VaD).

Dementia Disorders

In this section a brief introduction to the most common dementia disorders is given. We kindly refer to textbooks on the matter for more in-depth descriptions. Table 1.1 lists the most commonly applied diagnostic criteria for these disorders.

A Generic Disease Model of Neurodegenerative Dementia Disorders

Neurodegenerative dementia disorders are usually insidious in onset with a slowly progressive disease course. Heterogeneity regarding rate of progression exists within and across disorders, but in general (and ignoring rapidly progressive disorders such as spongiform encephalopathies) disease courses last years and progression is not evident from day to day, but rather over months or years. However, fluctuations from day to day (or even over shorter intervals) may occur.

A generic model of how neurodegenerative dementia disorders develop and from where they derive their unique clinical manifestation and course may be formulated (see Figs. 1.1 and 1.2). In AD, the specific pathophysiological mechanisms have been substantiated by findings from numerous studies [23, 24] but remain less well examined for the other neurodegenerative dementia disorders. An asymptomatic phase characterized by the accumulation of brain pathology is believed to precede clinical symptoms. In all neurodegenerative dementia disorders, specific proteins are known to accumulate in distinct brain regions, and it is generally believed that this accumulation begins in the asymptomatic phase, perhaps up to 2 or 3 decades prior to the emergence of the first symptoms. The preference of these presumed toxic proteins to accumulate in specific brain regions is believed to give rise to the clinical profile which is characteristic for each neurodegenerative dementia disorder. For example, tau accumulates (together with beta-amyloid) in the entorhinal cortex and hippocampus leading to early and prominent memory impairment in AD. Following this asymptomatic phase, patients will develop subtle cognitive impairments initially without impairments in the ability to perform ADL, and therefore will not fulfill criteria for dementia. In the 1990s, this predementia phase was coined mild cognitive impairment (MCI) and defines a transitional phase in which the patient or caregiver registers a change in cognition [3]. Further, the impairment

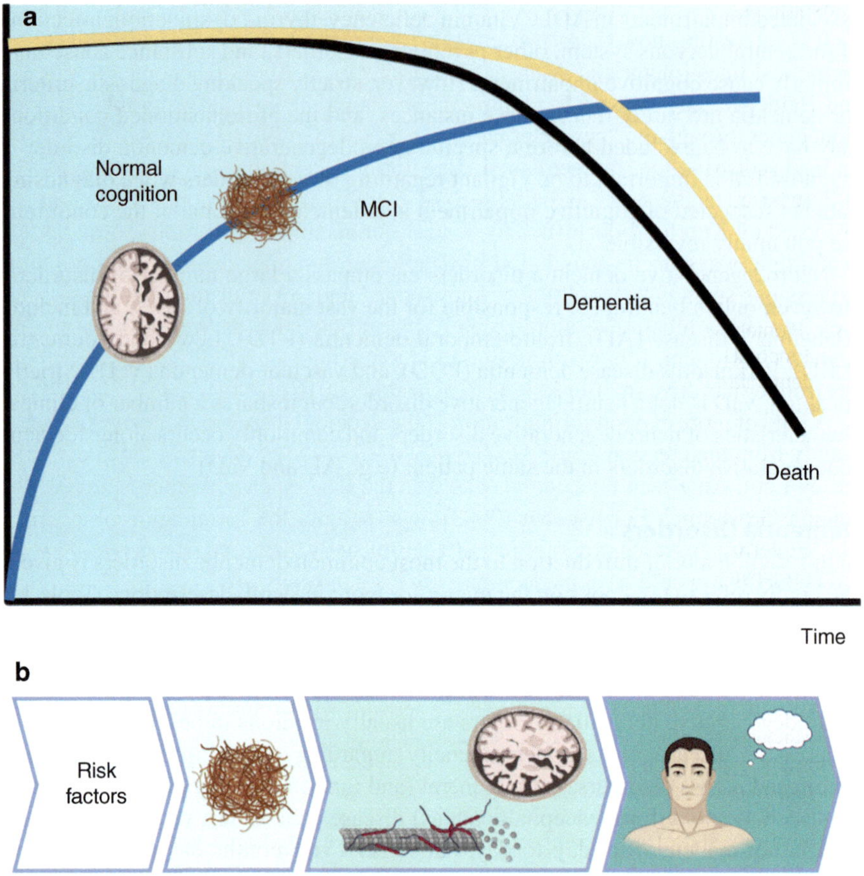

Fig. 1.1 Generic disease model for neurodegenerative dementia diseases. The figure depicts the various steps in the clinical and pathophysiological course of neurodegenerative dementias. Presumably, a number of interacting risk factors, including environmental and genetic factors interact to initiate and propagate the accumulation of pathological and toxic (to nerve cells and other brain cells) protein in isolated brain areas (predilection areas) (panel **b**). This occurs in the asymptomatic phase of the disease, where cognition will be normal (panel **a**). As protein accumulation spreads to other brain areas and neuronal dysfunction and frank cell death occurs, brain atrophy and subtle symptoms will develop. Onset is almost always insidious and slowly progressive through the various stages until the end-stage where the patient is bedridden, in need of 24-h care, and finally death ensues

is objectively measurable through cognitive assessment. Patients may only be affected on one cognitive domain as a reflection of the spatially limited deposition of protein and neuronal dysfunction it causes. In recent years it has been suggested that an additional phase should be interjected between the asymptomatic phase and the MCI phase [25]. This idea has in part been nurtured by the clinical observation that some patients complain of feeling cognitively impaired despite extensive neuropsychological assessment being unable to reveal any deficits. Nevertheless, a higher proportion of these patients may go on to develop MCI and dementia [26].

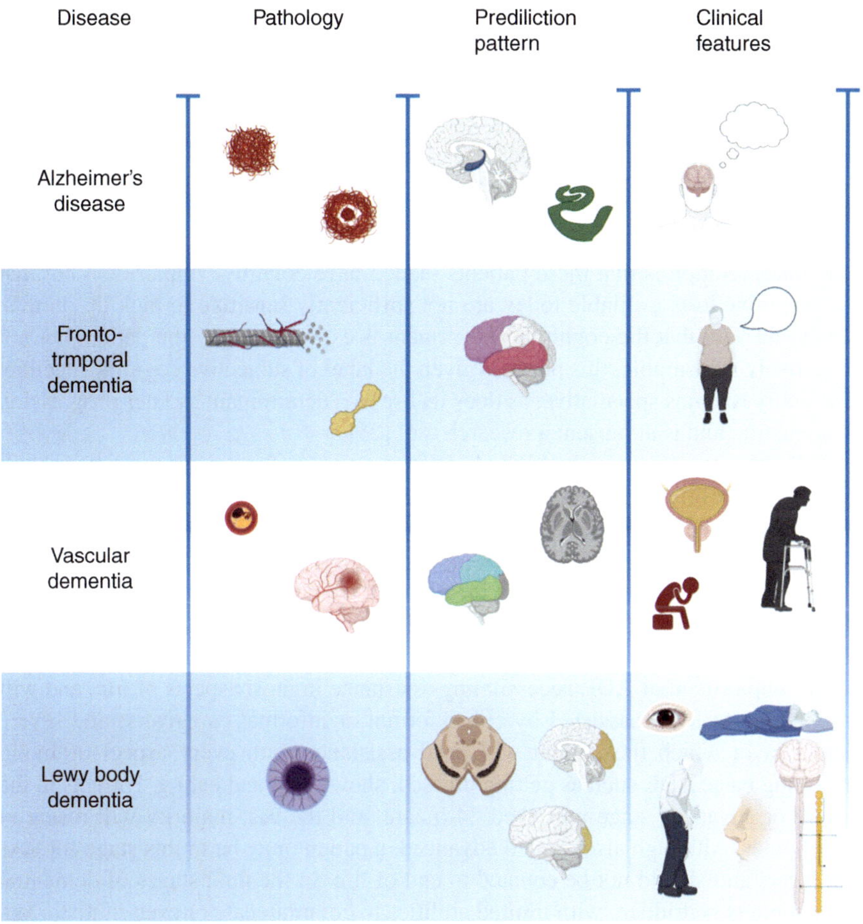

Fig. 1.2 Overview of neurodegenerative dementia disorders. The figure shows the pathological and clinical hallmarks of the four most common dementia disorders. AD: Accumulation of various species of beta-amyloid in extracellular plaques occurs as well as phosphorylated tau (intracellularly). Phosphorylated tau accumulation occurs in the early stages in the entorhinal cortex. This accumulation correlates well with symptoms. Beta-amyloid has a more widespread pattern of accumulation in all of the cortical areas, even in the asymptomatic stage. Atrophy of temporal and parietal cortical areas is a hallmark. Symptoms are cognitive and behavioral and include predominant impairment of episodic memory, but also language impairment and loss of semantic knowledge. FTD: Accumulating proteins leading to FTD include tau, fused in sarcoma protein, progranulin and TAR-DNA binding protein-43. Atrophy is prominent in frontal and temporal cortical areas. Symptoms include executive dysfunction and early and prominent behavioral symptoms such as apathy, inappropriate and disinhibited behavior, and anxiety. Language variants of FTD may present as pure motor speech disorders or with loss of semantic knowledge. VaD: Is caused by pathology of the cerebral vessels (e.g., stenosis or changes induced by hypertension), which leads to chronic microvascular lesions, lacunar infarcts, large-territory infarcts, hemorrhages (including microhemorrhages). Strategic infarcts in the thalamus may lead to dementia. Other common lesions are chronic vascular changes in the white matter (leukoaraiosis). For small vessel disease, a common clinical phenotype is one that includes decreased attention and executive dysfunction,

(continued)

depression, gait impairment, urge incontinence, and other neurological signs (e.g., slight hemiparesis). LBD: Accumulation of alpha-synuclein in Lewy bodies occur early on in brain stem areas. Hypometabolism in occipital regions is a common occurrence leading to visuocognitive impairments. Attentional and executive deficits are also common. A myriad of non-cognitive symptoms is often present with the obligatory presence of Parkinsonism. Other symptoms include REM-sleep behavior disorders, visual hallucinations, fluctuations, high risk of delirium, adverse reactions to anti-psychotics, autonomic dysfunction (e.g., obstipation and orthostatic hypotension), and anosmia.

One interpretation is that these patients indeed have cognitive impairment but that the cognitive tests available today are not sufficiently sensitive to pick up on this. Due to the fact that the cognitive impairment is experienced by the patient but not objectively measurable, this phase is given the label of subjective cognitive decline. The entity remains speculative, as does its use as a determinant of later progression to dementia, and is at present a research tool [25].

Patients may remain in the MCI phase for a number of years, whereas others will progress relatively fast to the dementia phase [27]. This will usually coincide with the spread of the accumulation of protein, neuronal dysfunction, and brain atrophy leading to more severe disease encompassing more cognitive domains and brain functions. Three phases are usually identified in the dementia phase: mild dementia in which the patient will have relatively mild impairment of ADL and able to function independently in some areas of everyday life; moderate dementia, with more severe impairment of ADL necessitating assistance in most aspects of life, and will not be able to live unassisted by either formal or informal caregivers; and severe dementia in which the patient will need assistance with every aspect of living including basic ADL such as getting dressed, showering, and eating. Patients in the severe or advanced stage will need 24-h care, and the vast majority will reside in care homes. Although also termed advanced, a patient may be in this stage for several years and should not be equated to end of life. In the final stages of dementia, the patient is bedridden, with limited abilities to communicate or even mutistic and unable to take food or drink. Neurodegenerative dementias are fatal diseases, and ultimately the patient will die from the disorder.

Alzheimer's Disease

AD is characterized by prominent and early episodic memory impairment. Patients may complain of forgetfulness regarding appointments, items when shopping, contents of conversations, etc. Usually, memories formed prior to the onset of the disease process will be preserved even in moderate stages, reflecting the relative affection of encoding of memories, but eventually, these memories will also erode. Semantic memory will also be affected, and a substantial number of patients will develop wordfinding problems and aphasia. Executive dysfunction and visuocognitive difficulties may also arise. The majority of patients with AD, as with other dementia disorders, will at some point have behavioral or psychiatric symptoms [28]. Depressive symptoms or outright depression, anxiety, irritability, and agitation are quite common, and aggression may develop [29]. Delusions may also arise in some patients which may vary in content, but believing to have been a victim of break-ins, stealing, or fraud is common, sometimes to account for mislaid objects, etc. Thoughts about a spouse's infidelity are also a common delusion. Capgras syndrome is the occurrence of a delusion that a loved one has been replaced by an impostor and may occur in patients with AD [30]. An important and prominent symptom is loss of insight and is almost always present in varying degrees. This may lead to considerable difficulty in getting the patient to accept the diagnosis, treatment, and the need for care, and thus may be a major source of caregiver burden.

As already previously alluded to, deposition of beta-amyloid and tau in cortical regions is believed to be pivotal in the pathophysiology of AD. The amyloid cascade hypothesis remains the backbone of the present understanding of the pathophysiology of AD [31]. The hypothesis states that deposition of beta-amyloid precedes downstream pathological events such as tau deposition, brain atrophy, and ultimately cognitive impairment. It has been suggested to define AD solely as a proteinopathy based on the amyloid cascade [9], but although a large volume of data supports the hypothesis, the repeated failures of phase 3 trials of drugs designed to reduce beta-amyloid to modify clinical symptoms have drawn the hypothesis into question [32]. It is indeed likely that other pathological processes such as immune responses play a role as well [33]. Aside from the deposition of proteins, hippocampal atrophy is an early sign of AD, although it is important to keep in mind that it may occur in other conditions such as depression [34]. Variants of AD include a frontal variant with more prominent executive dysfunction [35], a visual variant (posterior cortical atrophy) with prominent visuocognitive impairment including the occurrence of Balint's syndrome [36], a language impairment (logopenic aphasia) [37], and a parietal variant [38], exist. Moreover, AD may have an early onset (usually defined as below 65 years of age) [39]. Autosomal dominantly inherited AD caused by mutations in the gene coding amyloid precursor protein, a transmembrane protein, from which beta-amyloid is cleaved or presenilin 1 or 2, which is involved in the cleavage of the amyloid precursor protein, also exist [40]. Due to the fact that the amyloid precursor protein gene is located on chromosome 21, patients with Down's syndrome are at an increased risk of developing AD.

Case 1

Michael is a 75-year-old retired shopkeeper married to Judith for 50 year. They have three children. Both Michael and Judith are active retirees. Michael enjoys playing cards and golf with old friends, reading books, and spending time with the family. He has hypertension and was in an accident 7 years ago where he lost most of his vision on the left eye but is otherwise in good health. About a year ago, Judith started to notice that something had changed with Michael. It started by Michael apparently losing interest in reading. He also developed a "habit" of asking Judith about the same things more than once, for example, about appointments or what they were going to cook for dinner. About half a year ago, the couple went to their summer cottage, and on the 1-h drive there, Michael asked Judith three times where they were going, apparently forgetting what he had been told a few minutes before. On the same trip, he also got lost in a small wooded area where he usually goes for walks and wandered around for 2 h before finding his way back. He has also started to forget details from conversations he has had, and when reminded about the content of conversations, he is unable to remember or seem to pretend to remember. Michael has also stopped playing cards and is not as lively in social situations, where he withdraws to a quiet corner. When he is together with just 2 or 3 persons, Michael is more talkative. Michael has on occasion become worried and anxious if Judith has gone out alone. Michael still drives and plays golf. He helps around the house, but not as much as before, and he no longer cooks on his own, but still enjoys cooking together with Judith. Judith also now takes care of the financial side.

Judith confronts Michael with the changes, but Michael denies that something is wrong. He sometimes becomes annoyed when Judith brings up the subject and blames it on old age and that he has lost interest in doing things. Michael finally agrees to go to his GP, who refers him to a memory clinic, where Michael is diagnosed with AD.

Frontotemporal Dementia

FTD is associated with frontotemporal lobar degeneration, and two broad subtypes exist, namely behavioral variant FTD and language variant FTD.

Patients with behavioral variant FTD often present with changes in behavior and cognitive functions residing in frontal and temporal cortical areas. A very common change in behavior is apathy and lack of initiative, but disinhibitory behavior, socially inappropriate behavior, agitation, aggression, anxiety, echolalia, and utilization behavior (i.e., immediately using objects when presented to them) may also occur [41]. Executive dysfunction, impaired planning, and attentional deficits are common.

Case 2

Rachel works in a government office and is 59 years old. She has hypothyroidism. She is married to Ben, who is her second husband. They have no children together, but Rachel has a daughter from her previous marriage. About 1.5 years ago, the office where Rachel worked, was reorganized meaning that the workflow changed, and there were new coworkers who started working in the office. Rachel had difficulties handling the apparent extra workload, and she started to underperform. After about a half year, Rachel made a serious mistake and received a reprimand, after which she was sent home on sick leave. Her doctor diagnosed her with stress. Rachel started to become increasingly passive and did not take any initiative. She would become very anxious if Ben were not around. Rachel was not able to read as she was not able to concentrate on the text but enjoyed watching TV. She developed an extremely sweet tooth and would at times, eat all the candy she could find in the house. At times she would eat without restraint. On several occasions, Rachel's behavior was noticeably different than before. On one occasion, when the couple was invited for dinner, Rachel took eight pieces of meat, leaving only two pieces for the remaining three guests. When reprimanded by Ben, she did not acknowledge any wrongdoing and became very angry. On another occasion, she told a close friend that her dress was ugly and that she smelt. She also made sexual comments to a male friend and told a stranger that she was fat and should lose some weight. Eventually, Rachel was diagnosed with behavioral variant frontotemporal dementia.

As the word implies, patients with the language variant have impairments in language. Two distinct subtypes are usually recognized [13]. In semantic dementia, deficits in semantic memory are apparent such as loss of knowledge about things and concepts or loss of knowledge about pronunciation leading to surface dyslexia (i.e., difficulty in correctly pronouncing the word which does not follow the normal rules of pronunciation in a given language). Spontaneous speech will be fluent but empty and circumlocutory. Semantic dementia is usually associated with severe atrophy, and hypometabolism in the temporal lobe, specifically the temporal pole, and both the left or right side may be affected [42], giving rise to somewhat different symptoms. The second subtype is non-fluent primary progressive aphasia which differs from semantic dementia by principally being a speech motor problem rather than a language problem [13]. The patient may at first display a pure dysarthria underscoring the fact that the disease is a motor problem. Spontaneous speech will be forced and effortful. Both language variants may remain relatively isolated in the sense that other cognitive functions may stay unaffected, and thus dementia may be a misnomer for these conditions. Indeed, patients may have relatively preserved abilities regarding carrying out activities of daily living. However, other symptoms associated with impaired function of the frontal and temporal lobes may occur.

Case 3

To illustrate the differences between non-fluent primary progressive aphasia and semantic dementia, one can imaging asking the patient to name a picture of a zebra. A patient with semantic dementia may say, "Well I know it is an animal. Does it live in Asia or Africa? I forget. I think it eats grass. It looks like another animal which I forgot the name of, but this animal does not have stripes." The patient has clearly lost knowledge of what the name of the zebra is, and also knowledge of the zebra (i.e., whether zebras live in Asia or Africa) as well as knowledge of horses. Imagine asking a patient with non-fluent primary progressive aphasia to name the same picture of a zebra. The attempt may be as follows: "IIIt is a zzzzee....zzzzzeb.....zzzzeb...ra." It is clear that the patient is aware of the target word zebra, but it is laborious for the patient to pronounce the word reflecting the motor speech impairment.

The pathophysiology of FTD remains less well understood than in for example AD. No risk factors apart from genetic risk factors are known. Up to 30% of patients with FTD have been reported to have a strong family history with regards to FTD underscoring a genetic background for many if not all cases of FTD [43]. Nevertheless, only a small number of disease-causing genes are known, and for the majority of patients with FTD, a single genetic cause is not found. One of the common genetic causes of FTD is the hexanucleotide repeat C9ORF72, which may also cause amyotrophic lateral sclerosis, and both conditions may co-occur in individual patients [44], meaning that physicians caring for patients with FTD should be observant regarding symptoms suggesting motor-neuron disease.

Lewy Body Dementia and Parkinson's Disease Dementia

LBD is characterized by both cognitive and non-cognitive symptoms. Delineation between LBD and PDD is not straightforward in clinical practice, but a 1-year rule has been somewhat arbitrarily adopted in that if cognitive impairment ensues within one year of onset of motor symptoms, the patient has LBD. LBD and PDD share many features, and many patients with Parkinson's disease will develop cognitive impairment and progress to dementia [45]. It may be that LBD and Parkinson's disease represent different spectra of the same disease.

Visuocognitive impairments are common in LBD, reflecting the primary posterior affection of the brain, such as the occipital lobe and parietal regions [46]. A common finding on 18F-FDG-PET, a marker of neuronal metabolism, is hypometabolism of the occipital lobe, adjacent parietal regions, but relative sparing of the posterior cingulate gyrus, which lights up as an "island" of preserved metabolism in a "sea" of hypometabolism, and is aptly named "cingulate island sign" [47]. The origin of the "cingulate island sign" is uncertain but may reflect relative preservation of the hippocampus and the connections between the hippocampus and the posterior cingulate [48]. This is in line with the fact that hippocampal atrophy is not as commonly occurring in LBD as in AD and that memory impairments are less prominent, whereas deficits in attention are much more common [49]. One important caveat is, however, that many patients with LBD harbor pathological depositions of beta-amyloid, i.e., so-called co-pathology or dual pathology [50]. Cognitive fluctuations are often seen in patients with LBD, particularly fluctuations in attention. Fluctuations may last for seconds, minutes, or hours, where the patients are "zoned out," "not paying attention," "not there." This may also be observed during the consultation in the outpatient clinic as lapses in attention. It can be very dramatic, as reported in some case reports.

Case 4

Eric is 70 years old and has been diagnosed with LBD a year ago. Eric is a widower and has lived alone for 3 years. He was first seen by a dementia specialist about a year ago on the initiative of his two daughters, who had noticed changes in Eric's behavior. At the initial visit at the doctor's office, Eric's daughters reported changes over the preceding half a year or so, but when prompted by the doctor, Eric and his daughters were able to trace the first changes to about 2 years prior to the first visit. When asked, Eric reported that he and his late wife had not shared a bed for the last 5 year prior to her passing 3 years ago because Eric had developed "very uneasy sleeping" where he would thrash about in bed hitting his late wife. On a few occasions, he had fallen out of bed. Often in the morning, the bed sheets would be in complete disarray. When asked, Eric also reported the loss of smell for the last 10 years. Memory was not as impaired, but he would often lose focus, and he had visuospatial impairment. Eric also reported seeing shadows of passing figures in his peripheral vision. Fine motor skills had diminished, and he had developed a resting tremor. About half a year after the diagnosis, Eric started to complain about persons coming into his apartment unannounced. Sometimes they would sit on his sofa or wander around the home. He would ask them to leave but to no avail. It made Eric very uneasy, and he did not like being in his apartment. This led him to wander the streets for hours at a time. About 3 months ago, Eric was admitted to the hospital on the initiative of the professional carer, who had noticed that Eric would at times "zone out" and not be fully responsive. An EEG was performed, as were other investigations, but an experienced dementia expert recognized that these were cognitive fluctuations, as was confirmed by Eric's daughters by the information that "zoning out" was a "habit" that Eric had developed.

Non-motor symptoms include an array of symptoms and may be prominent and burdensome. Parkinsonism (bradykinesia, rigidity, tremor, postural instability) is almost always present. Visual hallucinations may be very prominent and extremely burdensome for the patient. Earlier findings indicated that visual hallucinations were often complex with the presence of family members in a tableau-type setting and not bothersome for the patient. However, this is rarely the case. More often, patients report seeing persons or animals, and a substantial number of persons report seeing shadows at the edge of the periphery of the visual field. REM-sleep behavior disorder is also common in which the patient "acts out" dreams and will develop aberrant motor activity during sleep, e.g., in the form of kicking or hitting the bed partner (if spouses do not share bedrooms, ask whether this is due to motor unrest during sleep), falling out of bed or waking with very ruffled bedsheets. Anosmia and autonomic symptoms may also be present [10]. Non-motor symptoms (excluding parkinsonism) may precede cognitive impairment for many years, e.g., REM-sleep behavior disorder or anosmia. Patients may not volunteer information about these symptoms, and it is therefore important to ask specifically about the symptoms. As is the case with Parkinson's disease, LBD is considered an alpha-synucleinopathy with involvement of cortical areas as well as the brainstem and substantia nigra.

Vascular Dementia

VaD is not a single disease but rather several different conditions that share the commonality that vascular lesions are the main cause of the dementia syndrome. Due to the plethora of vascular lesions which may give rise to VaD, the term vascular cognitive impairment has also been proposed encompassing all etiologies as well as the MCI and dementia stages [12].

Vascular lesions are common in populations with neurodegenerative diseases, especially in patients with AD [51], perhaps due to shared risk factors such as hypertension and diabetes. A diagnosis of VaD should be reserved for those patients where the main reason for dementia is vascular lesions and not simply a co-occurrence with other pathology. In patients where e.g. vascular and AD pathology are believed to contribute equally to the symptoms, a diagnosis of mixed dementia may be appropriate.

VaD may be classified by various characteristics. A common classification is whether the vascular lesions are due to small vessel or large vessel disease as this classification encompasses most patients and since pathology and clinical features generally align. In patients with small vessel disease, the disease trajectory may mirror that of neurodegenerative diseases with an insidious onset and being slowly progressive. Another presentation is a more stepwise progression [52]. This stepwise progression is usually associated with multiple infarcts. Another very common neuropathological lesion visible on structural scans are vascular white matter lesions (also termed leukoaraiosis) [53]. Microbleeds and enlarged perivascular spaces may also contribute, as may micro strokes, although the latter are usually only visible on ultra-high field MRI [54]. A stepwise progression may also be superimposed on a more generally downwards disease trajectory, reflecting a mixture of the two. Patients usually display a subcortical cognitive profile with executive dysfunction, attentional deficits, and reduced mental speed. Non-cognitive symptoms may include urge incontinence and depression as well as other symptoms and signs of stroke (e.g., slight hemiparesis or facial palsy, extensive plantar reflexes) [55]. In large vessel disease, the dementia syndrome usually develops more sudden after a more catastrophic event such as stroke (e.g., occlusion of the middle cerebral artery resulting in a media infarct) or hemorrhage including subarachnoid hemorrhage. Cognitive impairments may first become noticeable in the months following such events, as other symptoms may overshadow them.

Case 5

Mary-Beth is 83 years old and lives with her husband, George, 80. Mary-Beth has hypertension, type 2 diabetes, is slightly overweight (body mass index 27.5), and smoked 20 cigarettes a day until she was 70 years. Mary-Beth has trouble walking and uses a walking aid. She has also become increasingly forgetful. Before, she used to cook, but now George has taken over, and they live mostly on TV dinners. Mary-Beth has been referred to a dementia specialist by her GP. MMSE is 23, and ADL is affected. On questioning, Mary-Beth reports a history of urge incontinence for about 3 years. Moreover, Mary-Beth reports being sad and not very happy. She feels her energy levels are low, and she rarely looks forward to anything anymore. Sleep is disturbed as she has difficulties falling asleep. On examination, the gait is unsteady, and reflexes on the left side are brisk with an extensive plantar response. An MRI is performed revealing leukoaraiosis (Fazekas grade 3) and 2 lacunar infarcts on the right side (one in the thalamus). Mary-Beth is diagnosed with subcortical VaD.

As risk factors are shared between small vessel and large vessel disease, it is not surprising that the two may co-occur. Further, as strokes may occur in all brain regions, there may be great variability in symptoms. Stroke in some areas of the brain is however more likely to cause cognitive impairment in isolation such as strokes in the thalamus (so-called strategic infarcts) [56]. The existence of VaD underscores the importance of vascular care in patients with dementia, not only VaD patients, but also others, as the development of vascular pathology is likely to worsen cognitive impairment.

Other Causes of Dementia

A number of less common neurodegenerative disorders where cognitive impairment is often prominent but usually co-occur with motor manifestations also deserves mention. These include progressive supranuclear palsy, corticobasal degeneration, and multi-system atrophy. Spongiform encephalopathies of which Creutzfeldt-Jakob disease is the most common may manifest as an isolated rapidly progressive dementia disorder, but motor manifestations often develop prior to or in the months after cognitive impairment has become apparent [57]. We kindly refer the reader to other textbooks for further reading on these conditions.

A common clinical observation is patients with a phenotype congruent with AD, but not harboring beta-amyloid. These may sometimes be referred to as suspected non-Alzheimer pathology. Other less well-studied entities are primary age-related tauopathy (which some argue is a naturally occurring condition in aging), Limbic-predominant age-related TDP-43 encephalopathy (which may present with an Alzheimer-like phenotype) [15] and chronic traumatic encephalopathy associated with repeated minor head traumas (e.g., in boxers or combat soldiers) [58].

Conclusion

Dementia is a syndrome that may be caused by many different neurodegenerative diseases, but a handful underlie the majority of cases. These include AD, FTD, and LBD, as well as VaD, which, strictly speaking, is not a neurodegenerative disease. The disorders share commonalities in terms of disease course, but knowledge of the specific diseases is important. Dementia is a condition that affects almost all aspects of a patients' life as well as caregivers. Physicians will almost invariably come to manage patients with dementia, and therefore knowledge about dementia is important across specialties and settings.

References

1. International classification of diseases for mortality and morbidity statistics (11th Revision). World Health Organization; 2018.
2. Diagnostic and statistical manual of mental disorders. 5th edition. Washington, DC: American Psychiatric Association; 2013.
3. Petersen RC, Smith GE, Waring SC, Ivnik RJ, Tangalos EG, Kokmen E. Mild cognitive impairment: clinical characterization and outcome. Arch Neurol. 1999;56(3):303–8.

4. Winblad B, Palmer K, Kivipelto M, Jelic V, Fratiglioni L, Wahlund LO, et al. Mild cognitive impairment - beyond controversies, towards a consensus: report of the International Working Group on Mild Cognitive Impairment. J Intern Med. 2004;256(3):240–6.
5. Sperling RA, Aisen PS, Beckett LA, Bennett DA, Craft S, Fagan AM, et al. Toward defining the preclinical stages of Alzheimer's disease: recommendations from the National Institute on Aging-Alzheimer's Association workgroups on diagnostic guidelines for Alzheimer's disease. Alzheimers Dement. 2011;7(3):280–92.
6. Albert MS, DeKosky ST, Dickson D, Dubois B, Feldman HH, Fox NC, et al. The diagnosis of mild cognitive impairment due to Alzheimer's disease: recommendations from the National Institute on Aging-Alzheimer's Association workgroups on diagnostic guidelines for Alzheimer's disease. Alzheimers Dement. 2011;7(3):270–9.
7. McKhann GM, Knopman DS, Chertkow H, Hyman BT, Jack CR, Kawas CH, et al. The diagnosis of dementia due to Alzheimer's disease: recommendations from the National Institute on Aging and the Alzheimer's Association workgroup. Alzheimers Dement. 2011;7(3):263–9.
8. Dubois B, Feldman HH, Jacova C, Hampel H, Molinuevo JL, Blennow K, et al. Advancing research diagnostic criteria for Alzheimer's disease: the IWG-2 criteria. Lancet Neurol. 2014;13(6):614–29.
9. Jack CR, Bennett DA, Blennow K, Carrillo MC, Dunn B, Haeberlein SB, et al. NIA-AA research framework: toward a biological definition of Alzheimer's disease. Alzheimer's Dement. 2018;14(4):535–62.
10. Mckeith IG, Sci M, Boeve BF, Dickson DW, Halliday G, Taylor J-P, et al. Diagnosis and management of dementia with Lewy bodies Fourth consensus report of the DLB Consortium. Neurology. 2017;89(1):88–100.
11. McKeith IG, Ferman TJ, Thomas AJ, Blanc F, Boeve BF, Fujishiro H, et al. Research criteria for the diagnosis of prodromal dementia with Lewy bodies. Neurology. 2020;94(17):743–55. https://doi.org/10.1212/WNL.0000000000009323.
12. Sachdev P, Kalaria R, O'Brien J, Skoog I, Alladi S, Black SE, et al. Diagnostic criteria for vascular cognitive disorders: a VASCOG statement. Alzheimer Dis Assoc Disord. 2014;13:1–13.
13. Gorno-Tempini M, Hillis A, Weintraub S. Classification of primary progressive aphasia and its variants. Neurology;2011.
14. Rascovsky K, Hodges JR, Knopman D, Mendez MF, Kramer JH, Neuhaus J, et al. Sensitivity of revised diagnostic criteria for the behavioural variant of frontotemporal dementia. Brain. 2011;134(9):2456–77.
15. Nelson PT, Dickson DW, Trojanowski JQ, Jack CR, Boyle PA, Arfanakis K, et al. Limbic-predominant age-related TDP-43 encephalopathy (LATE): consensus working group report. Brain. 2019;142(6):1503–27.
16. Prince M, Wimo A, Guerchet M, Ali G, Wu Y, Prina M. The global impact of dementia: an analysis of prevalence, incidence, cost and trends. London: Alzheimer's Disease International. World Alzheimer Report 2015; 2015.
17. Dementia - a public health priority. WHO and Alzheimer's Disease International 2012 (www.who.int/mental_health/publications/dementia_report_2012/en).
18. Prince M, Ali G-C, Guerchet M, Prina AM, Albanese E, Wu Y-T. Recent global trends in the prevalence and incidence of dementia, and survival with dementia. Alzheimers Res Ther. 2016;8(1):23.
19. Erickson KI, Voss MW, Prakash RS, Basak C, Szabo A, Chaddock L, et al. Exercise training increases size of hippocampus and improves memory. Proc Natl Acad Sci U S A. 2011;108(7):3017–22.
20. Stephan BCM, Birdi R, Tang EYH, Cosco TD, Donini LM, Licher S, et al. Secular trends in dementia prevalence and incidence worldwide: a systematic review. J Alzheimers Dis. 2018;66(2):653–80.
21. Taudorf L, Nørgaard A, Islamoska S, Jørgensen K, Laursen TM, Waldemar G. Declining incidence of dementia: a national registry-based study over 20 years. Alzheimers Dement. 2019;15(11):1383–91.

22. Taudorf L, Nørgaard A, Waldemar G, Laursen TM. Mortality in dementia from 1996 to 2015: a national registry-based cohort study. J Alzheimers Dis. 2021;79(1):289–300.
23. Jack CR, Knopman DS, Jagust WJ, Petersen RC, Weiner MW, Aisen PS, et al. Updated hypothetical model of dynamic biomarkers. Lancet Neurol. 2013;12(2):207–16.
24. Bateman RJ, Xiong C, Benzinger TLS, Fagan AM, Goate A, Fox NC, et al. Clinical and biomarker changes in dominantly inherited Alzheimer's disease. N Engl J Med. 2012;367(9):795–804.
25. Jessen F, Amariglio RE, Van Boxtel M, Breteler M, Ceccaldi M, Chételat G, et al. A conceptual framework for research on subjective cognitive decline in preclinical Alzheimer's disease. Alzheimers Dement. 2014;10(6):844–52.
26. Slot RER, SAM S, Berkhof J, Brodaty H, Buckley R, Cavedo E, et al. Subjective cognitive decline and rates of incident Alzheimer's disease and non–Alzheimer's disease dementia. Alzheimer's Dement. 2018;15:465–76.
27. Hu C, Yu D, Sun X, Zhang M, Wang L, Qin H. The prevalence and progression of mild cognitive impairment among clinic and community populations: A systematic review and meta-analysis. Int Psychogeriatrics. 2017;29(10):1595–608.
28. Savva GM, Zaccai J, Matthews FE, Davidson JE, Mckeith I, Brayne C. Prevalence, correlates and course of behavioural and psychological symptoms of dementia in the population. Br J Psychiatry. 2009;194:212–9.
29. Sadak TI, Katon J, Beck C, Cochrane BB, Borson S. Key neuropsychiatric symptoms in common dementias: prevalence and implications for caregivers, clinicians, and health systems. Res Gerontol Nurs. 2015;7(1):44–52.
30. Pereira GCM, De Oliveira GC. Prevalence of capgras syndrome in Alzheimer's patients: a systematic review and meta-analysis. Dement e Neuropsychol. 2019;13(4):463–8.
31. Selkoe DJ, Hardy J. The amyloid hypothesis of Alzheimer's disease at 25 years. EMBO Mol Med. 2016;8(6):595–608.
32. Aisen PS. Editorial: failure after failure. What next in AD drug development? J Prev Alzheimer's Dis. 2019;6(3):150.
33. Heneka MT, Golenbock DT, Latz E. Innate immunity in Alzheimer's disease. Nat Immunol. 2015;16(3):229–36.
34. Cole J, Costafreda SG, McGuffin P, Fu CHY. Hippocampal atrophy in first episode depression: a meta-analysis of magnetic resonance imaging studies. J Affect Disord. 2011;134(1–3):483–7.
35. Woodward M, Jacova C, Black SE, Kertesz A, Mackenzie IR, Feldman H. Differentiating the frontal variant of Alzheimer's disease. Int J Geriatr Psychiatry. 2009;25(7):732–8.
36. Crutch SJ, Lehmann M, Schott JM, Rabinovici GD, Rossor MN, Fox NC. Posterior cortical atrophy. Lancet Neurol. 2012;11:170–8.
37. Henry ML, Gorno-Tempini ML. The logopenic variant of primary progressive aphasia. Curr Opin Neurol. 2010 Dec;23(6):633–7.
38. Marques IB, Tabuas-Pereira M, Milheiro M, Santana I. Biparietal variant of Alzheimer's disease: a rare presentation of a common disease. Case Reports. 2015;2015:bcr2014207011.
39. Rossor MN, Fox NC, Mummery CJ, Schott JM, Warren JD. The diagnosis of young-onset dementia. Lancet Neurol. 2010;9(8):793–806.
40. Bekris LM, Yu C-E, Bird TD, Tsuang DW. Review article: genetics of Alzheimer disease. J Geriatr Psychiatry Neurol. 2010;23(4):213–27.
41. Piguet O, Hornberger M, Mioshi E, Hodges JR. Behavioural-variant frontotemporal dementia: diagnosis, clinical staging, and management. Lancet Neurol. 2011;10(2):162–72.
42. Desgranges B, Matuszewski V, Piolino P, Chételat G, Mézenge F, Landeau B, et al. Anatomical and functional alterations in semantic dementia: a voxel-based MRI and PET study. Neurobiol Aging. 2007;28(12):1904–13.
43. Greaves CV, Rohrer JD. An update on genetic frontotemporal dementia. J Neurol. 2019;266(8):2075–86.
44. Rohrer JD, Isaacs AM, Mizielinska S, Mead S, Lashley T, Wray S, et al. C9orf72 expansions in frontotemporal dementia and amyotrophic lateral sclerosis. Lancet Neurol. 2015;14:291–301.

45. Janvin CC, Larsen JP, Aarsland D, Hugdahl K. Subtypes of mild cognitive impairment in parkinson's disease: progression to dementia. Mov Disord. 2006;21(9):1343–9.
46. Johnson DK, Morris JC, Galvin JE. Verbal and visuospatial deficits in dementia with Lewy bodies. Neurol Int. 2005;65(8):1232–8.
47. Gjerum L, Frederiksen KS, Henriksen OM, Law I, Anderberg L, Andersen BB, et al. A visual rating scale for cingulate island sign on 18F-FDG-PET to differentiate dementia with Lewy bodies and Alzheimer's disease. J Neurol Sci. 2020;410:116645.
48. Graff-Radford J, Murray ME, Lowe VJ, Boeve BF, Ferman TJ, Przybelski SA, et al. Dementia with Lewy bodies: basis of cingulate island sign. Neurology. 2014;83(9):801–9.
49. Calderon J. Perception, attention, and working memory are disproportionately impaired in dementia with Lewy bodies compared with Alzheimer's disease. J Neurol Neurosurg Psychiatry. 2001;70(2):157–64.
50. Maetzler W, Liepelt I, Reimold M, Reischl G, Solbach C, Becker C, et al. Cortical PIB binding in Lewy body disease is associated with Alzheimer-like characteristics. Neurobiol Dis. 2009;34(1):107–12.
51. De Reuck JL, Deramecourt V, Auger F, Durieux N, Florence CM, Charlotte P, et al. Cerebrovascular lesions in mixed neurodegenerative dementia: a neuropathological and magnetic resonance study. Eur Neurol. 2017;78(1–2):1–4.
52. Román GC, Erkinjuntti T, Wallin A, Pantoni L, Chui HC. Subcortical ischaemic vascular dementia. Lancet Neurol. 2002;1(7):426–36.
53. van der Flier WM, van Straaten ECW, Barkhof F, Verdelho A, Madureira S, Pantoni L, et al. Small vessel disease and general cognitive function in nondisabled elderly: the LADIS study. Stroke. 2005;36(10):2116–20.
54. De Reuck J. Frequency and topography of small cerebrovascular lesions in vascular and in mixed dementia: a post-mortem 7-tesla magnetic resonance imaging study with neuropathological correlates. Folia Neuropatol. 2017;55:31–7.
55. Erkinjuntti T. Subcortical vascular dementia. Cerebrovasc Dis Dis. 2000;13(2):58–60.
56. Jellinger KA. Pathology and pathogenesis of vascular cognitive impairment-a critical update. Front Aging Neurosci. 2013;5:17.
57. Zerr I, Parchi P. Sporadic Creutzfeldt–Jakob disease. Handb Clin Neurol. 2018;153:155–74.
58. Lesman-Segev OH, La Joie R, Stephens ML, Sonni I, Tsai R, Bourakova V, et al. Tau PET and multimodal brain imaging in patients at risk for chronic traumatic encephalopathy. NeuroImage Clin. 2019;24:102025.

Diagnosis and Support of Patients with Dementia: A Patient Perspective on Current Goals and Practice

2

Dianne Gove, Ana Diaz-Ponce, and Jean Georges

Abbreviation

AE Alzheimer Europe

Introduction

It is estimated that approximately nine million people in Europe have dementia [1]. Although the main symptoms of dementia are cognitive, dementia can affect all aspects of a person's life and their relationships with others. Each person is unique and may experience dementia in a different way. The symptoms that a person experiences may also differ depending on the type of dementia. With appropriate support, many people with dementia can live a good life.

Diagnosis is a key aspect of the management of dementia, in particular the way people affected by dementia (e.g. the patient and the carer) experience it. In addition, to ensure that people with dementia can carry on with their activities and live independently for as long as possible, appropriate and timely support should be provided to the patient and their family. This includes pharmacological as well as psycho-social treatments and interventions, as well as a supportive environment (e.g. inclusive communities where there is awareness and understanding of dementia, and patients with dementia feel safe and enabled to engage). In this chapter, we provide a brief overview of key issues related to timely diagnosis, disclosure of the diagnosis and care and support, followed for each topic by a reflection on the

D. Gove · A. Diaz-Ponce · J. Georges (✉)
Alzheimer Europe, Luxembourg, Luxembourg
e-mail: Dianne.Gove@alzheimer-europe.org; ana.diaz@alzheimer-europe.org; Jean.Georges@alzheimer-europe.org

K. S. Frederiksen, G. Waldemar (eds.), *Management of Patients with Dementia*,
https://doi.org/10.1007/978-3-030-77904-7_2

current situation, drawing on the findings of existing surveys carried out by Alzheimer Europe (AE) and with supporting commentaries from people with dementia.

Timely Diagnosis

Key Issues

A diagnosis can allow people to plan better for their future and to start treatments/interventions. It may help them to understand the condition better and to find ways of coping with the disease. Some patients with dementia and carers have described certain practical and psychological benefits of being diagnosed, such as putting an end to uncertainties and enabling them to access relevant support and care. Potential negative consequences of diagnosis include feeling distressed or experiencing stigma. "Therapeutic nihilism" may interfere with the diagnosis of dementia. This involves the belief held by some healthcare professionals that it is pointless to diagnose dementia as there is no treatment, a risk of stigma and as they feel they have nothing to offer [2–4].

Access to an early or timely diagnosis of dementia has become a policy and practice imperative [5], but the terms "early" and "timely" are often used interchangeably [6]. However, "timely" refers to a diagnosis that is made at the right time for a particular person, whereas "early" focuses on a diagnosis that is made early (i.e. in the chronological sense) [7]. According to Woods et al. [8, p. 321] timely diagnoses "prevent crises, facilitate adjustment and provide access to treatments and support." In most cases, an early diagnosis is also considered a timely diagnosis but in keeping with a person-centred approach, timely diagnosis is not linked to a particular disease stage but to its potential benefit to the individual patient [7]. It is therefore a very personal matter and raises the issue of whether and how to communicate a diagnosis of dementia, which is addressed in section "Disclosure of the diagnosis."

The underlying processes which result in dementia usually build up over several years, and it may take weeks, months or even years for a diagnosis to be made. Current research trends are moving in the direction of early, pre-clinical indicators of the pathological processes leading to, and underlying dementia. Indeed, the National Council on Ageing, Alzheimer's Association and the International Working Group promote the use of pre-clinical/asymptomatic biomarkers as accurate diagnostic tests, but as Rosin et al. [9] point out, this is primarily within a research framework, and more work is needed before they are incorporated into clinical practice. A key issue in relation to the management of dementia is therefore to agree on when the diagnostic procedure starts and how information that may be available about the risk of developing dementia is communicated to patients.

Another issue is that of equity. All citizens of Europe should have the opportunity to receive information about their risk status and to receive a timely diagnosis of dementia. This is currently not the case. In some countries, diagnosis and the detection of risk factors are fairly advanced. In others, people struggle to obtain a diagnosis at all, do not benefit from the latest scientific advances in diagnosis and/or are assessed using tools and instruments that are not suited to their needs and have not been validated on people with their characteristics (e.g. for many people from minority ethnic groups) [10]. This means that people do not all have access to the same potential benefits, including appropriate treatment and support and taking part in research. Such discrimination may be linked to a range of factors (e.g. attitudes of healthcare professionals, stigma, lack of resources, assumptions about the value of diagnosis, lack of training, etc.). There is still much to be done in order to achieve equity with regard to the diagnosis of dementia in Europe.

Practice and Perspectives

Currently, in Europe, many people affected by dementia still feel that diagnosis takes too long or is made too late. In a survey that AE carried out in 2006 in six European countries [11], carers reported that it had taken on average, 2 years and 2 months to get a diagnosis of dementia (i.e. from first symptoms to diagnosis). In addition, the survey also revealed important differences between countries, as carers in Germany reported on average 10 months to get a diagnosis whereas carers in the UK who had experienced a much longer timeframe (32 months on average). In a similar survey carried out in 2018, over a decade later [12], and involving 1409 carers in five European countries, carers reported an average length of time of 2.1 years between problems being noticed and the diagnosis being made, with the shorter times reported in the Czech Republic (1.6 years) and the longest in the Netherlands (2.6 years). These two surveys conducted a decade apart, showed that the length of time elapsing between the patient with dementia or carer noticing problems and a diagnosis being made had pretty much stayed the same.

The second survey [12] also showed that it often took more than 1 year for people to seek help since the first symptoms are noticed and that the decision to seek help is more likely to be made by a family member (64% in the AE survey) or in some cases, jointly by the patient with dementia and a family member (27%) (but only in 4% of the cases by the patient on his/her own). The quote below from a member of AE's European Working Group of People with Dementia (EWGPWD) refers to this time prior to diagnosis when first symptoms may be noticed but the patient often cannot make sense of them:

> My diagnosis came after a number of years of wondering what was wrong with me. At work the in-tray was not moving, I found myself at a Board meeting struggling for words. I thought I was losing my mind. (Helen Rochford-Brennan, Ireland)

Other important aspects include the stage of dementia at the time of diagnosis, and the perceived "timeliness" of the diagnosis. In the 2018 AE survey [12], 40% of people had been diagnosed at moderate or advanced stages of dementia and over half of the carers felt that the diagnosis should have been made earlier. Carers of people diagnosed at later stages tended to report more often that the diagnosis should have been made earlier and vice versa; when people with dementia had been diagnosed at a milder stage, carers tended to identify this as "the right time" for diagnosis. Still, more than a third of the people diagnosed at a mild stage would have preferred an earlier diagnosis.

The most frequent reasons mentioned by the carers in the survey for the late diagnosis were related to the carer's lack of awareness of dementia, the patient refusing to seek help, and the attitudes of the doctor (e.g. not considering that anything was wrong, or that it was worthwhile pursuing diagnosis). Also, waiting lists or long time needed for referral or assessments were highlighted as reasons for the delay. The excerpts below from two members of the EWGPWD provide examples of additional challenges and reasons for the delay of diagnosis experienced by people with dementia who are diagnosed before the age of 60 or with a less common form of dementia:

> Many people know of Alzheimer's disease only as disease of older people, and only of the last stage of the disease. They don't know about the different stages of the disease and that this disease can affect younger people. (Nina Baláčková, Czech Republic)

> I received a diagnosis of Frontotemporal dementia (FTD) at the age of 52 (…) Before the diagnosis of FTD I was diagnosed with depression. This is not unusual for people with dementia. Also, FTD is very rare in Finland and this made the diagnosis even more difficult (…) Several doctors were taking care of me, but they did not talk enough to each other. No one seemed to know what was happening to me. (..) (Petri Lampinen, Finland)

Disclosure of the Diagnosis

Key Issues

The potential benefits of a timely diagnosis are largely dependent on disclosure of the diagnosis, which is also linked to the ethical principle of autonomy. Some carers do not want the patient with dementia to be informed [13–15]. However, three recent systematic literature reviews of the diagnosis of dementia all report that the majority of people with and without cognitive impairment, within the primary care context as well as in memory clinics, prefer to be informed of a possible diagnosis of dementia [16–18]. Nevertheless, some people do not want to know and state this very clearly [19]. The right not to know is equally important, and for this to be a genuine choice, people need to understand fully what such a diagnosis means and hence what the implications of a diagnosis might be for them.

The practice of disclosing the diagnosis to carers and not to people with dementia used to be quite common [20]. Informing relatives of a diagnosis of dementia, but not the person who has dementia, could be considered as a failure to respect the autonomy and right of the latter to privacy and as breaching medical professionals' obligations with regard to confidentiality. It could be considered as running counter to the principles of beneficence and non-maleficence, although in some cases, disclosure to relatives may be considered justifiable (e.g. to ensure the care of a patient with very advanced dementia), provided that the patient had not clearly stated that certain people should not be informed. Disclosing the diagnosis solely to relatives makes them responsible for informing the patient even though they may lack the necessary information, understanding of the condition or skills to be able to carry out this task effectively and might not even be in favour of sharing the diagnosis.

Medical professionals should not inform carers of the diagnosis simply to avoid personal responsibility for disclosure of the diagnosis to the patient with dementia. Responsibility for the disclosure of the diagnosis must be clear and transparent. It should not be left to hazard or assumed to have been addressed by relatives and close friends of the person with dementia. People with dementia have a legal right to be informed (even if they choose not to be informed) and it should be documented whether and by whom the diagnosis was communicated. However, it should not be assumed that because someone has a diagnosis, they necessarily accept it or want to talk about having Alzheimer's disease, for example. Some people may be aware of their diagnosis but prefer to refer to the condition by a different name (e.g. preferring to talk about having "memory problems") [21].

Bailey, Dooley and McCabe [22] emphasise the need for doctors to tailor communication of the diagnosis to their patients' preferences and awareness, to consider which information can be discussed in the presence of carers and to create the right balance between honesty and hope when discussing prognosis and medication, bearing in mind how the cognitive impairment affects understanding. They point out that misunderstandings may limit the opportunities that people with dementia have to take an active role in decision making and hence in exercising their legal capacity, otherwise offered by timely diagnosis. According to Bailey et al. [22], disclosure is a delicate, complex and nuanced task, which can also be emotionally challenging, and for which many healthcare professionals would benefit from training and supervision.

It is considered unethical and illegal to treat or involve people in research who have not given informed consent (i.e. have not consented after having been provided with information that is suited to their ability to understand and that they have understood). With diagnosis, the same principle should apply. It might be argued that with diagnosis, there is no decision to be made and no issue of interference with a person's physical integrity. However, a diagnosis can be life changing and affect a whole range of future decisions, not least deciding whether to consent to symptomatic treatment that might be proposed. Clarity, precision, sensitivity and an understanding of people's current understanding of dementia are needed when informing people of a diagnosis. More research is needed into the psychological, emotional and social impact of receiving information about AD at all stages along the continuum (linked to pre-clinical, including at-risk status, prodromal AD or MCI due to AD and AD dementia).

Recent changes in the conceptualisation of Alzheimer's disease necessitate care and attention by healthcare professionals and researchers using such terms. Increasingly, laypeople have access to information on the Internet about dementia research where the use of the term "Alzheimer's disease" by professionals and academics does not necessarily correspond to their everyday use and understanding of that term. The use of euphemisms or non-medical terms by doctors to help patients understand diagnoses of dementia [23, 24] may further muddy the waters. Papers on the conceptual framework and lexicon (e.g. [25, 26]) are important for healthcare professionals and academics in clarifying conceptual changes and the accompanying terminology, but at the level of actual diagnosis and in society in general, it is important to address broader perceptions and understandings of disease, health and risk, the boundaries between the two and the implications of these for people's lives.

Additional attention is needed when discussing dementia and disclosing a diagnosis of dementia to people from minority ethnic groups, many of whom (but by no means all) may have limited knowledge of the national language, lower levels of education and different beliefs about the origin and nature of dementia (Alzheimer Europe 2018). In some ethnic communities, there is no word for dementia in everyday language and dementia is not seen as a medical condition. This has implications for preventive measures, diagnosis of dementia, disclosure of that diagnosis and subsequent access to care and support.

Practices and Perspectives

Disclosure and Quality

The AE 2018 survey [12] indicated that, although disclosing the diagnosis to the patient with dementia may have become a common practice in many countries, this is still not the case everywhere. People living in some countries may be less likely than others of being informed of their diagnosis. In the AE survey, whilst 99% of people living in Finland had been told their diagnosis, 59% of the Italian carers stated that the patient had not been informed of the diagnosis.

Overall, the reasons for not informing the patient with dementia included: the belief that they would not understand or were not aware, not wanting to upset them, or that the family thought it unnecessary, or the doctor had advised against telling the patient. In only a small proportion of cases (10%) had the decision to not inform been based on the expressed wish of the patient not to know.

The reasons for nondisclosure fell into four main categories: not wishing to upset the person, the person would not understand or was not aware, the family thought it unnecessary, and the doctor advised against telling the person.

Half of the carers stated that the patient with dementia had not been consulted in advance about who they would like to be present when the diagnosis would be disclosed. A carer had been present in the meeting where the diagnosis had been disclosed in 89% of the cases. Although in only a small proportion the carer had not been present during the disclosure, the following quote from a member of the EWGPWG highlights the relevance of this topic:

> A psychologist that I'd never met before was called in and she said "I'm sorry to tell you the scan has shown vascular dementia" (…) Nobody should be told they've got a serious illness alone (Carol Hargreaves, UK).

When the diagnosis was communicated, the experience of the carers in the survey tended to be quite positive, and many felt satisfied with the way diagnosis was communicated (i.e. 73% of the carers felt the doctor was well prepared and clear, and 62% felt the doctor had established a good relationship with the patient with dementia and the carer). Issues to improve in the disclosure to the carers, including the length of the meeting and opportunities for asking questions without the patient being present. There was also room for improvement in the disclosure to the patient with dementia as 28% of the carers thought the patient had not understood the diagnosis, and one in five stated that, during the meeting, the doctor had spoken mainly to them (rather than to the patient with dementia).

Reactions to Diagnosis

Some common reactions to the diagnosis are worry, uncertainty and sadness. In the 2018 AE survey [12], at the time of diagnosis, 74% of carers and around 30% of people with dementia felt worried about the future, and several were uncertain about the implications of the diagnosis. Over time, whilst many carers still felt worried about the future, acceptance was also very often reported. Feelings of sadness seemed common in both people with dementia and carers at the time of diagnosis and over time.

The results of the AE survey also suggested that the way the patient reacts to diagnosis may be linked to the timeliness of the diagnosis and the quality of the disclosure [6]. Carers who felt the diagnosis was not timely were more likely to report negative emotions and worries about the future at the time of diagnosis and 4 years later [6]. On the other hand, the survey also showed that a higher quality of diagnosis-sharing was associated with lower sadness and depression, despair, and greater acceptance and reassurance, both immediately after diagnosis and some time afterwards [6].

Sharing the Diagnosis with Others and Perceptions of Their Community

The decision to share the diagnosis with others is very important, as this may be an important step towards integrating dementia into the person's life. In the AE survey, only 2% of the carers said that no one else knew about the diagnosis. The people with whom carers had more often shared the diagnosis with were family members and, to a lesser extent, friends and neighbours. However, as the quote from a member of the EWGPWD describes below, telling people, even the closest ones is not always easy,

> After meeting with the doctor, I had to drive home over 60 miles and wondered how I was going to tell my husband and son (Helen Rochford-Brennan, Ireland)

The diagnosis was more rarely shared with other members of the community, such as members of clubs/churches attended by the person with dementia or local shopkeepers.

Overall, 38% did not agree with the statement about people in their community being aware of dementia; however nearly 60% felt that the patient with dementia was valued and respected by other people and continued to have an important role in his/her family and 44% felt that the patient was still part of their local community.

The quote below from a member of the EWGPWD describes the relevance, from the perspective of this person with dementia, of sharing the diagnosis with others and feeling included and part of the community where he lives,

> I was diagnosed with vascular dementia in 2010. (…) From early on it has been important for me to make other people aware of my situation. Whether I have lived in a large or small community my experience is that being open about my situation has made everyday life easier. People around me are accommodating and I feel included. Although my contributions may be somewhat limited at times, I experience that I still have a role to play and something to give, practically or in discussions and meetings. (Alv Orheim, Norway)

It is important also to consider, as in the examples provided by members of the EWGPWD below, that in some cases, people with dementia may feel that their freedom or their role in the family or in society may be restricted (e.g. not being allowed to do things on their own, not being asked or making decisions on their behalf, etc.)

> Two years after the diagnosis I had to return my driving license based on neuropsychological tests. I had been driving since I was 18 and it felt like I was deprived of my human rights. (Raoul Grönqvist, Finland)

> In the early days of my diagnosis, I jokingly said 'I'm not ready to give up my credit card just yet'. I said this because we know too often that a dementia diagnosis can mean a person is denied basic rights like the right to manage their own finance or the freedom to travel (Helen Rochford-Brennan, Ireland).

Care and Support

Key Issues

Receiving a timely diagnosis of dementia ideally opens the door to support, care and symptomatic treatment. Unfortunately, there are regional and national differences with regard to the availability of and access to post-diagnostic support. Sometimes, support is unavailable, too expensive, not suited to a person's needs or they are not entitled to it (e.g. if it is means tested, prioritised for people at a certain stage of dementia or restricted to certain age groups).

Where care or support is simply lacking, it could be asked whether this is linked to the lower value and priority attributed to older people, people with disabilities or people with mental health conditions (depending on how dementia is perceived in different societies), and thus a reflection of stigma. Stigma, linked to having the condition, or in some minority ethnic groups linked to whole families (based on the belief that dementia is a punishment or test from God), may also interfere with people's readiness to use available services because doing so would mean being associated with the condition and other people knowing about it. This issue also applies to seeking a diagnosis.

Other barriers to seeking post-diagnostic support and care include, amongst others, a distrust of healthcare professionals and the feeling that outside help would not be appropriate or is not yet needed. In some cases, people are not aware of available services or have difficulty navigating the complex healthcare system to benefit from them. Such barriers may be particularly common amongst, but in no way limited to, people from minority ethnic groups, especially those who have difficulties with the national language or who have experienced discrimination and prejudice in the past within the healthcare system [10]. Information about care and support needs to be communicated in different languages, in culturally appropriate places, by trusted members of the community and not solely in written form (so that people who have language or literacy problems, or visual impairments, can also benefit from such information).

This is a matter of equity in the provision of care and support, which applies to everyone. Particular groups of people risk discrimination and exclusion in the context of care and support not because of personal characteristics but because of historic, economic, political and social factors which result in the care and support available being less suited to their needs and preferences. The principles and practice of person-centred care and reasonable accommodation[1] should help ensure that care and support are provided which corresponds to each person's needs and preferences, and that they are involved in defining what these are. In keeping with the right to exercise their legal capacity, a full discussion about needs and preferences requires that people with dementia are informed of their diagnosis, understand the personal implications of it, and that they have the opportunity to benefit from shared or supported decision making if they so wish.

Practices and Perspectives

Information Received

Access to high-quality information at the time of diagnosis and over the course of the disease is essential for helping the individual adjust to dementia and to facilitate access to adequate support and services. The surveys carried out by AE in 2006 and 2018 [11, 12] suggested that some people with dementia and carers may not receive any information at the time of diagnosis. Although the surveys were conducted a decade apart, in both cases, 19% of the carers participating in the surveys reported that they had not received any information at the time of diagnosis. The following quote from a carer of a member of the EWGPWD describes this in a very powerful manner:

[1] Principle in the Convention on the Rights of Persons with Disabilities (2006), which states that reasonable adaptations should be made to ensure that people with disabilities enjoy the same rights and opportunities as other members of society.

> We were given the diagnosis, passed a few leaflets, and sent home. The silence was deafening. We didn't know who to turn to or where to go for information, for help, for solace. We each hit the internet separately, not wanting to upset the other, especially with what Dr Google told us. We had no hope (Jayne Goodrick, UK)

In the cases where information was provided, carers felt somewhat satisfied with the quality of the information received (i.e. 3.5 on average on a scale from 1 to 5). This information was most often related to the medical aspects of dementia (e.g. drug treatments, dementia and disease progression). Only around a quarter of the carers had received information on available services, support groups and healthy lifestyles. In all cases, the patient with dementia was less likely to receive information than the carer. Information about taking part in research was the type of information which fewest carers received. Topics, where carers would have appreciated further information, included practical advice about coping and living well with dementia, available services and disease progression. Other areas that were often neglected were information on care allowances, legal rights/issues and existing help and support groups.

The findings of the AE survey [12] also suggested that there were important differences in the type of information provided by country. For example the information received at the time of diagnosis in Italy and the Czech Republic tended to focus on medical aspects, whereas in the Netherlands, Finland and Scotland, carers were more often informed about Alzheimer's associations and available help/support groups.

In addition to the information received at the time of diagnosis, people affected by dementia often wish to keep up-to-date with issues related to dementia in order to better manage the disease. In the AE survey, the most popular sources of information were the Internet and Alzheimer's associations—with around two-thirds of the carers reporting these were the main sources of information used in their daily lives.

Care and Support

In the AE survey [12], the services which most carers were offered and which they used in the 6 months following diagnosis were contact with a named person or service ("case-manager" for signposting to services), day care and assessment of the needs of the patient with dementia. The information for which more carers took action included starting a drug treatment, arrangements for the management of the finances of the patient with dementia in the future and joining an Alzheimer association.

Services not offered but which carers would have liked to use included: assessment of needs, counselling/emotional support, education about living with dementia and memory training for the patient with dementia. The quote below from a member of the EWGPWD exemplifies the importance of receiving adequate support and interventions:

> My diagnosis led me to cognitive rehabilitation therapy, research through Trinity College and the Irish Dementia Working Group. (Helen Rochford-Brennan, Ireland)

Conclusions

There is widescale agreement about the importance of a timely diagnosis of dementia, but further work is still needed to address factors affecting the readiness to seek diagnosis, such as stigma, the normalisation of dementia, linguistic barriers, lack of health literacy and the belief that nothing can be done. Improvements are also needed with regard to disclosure and the provision of appropriate support and care following diagnosis. In the last decade, despite medical progress and better diagnostic procedures, as well as several national dementia strategies addressing the topic of diagnosis, there seems to be a lack of progress with regard to disclosure of the diagnosis to people with dementia. There is also an important gap in terms of equity and access to good quality post-diagnostic services and support across Europe. This is often even more challenging for people from minority ethnic groups. As Alzheimer's disease has been reconceptualised as a spectrum, careful attention needs to be paid during diagnosis as to how terms such as MCI, prodromal AD or AD dementia may be understood by patients.

Every person with dementia should have the opportunity to be informed about their diagnosis and the right not to be informed. People should be given the opportunity to be accompanied, if they so wish, by a relative, friend or person of their choice when being informed of the diagnosis. This should be communicated in a way that is clear and adapted to each person's needs, including written information and signposting about services and support. A diagnosis of dementia should be perceived as a process rather than a one-off exchange of information and should be followed by post-diagnostic support within a framework of advanced care planning.

References

1. Alzheimer Europe. The 2019 Alzheimer Europe yearbook: estimating the prevalence of dementia in Europe. Alzheimer Europe: Luxembourg; 2019.
2. Van Hout H, Vernooij-Dassen M, Bakker K, Blom M, Grol R. General practitioners on dementia: tasks, practices and obstacles. Patient Educ Couns. 2000;39:219–25.
3. Vernooij-Dassen M, Moniz-Cook ED, Woods RT, et al. Factors affecting timely recognition and diagnosis of dementia across Europe: from awareness to stigma. Int J Geriatr Psychiatry. 2005;20(4):377–86.
4. Gove D, Downs M, Vernooij-Dassen M, Small N. Stigma and GPs' perceptions of dementia. Aging Ment Health. 2016;20(4):391–400.
5. Campbell S. Living with uncertainty: mapping the transition from pre-diagnosis to a diagnosis of dementia. J Aging Stud. 2016;37:40–7.
6. Woods B, Arosio F, Diaz A, Gove D, Holmerová I, Kinnaird L, Mátlová M, Okkonen E, Possenti M, Roberts J, Salmi A, Buuse S, Werkman W, Georges J. Timely diagnosis of dementia? Family carers' experiences in 5 European countries. Int J Geriatr Psychiatry. 2019;34(1):114–21.
7. Dhedhi SA, Swinglehurst D, Russell J. 'Timely' diagnosis of dementia: what does it mean? A narrative analysis of GPs' accounts. BMJ Open. 2014;4:e004439.
8. Woods B, Moniz-Cook E, Iliffe S, Campion P, Vernooij-Dassen M, Zanetti O, Franco M. Interdem members. Dementia: issues in early recognition and intervention in primary care. J R Soc Med. 2003;96:320–4.

9. Rosin ER, Blasco D, Pilozzi AR, Yang LH, Huang X. A narrative review of Alzheimer's disease stigma. J Alzheimers Dis. 2020;78:515–28.
10. Alzheimer Europe. The development of intercultural care and support for people with dementia from minority ethnic groups. Alzheimer Europe: Luxembourg; 2018.
11. Georges J, Jansen S, Jackson J, Meyrieu A, Sadowsk A, Selmes M. Alzheimer's disease in real life--the dementia carer's survey. Int J Geriatr Psychiatry. 2008;23(5):546–51.
12. Alzheimer Europe. European Carers' Report 2018. Carers' experiences of diagnosis in five European countries. Luxembourg: Alzheimer Europe; 2018.
13. Shimizu MM, Raicher I, Yasumasa Takashashi D, Caramelli P, Nitrini R. Disclosure of the diagnosis of Alzheimer's disease: caregivers' opinions in a Brazilian sample. Arq Neuropsiquiatr. 2008;66(3B):625–30.
14. Quinn C, Jones IR, Clare L. Illness representations in caregivers of people with dementia. Aging Ment Health. 2017;21(5):553–61.
15. Zou Y, Song N, Hu Y, Gao Y, Zhang Y, Zhao Q, Guo Q, Li X, Li G, Xiao S, Chen S, Ren R, Wang G. Caregivers' attitude toward disclosure of Alzheimer's disease diagnosis in Urban China. Int Psychogeriatr. 2017;29(11):1849–55.
16. Werner P, Karnieli-Miller O, Eidelman S. Current knowledge and future directions about the disclosure of dementia: a systematic review of the first decade of the 21st century. Alzheimers Dement. 2013;9(2):e74–88.
17. van den Dungen P, van Kuijk L, van Marwijk H, van der Wouden J, Moll van Charante E, van der Horst H, van Hout H. Preferences regarding disclosure of a diagnosis of dementia: a systematic review. Int Psychogeriatr. 2014;26(10):1603–18.
18. Low L-F, McGrath M, Swaffer K, Brodaty H. Communicating a diagnosis of dementia: a systematic mixed studies review of attitudes and practices of health practitioners. Dementia. 2019;18(7–8):2856–905.
19. Marzanski M. Would you like to know what is wrong with you? On telling the truth to patients with dementia. J Med Ethics. 2000;26:108–13.
20. Van Hout HP, Vernooij-Dassen M, Jansen DA, Stalman WA. Do general practitioners disclose correct information to their patients suspected of dementia and their caregivers? A prospective observational study. Aging Ment Health. 2006;10(2):151–5.
21. Clare L, Quinn C, Jones IR, Woods RT. "I don't think of it as an illness": illness representations in mild to moderate dementia. J Alzheimers Dis. 2016;51(1):139–50.
22. Bailey C, Dooley J, McCabe R. How do they want to know? Doctors' perspectives on making and communicating a diagnosis of dementia. Dementia. 2018;18(7–8):3004–22.
23. Cody M, Beck C, Shue VM, Pope S. Reported practices of primary care physicians in the diagnosis and management of dementia. Aging Ment Health. 2002;6:72–6.
24. Downs M, Libbens RC, Rae C, Cook A, Woods R. What do general practitioners tell people with dementia and their families about the condition? A survey of experiences in Scotland. Dementia. 2002;1:47–58.
25. Dubois B. The emergence of a new conceptual framework for Alzheimer's disease. J Alzheimers Dis. 2018;62:1059–66.
26. Dubois B, Feldman H, Jacova C, Cummings J, et al. Revising the definition of Alzheimer's disease: a new lexicon. Lancet Neurol. 2010;9:1118–27.

3 Diagnostic Evaluation of Dementia

Amber Nous, Maxime Vande Vyver, Wietse Wiels, and Sebastiaan Engelborghs

Introduction

Dementia is an umbrella term, describing symptoms, consisting of cognitive decline that is severe enough to cause functional deficits. In almost all patients, dementia is associated with behavioral and personality changes. A patient with dementia depends on his or her caregiver to compensate for the functional deficits that affect activities of daily living (ADL). A dementia diagnosis does not imply an etiological diagnosis. Indeed, several brain disorders can cause dementia-like Alzheimer's disease (AD), vascular dementia (VaD), dementia with Lewy bodies (DLB), frontotemporal dementia (FTD), etc. Many patients have mixed causes, like, e.g., AD with cerebrovascular disease or DLB associated with AD co-pathology.

During the past decade, research has significantly improved the accuracy of an etiological dementia diagnosis. As AD is the most frequent cause of dementia, affecting up to 60–70% of dementia cases and exponentially increasing in

Amber Nous, Maxime Vande Vyver and Wietse Wiels contributed equally.

A. Nous · M. V. Vyver · S. Engelborghs (✉)
Department of Neurology, Universitair Ziekenhuis Brussel (UZ Brussel), Brussels, Belgium

Center for Neurosciences (C4N), Vrije Universiteit Brussel (VUB), Brussels, Belgium

Department of Biomedical Sciences, Reference Center for Biological Markers of Dementia (BIODEM), Institute Born-Bunge, University of Antwerp, Antwerp, Belgium
e-mail: Amber.Nous@uzbrussel.be; Maxime.VandeVyver@uzbrussel.be; Sebastiaan.Engelborghs@uzbrussel.be

W. Wiels
Department of Neurology, Universitair Ziekenhuis Brussel (UZ Brussel), Brussels, Belgium

Center for Neurosciences (C4N), Vrije Universiteit Brussel (VUB), Brussels, Belgium
e-mail: Wietse.Wiels@uzbrussel.be

K. S. Frederiksen, G. Waldemar (eds.), *Management of Patients with Dementia*,
https://doi.org/10.1007/978-3-030-77904-7_3

prevalence with age, most research has been performed with regard to improved early and differential diagnosis of AD.

Biomarker-Based Diagnosis of Alzheimer's Disease (AD)

The clinical diagnosis of AD was previously often based on the criteria from the National Institute of Neurological and Communicative Disorders and Stroke—Alzheimer's Disease and Related Disorders Association (NINCDS-ADRDA), originating from 1984 [1]. These criteria are based on the exclusion of other systemic and brain disorders that could account for cognitive deterioration and are confined to the dementia stage, at best resulting in a diagnosis of probable AD. A clinical diagnosis of probable AD achieves an average sensitivity and specificity of 81% and 70%, respectively [2]. A promising tool to increase the diagnostic accuracy of AD is the use of biomarkers that reflect the neuropathology of the disease.

Jack et al. [3] have modeled the biomarker changes across the continuum of AD in 2010. Since then, the model has been adapted several times [4], but its basis remained unchanged (Fig. 3.1). The last curve represents clinical function or activities of daily living. If functional deficits occur, a patient converts from mild cognitive impairment (MCI) to dementia due to AD. It is preceded by cognitive deficits, as objectified by a full neuropsychological examination. Cognitive deficits will appear as from the MCI stage on. Brain structure changes or brain atrophy result from neuronal degeneration and can be quantified by means of a brain magnetic resonance imaging (MRI) scan or a computerized tomography (CT) scan of the brain. Brain atrophy is preceded by functional changes in the brain that can be

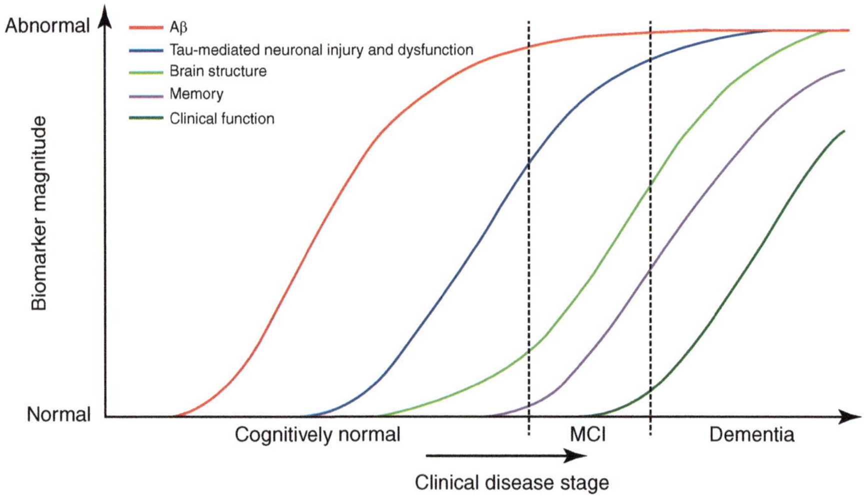

Fig. 3.1 Model of biomarker changes through the AD continuum (after Jack CR et al., Lancet Neurol. 2010;9(1):119–128

visualized through an 18-fluorodeoxyglucose (FDG) positron emission tomography (PET) scan. Functional changes are linked to neuronal injury and tau pathology, as can be analyzed in the cerebrospinal fluid (CSF). The first biomarker change consists of the abnormal processing of the β-amyloid peptide (Aβ), leading to the formation of amyloid plaques in the brain. The Aβ status can be determined through CSF analyses or by means of a PET scan. As the first amyloid plaques occur 10–20 years before symptom onset, Aβ is the earliest detectable biomarker change. This provides researchers an exceptional window for early diagnosis, future treatment, and prevention strategies.

Biomarker-based diagnosis has been introduced in daily clinical practice [5]. Biomarkers should always be interpreted as a panel, rather than individually, and in the light of the model of biomarker changes (Fig. 3.1). Moreover, biomarker changes should always be interpreted in the clinical context. Whereas hippocampal atrophy on a brain MRI scan is a rather unspecific finding in the elderly, it is suggestive of AD in the case of a patient with amnestic MCI who suffers from episodic memory problems. On the other hand, e.g., in case of differential diagnostic doubt between AD and FTD, the absence of hippocampal atrophy is supportive for ruling out AD [6]. This also implies that a search for (AD) biomarkers without having a clinical context is not done. E.g., analyzing the core AD CSF biomarkers in an asymptomatic individual is not part of daily clinical practice [5].

Timely Diagnosis of Dementia

Although AD and related disorders are still incurable, several treatment options exist [7]. Depending on the symptomatology and the needs of the patient and his/her surroundings, treatments might have beneficial effects on quality of life and can significantly delay nursing home placement, which is a wish of many patients. E.g., psycho-social education and early recognition and (non-)pharmacological treatment of behavioral changes like diurnal rhythm disturbances, depression, or agitation, and aggressiveness can significantly improve the quality of life of both patient and caregiver and thereby delay nursing home placement. Therefore, opting out a diagnostic work-up, will also limit the possible treatment options. Even symptomatic treatment options can have beneficial effects on quality of life, and the currently available treatment options are not solely pharmacological.

Do we need an early, biomarker-based diagnosis in every patient with cognitive deterioration? As long as no disease-modifying treatment options are available, it remains an option not to refer a patient to a memory clinic for an etiological (biomarker-based) diagnosis. As long as a patient has the intellectual capacity to take decisions, it is her/his right to refuse a diagnostic work-up that might lead to a diagnosis of an incurable disease like AD [8, 9]. In addition, how early a diagnosis should be made (e.g., in the MCI versus dementia stage of AD) primarily depends on the will of the patient. If a patient wants an early diagnosis in the MCI phase of AD in order to be able to take decisions with regard to his or her future (e.g., living will or advanced directives with regard to medical treatments), an early referral to a memory clinic is needed. On the other hand, if a patient at an advanced age is in a nursing home and has no troublesome symptoms, an etiological diagnosis will probably have no to very little therapeutic consequences.

The primary care physician is best placed to refer a patient with cognitive and/or behavioral signs and symptoms to a memory clinic for a diagnostic work-up, based on the wishes and needs of patient and caregiver and after discussing the possible options [10].

In what follows, the diagnostic steps are described, following a logical stepwise paradigm.

History Taking

Introduction

As the clinical picture of diseases causing cognitive impairment is often dominated by (or even limited to) cognitive decline and changes of behavior and/or personality, careful history taking is the cornerstone of the diagnostic evaluation. The clinician should aim to use clear, practical questions with a limited scope, adjusted to the patient's level of education and social context. General questions such as "How are you doing?" of "What can I do for you?" can obviously serve as polite conversation starters but rarely identify all the aspects involved in cognitive disorders.

The history taking should be driven by the standard clinical diagnostic criteria for dementia (see Chap. 1 for an overview of the most common diagnostic criteria). Corner stone of the history talking based on these diagnostic criteria is that there should be evidence of concern about a change in cognition or behavior, in comparison with the person's previous level [11]. This concern can be obtained from the patient, from an informant who knows the patient well, or from a skilled clinician observing the patient. Based on the diagnostic criteria, history taking will as well serve to detect potential mimics or exclusion criteria. E.g., in case of sudden onset, a clinical diagnosis of AD is improbable.

Based on the history taking, the primary care physician can decide (not) to refer a patient to a memory clinic [10]. In the memory clinic, the history taking will result in a differential diagnosis, which will guide the diagnostic process.

General Aspects of History Taking for Dementia Diagnosis

With Whom?

Although the physician's duty is first and foremost directed to his/her patient and symptoms are usually best understood from the patient's perspective, the nature of several cognitive disorders is such that certain symptoms (e.g., memory problems and/or confabulation, delusions that are not frankly absurd, insidious personality change, anosognosia, …) may only be recognized or fully understood through additional information from the patient's caregiver(s). Additionally, lack of insight is a common occurrence in many patients with dementia, which may mean that patients, even in the early stages, will neglect or under-report symptoms.

Medical History

Various disorders can mimic or even cause cognitive decline, especially in the elderly. These conditions should be ruled out and/or treated adequately before further diagnostic evaluation can be considered. Therefore, medical history taking is very important. Extensive questioning should therefore aim to identify all relevant active and past medical illnesses, hospitalizations, surgery, etc. Especially in the elderly, cognitive tests are highly influenced by active (severe) medical illnesses, a fortiori in the presence of delirium—which may have gone unrecognized. The effects of various prescription and illicit drugs, especially those with sedative or anti-cholinergic side effects, should not be underestimated and carefully evaluated. Ideally, the primary care physician provides the memory clinic staff with a clear overview of the individuals' medical and psychiatric history, which can be double checked with the patient (and his/her caregiver) during the first visit.

Social History and Life Style Habits

As acquired cognitive disorders and dementia are characterized by a change from a previous state of functioning, a general idea of the patient's educational and professional history is required. Furthermore, the selection of neuropsychological tests should be done in light of the patient's capacity to understand these tests (e.g., inability to read and write, language barrier). Formal education and the nature of professional activities should be enquired about.

As already mentioned, a patient with dementia depends on his or her caregiver to compensate for the functional deficits that affect ADL. Furthermore, to differentiate between MCI and dementia, assessment of ADL is required. These include the basic ADL and the instrumental ADL that comprises more complex activities such as using the telephone, shopping, preparing food, housekeeping, doing laundry, using transportation, handling medications, handling finances. Physicians should enquire whether and how the patient deals and has dealt with the more cognitively complex tasks of everyday life as dementia (as opposed to MCI) is characterized by impairment in one or more of these activities of daily living.

Lifestyle habits should be actively inquired too and should comprise the use of alcohol and recreational drugs, day-night rhythm, sleep quality, and dietary habits too.

Disease Course

The onset and disease course may provide further clues to a diagnosis. Was the onset sudden, e.g., after a stroke, a severe medical condition or surgery, or a psychologically difficult event? Do cognitive symptoms fluctuate more over time than should be expected from the good and bad days we all experience? Is there a progressive cognitive deterioration, or is it perceived as stepwise? How long have symptoms been present? Are there any "attacks," i.e., very sudden changes in behavior or conscience?

Family History

A detailed family history of neurodegenerative and cerebrovascular brain disorders is important in order to judge the risk of an autosomal dominant genetic etiology. The exact diagnosis should be asked for, as well as the age at disease onset as the risk of an autosomal dominant form increases when the age at onset is younger. It is also relevant to enquire about neurological symptoms in family members, as patients may not know the diagnosis of family members, or the family member may not have been diagnosed. Also, the age at and cause of death should be enquired for first and second-degree relatives; if a person died at a young age, before he/she was able to develop symptoms of dementia, it thus might result in a false-negative family history.

Cognitive Symptoms

Cognitive symptoms should be enquired systematically, checking the main cognitive domains. One should always bear in mind that changes to the previous level of functioning are important. Attention should be paid to the presenting symptom and the chronological order of the cognitive domains that were affected next. As most neurodegenerative brain diseases that cause dementia often start with subtle changes, the onset may be underestimated. What caregivers initially often report as disease onset is the moment when symptoms have become very overt, giving an impression of a rapid cognitive decline. Repeated and further questioning helps to identify more subtle cognitive changes.

Memory

Memory is the ability to receive, store, and retrieve information. The long-term memory is subdivided into several kinds, depending on the nature of the information stored: semantic, episodic (i.e., autobiographic), procedural. In patients with AD, storing new information in the episodic memory progressively gets more difficult and often starts insidiously. This will present as forgetfulness relating to everyday events that require storing new information: grocery shopping, retaining a telephone or bank account number, reiterating the events in a recently watched movie, what one had for dinner the previous day, etc. Repetitive question asking despite clear and repeated instruction suggests short-term memory deficits. These deficits may be masked by confabulations (honestly held erroneous beliefs to fill the amnestic gaps) or frank delusions (e.g., forgetting that one's spouse has gone to the hairdresser and suspecting infidelity). Simple recall tests (e.g., three everyday words) may serve as a quick screening tool. In most degenerative brain diseases, long-term memory is affected much later—especially considering fundamental autobiographical elements (one's date and place of birth, one's name). Sudden (e.g., overnight) and/or prominent loss of these autobiographical elements without affection of other components of memory often suggests psychiatric or functional disturbances. The deflection of simple personal questions towards one's attending spouse or caregiver (the "head turning sign") may be suggestive for memory problems due to neurodegenerative brain disease like AD.

Concentration and Attention

Concentration is generally regarded as the ability to focus one's thought and actions upon a single element or task, which is limited in time, requiring a break. Dividing attention is another aspect of attention (multitasking), which gets more difficult when one grows older. Although attention deficits are often reported by patients as "forgetfulness," these symptoms are not caused by a memory failure, and often the differentiation can be made by careful history taking. Although disorders of attention in (elderly) adults may have a medical cause (as a core symptom of delirium and of dementia), they are often caused by fatigue and sleep disorders, mood disturbances, and other circumstantial factors. Vice-versa, anosognosic patients may wave away their memory disturbances by claiming to be "distracted," "tired," or "absent-minded."

Orientation

Temporal and spatial orientation requires integrating different kinds of information and are often impaired in dementia. The ability to navigate and drive, find one's way in familiar as well as unfamiliar places should be inquired upon. Associated memory problems may contribute to an inability to realize the current day, date, or time of the year—as they may also impair spatial orientation ("how did I get here?").

Language

Language is a core element of everyday life and human interaction. Several cognitive domains are involved in the use of language.

The clinician should at first differentiate between a speech disorder (like dysarthria) and a language disorder. A language disorder (aphasia) can primarily affect speech production (so-called expressive aphasia) or the language comprehension (so-called receptive aphasia), or both. Especially in the case of receptive aphasia, reading or writing abilities will be impaired significantly. The clinician should observe and inquire about symptoms or signs of reduced verbal fluency, word-finding, and the general ability to make conversation. Often, the vocabulary gets reduced, as demonstrated by word-finding difficulties concerning less frequently used words. Secondary languages are affected first, but finally, also the primary language gets affected. Deterioration in reading or writing skills may be indirect clues to deficits of language. During a conversation, the clinician can observe the content and the style of conversation by the patient—speed, volume, articulation, and take note of several types of paraphasias (errors in spoken words). Furthermore, content should be observed for needlessly long explanations of an everyday concept, object, or story, which escapes the patient's memory (i.e., circumlocution).

Executive Disorders

Frontal lobe functions include integrating several mental functions in succession, as is required in planning and organization of complex tasks. Possible questions include asking whether any difficulties are experienced in technical activities or step-by-step endeavors such as cooking. Also in AD, executive functions get progressively impaired.

Behavioural and Psychological Signs and Symptoms of Dementia (BPSD)

The following categories of BPSD should systematically be enquired. In what follows, frequently occurring symptoms per category are described in order to help structuring the history taking.

Mood Disorders and Anxiety

Depressive symptoms are very frequent in patients with dementia [12]. Depression in the elderly can also mimic dementia, as depression in the elderly is more often associated with cognitive symptoms as compared to depressive disorders of earlier adulthood. On the other hand, depressive symptoms may also be the first clinical manifestation of dementia. It has been suggested that depression and dementia share common risk factors and thereby frequently occur together without being causally linked themselves, or those psychological symptoms may occur as a reaction to incipient decline in patients who are aware of their cognitive disturbances. The exact nature of the relationship between depressive symptoms and dementia in the elderly remains inconclusive, with multiple studies supporting both the risk factor and prodromal hypotheses. It seems unlikely that there is no connection at all [12, 13].

A thoughtful inventory of depressive symptoms (depressed mood, anhedonia, vegetative and sleep-related symptoms, suicidal thoughts, etc.) and symptoms of anxiety should be considered in all patients. Screening tools and rating scales may be helpful instruments to systematically enquire about these symptoms [13]. A very common feature of neurodegenerative brain diseases is apathy [14]. Although apathy may be a symptom of depression, further questioning may be helpful to differentiate between apathy as a syndrome versus a symptom that is part of depression. Apathy frequently does not alarm or bother the patient but may prove very stressful to family members and care providers.

Anxiety also frequently occurs and should be systematically enquired. One of the most frequent presentations of anxiety in patients with dementia is the fear of being left alone, which may result in "shadowing" of the main caregiver.

Sleep and Diurnal Rhythm Disturbances

Sleep quality should be systematically assessed as sleep disturbances are very burdensome for the caregiver and as poor sleep quality may have a negative impact on cognitive functioning. Moreover, sleep disturbances can sometimes be improved pharmacologically. When enquiring about sleep quality, signs, and symptoms of REM sleep behavior disorder (acting out dreams, nightmares) should be asked for.

Hallucinations and Delusions

Hallucinations and delusions are both frequent in dementia. Hallucinations should be characterized by the sensory modality they present in—generally visual as opposed to the typical auditory hallucinations of primary psychotic disorders.

Tactile and hallucinations in other sensory modalities may occur too but are very rare in dementia. As patients may or may not be aware of the hallucinatory nature of these events (especially when their content is relatively benign, e.g., a visiting family member or a dog in the garden), these often go unrecognized.

In AD, hallucinations are often not well defined and may be associated with (paranoid) delusions, occurring in the more advanced stages of the disease [15]. Patients with DLB may have well-formed complex hallucinations of people, animals, or objects that can occur in the earliest stages of the disease. Besides complex visual hallucinations, simple visual hallucinations and even visual illusions may occur in DLB, also in the periphery of the visual field. As the latter may as well occur briefly, they are often not perceived as visual hallucinations unless they are specifically asked for. The clinician should moreover be aware that (mild) hallucinations are quite frequent in general and can be provoked by a near endless list of medical conditions and (prescription or illicit) drugs. A frequent cause of visual hallucinations is the Charles-Bonnet syndrome, which is due to loss of visual acuity. As visual impairment is frequent in elderly patients, as is dementia, this is a frequent cause of visual hallucinations in elderly patients with dementia. In the Charles-Bonnet syndrome, patients are often aware of the false nature of these hallucinations, which is often not the case when the hallucinations are linked to dementia syndrome.

The combination of memory deficits and anosognosia may provoke paranoid delusions. Although not always in and of themselves entirely impossible (e.g., presumed adultery, relatives' financial interests, mislaid items having been stolen by intruders), their sudden prominence in patient's mental life and conversations with strangers may provide clues to their delusional nature. People with dementia may also suffer from the Capgras syndrome, also known as imposter syndrome, which is a delusion (and thus rather a symptom than a syndrome) that someone they know (e.g., spouse) has been replaced by an imposter.

Agitation and Aggressiveness

This category of BPSD becomes more frequent when dementia progresses [16, 17]. The same holds true for aberrant motor activity, which can be very burdensome for caregivers. Severity and frequency should be assessed, as well as provoking circumstances. The latter may help to develop a tailored non-pharmacological treatment strategy. If uncontrollable, these symptoms can be a reason for early nursing home placement.

Personality

Changes in personality is always worrisome and requires neuropsychiatric investigation. The patient should be evaluated for their general impression, grooming, and cleanliness. Is there a tendency towards harsh answers or inappropriate remarks, aggressiveness, impulsivity, and irritability? Even when taking possible marital or familial quarrels into account, caregiver history is often crucial in elucidating these aspects.

Motor Symptoms

Especially parkinsonian symptoms are frequent in neurodegenerative (and cerebrovascular) disorders that cause dementia. Bradykinesia, tremor, rigidity, and gait disturbances are frequent signs and symptoms that should be systematically questioned, the more so as they can also help to differentiate amongst causes of dementia. Given the frequency of the motor and parkinsonian symptoms, it is important to subject each patient to a physical and clinical neurological examination.

Physical Examination

A general physical examination should be performed in every patient in case of a dementia work-up. The general physical exam is needed to detect medical conditions that can cause dementia-like symptoms (e.g., heart failure, malignancy). The clinical neurological examination should focus on parkinsonian symptoms and gait disturbances, signs and symptoms of stroke (lateralization, focal neurological signs). FTD may be associated with amyotrophic lateral sclerosis, so the neurological exam should as well detect amyotrophy, signs of corticospinal tract involvement (paresis, hyperreflexia, …).

Blood Sampling, ECG, EEG

A blood sampling should be performed every time a dementia work-up is carried out. Blood analysis serves to rule out medical conditions that can cause dementia-like symptoms (e.g., renal failure, hepatic failure, hyper- or hypothyroidism, hypovitaminosis B12, folic acid deficiency) and should as well contain complete blood count and blood ionogram. In selected patients, additional serologic testing (HIV, Borrelia, syphilis) should be performed.

Both electrocardiography (ECG) and electro-encephalography (ECG) are worth considering. ECG is useful in selected patients (e.g., cardiovascular risk factors, cardiac comorbidity, bradycardia) before prescribing psychotropic medication. As some forms of epilepsy or a non-convulsive status may mimic some dementia symptoms, an EEG should be considered in selected patients.

Neuropsychological Examination

Introduction

A full neuropsychological examination is the cornerstone of the work-up of patients with dementia and is part of an integrative approach to the (differential) diagnosis of dementia [18]. Brief screening tests can be used to detect patients at risk for dementia [19]. The full neuropsychological examination should be performed by an experienced neuropsychologist and includes an array of different tests to investigate cognitive functioning. The latter has two major goals: [1] to detect cognitive decline and differentiate between normal aging and cognitive impairment and [2] to help in the differentiation between different causes of dementia. For the interpretation of the test results, the neuropsychologist takes into account the mood and mental status of the patient as well as his/her (neuropsychiatric) history. A neuropsychological evaluation thus as well consists of an expert clinical evaluation, besides the formal testing. As a dementia diagnosis cannot be made in a patient suffering from delirium and should be avoided in a patient suffering from major depressive symptoms, this clinical evaluation is of great importance. Furthermore, a neuropsychological exam can be used to stage the dementia syndrome and to monitor the cognitive decline in patients with dementia.

By use of careful history taking and a full neuropsychological examination, we are able to diagnose neurodegenerative (and cerebrovascular) brain diseases that cause dementia, even before the dementia stage is reached, the so-called MCI stage. Neuropsychological testing is furthermore useful in the differentiation of patients with MCI from those with mild dementia.

No single test is able to differentiate between different types of neurodegenerative and cerebrovascular diseases, which is why a panel of different neuropsychological tests should be used. The Diagnostic and Statistical Manual of Mental Disorders V (DSM-V) lists six cognitive domains, which might be affected in neurocognitive disorders, including complex attention, executive functions, learning and memory, language, perceptual motor functions, and social cognition [20]. Deficits in certain domains are more prevalent in different types of dementia [20]:

1. Complex attention includes sustained attention, divided attention, and selective attention.
2. Executive functions include planning, decision-making, working memory, responding to feedback, inhibition, and mental flexibility.
3. Learning and memory include free recall, cued recall, recognition memory, semantic and autobiographical long-term memory, and implicit learning.
4. Language includes object naming, word-finding, fluency, grammar, and syntax.
5. Perceptual motor function includes visual perception, visuoconstructional reasoning, and perceptual motor coordination.
6. Social cognition includes recognition of emotions, theory of mind, insight.

Cognitive Screening Tests

There are several cognitive screening tests used to identify adults at risk for dementia. These tests are also used to obtain a global index of cognitive functioning and in follow-up of patients with dementia. Benefits of these screening tests include being cheap, fast, and non-invasive. Most cognitive screening tests are sensitive to cultural background, premorbid intelligence, and education; results should always be treated with caution. The most commonly used screening test is the Mini-Mental State

Examination (MMSE) [21]. However, there are a lot of other cognitive screening tests available varying in assessment time between less than 5–21 min, including the Memory Impairment Screen [22], the phototest [23], Alzheimer Quick test [24], Quick Mild Cognitive Impairment screen [25], the Cognitive State test [26], Montreal Cognitive Assessment (MoCA) [27], Addenbrooke's Cognitive Examination—Revised [28] and others. These tests cover from one up to seven cognitive domains, including memory, language, orientation, executive functions, praxis, visuospatial abilities, and attention (e.g., MoCA) [19].

The most commonly used test, MMSE, tests patients on several cognitive aspects (attention and orientation, memory, registration, recall, calculation, language, and ability to draw) by use of 30 questions. A score of ≥25 is considered normal. However, a meta-analysis has shown that it has a very limited ability to differentiate between patients with MCI and healthy controls. It had the best value for ruling out a diagnosis of dementia in the community and primary care, but for other purposes should be combined with other neuropsychological tests [29]. As said before, early detection of patients with cognitive decline is important, making it a less interesting screening tool, which is why some reviewers suggest to replace the MMSE with more performant alternatives.

Most of the previously mentioned screening tests have been studied for use in a memory clinic setting but have not been validated in a population-based setting. According to recommendations based on a systematic review by De Roeck et al. [19], the MoCA test is the most suitable for overall population-based screening to detect MCI or AD dementia. Although these screening tests are cheap, fast, and non-invasive, clinicians and researchers should bear in mind that no screening test can be used in every setting, for all different neurodegenerative diseases, and for each population.

To conclude, the MoCA, testing seven different cognitive domains, is a promising screening instrument and is validated in a population-based setting, however, specificity to detect early AD is rather low. We should, however, bear in mind that the role of population-based screening for AD is debated. In the absence of disease-modifying drugs, population-based screening cannot be recommended.

A Dementia Diagnosis Requires a Full Neuropsychological Examination

In order to evaluate the extent of cognitive decline and to be able to differentiate between different causes of dementia, batteries of neuropsychological tests are used. Each test separately yields a score indexing the functioning on a certain or on several cognitive domains. This holds true for the MCI and early dementia stages; in more advanced stages of dementia, cognitive deficits tend to be global, which does not allow differentiating between AD and non-AD causes of dementia.

As mentioned before, neuropsychological testing can aid in the differentiation of patients with MCI and the healthy, ageing population. Important to mention is the fact that the boundaries between age-related cognitive changes and early dementia are more difficult to distinguish in patients aged 80 years or more, due to the fact that many of the structural and functional brain changes in AD overlap with changes observed in normal aging [18].

Different causes of dementia lead to distinguishable neuropsychological profiles (Table 3.1) [18]. In AD, the primary feature includes deficit in episodic memory (recall of experience that is personal to the patient), which is the earliest and most salient sign, with progression to problems with semantic memory (recall of general/lexical facts and impairment of language abilities). Episodic memory can be tested verbally and visually, by asking to remember a list of words (e.g., California Verbal Learning test) [30] or by asking to copy a figure and recall it at a later time (e.g., Visual Reproduction Test) [31] respectively. In a very early stage of AD, patients are particularly impaired on this delayed recall. Furthermore, patients with impairment of episodic memory (e.g., such as in AD) do not benefit from cueing. This is in contrast to patients with deficits of other cognitive domains (e.g., attentional deficits), which may also affect memory ability, and where cueing tends to improve

Table 3.1 Overview of typical cognitive deficits for some of the most common forms of dementia and of commonly used neuropsychological tests, typically used to detect these deficits

Disease	Cognitive impairment	Neuropsychological tests
AD	Episodic memory, semantic memory, language abilities, executive functions, visuospatial abilities	• Episodic memory: California Verbal Learning test, Visual Reproduction Test • Semantic memory, language: Verbal fluency, Boston Naming task • Executive functions: Tower of London, Part B of Trail Making test, Stroop test, Raven Progressive Matrices Task • Visuospatial abilities: Clock Drawing test, complex figure copying, Money Road Map test, segregation of overlapping figures
FTD	Executive functions, language, behavioural, and personality alterations	• Executive functions: Tower of London, Part B of Trail Making test, Stroop test, Raven Progressive Matrices Task, Frontal Assessment Battery • Semantic memory, language: Verbal fluency, Boston Naming task • Behaviour: neuropsychiatric questionnaire
DLB	Visuoperceptual/ visuoconstructive functions, executive functions, attention	• Visuospatial: Block Design Test, Clock Drawing Test, complex figure copying, segregation of overlapping figures • Executive functions: Tower of London, Part B of Trail Making test, Stroop test, Raven Progressive Matrices Task, Frontal Assessment Battery • Attention: Digit Span
VaD	Executive functions, visuoconstructional abilities	• Visuospatial: Block Design Test, Clock Drawing Test, complex figure copying, segregation of overlapping figures • Executive functions: Tower of London, Part B of Trail Making test, Stroop test, Raven Progressive Matrices Task, Frontal Assessment Battery

performance. Semantic memory can be tested by use of category fluency in which patients have to generate as much words belonging to a certain category as possible (e.g., category of animals), by use of picture naming tests (e.g., Boston naming task), or by testing the patients´ knowledge of conceptual hierarchies. With disease progression, AD patients also become impaired in executive functions (tested by use of tests like the Tower of London puzzle, Part B of the Trail Making Test, Raven Progressive Matrices Task, and Stroop Test) and visuospatial abilities (including visuoconstructional abilities tested by Clock Drawing test, complex figure copying and visuoperceptual abilities tested by Money Road Map Test) [32].

Episodic memory and visuospatial abilities are typically initially spared in FTD. Problems reported with memory in FTD are more likely linked to inattention, which can be examined with tests like Digit Span. FTD patients, and especially those suffering from semantic dementia or nonfluent primary progressive aphasia, also present with semantic memory impairments. FTD is furthermore characterized by problems with executive functioning, as well as behavioral changes. A commonly used test for detecting frontal dysexecutive phenotype is the Frontal Assessment Battery [33].

When it comes to cognitive domains affected, DLB is best delineated from AD by disproportionately severe visuospatial and visuoconstructive deficits in the former. This can be elucidated by tests for visuoperception (e.g., Money Road Map Test, segregation of overlapping figures), for visual search (parallel search tasks), and visuoconstructional abilities (e.g., drawing complex figures). They are often also more impaired in executive functions and attention than patients with AD [32].

VaD is characterized by greater deficits in executive functions and visuoconstruction, rather than memory and language. However, patients with vascular dementia exhibit a variable cognitive profile, which is a reflection of the extent and spatial location of the underlying pathology. They are usually less impaired regarding episodic memory.

Differential Diagnosis: Role of the Neuropsychological Examination

Next to the above-mentioned causes of dementia, some other causes might lead to cognitive impairment, e.g., depression or other psychiatric conditions, alcohol abuse, sleeping problems (e.g., obstructive sleep apnoea syndrome), multiple sclerosis, normal pressure hydrocephalus, and tumors. These conditions should be screened for during history taking (see above) and by use of supplementary investigations (see below), but screening for some of these conditions also takes part in the neuropsychological examination. Patients with multiple sclerosis have a slowing down of processing speed but might also get impaired on episodic memory, attention, or executive functions. Normal pressure hydrocephalus is characterized by executive dysfunction, psychomotor slowing, inattention, and mood symptoms, especially apathy.

Structural Imaging: Magnetic Resonance Imaging (MRI)

From Exclusion of Other Causes to Automated Volumetry

Structural imaging of the central nervous system has made incredible progress over the last 50 years and is indispensable in today's neurology practice. Computed tomography (CT) and magnetic resonance imaging (MRI) play a crucial role in the differential diagnosis of degenerative versus structural causes of cognitive impairment. Guidelines propose to perform structural imaging in all patients presenting with cognitive decline [34]. It enables exclusion of brain lesions such as brain neoplasms, strategic infarcts, subdural hematoma, and normal pressure hydrocephalus. These structural etiologies account for 2–5% of dementia cases and can be present in patients without suggestive history or without abnormalities on the clinical neurological examination [35].

To visualize the brain in detail, MRI is the preferred imaging modality because of its superior contrast of gray and white matter. Moreover, MRI is more performant to detect vascular pathology than CT scan, allows automated volumetry, which can be a helpful tool to detect (hippocampal) atrophy. In case of normal pressure hydrocephalus, prominent aqueductal flow void due to increased CSF velocity across the aqueduct is often seen on a specific sequences of a brain MRI scan. Certain patients will not be able to undergo an MRI, due to incompatible metal implants, claustrophobia, or the inability to lay still during the examination. If a patient is unable to undergo an MRI, CT can be sufficient for cognitive impairment work-up [36].

Different neurodegenerative disorders have characteristic signatures of brain atrophy that can be detected by structural imaging. Brain atrophy in AD generally follows the classic pattern described by Braak and Braak, with the hippocampus and entorhinal cortex affected first [37]. Scheltens and colleagues proposed a 5-point scale for visual assessment of medial temporal atrophy (MTA) on MRI [38]. The score is based on the coronal hippocampal height and width of the adjacent fissures. Hippocampal volume is lower compared to age-matched healthy controls in both dementia due to AD (20–30%) and MCI due to AD (15%) and a lower hippocampal volume in patients with MCI increases the risk to progress to the dementia stage [39]. With the increased availability of MRI, serial imaging to quantify the speed of volume loss over time in different brain regions seems interesting. Hippocampal volume reduces with age, but this reduction is twice as fast in AD compared to age-matched healthy controls and is even a predictor of evolution to the dementia stage in MCI [40]. With advancing computing power and MRI image quality (semi)automated volumetry of the hippocampus became feasible. Intuitively, the volumetric approach seems to have several advantages over visual MTA evaluation: lower to no interobserver variability, detection of more subtle changes, and a scale that is not limited to 5 discrete values. Automated extracted hippocampal volumes can differentiate between clinical diagnostic groups and may be a useful tool for characterizing and diagnosing AD, also in its prodromal stage [41]. Validation and harmonization exercises have been and are being performed [41, 42].

Limited Sensitivity and Specificity of Structural Imaging Biomarkers

Hippocampal atrophy is neither sensitive nor specific for AD. About one in ten AD patients has an atypical form of AD, with relatively preserved memory but impairment in other cognitive domains. These patients have a different pattern of brain atrophy, with relative sparing of the hippocampus and more prominent neocortical atrophy. The occipito-parietal cortex is most attained in posterior cortical atrophy, the left posterior temporal cortex in primary progressive aphasia, and the frontal lobes in the behavioral variant of AD [43]. The rate of hippocampal atrophy is not equal over the disease course of AD, but is inversely related to MMSE, with little volume loss earlier in the disease [44]. MCI may have a completely normal MRI for their age.

Specificity of hippocampal atrophy is also limited, since other non-AD neurodegenerative disorder causing dementia such as frontotemporal lobe degeneration, hippocampal sclerosis and the new entity limbic-predominant age-related TDP-43 encephalopathy are all associated with hippocampal atrophy [45–48].

PET Imaging

Introduction

Positron emission tomography (PET) is a nuclear imaging technique, using positron-emitting radionucleotides. These radionucleotides are fused with a molecule of choice and injected intravenously, after which they are transported through the bloodstream to specific organs or cells. Here they will decay and emit a positron that will almost immediately fuse with an electron, thereby emitting two photons in opposing directions that will be detected by cameras. These cameras attain a spatial resolution of 3–5 mm. PET allows the visualization of various molecular processes occurring in the body. The main disadvantages of the technique are the limited availability due to costs of hardware and the short half-life of relevant radionucleotides (The longest frequently used radionucleotide is fluorine-18 (F-18), with a half-life of 110 min) and thus the necessity to make them at the facility, or be in close proximity to a commercial dealer. As a PET scan involves radioactive tracers, there is exposure to radiation, albeit minimal. Altogether, PET imaging will not serve as a screening tool for dementia, but is a powerful diagnostic tool in selected subjects.

FDG-PET

^{18}-fluorodeoxyglucose (FDG) PET uses F-18 coupled to a 2-deoxy-glucose molecule as radiopharmaceutical. FDG has a similar uptake and metabolism as glucose. Glucose is the main energy source of the neuron and its uptake correlates well with synaptic activity. Most synapses in the brain are glumatergic, and FDG-PET is thus a proxy for local glutamatergic synaptic function. In neurodegenerative disorders, synaptic dysfunction is an upstream event of neuronal death, which enables earlier detection than techniques measuring atrophy [49]. A brain FDG-PET scan should be combined with structural imaging (mostly brain CT scan) in order to correct for brain atrophy and cerebrovascular disease

With aging, glucose metabolism of the brain decreases mainly in motor, parietal and anterior and middle cingulate cortex decreases in a symmetrical manner. The typical AD dementia pattern of hypometabolism in FDG-PET is early (possibly asymmetric) hypometabolism of the precuneus, posterior cingulate cortex (PCC), and temporoparietal cortex with sparing of the primary motor and sensory cortex. The hypometabolism may extend to frontal or occipital regions but is not more pronounced in these regions than in the PCC [49]. Atypical AD forms, with relatively preserved memory, have a different pattern with hypometabolism in occipital (PCA variant); left-sided posterior parietotemporal (logopenic variant); prefrontal, dorsolateral prefrontal and orbitofrontal (behavioral variant) or superior parietal cortex, contralateral to the most affected limbs (corticobasal syndrome due to AD) [50]. A meta-analysis of 119 studies in 2011 revealed a pooled sensitivity of 91% and specificity of 86% at differentiating AD dementia from healthy controls with FDG-PET [51]. Automated FDG-PET analysis seemed even more potent to answer this question, with a sensitivity of 99% and a specificity of 98% [52]. Only two studies used autopsy-confirmed cases and showed a pooled sensitivity of 89% and a specificity of 74% for discerning AD from healthy controls [53, 54]. In MCI due to AD, PCC seems to be most frequently affected, with other regions of the AD signature variably affected, but to a lesser extent than in AD dementia. The severity of hypometabolism is correlated with cognitive impairment in both MCI and dementia due to AD.

An important clinical question is whether FDG-PET can differentiate neurodegenerative disorders underlying dementia. DLB typically has lower metabolism in the occipital cortex, especially the primary visual and visual association cortex, while preserving regions commonly affected in AD, especially the PCC (known as "posterior cingulate island sign") [55]. The FDG-PET signature of frontotemporal lobar degeneration (FTLD) depends on the clinical variant: behavioral variant FTD has the involvement of frontal and anterior temporal lobes, semantic variant presents as bilateral but asymmetrical involvement of anterior temporal lobe, progressive nonfluent aphasia shows hypometabolism of the frontal opercular and temporal, insular cortex of the dominant hemisphere [56]. Patients with VaD typically show subcortical or focal cortical hypometabolism, corresponding to infarcted zones on structural imaging [56].

FDG-PET has found its way into the diagnostic criteria for AD, FTD, and DLB. Certain drawbacks exist for FDG-PET. High blood glucose levels in patients with uncontrolled diabetes mellitus mimic an AD signature in FDG-PET. Psychotropics and benzodiazepines, as well as alcohol, reduce overall glucose uptake, but without region-specific pattern [57].

Amyloid PET

Amyloid PET allows in vivo detection of one of the pathological hallmarks of AD: extracellular amyloid plaques. The first tracer was ^{11}C Pittsburgh-compound B (PiB), a thioflavin-T analog that at the concentrations used for PET only binds to the beta-sheets of amyloid plaques. The short half-life of ^{11}C led to the development of three approved equivalent ^{18}F tracers: florbetapir, flutemetamol, florbetaben that are, however, not all three available worldwide.

Since amyloid PET gives non-invasive in vivo information on one of the key players in AD, it is a useful diagnostic tool for AD. In autopsy-confirmed cases, amyloid PET imaging carried out on average 3 years before autopsy had a sensitivity of 91% and a specificity of 92% at differentiating AD from non-AD dementia [58]. The typical AD amyloid PET sequence shows uptake in the orbitofrontal and inferior temporal cortex, cingulate gyrus, and precuneus first, followed by prefrontal, lateral temporal, and parietal cortex [59]. In contrast to other imaging markers, atypical forms of AD present with a similar pattern. As holds true for all biomarkers, amyloid PET should only be used in the correct clinical context, especially given the high number of asymptomatic amyloid positive elderly. This makes amyloid PET an excellent instrument to rule out AD in individual subjects and to diagnose AD amongst individual younger patients. However, its positive predictive value might be less strong in individual elderly subjects due to the high number of asymptomatic amyloid positive subjects.

Amyloid PET is excellent at differentiating AD from a pure tauopathy as FTLD, with an accuracy of over 90% [60]. In DLB, however, up to 60% of patients have amyloid deposition following a similar pattern as AD, with a total amyloid load that is generally lower than patients with dementia due to AD. It was not thought possible to discriminate between both diseases based on amyloid PET, but a study published in 2020 on 39 autopsy-confirmed DLB and AD patients showed that a cut-off with 93% accuracy could be established in amyloid PET [61]. A meta-analysis concluded that patients with VaD have a similar percentage of amyloid positive scans as age-matched controls [62].

Defining amyloid positivity can be done in a qualitative or quantitative way. Standard uptake value (SUV) is a widely used quantifier to assess the activity of radioligand, corrected for weight and injected dose. For amyloid PET, an SUV ratio (SUVR) is calculated between regions with frequent amyloid deposition in AD and the cerebellum, where no amyloid deposition occurs. This value depends on the used tracer, pre- and postprocessing of images, and is difficult to generalize between centers. This problem is tackled by the "centiloid" measure, that corrects for these parameters by according a value to every scan, where 0 is no amyloid pathology, and 100 equals amyloid load in patients with mild dementia due to AD [63]. This enables to correctly interpret data from different centers within one study or to make shared databases easily interpretable.

CSF Biomarkers

Introduction

The CSF offers a window to the brain as the brain's metabolism and pathology is reflected in the CSF. To collect CSF, a lumbar puncture (LP) is needed, which is a safe and well-tolerated procedure. If performed correctly, LP has a low complication rate and a high diagnostic yield. While structural brain imaging studies may sometimes eliminate the need for a diagnostic LP, indications for diagnostic LP still remain, especially in cases of suspected infectious or immune-mediated inflammatory disorders of the nervous system. Moreover, diagnostic LP may be indicated in AD and other neurodegenerative disorders, Creutzfeldt-Jakob disease, normal pressure hydrocephalus. For the latter condition, evacuating LP is indicated.

As AD is the most frequent cause of dementia, most biomarker research focused on AD, resulting in several CSF biomarkers that increase the diagnostic accuracy of AD. Biomarkers that reflect the pathology of AD already show abnormal concentrations in the preclinical stage of AD, thus allowing early AD diagnosis. Although no CSF biomarkers for non-AD dementias are available for daily clinical practice yet, the core AD CSF biomarkers have an added diagnostic value for differential dementia diagnosis too.

Lumbar Puncture (LP)

An LP can be safely performed with a high acceptance rate and a high diagnostic yield. The most common complications of LP consist of post-LP back pain and post-LP headache (PLPH). Very rare (prevalence of <0.01%), but potential serious complications consist of post-LP infections, spinal and subdural cerebral hematoma, and cerebral venous thrombosis.

Although a substantial proportion (31%) of patients reported post-LP complaints in an international, multicenter LP feasibility study, these were mostly mild and transient [64]. Back pain, headache, and typical PLPH were reported by 17%, 19%, and 9% of subjects, respectively. Only 0.3% of the subjects needed a blood patch for PLPH, and in 0.7%, a hospitalization was required. The most important risk factors for post-LP complaints were related to patient characteristics: history of headache and fear of complications. A cutting bevel needle-type appeared to be the only procedure-related risk factor for typical PLPH. The number of LP attempts was related to post-LP back pain. A large needle diameter was a risk factor for severe headaches.

Based on the results of this international, multicenter LP feasibility study, as well as a literature review, consensus guidelines and recommendations for the LP procedure in adults were formulated [65]. These recommendations should minimize post-LP complications, the most frequent being PLPH and post-LP back pain.

Core AD CSF Biomarkers

The core AD CSF biomarkers are related to the three main pathological changes: amyloid-β deposition into extracellular amyloid plaques, intracellular neurofibrillary tangles formation, and neuronal loss. The β-amyloid peptide composed of 42 amino acids ($A\beta_{1-42}$) results from the cleavage of the transmembrane amyloid precursor protein. $A\beta_{1-42}$ is insoluble and aggregates into extracellular amyloid plaques, detected as decreased CSF $A\beta_{1-42}$ concentrations. Tau proteins are present in the cytosol of neurons, where they stabilize microtubules. In AD, a hyperphosphorylation of tau occurs, leading to the formation of neurofibrillary tangles. During the neurodegenerative process, tau and phosphorylated tau proteins are released into the extracellular space, resulting in increased CSF tau concentrations.

The first amyloid plaques occur at least 10 years, and probably 20–30 years before the first symptoms [3]; CSF $A\beta_{1-42}$ therefore is a very early marker of AD. CSF tau biomarkers change later in the pathophysiological process compared, and CSF tau is stronger correlated to cognitive decline than $A\beta_{1-42}$. CSF biomarkers give a complete overview of AD pathophysiology, and in addition, an LP is highly accessible with a low cost price, in contrast to the imaging-based markers used in AD diagnosis.

Core AD CSF Biomarkers for Early Diagnosis

The core AD CSF biomarkers $A\beta_{1-42}$, total protein tau (T-tau), and tau phosphorylated at threonine 181 (P-tau_{181}) are strongly associated with future development of AD dementia amongst patients with MCI, which was proven in a several prospective, longitudinal studies [5]. The core AD CSF biomarkers can in fact identify those MCI patients who have prodromal AD. In the study of Hansson et al., The combination of CSF $A\beta_{1-42}$ and T-tau at baseline yielded sensitivity and specificity levels of 95% and 83% for diagnosing prodromal AD in a heterogeneous MCI cohort [66].

Core AD CSF Biomarker for Differential Dementia Diagnosis

The core AD CSF biomarkers $A\beta_{1-42}$, T-tau, and P-tau_{181} can discriminate between AD and non-AD dementias, but they cannot be used to confirm another type of dementia [5]. Several other brain diseases can lead to changes of these CSF biomarker levels, causing possible misinterpretation of the biomarker results in the absence of clinical information. A marked increase in T-tau is also detected after stroke and in Creutzfeldt-Jakob's disease. For this reason,, P-tau_{181} is a very helpful marker for differential dementia diagnosis as it is a more specific marker for AD. Indeed, CSF levels of $A\beta_{1-42}$ and T-tau are often intermediate between normal control and abnormal AD values in non-AD patients, especially in DLB but also in FTD, VaD.

The addition of the most abundant Aβ isoform, $A\beta_{1-40}$ into an $A\beta_{1-42}/A\beta_{1-40}$ ratio diminishes inter-patient variability (to control for high or low $A\beta_{1-42}$ production, irrespective of AD pathology) and also improves differential dementia diagnosis in patients with intermediate P-tau_{181} levels [67]. Increased concordance between amyloid markers (amyloid PET scan and CSF Aβ) was found in two studies when the $A\beta_{1-42}/A\beta_{1-40}$ ratio was applied compared to a CSF $A\beta_{1-42}$ concentration alone [68]. Therefore, the $A\beta_{1-42}/A\beta_{1-40}$ ratio has become part of the core AD CSF biomarkers.

Other CSF biomarkers are under development and may, following validation and standardization, be used in daily clinical practice, like neurofilament light to diagnose FTD.

Conclusions

In the past, the diagnosis of AD could only be suggested when the dementia stage was reached. Due to major advances in biomarker-based research, it is now possible to detect AD-related changes at the first clinical symptoms.

If a timely diagnosis is desirable, history taking and a full neuropsychological examination are the cornerstone of a dementia diagnosis. Specific biomarkers can be applied to increase the early and differential diagnostic accuracy.

References

1. McKhann G, Drachman D, Folstein M, Katzman R, Price D, Stadlan EM. Clinical diagnosis of Alzheimer's disease: report of the NINCDS-ADRDA Work Group under the auspices of Department of Health and Human Services Task Force on Alzheimer's Disease. Neurology. 1984;34(7):939–44. https://doi.org/10.1212/wnl.34.7.939.
2. Knopman DS, DeKosky ST, Cummings JL, Chui H, Corey-Bloom J, Relkin N, et al. Practice parameter: diagnosis of dementia (an evidence-based review). Report of the Quality Standards Subcommittee of the American Academy of Neurology. Neurology. 2001;56(9):1143–53. https://doi.org/10.1212/wnl.56.9.1143.
3. Jack CR Jr, Knopman DS, Jagust WJ, Shaw LM, Aisen PS, Weiner MW, et al. Hypothetical model of dynamic biomarkers of the Alzheimer's pathological cascade. Lancet Neurol. 2010;9(1):119–28. https://doi.org/10.1016/S1474-4422(09)70299-6.
4. Jack CR Jr, Holtzman DM. Biomarker modeling of Alzheimer's disease. Neuron. 2013;80(6):1347–58. https://doi.org/10.1016/j.neuron.2013.12.003.
5. Somers C, Struyfs H, Goossens J, Niemantsverdriet E, Luyckx J, De Roeck N, et al. A decade of cerebrospinal fluid biomarkers for Alzheimer's Disease in Belgium. J Alzheimers Dis. 2016;54(1):383–95. https://doi.org/10.3233/JAD-151097.
6. Gossye H, Van Broeckhoven C, Engelborghs S. The use of biomarkers and genetic screening to diagnose frontotemporal dementia: evidence and clinical implications. Front Neurosci. 2019;13:757. https://doi.org/10.3389/fnins.2019.00757. eCollection 2019
7. Joe E, Ringman JM. Cognitive symptoms of Alzheimer's disease: clinical management and prevention. Br Med J. 2019;367:l6217. https://doi.org/10.1136/bmj.l6217.
8. Frederiksen KS, Nielsen TR, Winblad B, Schmidt R, Kramberger MG, Jones RW, et al. European Academy of Neurology/European Alzheimer's Disease Consortium position state-

ment on diagnostic disclosure, biomarker counseling, and management of patients with mild cognitive impairment. Eur J Neurol. 2020. doi: https://doi.org/10.1111/ene.14668.
9. De Roeck EE, Engelborghs S, Dierckx E. Next generation brain health depends on early Alzheimer Disease diagnosis: from a timely diagnosis to future population screening. J Am Med Dir Assoc. 2016;17(5):452–3. https://doi.org/10.1016/j.jamda.2016.02.015.
10. Liss JL, Seleri Assunção S, Cummings J, Atri A, Geldmacher DS, Candela SF, et al. Practical recommendations for timely, accurate diagnosis of symptomatic Alzheimer's disease (MCI and dementia) in primary care: a review and synthesis. J Intern Med. 2021. doi: https://doi.org/10.1111/joim.13244.
11. Albert MS, DeKosky ST, Dickson D, Dubois B, Feldman HH, Fox NC, et al. The diagnosis of mild cognitive impairment due to Alzheimer's disease: recommendations from the National Institute on Aging-Alzheimer's Association workgroups on diagnostic guidelines for Alzheimer's disease. Alzheimers Dement. 2011;7(3):270–9. https://doi.org/10.1016/j.jalz.2011.03.008.
12. Wiels W, Baeken C, Engelborghs S. Depressive symptoms in the elderly-an early symptom of dementia? A systematic review. Front Pharmacol. 2020;11:34. https://doi.org/10.3389/fphar.2020.00034. eCollection 2020
13. Van der Mussele S, Fransen E, Struyfs H, Luyckx J, Mariën P, Saerens J, et al. Depression in mild cognitive impairment is associated with progression to Alzheimer's disease: a longitudinal study. J Alzheimers Dis. 2014;42(4):1239–50. https://doi.org/10.3233/JAD-140405.
14. Vloeberghs R, Opmeer EM, De Deyn PP, Engelborghs S, De Roeck EE. Apathy, depression and cognitive functioning in patients with MCI and dementia. Tijdschrift Gerontologie Geriatrie. 2018;49(3):95–102. https://doi.org/10.1007/s12439-018-0248-6.
15. Van der Mussele S, Mariën P, Saerens J, Somers N, Goeman J, De Deyn PP, et al. Psychosis associated behavioral and psychological signs and symptoms in mild cognitive impairment and Alzheimer's dementia. Aging Ment Health. 2015;19(9):818–28. https://doi.org/10.1080/13607863.2014.967170.
16. Van der Mussele S, Mariën P, Saerens J, Somers N, Goeman J, De Deyn PP, et al. Behavioral syndromes in mild cognitive impairment and Alzheimer's disease. J Alzheimers Dis. 2014;38(2):319–29. https://doi.org/10.3233/JAD-130596.
17. Van der Mussele S, Le Bastard N, Saerens J, Somers N, Mariën P, Goeman J, et al. Agitation-associated behavioral symptoms in mild cognitive impairment and Alzheimer's dementia. Aging Ment Health. 2015;19(3):247–57. https://doi.org/10.1080/13607863.2014.924900.
18. Salmon DP, Bondi MW. Neuropsychological assessment of dementia. Annu Rev Psychol. 2009;60:257–82. https://doi.org/10.1146/annurev.psych.57.102904.190024.
19. De Roeck E, De Deyn PP, Dierckx E, Engelborghs S. Brief cognitive screening instruments for early detection of Alzheimer's disease: a systematic review. Alzheimers Res Ther. 2019;11(21):1–14. https://doi.org/10.1186/s13195-019-0474-3.
20. American Psychiatric Association. Diagnostic and statistical manual of mental disorders. 5th ed. Arlington, VA: American Psychiatric Association; 2013.
21. Folstein MF, Folstein SE, McHugh PR. Mini-mental state: a practical method for grading the cognitive state of patients for the clinician. J Psychiatr Res. 1975;12:189–98. https://doi.org/10.1016/0022-3956(75)90026-6.
22. Buschke H, Kuslansky G, Katz M, Stewart WF, Sliwinski MJ, Eckholdt HM, et al. Screening for dementia with the memory impairment screen. Neurology. 1999;52:231–8. https://doi.org/10.1212/wnl.52.2.231.
23. Carnero-Pardo C, Espejo-Martínez B, López-Alcalde S, Espinosa-García M, Sáez-Zea C, Hernández-Torres E, et al. Diagnostic accuracy, effectiveness and cost for cognitive impairment and dementia screening of three short cognitive tests applicable to illiterates. PLoS One. 2011;6:1–6. https://doi.org/10.1371/journal.pone.0027069.
24. Wiig EH, Nielsen NP, Minthon L, et al. Alzheimer's quick test: assessment of parietal function. Harcourt Assessment: San Antonio, TX; 2002.
25. O'Caoimh R, Gao Y, Gallagher PF, Eustace J, McGlade C, Molloy DW. Which part of the Quick mild cognitive impairment screen (Qmci) discriminates between normal cognition, mild

cognitive impairment and dementia? Age Ageing. 2013;42:324–30. https://doi.org/10.1093/ageing/aft044.
26. Babacan-Yildiz G, Isik AT, Ur E, Aydemir E, Ertas C, Cebi MC, et al. OST: Cognitive State Test, a brief screening battery for Alzheimer disease in illiterate and literate patients. Int Psychogeriatr. 2013;25:403–12. https://doi.org/10.1017/S1041610212001780.
27. Nasreddine ZS, Phillips NA, Bedirian V, Charbonneau S, Whitehead V, Collin I, et al. The Montreal Cognitive Assessment, MoCA: a brief screening tool for mild cognitive impairment. J Am Geriatr Soc. 2005;53:695–9. https://doi.org/10.1111/j.1532-5415.2005.53221.x.
28. Mioshi E, Dawson K, Mitchell J. The Addenbrooke's cognitive examination revised (ACE-R): a brief cognitive test battery for dementia screening. Int J Geriatr Psychiatry. 2006;21:1078–85. https://doi.org/10.1002/gps.1610.
29. Mitchell AJ. A meta-analysis of the accuracy of the mini-mental state examination in the detection of dementia and mild cognitive impairment. J Psychiatr Res. 2009;43(4):411–31.
30. Elwood RW. The California Verbal Learning Test: psychometric characteristics and clinical application. Neuropsychol Rev. 1995;5(3):173–201. https://doi.org/10.1007/BF02214761.
31. Hori T, Sanjo N, Tomita M, Mizusawa H. Visual reproduction on the Wechsler Memory Scale-Revised as a predictor of Alzheimer's disease in Japanese patients with mild cognitive impairments. Dement Geriatr Cogn Disord. 2013;35(3–4):165–76. https://doi.org/10.1159/000346738.
32. Lezak MD, Howieson DB, Bigler ED, Tranel D. Neuropsychological assessment. 5th ed. New York: Oxford University Press; 2012.
33. Dubois B, Slachevsky A, Litvan I, Pillon B. The FAB. A frontal assessment battery at bedside. Neurology. 2000;55:1621–6. https://doi.org/10.1212/wnl.55.11.1621.
34. Sorbi S, Hort J, Erkinjuntti T, Fladby T, Gainotti G, Gurvit H, et al. EFNS-ENS Guidelines on the diagnosis and management of disorders associated with dementia. Eur J Neurol. 2012;19:1159–79.
35. Chui H, Zhang Q. Evaluation of dementia: a systematic study of the usefulness of the American Academy of Neurology's Practice Parameters. Neurology. 1997;49(4):925–35. https://doi.org/10.1212/WNL.49.4.925.
36. Frisoni GB, Rossi R, Beltramello A. The radial width of the temporal horn in mild cognitive impairment. J Neuroimaging. 2002;12(4):351–4. https://doi.org/10.1111/j.1552-6569.2002.tb00143.x.
37. Pennanen C, Kivipelto M, Tuomainen S, Hartikainen P, Hänninen T, Laakso MP, et al. Hippocampus and entorhinal cortex in mild cognitive impairment and early AD. Neurobiol Aging. 2004;25(3):303–10. https://doi.org/10.1016/S0197-4580(03)00084-8.
38. Scheltens P, Leys D, Barkhof F, Huglo D, Weinstein HC, Vermersch P, et al. Atrophy of medial temporal lobes on MRI in 'probable' Alzheimer's disease and normal ageing: diagnostic value and neuropsychological correlates. J Neurol Neurosurg Psychiatry. 1992;55(10):967–72. https://doi.org/10.1136/jnnp.55.10.967.
39. Ottoy J, Niemantsverdriet E, Verhaeghe J, De Roeck E, Struyfs H, Somers C, et al. Association of short-term cognitive decline and MCI-to-AD dementia conversion with CSF, MRI, amyloid- and 18 F-FDG-PET imaging. NeuroImage: Clin. 2019;22:101771. https://doi.org/10.1016/j.nicl.2019.101771.
40. Tabatabaei-Jafari H, Shaw ME, Cherbuin N. Cerebral atrophy in mild cognitive impairment: a systematic review with meta-analysis. Alzheimer's Dement. 2015;1(4):487–504. https://doi.org/10.1016/j.dadm.2015.11.002.
41. Niemantsverdriet E, Ribbens A, Bastin C, Benoit F, Bergmans B, Bier JC, et al. A retrospective Belgian multi-center MRI biomarker study in Alzheimer's Disease (REMEMBER). J Alzheimers Dis. 2018;63(4):1509–22. https://doi.org/10.3233/JAD-171140.
42. Bosco P, Redolfi A, Bocchetta M, Ferrari C, Mega A, Galluzzi S, et al. The impact of automated hippocampal volumetry on diagnostic confidence in patients with suspected Alzheimer's disease: a European Alzheimer's Disease Consortium study. Alzheimers Dement. 2017;13(9):1013–23.

43. Dubois B, Feldman HH, Jacova C, Hampel H, Molinuevo JL, Blennow K, et al. Advancing research diagnostic criteria for Alzheimer's disease: the IWG-2 criteria. Lancet Neurol. 2014;13(6):614–29.
44. Sabuncu MR, Desikan RS, Sepulcre J, Yeo BT, Liu H, Schmansky NJ, et al. The dynamics of cortical and hippocampal atrophy in Alzheimer disease. Arch Neurol. 2011;68(8):1040–8. https://doi.org/10.1001/archneurol.2011.167.
45. Nelson PT, Dickson DW, Trojanowski JQ, Jack CR, Boyle PA, Arfanakis K, et al. Limbic-predominant age-related TDP-43 encephalopathy (LATE): consensus working group report. Brain. 2019;142(6):1503–27. https://doi.org/10.1093/brain/awz099.
46. Wirth M, Villeneuve S, Haase CM, Madison CM, Oh H, Landau SM, et al. Associations between Alzheimer disease biomarkers, neurodegeneration, and cognition in cognitively normal older people. JAMA Neurol. 2013;70(12):1512–9. https://doi.org/10.1001/jamaneurol.2013.4013.
47. Zarow C, Wang L, Chui HC, Weiner MW, Csernansky JG. MRI shows more severe hippocampal atrophy and shape deformation in hippocampal sclerosis than in Alzheimer's disease. Int J Alzheimers Dis. 2011;2011:483972. https://doi.org/10.4061/2011/483972.
48. van de Pol LA, Hensel A, van der Flier WM, Visser PJ, Pijnenburg YA, Barkhof F, et al. Hippocampal atrophy on MRI in frontotemporal lobar degeneration and Alzheimer's disease. J Neurol Neurosurg Psychiatry. 2006;77(4):439–42. https://doi.org/10.1136/jnnp.2005.075341.
49. Laforce R Jr, Soucy JP, Sellami L, Dallaire-Théroux C, Brunet F, Bergeron D, et al. Molecular imaging in dementia: past, present, and future. Alzheimers Dement. 2018;14(11):1522–52. https://doi.org/10.1016/j.jalz.2018.06.2855.
50. Sala A, Caprioglio C, Santangelo R, Vanoli EG, Iannaccone S, Magnani G, et al. Brain metabolic signatures across the Alzheimer's disease spectrum. Eur J Nucl Med Mol Imaging. 2020;47(2):256–69. https://doi.org/10.1007/s00259-019-04559-2.
51. Bloudek LM, Spackman DE, Blankenburg M, Sullivan SD. Review and meta-analysis of biomarkers and diagnostic imaging in Alzheimer's disease. J Alzheimers Dis. 2011;26(4):627–45. https://doi.org/10.3233/JAD-2011-110,458.
52. Mosconi L, Tsui WH, Herholz K, Pupi A, Drzezga A, Lucignani G, et al. Multicenter standardized 18F-FDG PET diagnosis of mild cognitive impairment, Alzheimer's disease, and other dementias. J Nucl Med. 2008;49(3):390–8. https://doi.org/10.2967/jnumed.107.045385.
53. Silverman DH, Small GW, Chang CY, Lu CS, Kung De Aburto MA, Chen W, et al. Positron emission tomography in evaluation of dementia: Regional brain metabolism and long-term outcome. J Am Med Assoc. 2001;286(17):2120–7. https://doi.org/10.1001/jama.286.17.2120.
54. Jagust W, Reed B, Mungas D, Ellis W, DeCarli C. What does fluorodeoxyglucose PET imaging add to a clinical diagnosis of dementia? Neurology. 2007;69(9):871–7. https://doi.org/10.1212/01.wnl.0000269790.05105.16.
55. Yousaf T, Dervenoulas G, Valkimadi PE, Politis M. Neuroimaging in Lewy body dementia. J Neurol. 2019;266(1):1–26. https://doi.org/10.1007/s00415-018-8892-x.
56. Shivamurthy VK, Tahari AK, Marcus C, Subramaniam RM. Brain FDG PET and the diagnosis of dementia. Am J Roentgenol. 2015;204(1):W76–85. https://doi.org/10.2214/AJR.13.12363.
57. Salmon E, Bernard Ir C, Hustinx R. Pitfalls and limitations of PET/CT in brain imaging. Semin Nucl Med. 2015;45(6):541–51. https://doi.org/10.1053/j.semnuclmed.2015.03.008.
58. Fink HA, Linskens EJ, Silverman PC, McCarten JR, Hemmy LS, Ouellette JM, et al. Accuracy of biomarker testing for neuropathologically defined Alzheimer disease in older adults with dementia. Ann Intern Med. 2020;172(10):669–77.
59. Klunk WE, Engler H, Nordberg A, Wang Y, Blomqvist G, Holt DP. Imaging brain amyloid in Alzheimer's disease with Pittsburgh Compound-B. Ann Neurol. 2004;55(3):306–19. https://doi.org/10.1002/ana.20009.
60. Rabinovici GD, Rosen HJ, Alkalay A, Kornak J, Furst AJ, Agarwal N, et al. Amyloid vs FDG-PET in the differential diagnosis of AD and FTLD. Neurology. 2011;77(23):2034–42. https://doi.org/10.1212/WNL.0b013e31823b9c5e.
61. Kantarci K, Lowe VJ, Chen Q, Przybelski SA, Lesnick TG, Schwarz CG, et al. β-Amyloid PET and neuropathology in dementia with Lewy bodies. Neurology. 2020;94:e282–91. https://doi.org/10.1212/WNL.0000000000008818.

62. Ossenkoppele R, Jansen WJ, Rabinovici GD, Knol DL, van der Flier WM, van Berckel BN, et al. Prevalence of amyloid PET positivity in dementia syndromes: a meta-analysis. J Am Med Assoc. 2015;313(19):1939–49.
63. La Joie R, Ayakta N, Seeley WW, Borys E, Boxer AL, DeCarli C, et al. Multi-site study of the relationships between ante mortem [11C]PIB-PET Centiloid values and post mortem measures of Alzheimer's disease neuropathology. Alzheimers Dement. 2019;15(2):205–16.
64. Duits FH, Martinez-Lage P, Paquet C, Engelborghs S, Lleó A, Hausner L, et al. Performance and complications of lumbar puncture in memory clinics: results of the multicenter lumbar puncture feasibility study. Alzheimers Dement. 2016;12(2):154–63. https://doi.org/10.1016/j.jalz.2015.08.003.
65. Engelborghs S, Niemantsverdriet E, Struyfs H, Blennow K, Brouns R, Comabella M, et al. Consensus guidelines for lumbar puncture in patients with neurological diseases. Alzheimers Dement. 2017;8:111–26. https://doi.org/10.1016/j.dadm.2017.04.007.
66. Hansson O, Zetterberg H, Buchhave P, Londos E, Blennow K, Minthon L. Association between CSF biomarkers and incipient Alzheimer's disease in patients with mild cognitive impairment: a follow-up study. Lancet Neurol. 2006;5(3):228–34. https://doi.org/10.1016/S1474-4422(06)70355-6.
67. Slaets S, Le Bastard N, Martin JJ, Sleegers K, Van Broeckhoven C, De Deyn PP, et al. Cerebrospinal fluid Aβ1–40 improves differential dementia diagnosis in patients with intermediate P-tau181P levels. J Alzheimers Dis. 2013;36(4):759–67. https://doi.org/10.3233/JAD-130107.
68. Niemantsverdriet E, Ottoy J, Somers C, De Roeck E, Struyfs H, Soetewey F, et al. The cerebrospinal fluid Aβ1–42/Aβ1–40 ratio improves concordance with amyloid-PET for diagnosing Alzheimer's disease in a clinical setting. J Alzheimers Dis. 2017;60(2):561–76. https://doi.org/10.3233/JAD-170327.

Disclosure of Diagnosis in MCI and Dementia

4

Kristian Steen Frederiksen and Gunhild Waldemar

List of Abbreviations

AD Alzheimer's disease
MCI mild cognitive impairment

Introduction

Case 1

My name is Chris Roberts. I am 59 years old. I have 5 children and two grandchildren. You now know more about me than anyone ever did during and after my initial diagnosis.

I have a diagnosis of mixed dementia. I was first diagnosed with vascular and a few months later, with Alzheimer's as well. It took 13 months, but I did not mind, because I wanted a correct diagnosis, a reason for my behaviour and problems. It was a very negative experience, but I did feel relieved that I now had a label and a diagnosis of something at last. But before the diagnosis, there was a length of time when we had nothing, no information, no support, no offer of counselling and my life was on hold. We felt we were in limbo; this is when the damage to one's quality of life is mostly felt and impacted. Jobs

K. S. Frederiksen (✉) · G. Waldemar
Danish Dementia Research Centre, Department of Neurology, Rigshospitalet, University of Copenhagen, Copenhagen, Denmark
e-mail: Kristian.steen.frederiksen@regionh.dk

K. S. Frederiksen, G. Waldemar (eds.), *Management of Patients with Dementia*,
https://doi.org/10.1007/978-3-030-77904-7_4

can be lost, marriages broken, a time of arguments with anger, fear, guilt, and loss, which in turn, can have detrimental effects on daily living. Combine all that with an eventual diagnosis which looks, sounds, and feels like a death sentence, usually down to stigma, lack of knowledge and misconceptions … is it then any wonder people contemplate ending their lives? I certainly did.

How a delivery of a life changing diagnosis is given can be as disempowering as the diagnosis itself. We had no clue about services, support or respite, for me or for my wife Jayne. "Stage appropriate" and tailored services should have been correctly signposted. If you can understand your illness, its problems and deficits, then you can feel more able to embrace it and live again, to find your own strategies, your own management of your cognitive challenges.

At first, it was easier not to talk about my diagnosis, the stigma, and misconceptions, added with a lack of understanding, do not give any confidence to discuss it with anyone. I felt ashamed and embarrassed.

But, by coming out, as it were, talking about it and having honest conversations, really did … and does … help. By hiding away and not speaking about dementia, we are perpetuating the very stigma that we do not want. Plus, nobody should have the added stress of keeping secrets. This dark hole in our lives, then led to fear. I was not just living with dementia, I was also living with guilt. Guilt about how my diagnosis was going to affect my wife and my children, I felt I had let them down. That is also when depression also started to share my life. But my diagnosis is not just about me, it affects my family much more than myself, it affects everyone around you, even your friends and neighbours. You need to prepare, plan, and make adaptations, you need to be enabled, not disabled. We now, over time, have the information we all so needed back then. We all have a new life. It is not as good as the old one but I am still here and that is much better than the alternative. We had been "husband and wife", we then became "patient and carer", but are now back to what we do best, "husband and wife", we are a team again. My wife has become my enabler, my supporter, and my, "cognitive bridge", the link to normal life. She is there to "look out" for me, just, as I, used to look out for her. We have always cared for each other and continue to do so, we are, at the moment, "living with dementia, not dying from it".

A diagnosis of dementia is for many people a feared message to receive [1]. Symptoms such as forgetting one's children or one's own name are often reported anecdotally as a dreaded consequence of Alzheimer's disease (AD). Dementia disorders are at present incurable and associated with significant social stigma as Chris in case 1 mentions. Further, in a German study, between 25% and 50% of respondents reported fearful reactions towards people with dementia [2]. Despite the many negative emotions expressed by the patients in the cases, it is also clear that there is a wish to get an explanation for the change in memory and other cognitive functions patient's experience [3–8]. In a systematic review, it was found that 90.7% of persons without cognitive impairment and 84.8% of patients referred for diagnostic evaluation in a memory clinic wished to have a possible diagnosis of dementia disclosed [9]. Further reasons for wanting to have a diagnosis of mild dementia disclosed include the right to know, confirmation of suspicions and better understanding; allowing opportunities for future care planning, facilitating a focus on the abilities rather than disabilities of the person with dementia, positive adaptations within family and spouse relationships, access to early treatments, both pharmacological and psychological, and participation in research studies [3–5, 7, 8].

Although receiving a diagnosis of a dementia disorder may have great impact, the way the diagnosis is delivered also has great impact. As Chris in case 1 puts it *"How a delivery of a life changing diagnosis is given can be as disempowering as the diagnosis itself"*. That is, the way in which a diagnosis of dementia is delivered is not trivial and may shape the way the patient perceives and adjusts to the diagnosis. In a study of how disclosure of a diagnosis of dementia was carried out, it was found that a "warning" by the physician of an impending diagnosis of dementia before it was made "official" was perceived to lessen the shock for the patient [4]. That this is not trivial is indicated by the findings in a qualitative study of the emotional reactions of patients receiving a diagnosis of dementia. It was found that the emotional stress impeded the cognitive processing and retention of information given at the diagnostic disclosure meeting [10]. A sense of shock is also revealed in the four cases in this chapter. A sense of emptiness is reported by Stefan in case 4. Helen in case 2 writes that *"The diagnosis was like jumping off a cliff"* clearly indicating the emotional toll experienced by patients when a diagnosis of dementia is delivered.

Mild Cognitive Impairment: Dealing with an Uncertain Label

Case 2

Helen Rochford-Brennan, Ireland. My diagnosis took a long time, was it MCI or Alzheimer's dementia? But living with that uncertainty and fear of Alzheimer's was worse. The neurologist and other doctors disagreed and there was some delay as a result. Once diagnosis came, I felt a relief—at least I knew what it was. I received information but it was not sufficient. I drove home feeling absolute despair and I believe quality information would have lessened that despair. There is more information available now—we are much more aware today and I believe that is a very good thing.

I got my diagnosis alone and had to drive two hours home to tell my family, I would advise anyone going to an appointment to bring support. I believe my medical team did their best, they were kind and well-intentioned but they did not have the supports to offer me. The diagnosis was like jumping off a cliff.

The fact that there was very little information at the moment of diagnosis certainly shaped my view of the disease—I filled in the blanks myself, I went home and look up the internet. Dr. Google is always frightening but it was Dr. Google or nothing. Quality information would have made a big difference. I also believe increased information about medication options, side effects, and benefits would have been helpful.

My diagnosis was not the end of my life it was the beginning of a different life but I had to find that different life myself. I hope there will be a pathway to support people on that journey in the future. I was glad I was told—I felt confused and was finding it difficult to remember basic things and struggling at work, it was a relief to know there was a name for what I was feeling. There is a fine line between Mild Cognitive Impairment (MCI) and early onset dementia. We need more clarity and more information. Brain disease may not be MCI and may not be Alzheimer's dementia. I hope in the future more research will be done into both MCI and the impact of giving a person that diagnosis. Every person must be supported in whatever way is best for them.

There was not a significant discussion on progression. For example, driving was not mentioned and as a person living in a rural area that was significant—driving means independence and connection and community. The biggest thing lacking in my diagnosis was hope. Hope is so important, and I would encourage anyone diagnosed to, get in touch with your local Alzheimer's group. Hope and support will be a balm to your panic.

In recent decades, the diagnostic threshold in terms of disease severity has been lowered, meaning that patients are more often than previously diagnosed with AD or other neurodegenerative dementia disorders prior to the dementia stage. This predementia stage is often labelled mild cognitive impairment (MCI). MCI was first introduced into medical literature in the 1980s [11], but not popularized until the 1990s with the publication of diagnostic criteria for MCI [12]. The basic premise was to capture the predementia stage of AD and hence the diagnosis was heavily skewed towards memory impairment. Later on, criteria for multidomain MCI and non-memory single domain MCI has been developed to better reflect the clinical reality of patients with diverse cognitive profiles and to develop criteria for the predementia stage for other neurodegenerative dementia disorders such as vascular dementia and Lewy body disease [13]. A patient with MCI will display cognitive impairment but no or only very mild impairment in activities of daily living, and according to the aforementioned be at a higher risk of (or destined to) progress to dementia. Although envisioned as diagnostic criteria for research, the diagnosis of MCI has slowly diffused into clinical practice in many centres. This may be seen as an inevitable evolution for "only in research" criteria but may also be a consequence of a need to diagnose patients in the predementia stage, and a means to convey to the patients that they do not have dementia.

Despite the fact that the diagnosis of MCI may have value in the clinic, it has also brought further complexity to the diagnosis and disclosure of neurodegenerative disorders. Some of these issues have been further compounded by the introduction of biomarkers into clinical routine and incorporation of these biomarkers into the diagnostic criteria for MCI (often labelled as either MCI due to AD or prodromal AD) [14, 15]. As mentioned previously, patients with MCI were hypothesized to be at an increased risk of progression to dementia. Indeed, this has also been shown to be the case with an incremental risk of progression with an increasing number of positive biomarkers [16]. On the other hand, observational studies have also clearly demonstrated that taken at a group level, patients with MCI are a heterogenous group with diverse underlying conditions. This includes non-neurodegenerative disorders, which are not associated with progression to dementia. This is also likely to be one of the factors for the relatively high, although varying, rates of reversion back to normal cognition in cohorts of patients with MCI [17]. The clinician thus faces the issue of diagnosing patients in the MCI stage, some of whom will progress to dementia, whereas others will not. At present, it is possible to predict with a moderate to high accuracy which patients at a group level are at an increased risk of progressing to dementia [18]. However, the clinician deals with patients at an individual level, and will have to extrapolate from group level to the individual patient level, which will add uncertainty in terms of the accuracy of progression prediction. In other words, the clinician will be faced with diagnosing neurodegenerative diseases such as AD in very early stages (i.e. MCI stage) for which there is no disease-modifying therapy and where predicting who will progress is associated with some uncertainty. Indeed, in a small study of patients with MCI, the uncertainty of prognosis was one of the factors identified that patients with MCI had to cope with [19]. As a further indicator of the uncertainty of the diagnostic label of MCI, patients often reported perceiving multiple reasons for their cognitive impairment such as personality traits and information overload [19]. It may therefore be relevant to consider whether disclosing a diagnosis of MCI may always be warranted. As demonstrated by Helen in case 2, she felt a great relief by the diagnosis, because despite being at an early stage of the disease, she clearly felt that something had change, and now had an explanation. Helen's wish for disclosure may be in line with the majority of patients with mild cognitive symptoms. In a study of mild dementia 96% of patients reported wanting to be informed of the diagnosis, and 98% of carers reported wanting to be informed if they developed dementia [3]. However, this proportion may be lower in MCI patients, and regardless of the fact that the vast majority of patients wishes to be informed, an individual approach is advisable to also accommodate those patients who may not wish to be informed. Helen's case demonstrates a second issue when it comes to the MCI label in clinical practice. Helen writes "*...was is Alzheimer's or MCI*". This clearly demonstrates the difficulty for patients to understand the difference between a label describing the severity of symptoms versus the underlying cause of the symptoms. This is likely to be rooted in several factors including the quality of and amount of information given by the clinician when disclosing a diagnosis of MCI.

Some special instances with regard to interpretation of biomarkers deserves mention in order to illustrate the complexity of biomarker interpretation. Due to the prevalence of the disease, the most mature biomarkers are related to AD for which it is possible to perform a molecular diagnosis. Specifically, this can be done by measurements of beta-amyloid and phosphorylated tau in the cerebrospinal fluid and amyloid and tau positron emission tomography brain scans. Deposition of beta-amyloid and phosphorylated tau are hypothesized to be central to the pathophysiology of AD, which is why the presence of abnormal deposition in the brain of these proteins are often taken as a sign of AD. However, studies have clearly demonstrated that beta-amyloid is present in a high proportion of older adults without cognitive symptoms [20]. This prevalence is age-dependent and is over 20% in persons over 80 years [21]. Furthermore, beta-amyloid is prevalent in patients with disorders not associated with beta-amyloid or may occur as co-pathology [22]. These and other observations warrant a certain degree of caution and careful consideration when interpreting biomarkers.

In a systematic review of the ethical issues of a biomarker-based diagnosis of AD, including in the MCI stage, the uncertainty of predicting the disease course for individual patients was raised as an issue, together with the right to know and the right not to know [23]. As always, an individual approach should be adopted, and there are at present efforts underway to develop models for individual prognostication based on predictive factors, but the method needs further development and clinical validation. In patients with dementia, accurate diagnosis and precise prognostication remains important, as does the process of diagnostic disclosure. Nevertheless, since patients in the dementia stage often have a larger need for support, diagnostic disclosure will have a more immediate and obvious impact on the life of the patient.

Case 3

My story—When I got told I had Alzheimer's—Stefan Eriksson, 55. My wife and I sat in front of the doctor. The moment he told us about my diagnosis I felt empty. We were sure I did not have Alzheimer's. No one gets Alzheimer's at my age … at 50. I was young! I loved to work, to travel, to take care of my family and to live. Now the doctor is telling me that the test results are indicating that I have Alzheimer's. He told me I would not be able to ever work again. He took my driving license from me and sent us to a room with a psychologist. It felt like the whole world was falling apart and he just took everything from me. Even my freedom, with driving. We were just so shocked. Our minds stood still and since we did not find any questions to ask the psychologist, she did not have anything to answer. She did not give us any advice, any numbers to call, any information about the illness. Nothing. We knew nothing about Alzheimer's more than that we thought only old people got it and that you lose your memory. We were so wrong. We had, for example, no idea your motor skills and self-esteem would be affected or how stress would affect you. The psychologist should be used to this, shocked individuals who are there to be guided through this. We needed her help but we got nothing. The psychologist just told us "You can still live a pretty good life" and then she sent us home. Home to what?

For weeks I sat in my house, looking out of the window. My wife had to work, I was not allowed to. Since I was so "young" our town did not have anything to offer me to do during the day. My wife finally found a dementia nurse on Google and we booked a meeting. We had to fight for everything. We had pretty much to fight for my right to fit into society. The town finally agreed to open up a daily activity centre for me and two other people around my age with similar problems.

What I learned along the way is that you will lose pretty much everything you thought you had in society, freedom, respect, friends, and more. But it is so important to accept your illness. It is what it is. Once you accept it you will be able to move on and to see the positive things in life. My kids and their mentality "come on dad, look on the bright side, we will be able to hang out way more than before, you can still do things you love, find new hobbies, and so on", that gave me light in my life when I needed it the most. My friends that are still with me today also means so much to me. They dare to ask how I feel and they treat me just like before and like I'm me, Stefan, not a person with Alzheimer's.

Is It Safe to Disclose a Diagnosis of MCI and Mild Dementia?

All the patients in this chapter describe a sense of shock at the diagnosis and a number of negative feelings such as despair, emptiness, loneliness, unpreparedness. It is perhaps not surprising that a diagnosis of a serious brain disorder elicits such emotions and may be difficult to eliminate and may be viewed as a part of a normal process of adjusting. A number of factors have been cited in the literature that are perceived by patients and caregivers as possibly negative consequences of receiving a diagnosis of mild dementia. These include emotional upset, rejection by family and friends as well as social stigma and embarrassment, no effective medical treatment, suicidal ideation in patients, and not wishing to cause burden to family [3, 5–8]. These factors which are perceived as negative needs to be balanced against those factors perceived as positive, which have already been mentioned previously in the chapter. Nevertheless, it raises the issue of whether disclosing a diagnosis of MCI or mild dementia is safe. Carpenter el al investigated the impact of receiving a diagnosis of very mild dementia (Clinicians' dementia rating = 0.5), mild dementia (Clinicians' dementia rating = 1) and no cognitive impairment in a group of patients referred for evaluation for memory complaints on various measures of emotional distress [24]. The authors found that anxiety was significantly reduced following disclosure independently of which diagnosis was disclosed, and no change in depressive symptoms [24]. This finding is somewhat corroborated by a small retrospective study in which none out of 50 patients diagnosed with dementia had developed catastrophic thoughts or suicide 1 year after diagnosis [3]. However, in a large survey, 55% of caregivers reported that disclosure of a dementia diagnosis had caused depressive symptoms in their family member who had received a diagnosed [25]. In a US study of suicide in patients with a dementia diagnosis over a 5-year period, a total of 241 suicides (out of a study population of 294,952) occurred. Risk factors included prior inpatient psychiatric treatment, depression, prescription fills of anxiolytic and anti-depressants, and younger age. Importantly, 75% of suicides occurred in those with a new diagnosis of dementia [26]. The rate of suicide is comparable in the population without dementia, and as such does not warrant extra vigilance in patients with dementia, but in those patients with prior psychiatric disease risk of suicide should be considered especially around the time of diagnosis.

A number of studies have examined the impact of disclosing biomarker status in different patient populations. In a group of persons with subjective cognitive complaints undergoing amyloid PET, of which 11 out of a total of 63 participants had a positive amyloid scan, there were no significant changes in mood or significant emotional impact, or perceived risk of developing AD. Nor was this associated with significant emotional impact, regardless of amyloid status.[28] These findings seem to be stable over time (at 1 year follow-up) [27]. On the positive side, participants with a positive scan were more likely to make positive changes to their lifestyle [28]. These findings are in line with another study. In a qualitative study in patients with amnestic MCI, some emotional stress was detected in a minority of patients at 6-month follow-up, but the importance of the finding remains uncertain [29].

Physician's Practices and Attitudes Regarding Diagnostic Disclosure in MCI and Mild Dementia

A number of surveys have examined the knowledge and attitudes of physicians on MCI and dementia. In a sample of neurologists, geriatricians, and psychiatrists in memory clinics, 89.5% of respondents found that MCI was very or somewhat useful [30]. In a sample of geriatricians who reported practicing in various settings, 70% reported that it was important to separate MCI from dementia [31]. Finally, Werner et al. sampled family physicians, but did not ask about the attitude of physicians in regards to the usefulness of MCI as a diagnostic label, but did report that 70% thought that MCI was due to normal ageing [32]. In family physicians, the knowledge of MCI was relatively low, and the diagnostic tests perceived as most useful were blood sampling for T3, T4, and TSH, whereas neuropsychological assessment, MRI and SPECT scans were found less useful [32]. In contrast, physicians in memory clinics reported frequent use of PET, MRI, and lumbar puncture [30].

The practices regarding disclosure of MCI may vary as reported in different studies [30, 33, 34], but a majority always or almost always disclosed the diagnosis [30, 34] as well as the risk of progression, although to a lesser degree, but not rate of progression [30]. In a semi-qualitative study, it was found that physicians expressed several different uncertainties when disclosing a diagnosis of MCI, of which half of the uncertainties were related to predictions of future disease course [35]. Physicians were also more likely to discuss the probability of progression regardless of whether the patient asked, whereas they tended to more often only discuss possible rate of progression and future symptoms if specifically asked, although this was the same for MCI and dementia [30]. A number of physician-related factors were also associated with differences in disclosure practices. For example, if the physician recruited patients with MCI for research he/she was more likely to discuss the diagnosis more in-depth with patients with MCI, and to discuss the underlying cause of MCI [30]. Lastly, physicians were more likely to use visual aids and to show scans when disclosing the diagnosis in MCI patients.

The Process of Diagnostic Disclosure

Setting the Stage: The Initial Visit at the Doctor's Office

Case 4

My experience of diagnosis. I am Nina Baláčková from the Czech Republic and I wish to share my experience of my diagnosis of "atypical young onset Alzheimer's".

When I was 46, I realized that my memory was bad and I felt tired. At that time, I was thinking about Alzheimer's disease as my mom had it, but the neurologist played down my lapses of memory saying that she herself was forgetting things too: "It is normal after the forties...".

I worked as an accountant but at the age of 48, I was having serious problems in my job because I could not work as fast as usual. I also had problems with counting and logical thinking but just felt great fatigue and forgetfulness. I thought that I had got older, so such problems were normal. For a few months, I worked from early morning till late afternoon, and later on, went into the office on Saturdays so others would not know about it. After several months, I was no longer able to work. Then I decided to go and see my GP who sent me to a neurologist. But this time, I chose a different one.

The neurologist asked me if anybody in my family had Alzheimer's. I answered her calmly that my mom had it because I had no idea that I might have it too. Then I did a "clock test". She saw it and immediately wrote a referral to a psychiatrist, and gave it to me, saying: "You know, for Alzheimer's, you need to see a psychiatrist". This was how I learnt about my diagnosis!!! That doctor was really good at diagnosis but her way of informing me about such a serious diagnosis was very strange.

After that, I fell into a deep depression. I was divorced, with two children studying at university and I had financial problems. I did not know much about this disease. I imagined that soon, I would not be able to recognize my children and would become a heavy burden for them. I went to see the psychiatrist with depression. I found information about this disease on the Internet. I read that people sometimes get confused, lost in time or place... When I read it, I realized that many of things that were written there were my own problems. When I saw the doctors later on, I told them I had problems with logical thinking, counting and time, and that I got lost going to the post office.

The doctor diagnosed depression but did not want to know where it came from. She told me that I was too young for Alzheimer's. My GP was very clever and advised me to see another psychiatrist, who told me at the first appointment that it looked like Alzheimer's and that we needed to do some tests. It was important to start taking the right medicine as soon as possible. I bought it and my problems decreased in 3 weeks. Unfortunately, this doctor had to finish her job and transferred me to her colleague who sent me to psychiatric clinic for one month's observation. It felt like a holiday as at that time, my life was very difficult for me (dressing, shopping, cooking), but when I returned home, I still did not know if I had Alzheimer's or not. They sent me to one of our top neurologists specialized in dementia. It took 3 more months and many examinations including genetic tests and MRI. I have now got a diagnosis: atypical form of young onset Alzheimer's. So I got my final diagnosis after 9 months even though it could have been done in one!!!

The majority of patients who are evaluated for cognitive impairment, will have sought medical attention because they feel something has changed with regard to their ability to remember or problems in other cognitive areas. However, by mapping the motives for why the patient ends up in the physician's office may uncover other reasons (Table 4.1). For example, the patient may not acknowledge that something has changed due to the lack of insight or perhaps because of embarrassment

Table 4.1 Suggested items for the diagnostic disclosure in MCI and mild dementia

At the initial diagnostic evaluation	Map motives of the patient for seeking medical evaluation
	Map social and cultural perceptions in relation to the disorder
	Map the wishes of the patient in terms of information given if diagnostic tests are undertaken
	Be mindful of communication to allow for adjustments due to cognitive impairment or other factors
	Inform about the process of diagnostic evaluation
	Inform about the aims of possible diagnostic evaluations, possible outcomes, uncertainties in interpretation and prognostication
	Inform about possible alternatives to biomarker sampling (e.g. accepting a higher diagnostic uncertainty or "watchful waiting")
At the diagnostic disclosure consultation	Inform according to the wishes of the patient
	Inform about the outcome of biomarkers and be open about uncertainties
	In case of diagnostic uncertainty, consider further diagnostic evaluation and second opinion consults
	Inform about treatment options including brain-healthy advice, which should always be given
	Always supply a plan for follow-up or post diagnostic care
	If possible, also give information in writing (e.g. hand-outs)

or being afraid of what may be discovered in terms of possible diseases. In those instances, it may have been the caregiver who has been the main facilitator for the diagnostic evaluation to have been set in motion, and it is important to affirm that the patient consents to the diagnostic evaluation. It may also be that a patient is convinced that nothing is wrong and their motivation for seeking medical evaluation is to have this confirmed. Confirmation of the presence of a brain disorder may therefore be unwanted information.

By discussing the possible diagnostic procedures as well as the possible outcomes with the patient and caregiver, the patient is able to make an informed decision about whether or not to proceed. This may include informing about the possibility of diagnosing a serious and progressive brain disorder with no curable treatment. However, it is important as a physician also to keep in mind that the diagnostic process is not only a matter of whether the patient does or does not have a neurodegenerative disease, but also to be vigilant and inform about the possibility of diagnosing potentially reversible conditions such as depression, normal pressure hydrocephalus, vitamin deficiency, and other medical conditions. Likewise, management of comorbidities (e.g. hypertension, hypercholesteroemia), other risk factors (e.g. sedentary lifestyle, alcohol overuse) and associated symptoms (e.g. depression, epilepsy) in patients with neurodegenerative dementia diseases is important and may reduce the risk of progression and increase quality of life [36].

Delineating MCI from mild dementia can in clinical practice be difficult. In relationship to diagnostic efforts, the stage of the disease may impact on how and to what end diagnostic procedures are undertaken. In terms of the aforementioned reversible conditions, it is of no consequence whether the patient has MCI or mild dementia, but in terms of diagnosing an underlying neurodegenerative disorder, it may have. For example, in patients with dementia, support in terms of a case manager, referral to a day care centre, and support for the caregiver will be necessary for many patients, and in the case of AD, treatment with acetylcholinesterase inhibitors and memantine, may be offered. On the other hand, in patients with MCI, and per definition, they function independently with no or very little need for help in activities of daily living. This means that a diagnosis of MCI will have fewer practical consequences. That is not to say that diagnosing MCI may not have any consequences. Moreover, patients with MCI may have a high need for further information and may want to plan for the future in terms of advance directives, wills and other legal arrangements. Moreover, diagnosing patients in the MCI stage may empower patients to actively try to mitigate their risk of progression (e.g. taking up a more active life, reducing alcohol consumption). Furthermore, it is important that MCI is a syndrome and not a specific disease, and therefore from a purely bio-medical point of view should not represent the final diagnosis, unless all reasonable diagnostic avenues have been tried.

Throughout the diagnostic process, it is important to keep in mind that communication needs to be adjusted to the abilities of the patient and take into account not only the cognitive impairment but also social and cultural aspects of the patients´ life.

Pre-Biomarker Sampling Counselling

Most patients are likely to readily accept blood sampling and a structural scan as these investigations primarily aims to detect the potentially reversible conditions mentioned earlier on. However, lumbar puncture (with the aim to sample markers of neurodegeneration and AD), 18F-FDG-PET, amyloid, and tau PET may not be acceptable for all patients. Although these investigations may be associated with minor physical discomfort, the main reason may be that these biomarkers aim, for all practical purposes and in the present setting, specifically at diagnosing neurodegenerative dementia disorders.

Before initiating the process of counselling, it is essential to determine clinical competency of the patient. Usually, most patients with MCI will have the appropriate capacity, however, in some neurodegenerative disorders, e.g. frontotemporal dementia, it may be impaired early on. In patients with dementia, risk of reduced competency is likely to be higher. Four core components of clinical competency need to be considered [37]: (1) understanding—i.e., the ability to comprehend information relevant to a decision; (2) appreciation—i.e., the ability to apply that information to one's own situation; (3) reasoning– i.e., the ability to evaluate the potential consequences of one's own decisions; and (4) expression of choice—i.e., the ability to communicate one's own choices. Clinical competency may be evaluated by specific interviews, vignette methods, neuropsychological tests [38–43], but also by general clinical judgement taking into consideration the aforementioned core components. Factors such as cultural, social and educational background, and psychiatric comorbidities should also be considered.

Pre-biomarker counselling may include information about the purpose and aim, limitations and possible benefits and disadvantages. As in all phases, an individualized approach is necessary as these factors will vary from patient to patient. In terms of purpose and outcome, biomarker sampling aim to diagnose underlying causes of the syndrome, to increase the diagnostic accuracy and to increase the ability to predict progression. In MCI patients, the latter will take the forefront. It is important at this stage to discuss this aspect as diagnosing a neurodegenerative disorder at the MCI stage may be unwanted by some patients, and as patients will have the right to know, there is an equal right not to know [23]. Discussing the possible outcome and benefit of biomarker sampling will also help to ensure that the patient does not have unrealistic expectations (e.g. that biomarker sampling will open up for the possibility of treatment or even a cure) of the outcome of the investigations. To ensure that the physician enables the patient to make a truly informed and conscious choice in the matter, information should be delivered faithfully and as neutral as possible. Moreover, it is not a real choice unless alternative approaches are presented. Diagnosing neurodegenerative diseases without the use of biomarkers is possible with an acceptable diagnostic accuracy and certainty. Another possibility would be to follow the patient over time to ascertain the disease course, and ultimately in some instances, the diagnosis.

Pre-biomarker sampling counselling should also help to "set the stage" for the diagnostic disclosure. By informing about the purpose of biomarker sampling (which will include possibly diagnosing a neurodegenerative brain disorder) this may serve as a forewarning to the patient of what may come, and enable the patient to prepare and possibly to discuss the possibility with, e.g. a spouse or another family member or friend. It is also important that there is continuity between the pre-biomarker sampling counselling and the information given when the diagnosis is disclosed. For example, if the patient has been informed that a definitive diagnosis will be possible after biomarker sampling, a less certain diagnosis may be a disappointment. In this vein it is obvious that optimally it should be the same physician who delivers the pre-biomarker sampling counselling and discloses the diagnosis or that what has been said is communicated to the physician disclosing the diagnosis (e.g. through case notes or a nurse present at both appointments). Moreover, a physician knowledgeable about biomarkers and neurodegenerative dementia disorders should undertake the biomarker counselling and diagnostic disclosure.

Disclosing the Diagnosis

As reported by almost all of the patients in the cases in this chapter, the diagnosis came as a surprise or even a shock. Stefan in case 3 writes: "*The moment he told us about my diagnosis I felt empty. We were sure I didn't have Alzheimer's. No one gets Alzheimer's at my age ... at 50. I was young!*" The diagnostic disclosure left him blindsided. To Nina in case 4, the diagnosis was delivered very bluntly and almost, it seems, in passing: "*She saw it and immediately wrote a referral to a psychiatrist, and gave it to me, saying: 'You know, for Alzheimer's, you need to see a psychiatrist'. This was how I learnt about my diagnosis!!! That doctor was really good at diagnosis but her way of informing me about such a serious diagnosis was very strange*". It is obvious from these quotes that although the outcome of the disclosure process in terms of the diagnosis being delivered does not change, the way it is done, does matters.

When disclosing a diagnosis, it is a good idea to have the patient be accompanied by a caregiver to offer support and to be an extra pair of ears. As always, communication should be adjusted to the individual patient, and the wishes in terms of level of information, should be respected. Information should preferably also be provided in writing to support remembering and may also be used as a starting point for discussions in the family. Explanations about biomarkers and their interpretation may be difficult. A large body of evidence exists on how to convey risk to patients in a spectrum of diseases, and it can be beneficial for the physician to consider applying these when communicating results of biomarkers to the patient. The physician should be open about the uncertainty in biomarker interpretation. As already discussed earlier on, biomarkers may not give a definite prognosis in MCI regarding progression to dementia. It may therefore be advisable to avoid a deterministic interpretation (i.e. patients with MCI and one or more biomarkers will inevitably progress to dementia) and instead adopt a probabilistic interpretation (i.e. patients with MCI and one or more biomarkers are at an increased risk of progressing to dementia). If the diagnosis is uncertain, a discussion of further diagnostic evaluation may be relevant or offering the option of a second opinion evaluation.

When disclosing a diagnosis of dementia or MCI, the patient should always be given information about follow-up and post diagnostic care. This will vary widely between patients, but a clearly communicated plan for the near future should be given. For some patients with MCI, this may include instructions to contact their GP if they feel symptoms are getting worse, whereas for patients with a neurodegenerative dementia disorder, follow-up should be in a clinic which offer specialized care and a multiprofessional setting. Advise on brain-healthy behaviour and attention to modifiable risk factors is almost always relevant and will often help to empower the patient to do something themselves to influence the disease course. Discussion of advance directives, wills, and other legal matters may also be relevant.

Conclusion

Patients who seek out medical attention for cognitive complaints are individuals, and the diagnostic process and information should have this as its starting point. The physician should map motives for seeking evaluation and communicate the possibilities in terms of diagnostic assessments and possible outcomes. This will often require specialist knowledge of biomarkers and of neurodegenerative diseases. Diagnostic evaluation may uncover incurable brain disorders but may similarly reveal potentially reversible causes of the diagnostic evaluation and this and other aspects such as uncertainties regarding interpretation of biomarker should be communicated to the patient. Although neurodegenerative diseases are incurable, symptoms, and comorbidities are manageable and may reduce progression rates and improve functioning and quality of life. Following diagnosis, a plan for follow-up and post-diagnostic care should always be communicated.

References

1. Hajek A, König H-H. Fear of Dementia in the general population: findings from the German socio-economic panel (GSOEP). J Alzheimers Dis. 2020;75(4):1135–40. https://doi.org/10.3233/JAD-200106.
2. Von Dem Knesebeck O, Angermeyer MC, Lüdecke D, Kofahl C. Emotional reactions toward people with dementia - results of a population survey from Germany. Int Psychogeriatr. 2014;26(3):435–41. https://doi.org/10.1017/S1041610213002056.
3. Pinner G, Bouman WP. Attitudes of patients with mild dementia and their carers towards disclosure of the diagnosis. Int Psychogeriatr. 2003;15(3):279–88.
4. Byszewski AM, Molnar FJ, Aminzadeh F, Eisner M, Gardezi F, Bassett R. Dementia diagnosis disclosure. Alzheimer Dis Assoc Disord. 2007;21(2):107–14. https://doi.org/10.1097/WAD.0b013e318065c481.
5. Connell CM, Boise L, Stuckey JC, Holmes SB, Hudson ML. Attitudes toward the diagnosis and disclosure of dementia among family caregivers and primary care physicians. Gerontologist. 2004;44(4):500–7. https://doi.org/10.1093/geront/44.4.500.
6. Derksen E, Vernooij-Dassen M, Gillissen F, Olde Rikkert M, Scheltens P. Impact of diagnostic disclosure in dementia on patients and carers: qualitative case series analysis. Aging Ment Health. 2006;10(5):525–31. https://doi.org/10.1080/13607860600638024.

7. Derksen E, Vernooij-Dassen M, Gillissen F, Olde-Rikkert M, Scheltens P. The impact of diagnostic disclosure in dementia: a qualitative case analysis. Int psychogeriatr. 2005;17(2):319–26. https://doi.org/10.1017/s1041610205001316.
8. Elson P. Do older adults presenting with memory complaints wish to be told if later diagnosed with Alzheimer's disease? Int J Geriatr Psychiatry. 2006;21(5):419–25. https://doi.org/10.1002/gps.1485.
9. Van Den Dungen P, Van Kuijk L, Van Marwijk H, et al. Preferences regarding disclosure of a diagnosis of dementia: a systematic review. Int Psychogeriatr. 2014;26(10):1603–18. https://doi.org/10.1017/S1041610214000969.
10. Aminzadeh F, Byszewski A, Molnar FJ, Eisner M. Emotional impact of dementia diagnosis: exploring persons with dementia and caregivers' perspectives. Aging Ment Health. 2007;11(3):281–90. https://doi.org/10.1080/13607860600963695.
11. Reisberg B, Ferris SH, de Leon MJ, et al. The stage specific temporal course of Alzheimer's disease: functional and behavioral concomitants based upon cross-sectional and longitudinal observation. Prog Clin Biol Res. 1989;317:23–41.
12. Petersen RC, Smith GE, Waring SC, Ivnik RJ, Tangalos EG, Kokmen E. Mild cognitive impairment: clinical characterization and outcome. Arch Neurol. 1999;56(3):303–8. https://doi.org/10.1001/archneur.56.3.303.
13. Winblad B, Palmer K, Kivipelto M, et al. Mild cognitive impairment - beyond controversies, towards a consensus: report of the International Working Group on Mild Cognitive Impairment. J Intern Med. 2004;256(3):240–6. https://doi.org/10.1111/j.1365-2796.2004.01380.x.
14. Albert MS, DeKosky ST, Dickson D, et al. The diagnosis of mild cognitive impairment due to Alzheimer's disease: recommendations from the National Institute on Aging-Alzheimer's Association workgroups on diagnostic guidelines for Alzheimer's disease. Alzheimers Dement. 2011;7(3):270–9. https://doi.org/10.1016/j.jalz.2011.03.008.
15. Dubois B, Feldman HH, Jacova C, et al. Advancing research diagnostic criteria for Alzheimer's disease: the IWG-2 criteria. Lancet Neurol. 2014;13(6):614–29. https://doi.org/10.1016/S1474-4422(14)70090-0.
16. Gramkow MH, Gjerum L, Koikkalainen J, et al. Prognostic value of complementary biomarkers of neurodegeneration in a mixed memory clinic cohort. PeerJ. 2020;8:e9498. https://doi.org/10.7717/peerj.9498.
17. Overton M, Pihlsgård M, Elmståhl S. Diagnostic stability of mild cognitive impairment, and predictors of reversion to normal cognitive functioning. Dement Geriatr Cogn Disord. 2020. doi:https://doi.org/10.1159/000506255.
18. van Maurik IS, Vos SJ, Bos I, et al. Biomarker-based prognosis for people with mild cognitive impairment (ABIDE): a modelling study. Lancet Neurol. 2019;18(11):1034–44. https://doi.org/10.1016/S1474-4422(19)30283-2.
19. Joosten-Weyn Banningh L, Vernooij-Dassen M, Rikkert MO, Teunisse J-P. Mild cognitive impairment: coping with an uncertain label. Int J Geriatr Psychiatry. 2008;23(2):148–54. https://doi.org/10.1002/gps.1855.
20. Jansen WJ, Ossenkoppele R, Tijms BM, et al. Association of cerebral amyloid-β Aggregation with cognitive functioning in persons without dementia. JAMA Psychiat. 2018;75(1):84–95. https://doi.org/10.1001/jamapsychiatry.2017.3391.
21. Jansen WJ, Ossenkoppele R, Knol DL, et al. Prevalence of cerebral amyloid pathology in persons without dementia. JAMA. 2015;313(19):1924. https://doi.org/10.1001/jama.2015.4668.
22. Bergeron D, Gorno-Tempini ML, Rabinovici GD, et al. Prevalence of amyloid-β pathology in distinct variants of primary progressive aphasia. Ann Neurol. 2018;84(5):729–40. https://doi.org/10.1002/ana.25333.
23. Vanderschaeghe G, Dierickx K, Vandenberghe R. Review of the ethical issues of a biomarker-based diagnoses in the early stage of Alzheimer's disease. J Bioeth Inq. 2018;15(2):219–30. https://doi.org/10.1007/s11673-018-9844-y.
24. Carpenter BD, Xiong C, Porensky EK, et al. Reaction to a dementia diagnosis in individuals with Alzheimer's disease and mild cognitive impairment. J Am Geriatr Soc. 2008;56(3):405–12. https://doi.org/10.1111/j.1532-5415.2007.01600.x.

25. Laakkonen M-L, Raivio MM, Eloniemi-Sulkava U, et al. How do elderly spouse care givers of people with Alzheimer disease experience the disclosure of dementia diagnosis and subsequent care? J Med Ethics. 2008;34(6):427–30. https://doi.org/10.1136/jme.2007.021956.
26. Seyfried LS, Kales HC, Ignacio RV, Conwell Y, Valenstein M. Predictors of suicide in patients with dementia. Alzheimers Dement. 2011;7(6):567–73. https://doi.org/10.1016/j.jalz.2011.01.006.
27. Wake T, Tabuchi H, Funaki K, et al. Disclosure of amyloid status for risk of Alzheimer disease to cognitively normal research participants with subjective cognitive decline: a longitudinal study. Am J Alzheimers Dis Other Dement. 2020;35:1–9. https://doi.org/10.1177/1533317520904551.
28. Wake T, Tabuchi H, Funaki K, et al. The psychological impact of disclosing amyloid status to Japanese elderly: a preliminary study on asymptomatic patients with subjective cognitive decline. Int Psychogeriatr. 2018;30(5):635–9. https://doi.org/10.1017/S1041610217002204.
29. Vanderschaeghe G, Schaeverbeke J, Bruffaerts R, Vandenberghe R, Dierickx K. Amnestic MCI patients' experiences after disclosure of their amyloid PET result in a research context. Alzheimers Res Ther. 2017;9(1):1–16. https://doi.org/10.1186/s13195-017-0321-3.
30. Frederiksen KS, Nielsen TR, Appollonio I, et al. Biomarker counseling, disclosure of diagnosis and follow-up in patients with mild cognitive impairment: A European Alzheimer's disease consortium survey. Int J Geriatr Psychiatry. 2020. doi:https://doi.org/10.1002/gps.5427
31. Mitchell T, Woodward M, Hirose Y. A survey of attitudes of clinicians towards the diagnosis and treatment of mild cognitive impairment in Australia and New Zealand. Int Psychogeriatr. 2008;20(1):77–85. https://doi.org/10.1017/S1041610207005583.
32. Werner P, Heinik J, Kitai E. Familiarity, knowledge, and preferences of family physicians regarding mild cognitive impairment. Int Psychogeriatr. 2013;25(5):805–13. https://doi.org/10.1017/S1041610212002384.
33. Bertens D, Vos S, Kehoe P, et al. Use of mild cognitive impairment and prodromal AD/MCI due to AD in clinical care: A European survey. Alzheimers Res Ther. 2019;11(1):1–12. https://doi.org/10.1186/s13195-019-0525-9.
34. Nielsen TR, Svensson BH, Rohr G, et al. The process of disclosing a diagnosis of dementia and mild cognitive impairment: a national survey of specialist physicians in Denmark. Dementia. 2020;19(3):547–59. https://doi.org/10.1177/1471301218777443.
35. Visser LNC, Pelt SAR, Kunneman M, et al. Communicating uncertainties when disclosing diagnostic test results for (Alzheimer's) dementia in the memory clinic: the ABIDE project. Health Expect. 2020;23(1):52–62. https://doi.org/10.1111/hex.12964.
36. Frederiksen KS, Cooper C, Frisoni GB, et al. A European Academy of Neurology guideline on medical management issues in dementia. Eur J Neurol. 2020;27(10):1805–20. https://doi.org/10.1111/ene.14412.
37. Appelbaum PS. Assessment of patients' competence to consent to treatment. N Engl J Med. 2007;357(18):1834–40. https://doi.org/10.1056/NEJMcp074045.
38. Appelbaum P, Grisso T. MacCAT-CR: MacArthur competence tool for clinical research. Sarasota, FL: Professional Resource Press; 2001.
39. Joffe S, Cook EF, Cleary PD, Clark JW, Weeks JC. Quality of informed consent: a new measure of understanding among research subjects. J Natl Cancer Inst. 2001;93(2):139–47. https://doi.org/10.1093/jnci/93.2.139.
40. Jeste DV, Palmer BW, Appelbaum PS, et al. A new brief instrument for assessing decisional capacity for clinical research. Arch Gen Psychiatry. 2007;64(8):966. https://doi.org/10.1001/archpsyc.64.8.966.
41. Gurrera RJ, Moye J, Karel MJ, Azar AR, Armesto JC. Cognitive performance predicts treatment decisional abilities in mild to moderate dementia. Neurology. 2006;66(9):1367–72. https://doi.org/10.1212/01.wnl.0000210527.13661.d1.
42. Stormoen S, Almkvist O, Eriksdotter M, Sundström E, Tallberg I-M. Cognitive predictors of medical decision-making capacity in mild cognitive impairment and Alzheimer's disease. Int J Geriatr Psychiatry. 2014;29(12):1304–11. https://doi.org/10.1002/gps.4114.
43. Gambina G, Bonazzi A, Valbusa V, et al. Awareness of cognitive deficits and clinical competence in mild to moderate Alzheimer's disease: their relevance in clinical practice. Neurol Sci. 2014;35(3):385–90. https://doi.org/10.1007/s10072-013-1523-5.

Anti-dementia Medication

5

Vesna Jelic and Bengt Winblad

List of Abbreviations

ADL	Activities of daily living
AEs	Adverse events
AD	Alzheimer's disease
ADAS-Cog	Alzheimer's Disease Assessment Scale Cognitive Subscale
ACh	Acetylcholine
AChEI	Acetylcholinesterase inhibitor
APOE	Apolipoprotein E
APOE-ε4	Apolipoprotein E epsilon 4
Aβ	Amyloid beta
BuChE	Butyrylcholinesterase
CYP	Cytochrome group of enzymes P450
DLB	Dementia with Lewy bodies
FDA	Food and Drug Administration

V. Jelic (✉)
Clinic for Cognitive Disorders, Theme Aging and Inflammation, Karolinska University Hospital-Huddinge, Stockholm, Sweden

Division of Clinical Geriatrics, Department of NVS, Karolinska Institutet, Neo, Plan 7, Stockholm, Sweden
e-mail: vesna.jelic@ki.se

B. Winblad
Clinic for Cognitive Disorders, Theme Aging and Inflammation, Karolinska University Hospital-Huddinge, Stockholm, Sweden

Division of Neurogeriatrics, Department of NVS, Center for Alzheimer Research, Karolinska Institutet, BioClinicum J9:20, Stockholm, Sweden
e-mail: bengt.winblad@ki.se

K. S. Frederiksen, G. Waldemar (eds.), *Management of Patients with Dementia*,
https://doi.org/10.1007/978-3-030-77904-7_5

LBD	Lewy body dementia
MRI	Magnetic resonance imaging
MCI	Mild cognitive impairment
PDD	Parkinson disease dementia
REM	Rapid eye movement
DOMINO-AD	UK Donepezil and Memantine in moderate to severe AD
VaD	Vascular dementia

Introduction

The most common aetiology of dementia is a neurodegenerative process in the brain triggered by various proteinopathies and consequent differences in pathophysiological, clinical and biomarker phenotypes that are summarised under specific diagnoses (Chap. 2). The core trigger of neurodegeneration in the most common sporadic forms of primary degenerative dementias is still unknown (or under debate) and starts years before the clinical symptoms of the disease. As a result, there are currently no specific preventive strategies or disease-modifying therapeutics available. Clinical symptoms of dementia are due to a progressive loss of neuronal function that is mediated by signal substances or neurotransmitters in the brain cells' synapses. In the early 1990s this was one of the underlying ideas behind the first specific anti-dementia treatment for the most common form of dementia: Alzheimer's disease (AD). Today it continues to be the only evidence-based, first-line treatment approach. A limited and transient symptomatic effect of current medications without substantial and sustained long-term benefit is driving research efforts towards new treatment strategies in the hope of achieving disease-modifying effects. In this context drug targets are changing, and the amyloid cascade hypothesis occupies a key role in the development of new drugs. Accordingly, focus on target patient population further to the "left" on the clinical trajectory of disease evolution, i.e. towards early or prodromal stages of AD such as mild cognitive impairment (MCI), preferably well phenotyped with molecular and imaging AD biomarkers.

History of Pharmacological Treatment of Dementia

Current anti-dementia medications stem from the anticholinergic hypothesis of AD [1], which is based on converging evidence of reduced choline uptake and acetylcholine (ACh) release, degeneration of cholinergic cells in the nucleus basalis of Meynert with consequent loss of neocortical cholinergic innervation [2, 3]. In parallel, experimental studies demonstrated the role of ACh in learning and memory [4].

In 1993 tacrine was the first centrally acting cholinesterase inhibitor approved for the treatment of AD. Though the initial reports on the efficacy of the drug were very good, it was quickly taken off the market due to its hepatotoxicity. Tacrine caused elevated hepatic enzymes and its metabolite was cytotoxic [5].

In 1996 donepezil was approved for the treatment of mild to moderate AD, supported by the outcomes of 19 randomised clinical trials (RCTs) (three in severe stages of the disease and 16 in the mild to moderate stage) designed to assess treatment efficacy on cognition, function and/or behaviour and neuropsychiatric symptoms [6, 7].

In 2006 the US Food and Drug Administration (FDA) approved donepezil for the treatment of severe AD just 1 month after data from a Swedish study on severe AD in nursing home settings were published [8, 9].

Rivastigmine entered market in 2000, supported by the outcomes of six RCTs showing its efficacy in terms of the three above-mentioned symptom domains in mild to moderate AD. One RCT was performed in severe stages of the disease [10]. Due to a higher frequency of adverse events (AE), in particular gastrointestinal (GI) ones, the rivastigmine transdermal patch with gradual release over 24 h was developed in 2007 [11, 12]. In 2013 the FDA expanded the approved indication for the rivastigmine patch (13.3 mg/24 h) to include the severe stages of AD.

Approved in 2001, galantamine is the most recent acetylcholinesterase inhibitor (AChEI) used in treating AD, also mild to moderate AD, its efficacy assessed in eight RCTs (one in severe stages of the disease and seven in mild to moderate stages) [10]. Due to faster elimination, a half-life extended-release oral product was developed to permit single instead of the original twice-daily intake.

In 2003 the FDA approved memantine for the treatment of patients with moderate to severe probable AD, its efficacy assessed in six clinical trials (three in moderate to severe AD and three in mild to moderate) [10].

In 2014 the FDA approved donepezil-memantine as an extended-release capsule for patients stabilised on daily dose of donepezil 10 mg and not currently on memantine. The recommended starting dose is 7 mg/10 mg, taken once a day in the evening, which should be increased in 7 mg increments until reaching the recommended maintenance dose of 28 mg/10 mg once daily [13]. This drug formulation is not approved in Europe (Table 5.1).

Table 5.1 Six-month randomised double-blind clinical trials of AChEI and memantine efficacy in AD patients (Data from Cochrane Database of Systematic Reviews)

Drug	Legislation (year)	Indication	6-month RCTs[a] number (year)	No. of patients	MMSE (range)	Efficacy			
						Cognition	Global change	Function	Behaviour
Donepezil	1996 (USA) 1997 (Europe)	Mild to moderate AD	6 (1998–2011)[a]	1893	17–22	+	+	+	-
	2005	Moderate to severe AD	8 (2001–2017)[b]	3522	1–14	+/–	+	+	-
23 mg ER tablet	2010 (USA)	Moderate to severe AD	Evaluated in 2 of 8 studies						
Rivastigmine	1998 (Europe)	Mild to moderate AD	7 (2000–2011)	4938	10–26	+	+	+	-
	2000 (USA)	Severe AD (capsules)	1 (2005)	218	5–12				
	2013	Severe AD 13.3 mg (transdermal patch)							
Galantamine	2000 (Europe)	Mild to moderate AD	5[c] (1997–2005)	3792	10–24	+	+	+	+/–
	2001 (USA)	Severe AD	1 (2009)	505	5–12	+	-	-	-
Memantine	2002 (Europe)	Moderate to severe AD	11 (2003–2011)	3732	3–14	+/–	+/–	+/–	+/–
	2003 (USA)	Mild to moderate	4 (2004–2011)	1672	10–23	+/–	+/–	+/–	+/–

In the Efficacy column, treatment-related change in domain-specific outcomes across the RCTs has the following annotations: + positive change; - absence of change or negative trends; +/- no conclusive evidence across the studies

AChEI acetylcholinesterase inhibitor, *AD* Alzheimer's disease, *ER* extended release, *MMSE* mini-mental state examination, *RCT* randomised controlled trial

[a]Only late-stage 6-month RCTs using minimal effective dose of donepezil 5 mg reporting sufficient data and at least two out of four domains included as primary outcomes (according to Birk 2018).

[b]Tariot et al. study [7] was included for moderate to severe AD since patients were nursing home residents with a mean MMSE of 14.4, broad score range of 5–26

[c]Five- and seven-month RCTs also included

Pharmacodynamics and Pharmacokinetics: Relevant Information for Clinicians

The pharmacodynamics of drugs refers to the underlying mechanism of its biological effect and biochemical and molecular interactions. An important aspect of pharmacodynamics involves identifying which intrinsic and extrinsic variables affect the relationship between the concentration and effect of the drug [14].

The pharmacokinetic characteristics of drugs, such as release, absorption, distribution, bioavailability, metabolism and excretion are crucial for determining a daily effective dose, minimum and maximum dose, dosage regimen and form of administration [14] (Table 5.2).

Acetylcholinesterase Inhibitors

The three AChEIs currently in use decrease the breakdown of acetylcholine (ACh) in the synaptic cleft, potentiating the effect in the synapse of ACh by inhibiting the enzyme cholinesterase, which has two major forms: AChE and butyrylcholinesterase (BuChE). The former is highly selective to ACh and hydrolysing it to acetate and choline terminates its action in the synapse. Contrary to AChE, BuChE also metabolises other endogenous and exogenously applied molecules, such as certain neuropeptides, and centrally active substances such as organophosphates.

Although the main mode of action of donepezil, rivastigmine and galantamine is similar, their pharmacological properties differ (Table 5.1). Non-competitive inhibition of donepezil and rivastigmine means that they bind and inhibit AChE irrespective of whether it has already been bound to its substrate ACh, in contrast to galantamine, which competes with ACh for the binding site on AChE. The reversibility of enzyme inhibition is a major requirement for the therapeutic non-toxic effect of AChEI.

AChE exists in two isoforms in the nervous system, G1, which is selectively present in the cortex and hippocampus, while the G4 isoform is predominant in the motor endplate in the peripheral nervous system (Weinstock, 1999). The higher selectivity of rivastigmine to the G1 isoform explains the absence of peripheral cholinergic effects, such as muscle cramps and weakness, described as side effects of donepezil and galantamine. An additional advantage of rivastigmine compared to the other AChEIs is that AChE activity, particularly its G4 isoform, decreases during the disease course and G1 isoform is probably mainly responsible for hydrolysing ACh. Furthermore, rivastigmine is not specific for AChE over BuChE [15], the latter less affected by the disease or even increased [16]. However, rivastigmine has a noticeably short elimination half-life compared to donepezil and galantamine, which requires two oral daily doses to reach a steady-state concentration in the plasma. More than one daily dose of a drug compromises compliance with treatment in patients with dementia. Another disadvantage of rivastigmine is that plasma concentration of the drug increases more than proportionally when the dose increases. Nonlinear pharmacokinetics results in more side effects in comparison

Table 5.2 Pharmacodynamic and pharmacokinetic properties of acetylcholinesterase inhibitors

Properties	Donepezil	Galantamine	Rivastigmine	Memantine
Mode of action	Non-competitive, rapidly reversible inhibitor	Competitive, rapidly reversible + nAChR modulation	Non-competitive, slowly reversible	Non-competitive, low-affinity, NMDA receptor antagonist
AChE/BuChE selectivity	300	50	1	
Brain vs peripheral selectivity	Yes	No	Yes	
Formulation	Tablets (ER) (5, 10, 23 mg)	Tablets (ER) (8, 16, 24 mg) Oral solution (2 mg/ml)	Capsules (1.5, 3, 4.5, 6 mg) Oral solution (2 mg/ml) Transdermal patch (4.6, 9.5, 13.3 mg/24h)	Tablets (10, 20 mg)
Effective dose(s)	5–10, 23[a] mg (once daily)	16–24 mg (once daily)	6–12 mg (divided into two daily doses)	10–20 mg (once daily)
Absorption affected by food	No	Yes	Yes	No
Bioavailability (%)	100	100	35 (3mg), 70 (6mg)	100
Time to reach $C_{max,ss}$ (h) (t_{max})	6	4–5	1 (capsule), 8 (patch)	3–8
Elimination half-life (h) ($t_{½}$)	73	6–8	1.5–2 (capsule), 3.4 (patch)	60–70
Metabolism	Hepatic (CYP2D6, CYP3A4, UGT)	Hepatic (CYP2D6, CYP3A4, UGT)	Esterases in liver and intestine	Mainly unmetabolised
Renal excretion (%)	17	50	Metabolite	57–82 (pH dependent)
Kinetics	Linear	Linear	Nonlinear	Linear
Steady state (days)	14–21	6	1	11

nAChR nicotinic acetylcholine receptors, *NMDA* *N*-Methyl-D-aspartate, *AChE* acetylcholinesterase, *ER* extended release, $C_{max,ss}$ maximum steady-state plasma drug concentration during a dosage interval, *CYP* cytochrome P450, *UGT* uridine 5'-diphospho-glucuronosyltransferase
[a]Donepezil ER 23 mg only approved in USA

with donepezil and galantamine. The rivastigmine patch has considerably better tolerability since it gradually releases the drug over 24 h [17, 18].

A further distinctive pharmacokinetic characteristic of galantamine is its dual mode of potentiating cholinergic transmission by additional interaction with nicotinic receptors. This effect was expected to be extra beneficial since the severity of cognitive impairment in AD correlates with loss of nicotinic receptors [19].

An important aspect of pharmacokinetics is an effect of renal and hepatic metabolism on drug elimination, which differs among AChEI with consequent effect on drug interactions and frequency of adverse effects of treatment [20].

Donepezil is metabolised in the liver by the cytochrome group of enzymes P450 (CYP) (Table 5.1), and the primary route of elimination is renal. No dose adjustments are needed in subjects with moderate renal dysfunction. However, even in mild to moderate liver impairment, the recommended 5 mg dose should be maintained. There is only one active metabolite with low affinity and negligible effect on AChE inhibition and pharmacological effect of the drug. Drugs that are potent CYP inhibitors (ketoconazole, cimetidine) influence plasma concentrations of donepezil considerably.

Rivastigmine is mainly metabolised by cholinesterase-mediated hydrolysis in the liver and to negligible extent in the intestines, to inactive metabolites (Table 5.1). CYP enzymes are not significantly involved in the rivastigmine metabolism, making drug interactions unlikely. Renal excretion is also a primary route of elimination, with no need for dose reduction in mild to moderate renal impairment. Since dose titration to tolerability is the basis for individually determining the maximum treatment dose, even in moderate liver cirrhosis, there is no general recommendation about the maximum dose.

Up to 30% of galantamine is excreted unmetabolised in the urine, while the rest is metabolised through various pathways, e.g. as CYP enzymes and glucuronidation, which provides active metabolites, though in low concentrations, in the plasma and a doubtful contribution to the pharmacological effect of the drug. Use of galantamine in patients with moderate to severe hepatic dysfunction is not recommended due to an up to 60% reduction in metabolic clearance.

Memantine

Memantine is a non-competitive, low-affinity antagonist of the *N*-methyl-D-aspartate (NMDA) ionotropic channel receptor, which is a binding site for a major excitatory neurotransmitter glutamate. Pathologically increased NMDA receptor activity has been demonstrated in AD, as well as impairment of learning and memory, with their blockade [21]. Memantine's low-binding affinity restores homeostasis in the glutamatergic system without accumulation in ion channels or blocking of synaptic neurotransmission [22]. Memantine is believed to have both a symptomatic treatment effect and neuroprotective properties [23].

CYP enzymes do not contribute significantly to metabolism of memantine to its inactive metabolites; however, memantine seems to be both a potent and selective inhibitor of CYP2B6 enzyme in its therapeutic doses, which might have clinical relevance in terms of drug interactions [24]. Since memantine and its metabolites are excreted renally by tubular secretion, concomitant therapy with drugs with a similar route of elimination could lower clearance of memantine. However, the widely used oral antidiabetic metformin did not have pharmacokinetic interactions with memantine during a single-dose, 6-day treatment in healthy volunteers, despite the similar route of elimination [25]. In patients with severe renal impairment only half of a maximum daily dose is recommended, while in moderate renal insufficiency tolerance during the titration phase with 10 mg is the guiding principle in determining the individual maximum dose.

Pharmacogenetics: Towards a Personalised Treatment

Genetic variations in drug metabolising enzymes as well as AChEs could contribute to the individual therapeutic failures and different side effects or AEs across the different compounds from the same class, Table 5.2. Different profiles of common genetic risk factors for AD, such as DNA apolipoprotein E epsilon 4 (APOE-e4) genotype, might also have impact on treatment response in AChEIs. A number of studies performed on genetic polymorphisms in cytochromes [20], in particular CYP2D6, for AChEI treatment identified several groups of metabolisers: 5–10% of poor metabolisers, 10–17% of intermediate, 70–80% of extensive and 3–5% of ultra-rapid metabolisers [26]. These genetically determined metabolic phenotypes result in different plasma concentrations of the drugs, from almost toxic levels in poor metabolisers to much below therapeutic levels in the ultra-rapid group. To date pharmacogenetic studies on response to AChEI treatment in AD are discrepant, partly due to different number of patients included, follow-up periods and definition of responders vs non-responders. Ten studies on patient populations ranging from 27 to 396 individuals treated with either donepezil, galantamine or rivastigmine were performed analysing treatment response for different phenotypes of cytochromes, mostly CYP2D6 [20]. A study investigating the effects of 16 functional polymorphisms of CYP2D6 on treatment effect in 57 AD patients treated with donepezil reported significantly higher frequencies of gene variants in responders that contribute to decreased or absent enzyme activity [27]. An Italian prospective study that included 171 patients treated with one of the three AChEIs, however, found no effect of different CYP2D6 and BChE genotypes after 1 year of treatment, irrespective of the medication used [28].

The number of published scientific studies on the influence of different genotypes of cholinergic markers (AChE, BChE and choline acetyltransferase) is growing. The BChE genotype affected treatment effect in both rivastigmine and memantine add-on therapy [29]. A deleterious effect of the BChE-K variant in donepezil treatment of MCI over 3 years was reported in a case–control study [30]. The interaction between the BChE-K genotype and donepezil response on cognitive function in this study was significantly associated with the duration of treatment. Furthermore, homozygous BChE-K carriers displayed a steeper cognitive decline on Mini-Mental State Examination (MMSE) and Clinical Dementia Rating—Sum of Boxes in donepezil-treated subjects carrying APOE-ε4 allele.

A possible explanation is that parallel pharmacological inhibition of AChE by donepezil treatment and inhibition of BChE due to polymorphism in BChE-K-variant of the enzyme cause toxic overload of acetylcholine [31, 32]. Thus, BChE genotyping represents a promising tool in selecting non-responders for AChEI therapy when eventual treatment of AD patients with a prodromal phase of the disease is considered on a case-by-case basis.

The APOE-ε4 allele is associated with an increased risk for developing late-onset sporadic AD. The majority of RCTs, three performed with donepezil, three with galantamine and two with rivastigmine (*n* = 2462 patients with AD), reported no influence of the apolipoprotein E (APOE) genotype on treatment response [20]. In one study on the effects of long-term treatment with donepezil in 40 patients, APOE-ε4 carriers demonstrated a poorer response on the Alzheimer's Disease Assessment Scale Cognitive Subscale (ADAS-cog) score after 3 years therapy [33]. In a case–control study on 81 patients, in contrast, after 12–16 months of treatment, there was a better response in specific cognitive domains of attention and memory and on MMSE in APOE-ε4 carriers [34].

Although APOE polymorphism does not seem to have an independent effect on AChEI clinical response, patients with the APOE-ε4 and CYP2D6 genotype with decreased function alleles demonstrated an increased frequency of treatment non-response [35].

Models built on the likely beneficial or detrimental effect of long-term AChEI treatment, incorporating relevant modifying factors such as age, sex and BuChE-K and APOE-ε4 polymorphism were suggested [36]. This approach might optimise treatment outcomes in future but it does not presently guide the therapeutic decisions of clinicians. With respect to optimising treatment efficacy, more complex, different neurodegenerative phenotypes will likely be defined in the future based on genetic and biomarker profiles.

Translation of Clinical Trial Outcomes to Relevant Benefits in Clinical Practice

A large number of RCTs were performed with AChEIs to evaluate their efficacy, usually against placebo treatment in AD (Table 5.1). How long trials lasted was based on their outcomes: 6–12 months if symptom improvement was intended or 18–24 months if modification of clinical course was expected [37]. Three-month trials were considered too short to demonstrate a clinically meaningful effect [37]. The most relevant clinical outcomes in the RCTs are improvement in cognitive performance, various aspects of activities of daily living (ADL), severity rating of the disease and the clinician's global impression of change compared to baseline performance [38]. Outcomes across different domains in RCTs with patients with AD are quantified by representative scales, such as: MMSE [39] and ADAS-Cog [40] for global and domain-specific cognitive status; Disability Assessment for Dementia Scale [41] and Progressive Deterioration Scale [42] for ADL; Clinician's Interview-Based Impression of Change Plus Caregiver Input (CIBIC-Plus) [43] and Gottfries-Bråne-Steen Scale [44] for global clinical state; and Neuropsychiatric Inventory (NPI) [45] for neuropsychiatric symptoms. In trials in severe AD due to floor effect on MMSE and ADAS-Cog, the Severe Impairment Battery (SIB) [46] was used to assess cognitive decline.

A clinically relevant change is difficult to reconstruct based on minor changes or cut-off scores on individual assessment scales used across domains as trial outcomes. The change has to be relevant for both patient and caregiver in real life. Applied in a standardised way by a clinician and caregiver, the CIBIC-Plus uses a composite score, showing if there was meaningful improvement based on criteria relevant to the patients and their carer.

Pooled data from both RCTs and observational studies make it possible to assess not only efficacy through meta-analyses but also the occurrence and profile of AEs on a large scale, not to mention differences in outcomes based on the characteristics of the patient population at baseline. For example, in the meta-database from the Alzheimer's Disease Cooperative Study and the Alzheimer's Disease Neuroimaging Initiative (n = 2793 participants) conducted from 1993 to 2012 older individuals with AD dementia enrolled in clinical trials with AChEI showed substantially less cognitive worsening measured with the ADAS-cog or MMSE than younger individuals [47].

It could be argued that the isolated small effect on cognition without effect on functional decline cannot be considered as clinically relevant. Similarly, improved or stabilised performance of ADL may not have enough of an effect to have an impact on outcomes of institutionalisation, carer impact or quality of life [48]. A systematic review and meta-analysis of the effectiveness of all commonly used pharmacological interventions to improve quality of life and well-being in people with dementia did not find consistent evidence [49]. However, only 12- to 24-week AChEI RCTs on donepezil were included in this review, since comparable trials with rivastigmine or galantamine did not report quality of life outcomes. Thus, it is still unclear whether improvements in quality of life can be expected to continue beyond short-term RCTs.

Donepezil

The main findings of RCTs on donepezil are similar in both mild to moderate and moderate to severe disease, with donepezil showing benefits compared with placebo at 26 weeks (6 months) for cognitive function, ADL and the clinician-rated global impression scales (Table 5.1). There were no differences on measures of behavioural symptoms or quality of life. AEs and withdrawal from the study were dose-related, occurring more often in patients treated with 10 and 23 mg/day [6]. Slow-release donepezil formulation of 23 mg/day did not show any advantages compared to 10 mg/day [50, 51].

Only 11% of patients with probable AD were eligible for RCTs sponsored by pharmaceutical companies due to restricted inclusion criteria [52]. Given the moderate improvements in individual domain-specific rating scales during a relatively short evaluation time in such highly selected patient populations, there was a need for more real-life outcomes in typical real-life patients with common comorbidities.

A large-scale UK-based trial called AD 2000, which did not receive any funding from pharmaceutical companies [53], was initially designed to address relevant clinical and social benefits and economic outcomes during long-term treatment.

Although the trial aimed to recruit 3000 patients referred to a memory clinic, only 566 individuals with AD and with or without cerebrovascular disease and vascular dementia (VaD) diagnosis were randomised. The trial had a modified cross-over design since patients were randomised to donepezil 5 mg/day or placebo in the initial 12 weeks and then re-randomised to 5 or 10 mg/day or placebo. The trial aimed to "determine whether donepezil produces worthwhile improvements in disability, dependency, behavioural and psychological symptoms, carers' psychological well-being, or delay in institutionalisation and if so, which patients benefit, from what dose, and for how long" [6, 53]. The first 2 years of treatment showed small improvements on tests of cognitive (MMSE) and functional (Bristol ADL Scale) ability but there was no significant delay in entry to institutional care or progression of disability, which were two primary outcome measures.

The study was criticised for various methodological limitations, for example repeated washouts that could have been associated with a loss of benefits of donepezil treatment. In addition, 48% of patients had discontinued the trial within 1 year and <20% remained by the end of the second year.

Galantamine

RCTs on galantamine that mainly included patients with mild to moderate AD [54], treatment showed significant improvements in cognition irrespective of daily dose (8–32 mg/day) or drug formulation (bi-daily vs extended-release tablets) (Table 5.1). On CIBIC, improvement or stabilisation was observed at all daily doses, except for 8 mg/day. Trials that reported changes in ADL and the Neuropsychiatric Inventory scale as outcomes showed significant treatment effect on function and behaviour [55–57]. The 6-month RCT with galantamine in patients with severe AD residing in a nursing home reported an improvement in cognitive function but there was no significant effect on ADL, which is a desirable treatment effect in advanced dementia [58]. An international, 7-month multi-centre RCT reported efficacy across all core domains in patients with comorbid AD and cerebrovascular disease [59].

Rivastigmine

A 26-week RCT reported that oral rivastigmine taken in 6 and 12 mg divided into two daily doses and a rivastigmine transdermal patch 9.5 mg/day showed benefits compared to placebo on measures of cognitive function, ADL and the physician-rated global impression of change scales, but there was no difference with respect to behavioural symptoms in mild to moderate AD (Table 5.1) [60]. Effect on cognition was rather small and thus probably not clinically relevant. Significant improvements compared to placebo on GCI scale were shown at the 26-week assessment but not at earlier time points. The transdermal patch (9.5 mg/day) seems to be as effective as peroral capsules, as suggested in the IDEAL study [61].

Memantine

In contrast to AChEI, memantine treatment led to functional improvement and reduced care dependence in severely demented patients in one initial 3-month RCT [62] and showed some beneficial effect in moderate to severe or severe AD in RCTs lasting 6 months or more (Table 5.1). Most of these studies (five RCTs listed in Table 5.1) compared the efficacy and safety of memantine (versus placebo) in patients already receiving stable treatment with donepezil [63]. Memantine was marginally superior to placebo on outcomes measuring cognitive function, ADL, behaviour and mood in mild to moderate and moderate to severe AD. A systematic review and meta-analysis of nine studies including monotherapy showed minor clinical benefits across all outcomes, including clinical global impression of improvement [64]. A meta-analysis and meta-regression of 18 RCTs involving 5004 patients reported that memantine was only slightly superior to placebo in outcomes measuring cognitive function, neuropsychiatric symptoms, global clinical assessment and discontinuation due to inefficacy, and showed no improvement in functional ability [65]. The authors concluded that the clinical relevance of memantine's efficacy in AD is doubtful. They also argued that the conclusions in several previous, optimistic meta-analyses [64, 66, 67] overlooked the relevance of the intervention effect size, which was very small across all efficacy domains [68].

Comparative Evidence of Efficacy

Head-to-head trials directly comparing efficacy of different AChEIs are sparse and limited since the majority of them used open-label design, different measurement scales for assessing outcomes and a range of fixed and flexible doses of the drugs being tested [69]. Four trials providing direct comparison of two AChEIs are frequently cited in the literature: one 52-week [70] and one 12-week open-label trial [71] compared donepezil with galantamine, and one 12-week open-label [72] and one 2-year double-blinded randomised trial [73] compared donepezil with rivastigmine. While shorter, the 12-week trials found statistically significant differences in efficacy on cognitive and functional outcomes in favour of donepezil over galantamine, while the longer 52-week trial did not find significant differences in efficacy [69]. Both trials comparing directly donepezil and rivastigmine found a similar effect on cognitive measures, while the double-blind study demonstrated even a small, statistically significant effect on functional measures in favour of rivastigmine over donepezil. Regarding positive effect on measures of change in behaviour, donepezil was significantly better than galantamine.

A network meta-analysis is another option for comparing the efficacy of two treatments and indirectly estimates differences between the effects of two drugs tested in separate RCTs by making an inference based on their efficacy versus placebo, which is a common comparator [74].

Safety and Tolerability

Most side effects of AChEI are due to cholinergically mediated GI symptoms. Across all RCTs on AChEI the most common reasons for trial discontinuation were nausea (2–8%) and vomiting (1–5%) [75]. Transdermal administration of rivastigmine has considerably improved tolerance of the drug [76]. The meta-analysis of memantine trials found no differences between memantine and placebo for both all-cause treatment discontinuation and for treatment discontinuation due to AEs [65]. A slight reservation about this conclusion is that patients with severe AD might underreport AE, possibly leading to safety overestimation of memantine prescribed in this disease stage. Table 5.3, which summarises AEs reported in anti-dementia drug RCTs, is based on Alva and Cummings' 2008 review [75], which compiled and analysed odds ratio data on AEs listed in manufacturers' patient information leaflets for donepezil, galantamine, rivastigmine and memantine. It is worth

Table 5.3 Adverse events reported in clinical trials with anti-dementia drugs

	Significant odds ratios	Non-significant odds ratios
Donepezil	Anorexia[a], diarrhoea[a], muscle cramps, nausea[a], vomiting[a]	Abnormal dreams, accidents, arthritis, back pain, chest pain, confusion, ↑ dehydration, *depression*, dizziness, ecchymosis, eczema, emotional lability, fatigue, fever, frequent urination, *hallucinations*, headache, haemorrhage, hostility, hyperlipidaemia, hypertension, infection, insomnia, nervousness, pain, personality disorder, somnolence, syncope, urinary incontinence, weight loss
Rivastigmine		
Oral administration (capsule)	Abdominal pain, anorexia[a], anxiety, asthenia, depression, diarrhoea, dizziness[a], dyspepsia, fatigue, flatulence, headache, malaise, nausea[a], sweating, tremor, vomiting[a], weight loss	Abdominal pain, accidental trauma, aggression, confusion, constipation, eructation, hallucinations, hypertension, influenza-like symptoms, insomnia, rhinitis, syncope, urinary tract infection, vertigo
Transdermal patch	*Same AEs profile, no significant odds ratios*	
Galantamine	Anorexia[a], dizziness[a], dyspepsia, fatigue, headache, nausea[a], vomiting[a], weight loss	Abdominal pain, anaemia, bradycardia, *depression*, diarrhoea, haematuria, insomnia, rhinitis, somnolence, syncope[a], tremor, urinary tract infection
Memantine	Constipation, headache, hypertension, pain	Back pain, confusion, coughing, *dizziness, dyspnoea, fatigue,* hallucinations, somnolence, vomiting

AE adverse events, AEs reported by at least 2% of patients receiving different therapeutic dosages and occurring at least twice the frequency seen in placebo-treated patients

[a]Most frequent AEs leading to discontinuation of treatment. Italics indicate AEs with odds ratios close to marginal significance. Based on Alva and Cummings [74]

mentioning to patients that most of the common GI side effects disappear in one to a few days.

In most cases typical GI cholinomimetic AEs are mild and transient and can be reduced by longer titration to the target dose, e.g. the recommended 6-week titration of donepezil from 5 to 10 mg/day. While donepezil does not have to be taken with food to reduce the frequency of GI AEs, it is recommended that galantamine and rivastigmine are administered with food. Adding anti-emetic medication and adequate fluid intake can ease nausea, which in a minority of patients taking galantamine, and even donepezil, was experienced for more than a week. To avoid nausea, donepezil is usually prescribed for the night. However, if lucid dreams develop, the patient is advised to take donepezil in the morning.

Both donepezil and galantamine treatment may reduce rapid eye movement (REM) sleep latency and lead to decreased slow-wave sleep [77]. Insomnia in RCTs was two to threefold more frequent in patients treated with donepezil than in those on placebo. Rivastigmine increases REM density and does not affect REM sleep latency. Lack of sleep was reported in patients treated with rivastigmine diagnosed with AD, dementia with Lewy bodies (DLB) or Parkinson's disease dementia (PDD) [78].

While AEs leading to discontinuation in RCTs were similar for both oral and transdermal administration of rivastigmine, their safety and tolerability profiles are different. The 9.5 mg/24 h rivastigmine transdermal patch had similar efficacy to the rivastigmine capsule (12 mg/day), with one-third of the incidence of GI side effects [11].

Interestingly, skin irritation related to the rivastigmine patch had low incidence in clinical trials, was not related to the dose and could be avoided by omitting application of the patch on the same site within 14 days. In clinical practice common notification of skin irritation is often related to various manufactures and differences in adhesive substances. Low body weight is a risk factor for experiencing more severe AEs, particularly the GI profile. Body weight of less than 50 kg is a warning sign that the patient will probably discontinue treatment with either rivastigmine capsules or patch due to AEs. Thus, weight monitoring during treatment is obligatory, and this refers to all compounds in the AChEI class. Frail older patients risk developing slight nausea and subsequent loss of appetite that may continue unnoticed for some time, resulting in weight loss over a longer period.

In the FDA Adverse Event Reporting System database serious AEs associated with AChEI are rhabdomyolysis, convulsions, falls, loss of consciousness, syncope, pneumonia and death. Other severe complications are increased gastric acid secretion, GI bleeding, urinary obstruction, deterioration of symptoms of asthma or obstructive pulmonary disease, seizures and exacerbation of extrapyramidal symptoms in Parkinsonism.

When data from unpublished studies on the use of galantamine in people with MCI at risk of developing AD were pooled, researchers found a significantly higher rate of unexplained death in the patient group treated with active drugs [54]. The studies combined included 2048 people >50 years of age with MCI. The difference in death rates between the drug groups and the placebo became apparent within the first 3 months of treatment of patients with MCI, whereas in placebo-controlled studies of up to 6 months among patients with dementia, death rates did not differ between galantamine and placebo [79, 80]. The deaths in the galantamine MCI trials were mostly due to cerebrovascular or cardiovascular causes.

In a real-life setting it is important to be aware of frailty, comorbidities and polypharmacy in individual patients. In particular the physician should be aware of the vagotonic effect of AChEIs on sinoatrial and atrioventricular nodes causing bradycardia and heart block. A population-based study showed that recent initiation of cholinesterase inhibitors was associated with approximately a doubling of the risk of hospitalisation for bradycardia [81]. Absolute contraindications to AChEI are second or third-degree heart block in an unpaced patient; QT prolongation; and bradycardia <50 bpm. Beta-blockers are commonly prescribed drugs, and AChEIs should be prescribed cautiously if the pulse rate is between 50 and 60 bpm, even in an asymptomatic patient.

Memantine is well tolerated, but dose adjustments are needed in more severe renal impairment. AEs could be provoked by alkalinisation of the urine and therefore sodium bicarbonate and carbonic anhydrase inhibitors should be avoided.

Open-label extension and observational studies have reported good tolerability with prolonged memantine therapy, although there is a substantial dropout and survivor bias [82, 83], just as there is a risk confusion and/or having hallucinations.

Possible Beneficial Effects of AChEIs on Comorbidities in AD Patients

Evidence in the literature indicates that AChEIs can also have a beneficial effect on comorbidities as well as reduce cardiac morbidity and mortality in AD patients [84]. While bradycardia is a non-favourable and potentially serious side effect of AChEI treatment, particularly during treatment with donepezil [85], AChEIs can slow the heart rate in patients with atrial fibrillation and other causes of tachycardia. A number of studies reported a possible cardio-protective effect of AChEI [86]. A cohort study with 7073 patients from the Swedish Dementia Registry found, after accounting for confounders, that patients with AD or mixed dementia who used AChEI had a 34% lower risk of either myocardial infarction or death compared to those who did not [87]. AChEI can improve GI motility and reduce the need for laxatives in the elderly population with AD. An increase in parasympathetic innervation to the eye during AChEI therapy can reduce intraocular pressure in comorbid glaucoma in patients with AD. Furthermore dry-mouth and atonic bladder can benefit from AChEI treatment in this patient population. However, evidence from RCTs is lacking and is mostly based on real-life observational and case studies in patients who are not usually recruited in trials [84]. Nevertheless, this puts emphasis on the importance of monitoring comorbidities, polypharmacy and adjusting treatment with other drugs if a pleiotropic effect of AChEI is expected.

Treatment Efficacy Beyond the AD

Lewy body dementia (LBD) is the second most common form of neurodegenerative dementia after AD. It includes dementia with Lewy bodies (DLB) and Parkinson's disease dementia (PDD). Similar to patients with AD, patients with LBD show marked cholinergic deficits, but the deficits are more severe in LBD compared to AD and occur earlier in the course of the disease. Six RCTs examining LBD and cognitive impairment with no dementia in Parkinson's disease (CIND-PD) that included 1236 patients showed a positive impact on global assessment, cognitive function and neuropsychiatric symptoms such as hallucinations, apathy, anxiety and sleep disorders, and on ADL rating scales [88]. Among studies included in this meta-analysis donepezil was used as intervention drug in three studies with PDD and one with CIND-PD, while rivastigmine was used in one study with PDD and one with DLB patients. Two 24-week RCTs using memantine in a mixed study population of both DLB and PDD patients showed a significant benefit overall on clinical global impression of change but could not demonstrate a consistent pattern of treatment response in clinical subtypes of LBD with regard to cognition and non-cognitive neuropsychiatric symptoms [89, 90]. Both 24-week trials reported that memantine was well tolerated. However, there are case reports of severe states of confusion in conjunction with the introduction of memantine in patients with LBD [91, 92].

A large-scale UK study in Oxfordshire that monitored treatment with AChEI collected over 4 years data on 1250 patients, supplementing the data with an examination of retrospective case notes [93]. Patients were reassessed after a mean period of 4 months to evaluate clinical and cognitive response to therapy. The study defined clinical response as improvement sufficient to merit continuation of therapy, while an MMSE improvement of two or more points was defined as cognitive response. Patients with DLB and PDD had a better clinical and cognitive response compared to patients with AD. Cognitive but not clinical response was more likely in patients with moderate dementia than in those with mild dementia.

Vascular cognitive impairment (VCI) covers a range of cognitive and behavioural changes associated with vascular pathology. Evaluating the treatment effect using one common test battery is difficult in an etiologically heterogeneous patient group that includes both small- and large-vessel disease, either cortical or subcortical strategic infarctions, comorbidity with AD pathology (i.e. mixed dementia) or LBD. All three AChEI drugs and memantine were evaluated for their effects in vascular cognitive impairment diagnosed according to the NINDS-AIREN criteria [59, 94–97]. Only slight cognitive improvements were reported for donepezil, galantamine and memantine treatment in vascular cognitive impairment. There was evidence that in mixed dementia, galantamine could improve both cognition and global functioning [59, 95]. Two 6-month RCTs using galantamine in patients with both AD and VaD that included 1378 participants had a significantly higher patient dropout rate, mainly due to GI side effects. A meta-analysis conducted by Kavirajan and Schneider [98] included placebo-controlled RCTs with all three AChEI and memantine in VaD. They concluded that current anti-dementia treatment led to small benefits in cognition of uncertain clinical significance in patients with mild to moderate VaD. In post-hoc analyses of the original RCTs, donepezil and galantamine showed greater improvement in patients with cortical and multiple territorial lesions compared to those with subcortical lesions.

Delirium or confusion is frequent in elderly, cognitively impaired patients, and it is hypothesised that it could be induced by a lack of acetylcholine in the brain. An open-label 24-month study of 246 patients aimed to determine whether rivastigmine had any effect on delirium in VaD [99] suggested that rivastigmine may help reduce the frequency of delirium episodes and help shorten their duration.

A hypothesis that treatment with AChEI could result in clinical improvement in some rare dementias associated with neurological conditions was tested in eight 12- to 24-week RCTs with 567 participants who received ether an active drug or placebo [100]. One study with donepezil and one with rivastigmine treatment were performed on dementia due to Huntington's disease, one study included patients with cerebral autosomal dominant arteriopathy with subcortical infarcts and leuko-encephalopathy (CADASIL) treated with donepezil, galantamine was applied in one study on frontotemporal dementia, two studies evaluated donepezil and two rivastigmine in multiple sclerosis. One 6-week RCT on donepezil was performed in progressive supranuclear palsy [101]. No firm evidence can be drawn from these trials since the sample size is small and the effect on outcomes is either small or too insufficient to be considered as clinically relevant. In four trials that included patients with multiple sclerosis, the effect of AChEI on cognitive function was observed indirectly in the clinician's impression of cognitive change in three of the four trials [100]. In one RCT that included patients with CADASIL there was a beneficial effect on measures of cognitive functions [102]. An open-label study in frontotemporal dementia reported that patients treated with rivastigmine were less behaviourally impaired and that caregiver burden was reduced after 12 months of treatment [103]. In the progressive supranuclear palsy trial using donepezil, patients' memory test scores improved, whereas their ADL and mobility scores significantly worsened [101].

AChEIs in chronic traumatic brain injury due to post-traumatic cognitive impairments, particularly memory impairments, have also been evaluated in a short-term RCT with rivastigmine [104]. There was only a weak trend favouring rivastigmine in computerised neuropsychological testing but not in the standardised clinical interviews used to assess the outcome. Interestingly, the patients with more severe injuries, possibly also showing significant focal lesions and without the APOE-ε4 genotype, were most likely to respond.

Four additional RCTs evaluated donepezil and galantamine as adjunctive therapy for depression in non-demented elderly, but there was no benefit in terms of cognitive outcomes or improvement of depressive symptoms [105]. One study even reported that there was increased depression recurrence when depressed patients in remission were treated with donepezil [106].

Health-Economic Issues

Health technology assessment agencies assess the effectiveness or cost-effectiveness of drugs approved for AD from various perspectives, such as those of clinicians, patients and their representatives, drug companies, researchers and public funding and healthcare resources [107]. The cost-effectiveness of current anti-dementia drugs is difficult to assess since there are either small or non-existing benefits in terms of functional improvement, and there is no disease-modifying effect. Furthermore, outcomes driving decision-making are mainly based on clinical scales that are questioned in terms of their relevance for patients and their caregivers. Economic modelling addresses these challenges, including resource use, healthcare costs and quality-adjusted life years of patients [108].

Evidence weighing clinical effectiveness versus cost-effectiveness is also needed to guide the reimbursement of payors. The main issue regarding cost-effectiveness of AChEI prescription is not drug costs per se, but the impact across different sectors such as delay to the institutional care [109].

A study that attracted a great deal of attention in this context was the UK Donepezil and Memantine in moderate to severe AD (DOMINO-AD) study in patients with an MMSE score of 5–13 who were on a stable dose of long-term donepezil treatment. These patients were randomised in four arms: continuation of donepezil, discontinuation, change to memantine or addition of memantine. Over 12 months, groups treated with donepezil or memantine in mono or combination therapy showed cognitive and functional benefits [110]. Secondary and post-hoc analyses of the data from the DOMINO-AD study showed that treatment with donepezil but not memantine monotherapy may delay admission to residential and nursing home care by up to 6 months [111, 112].

State-of-the-Art Management: Key Issues in Clinical Practice

When to Start?

Intuitively, the treatment should be beneficial if started early in the course of the disease. This means that hypothetically the best target populations are symptomatic individuals at high risk of developing AD but without advanced cognitive impairment or manifest dementia and who still have functional cholinergic synapses, even in the presence of wide-spread molecular pathology of the disease. However, there is no evidence to suggest that AChEI and memantine efficacy is dependent on the presence of amyloid pathology, as all of the RCTs were conducted before biomarkers of amyloid beta (Aβ)-42 pathology were widely available and thus could not be included in large-scale RCTs.

A Cochrane systematic review analysed the results of AChEI treatment for MCI in nine studies that included 5149 individuals with MCI [113]. The authors performed a meta-analysis of the three studies that were comparable that reported on conversion to dementia and none of them provided strong evidence of a beneficial effect of AChEI (donepezil and galantamine) on the progression to dementia at 1, 2 or 3 years [114, 115]. Apart from conversion to dementia, there was no effect on the cognitive test scores used as outcome measures either. All nine studies from the Cochrane review reported a significantly higher frequency of adverse drug reaction as well as higher dropout rate in the active drug arm, with the highest rate of discontinuation occurring early on.

Early RCTs with AChEI in MCI recruited an extremely heterogeneous group of patients based on clinical definition and, while they certainly included some patients with a neurodegenerative process consistent with AD, they probably also included many patients who would not decline over time and who remained stable cognitively irrespective of any intervention.

In clinical settings clinicians meet patients with symptoms consistent with early or prodromal AD, such as individuals with MCI or those with persistent subjective cognitive decline [116, 117]. Occasionally, even only "worried well" people without any symptoms of the disease ask for a full assessment and in case of biomarker-positive findings they expect treatment with currently marketed drugs for dementia due to AD. However, do these individuals benefit from treatment usually prescribed in subjects with AD dementia? Is it ethical to treat an individual who has no predictable trajectory of decline in terms of clinically manifesting AD dementia?

Two logistic regression models including demographic, clinical and imaging test information with and without cerebrospinal fluid AD biomarkers demonstrated in a multi-centre European study that an estimate of the individual person's risk of progression from MCI to dementia the 26 months the study lasted can be improved in 65% of subjects by inclusion of cerebrospinal fluid AD biomarkers in addition to the recommended standard assessment battery with clinical and imaging tests [118].

Biomarker-based preclinical detection of AD has opened a debate on how early during the course of the disease treatment should be initiated given the uncertainty of clinical progression [119, 120]. In a recent European Alzheimer's Disease Consortium survey 23.6% of physicians offer AChEI treatment to individuals with MCI, while 50% of respondents seldom or never treat subjects with MCI [121].

A 2015 online survey of 102 members of the European Academy of Neurology and the European Alzheimer's Disease Consortium found that over 70% of the physicians considered that a biomarker-based diagnosis of prodromal AD/MCI due to AD had added value in terms of the MCI diagnosis [122]. Among the respondents 36% prescribed AChEI routinely and 39% sometimes.

At the moment no regulatory agencies recommend treatment of prodromal AD or MCI with either AChEI or memantine [123].

Who Should Prescribe the Treatment?

AChEIs are mostly prescribed by secondary care medical specialists, such as psychiatrists, geriatricians and neurologists, depending on healthcare organisation in different countries. Usually, a dementia specialist does the diagnostic disclosure in the very early stage of the disease because the diagnosis of prodromal AD (MCI due to AD) is dependent on biomarkers [124]. Therefore, careful counselling throughout the diagnostic process [125], individual approach to treatment initiation and adequate follow-up on AEs and the treatment effect are of utmost importance [122].

AChEI treatment comprises two stages, dose escalation to the clinically effective dose, usually during the first 4 weeks, and then the maintenance phase or sustained treatment with the optimal therapeutic dose. This regime requires frequent monitoring of AEs with escalation of AChEI dose, which can be monitored by specialist nurses on staff at the memory clinic who are trained and experienced in establishing close contact with both a patient and a caregiver.

In most countries in Europe, primary care physicians with expertise in diagnosing and treating AD can also prescribe AChEIs. However, patients with MCI/prodromal, early-onset disease and atypical clinical presentations of AD should be reviewed regularly at the specialist level regardless of whether AChEI treatment or treatment with memantine is initiated. Late-onset sporadic AD cases can either be recommended by a specialist for initiation of AChEI treatment in primary care or the treatment can be initiated by a specialist and transferred to primary care once the patient is stabilised on the optimal maintenance dose.

When to Switch or Combine?

Comparative trials could not demonstrate a consistent significant difference in efficacy between the three currently marketed AChEIs [126]. Frequency and type of AEs seem to be the main difference across the various AChEIs.

Switching between AChEIs is called for when one specific AChEI is not tolerated. It is known that up to 50% of patients can tolerate another AChEI and also show a benefit from continued treatment [127]. In clinical practice the most common scenario is a switch from oral donepezil, galantamine or rivastigmine to the rivastigmine patch. A multi-centre open-label Japanese study investigated the efficacy and safety of switching to the rivastigmine transdermal patch in patients with AD who had a poor response to or experienced difficulty in continuing donepezil or galantamine [128]. After 8 weeks in the titration period and 16 weeks in a maintenance period, MMSE scores were unchanged, mainly in the patients in a mild stage of the disease. In total, 30.5% of patients showed local skin irritation, 22.0% in the titration period, and in 10.2% in the maintenance period.

Due to its short half-time, a break of more than 3 days in rivastigmine treatment requires starting with an oral or transdermal dose of 1.5 mg twice daily or 4.6 mg/24 h, with subsequent re-titration after 3–4 weeks. When switching from oral to transdermal administration, the patch should be applied on the day following the last oral dose: (a) from a 3–6-mg oral daily dose to 4.6 mg/24-hour patch; (b) from a stable 9-mg oral daily dose to 9.5 mg/24-h patch; and (c) if a 9 mg oral dose was not stable or well tolerated, switching to a 4.6 mg/24-h patch is recommended.

When to End Treatment?

There is still no universal recommendation about the termination of AChEI treatment once the disease reaches advanced stages, particularly when the patient moves to residential care. The rule of thumb is to reduce overall polypharmacy in frail people with advanced dementia or those in palliative care, since an already modest therapeutic effect on cognition and function fades. Furthermore frequency of AEs increases in the frail elderly patient population [81, 129]. On the other hand, patients' caregivers and relatives might insist on continued treatment as an indicator of their persistent loving care for the patient and a remaining hope for some treatment benefit. Most AChEIs are available in a generic form and thus affordable, but cost of questionably beneficial long-term treatment in patients with advanced dementia remains an issue.

A meta-analysis summarised five RCTs on the discontinuation of AChEIs in outpatients with possible or probable AD [130]. An additional RCT examined discontinuation among institutionalised patients with probable moderate to severe AD [131]. Due to various designs and outcomes it was difficult to draw general conclusions about the discontinuation of the treatment. While outpatient studies reported poorer cognitive outcomes among those who discontinued AChEIs, the inpatient study did not report a significant difference between continuation and discontinuation. A recent systematic review of practice guidelines and recommendations on the discontinuation of AChEI in dementia reported that 11 out of the 16 professional guidelines examined recommended discontinuation under specific circumstances, while of the remaining five, three offered no recommendation regarding discontinuation and two recommended against discontinuing AChEI treatment [132]. Even the guidelines that advocate discontinuation leave the decision to the clinician, who should weigh cost and benefit with regard to lack of treatment response or loss of treatment effectiveness, side effects or AEs, issues with patient/caregiver compliance, severity of cognitive and/or functional impairment, behavioural disturbances, overall medical condition, institutionalisation and the family or caregiver's preferences. The Canadian guidelines operationalised the decision to discontinue and recommended stopping treatment in patients with accelerated decline over 6 months, as measured by a decrease of three or more points on MMSE [133]. On the other hand, the UK recommendation approaches MMSE cut-offs with caution, instead suggesting that the level of overall disease severity should be considered [134].

In summary, there is no strict, evidence-based algorithm or standardised recommendations in terms of duration or the discontinuation of treatment. The sound judgement of a clinician and common sense indicate that an institutionalised patient who makes the transition from active to end of life care, who cannot interact meaningfully with others and who cannot perform basic ADLs will not benefit from continued treatment with AChEI.

Table 5.4 Level of evidence and strength of recommendation.

	AD	LBD	Mixed dementia	VaD	FTD	MCI
AChEI	I A	I A	I A	I A	I A	I A
• *Donepezil*	√	√	√	×	×	×
• *Rivastigmine*	√	√	√	×	×	×
• *Galantamine*	√		√	×	×	×
Memantine	I A	I B	I B	I A	I A	I A
	√	√	√	×	×	×
Combination Therapy	I B					
	√					

AD Alzheimer's disease, *LBD* Lewy body dementia, *VaD* vascular dementia, *FTD* frontotemporal dementia, *MCI* mild cognitive impairment, *AChEI* acetylcholinesterase inhibitor, I A: recommendation (A) is directly based on evidence from meta-analysis or at least one large good-quality RCT (I); I B: recommendation (B) is based on evidence from small, non-replicated RCTs or at least one controlled study with randomisation (II) or extrapolated data from evidence level I; √: treatment recommended; ×: treatment not recommended. Based on O'Brien et al. [122]

Regulatory Recommendations

The strength of treatment recommendation for clinical practice is derived from four categories of evidence for causal relationships and treatment according to standard criteria [123]. Table 5.4 provides a state-of-the-art overview of strength of recommendations for clinical practice based on a review of guidelines published by European regulatory bodies [123, 135, 136].

Future Treatments and How Close Are They?

Intervention in amyloid and/or tau processing is the mainstream of research towards disease-modifying treatments, some of which have reached phase-III clinical trials.

In parallel, new diagnostic research guidelines for AD recommend enrichment of study populations for clinical trials in prodromal AD by including Aβ42-positive biomarkers besides the amnestic MCI phenotype [137]. The dynamics of biomarker changes are also included in trial outcomes of disease-modifying interventions [37].

Many attempts have been made to reduce the burden of Aβ aggregates that form the intraparenchymal senile plaques. The large majority of trials are immunotherapy based, i.e. they use antibodies directed against the fibrils forming the senile plaques. Most trials use passive immunotherapy, where antibodies to Aβ are formed in mice, humanised and given intravenously to patients every 2–4 weeks.

Passively administered human IgG1 monoclonal antibody, aducanumab (BIIB037) was originally derived from healthy elderly donors without any cognitive problems. This antibody binds aggregated forms of Aβ, but not to monomers. In successful phase-IIB studies, aducanumab was shown to remove amyloid from the brain and to slow cognitive decline in patients with mild or prodromal AD after 1 year of monthly intravenous infusions in the PRIME study [138]. Aducanumab was then directly tested in two phase-III trials, EMERGE and ENGAGE. Planned to run for 18 months, each study enrolled more than 1600 patients but the trials were stopped in March 2019 after about half of the patients had been enrolled. The reason given was that EMERGE and ENGAGE would miss their primary endpoints. In October 2019, the company sponsoring the trials announced that the earlier interim futility analysis was wrong, and a reanalysis of a larger dataset was positive and showed that the treatment reduced cognitive decline when the highest dose 10 mg/kg populations from the two studies were merged. The company has now filed for conditional approval. Side effects, mainly amyloid-related imaging abnormalities and especially in APOE-ε4 carriers, were declared manageable. The mechanism behind these signal changes on MRIs is probably cerebral vasogenic oedema or micro-haemorrhages induced by Aβ immunotherapy [139, 140]. These AEs were observed in 37–47% of patients who received higher doses of aducanumab.

The extent of tau pathology correlates with severity of cognitive impairment and the neurofibrillary tangle pathology – as seen in tau positron emission tomography and is predictive of future brain atrophy [141]. The extraneuronal tau plays a crucial role in the propagation of tau pathology. More accessible to drugs, the extracellular pool is a promising treatment target for immunotherapy with vaccines and humanised antibodies in clinical development [142]. Other drug development programmes are pursuing tau aggregation inhibitors and molecules with other modes of action.

Different pathophysiological pathways contribute to the multifactorial nature and heterogeneity of AD, which is why it is plausible to pursue multiple targets in search of new treatments that might be more effective when combined. Simultaneous intervention in multiple pathways, such as neuroinflammation, microglial activation and lipid metabolism, together with amyloid/tau-based therapies, might be more effective than a single-target approach [143].

Instead of Summary Supplemental Cases

Case 1

A 69-year-old male is referred for cognitive assessment due to a subjectively experienced increase in memory difficulties in the last year. Highly educated, he is physically vital with an unremarkable medical history, except possible late-onset AD in his mother. He does not have any practical difficulties in daily life, including instrumental ADL, which is confirmed by his spouse, who is nonetheless concerned about her husband's memory problems.

The Montreal Cognitive Assessment test is 25/30 (loss of point for correct date and four points on delayed recall). Extended neuropsychological test battery confirms amnestic MCI profile. MRI did not reveal considerable structural brain pathology. Medial temporal atrophy was grade 1 bilaterally. DNA APOE genotype is 3/4, and in the cerebrospinal fluid there is significantly lower Aβ42, Aβ42/40 and increased p-tau and total-tau protein.

How would you explain the diagnosis and prognosis to the patient?

What decision should you take about treatment?

Case 2
An 80-year-old widow living alone has mild to moderate late-onset AD and was tolerating the initial dose of donepezil 5 mg well. During the dose escalation phase she developed GI AEs with diarrhoea and continued nausea. She has no significant polypharmacy and, in addition to donepezil, she takes levothyroxine to substitute her hypothyreosis.

What is your decision about continued treatment?

Case 3
You receive a phone call from the relatives of a former patient, an 84-year-old male diagnosed with moderate to severe AD who recently moved to residential care in a nursing home due to both functional deterioration and behavioural and psychiatric symptoms in dementia. He has increased anxiety and hallucinations and is periodically agitated. He is generally oriented to people and has preserved autonomy regarding basic ADL. The nursing home doctor told the relatives that he planned to discontinue the donepezil 10 mg that the patient had been receiving for the last 3 years and would instead introduce a low dose of atypical neuroleptics.

The relatives ask for a second opinion. What do you suggest?

Case 4
A 55-year-old female with early-onset AD diagnosed 2 years ago is treated with donepezil 10 mg, which she tolerates well. During follow-up her MMSE decreased by two points for current score of 24/30. Her husband said that the patient was seen at the emergency department 2 days ago due to an episode of unprovoked generalised epileptic seizure. Donepezil was discontinued and treatment with levetiracetam 500 mg was initiated.

The patient and caregiver would like to know if donepezil or some other anti-dementia drugs will be prescribed in the future. What is your reply?

Case Comments

Case 1

This is a highly functional individual in an early clinical phase of the disease according to the National Institute on Aging and Alzheimer's Association's biological classification of AD based on positive biomarkers of amyloid pathology and neurodegeneration [144]. The patient was seeking assessment due to subjectively experienced memory problems, as also observed by his long-term spouse. Provide information about the MCI diagnosis and the risk of developing AD dementia. Treatment counselling should start with information about symptomatic treatment and, if they are highly motivated to do treatment, offer AChEI.

Case 2

Since the patient tolerated donepezil 5 mg, a therapeutic dose, well, it should remain the target dose for at least the 4–6 months before the next clinical follow-up. Then depending on eventual deterioration, try to escalate again to 10 mg, since a tolerance for higher doses may increase with a longer titration period. If the treatment with donepezil 5 mg lacks efficacy and repeated AEs occur after the new trial with 10 mg, consider switching to another AChEI.

Case 3

The patient still has some remaining functional capacity and there is no reason to discontinue donepezil. If there is increased anxiety or agitation, add memantine or selective serotonin reuptake inhibitors, or in case of psychotic symptoms, consider a low dose of atypical/second-generation neuroleptics with regular evaluations of both efficacy and tolerance.

Case 4

Incidence of epilepsy in sporadic AD is higher than in healthy population and the relative risk of unprovoked seizures increases in patients with early-onset AD [145]. Theoretically, AChEIs might lower the seizure threshold but, based on data from drug registries, they rarely provoked seizures [146]. If the patient is put on prophylactic antiepileptic treatment, donepezil treatment can be reinitiated. Dose escalation is recommended. Continued treatment with AChEI is recommended in this patient since she seems to respond to therapy and has a stable course of the disease. Interestingly, there is experimental evidence that levetiracetam can improve cognition in AD [147].

References

1. Francis PT, et al. The cholinergic hypothesis of Alzheimer's disease: a review of progress. J Neurol Neurosurg Psychiatry. 1999;66(2):137–47.
2. Davies P, Maloney AJ. Selective loss of central cholinergic neurons in Alzheimer's disease. Lancet. 1976;2(8000):1403.
3. Whitehouse PJ, et al. Alzheimer disease: evidence for selective loss of cholinergic neurons in the nucleus basalis. Ann Neurol. 1981;10(2):122–6.

4. Drachman DA, Leavitt J. Human memory and the cholinergic system. A relationship to aging? Arch Neurol. 1974;30(2):113–21.
5. Watkins PB, et al. Hepatotoxic effects of tacrine administration in patients with Alzheimer's disease. JAMA. 1994;271(13):992–8.
6. Birks JS, Harvey RJ. Donepezil for dementia due to Alzheimer's disease. Cochrane Database Syst Rev. 2018;6(6):Cd001190.
7. Tariot PN, et al. A randomized, double-blind, placebo-controlled study of the efficacy and safety of donepezil in patients with Alzheimer's disease in the nursing home setting. J Am Geriatr Soc. 2001;49(12):1590–9.
8. Winblad B, et al. Donepezil in patients with severe Alzheimer's disease: double-blind, parallel-group, placebo-controlled study. Lancet. 2006;367(9516):1057–65.
9. Jelic V, et al. Donepezil treatment of severe Alzheimer's disease in nursing home settings. A responder analysis. Dement Geriatr Cogn Disord. 2008;26(5):458–66.
10. Di Santo SG, et al. A meta-analysis of the efficacy of donepezil, rivastigmine, galantamine, and memantine in relation to severity of Alzheimer's disease. J Alzheimers Dis. 2013;35(2):349–61.
11. Winblad B, et al. IDEAL: a 6-month, double-blind, placebo-controlled study of the first skin patch for Alzheimer disease. Neurology. 2007;69(4 Suppl 1):S14–22.
12. Winblad B, Machado JC. Use of rivastigmine transdermal patch in the treatment of Alzheimer's disease. Expert Opin Drug Deliv. 2008;5(12):1377–86.
13. Deardorff WJ, Grossberg GT. A fixed-dose combination of memantine extended-release and donepezil in the treatment of moderate-to-severe Alzheimer's disease. Drug Des Devel Ther. 2016;10:3267–79.
14. Jann MW, Shirley KL, Small GW. Clinical pharmacokinetics and pharmacodynamics of cholinesterase inhibitors. Clin Pharmacokinet. 2002;41(10):719–39.
15. Giacobini E. Selective inhibitors of butyrylcholinesterase: a valid alternative for therapy of Alzheimer's disease? Drugs Aging. 2001;18(12):891–8.
16. Wilkinson DG, et al. Cholinesterase inhibitors used in the treatment of Alzheimer's disease: the relationship between pharmacological effects and clinical efficacy. Drugs Aging. 2004;21(7):453–78.
17. Kurz A, Farlow M, Lefèvre G. Pharmacokinetics of a novel transdermal rivastigmine patch for the treatment of Alzheimer's disease: a review. Int J Clin Pract. 2009;63(5):799–805.
18. Emre M, et al. Drug profile: transdermal rivastigmine patch in the treatment of Alzheimer disease. CNS Neurosci Ther. 2010;16(4):246–53.
19. Kadir A, et al. PET imaging of cortical 11C-nicotine binding correlates with the cognitive function of attention in Alzheimer's disease. Psychopharmacology. 2006;188(4):509–20.
20. Noetzli M, Eap CB. Pharmacodynamic, pharmacokinetic and pharmacogenetic aspects of drugs used in the treatment of Alzheimer's disease. Clin Pharmacokinet. 2013;52(4):225–41.
21. Parsons CG, Stöffler A, Danysz W. Memantine: a NMDA receptor antagonist that improves memory by restoration of homeostasis in the glutamatergic system--too little activation is bad, too much is even worse. Neuropharmacology. 2007;53(6):699–723.
22. Parsons CG, Gilling K. Memantine as an example of a fast, voltage-dependent, open channel N-methyl-D-aspartate receptor blocker. Methods Mol Biol. 2007;403:15–36.
23. Danysz W, Parsons CG. The NMDA receptor antagonist memantine as a symptomatological and neuroprotective treatment for Alzheimer's disease: preclinical evidence. Int J Geriatr Psychiatry. 2003;18(Suppl 1):S23–32.
24. Micuda S, et al. Inhibitory effects of memantine on human cytochrome P450 activities: prediction of in vivo drug interactions. Eur J Clin Pharmacol. 2004;60(8):583–9.
25. Rao N, et al. Investigation of the pharmacokinetic and pharmacodynamic interactions between memantine and glyburide/metformin in healthy young subjects: a single-center, multiple-dose, open-label study. Clin Ther. 2005;27(10):1596–606.
26. Zhou SF, Liu JP, Chowbay B. Polymorphism of human cytochrome P450 enzymes and its clinical impact. Drug Metab Rev. 2009;41(2):89–295.

27. Seripa D, et al. Role of cytochrome P4502D6 functional polymorphisms in the efficacy of donepezil in patients with Alzheimer's disease. Pharmacogenet Genomics. 2011;21(4):225–30.
28. Chianella C, et al. BCHE and CYP2D6 genetic variation in Alzheimer's disease patients treated with cholinesterase inhibitors. Eur J Clin Pharmacol. 2011;67(11):1147–57.
29. Han HJ, et al. Effect of rivastigmine or memantine add-on therapy is affected by butyrylcholinesterase genotype in patients with probable Alzheimer's disease. Eur Neurol. 2015;73(1–2):23–8.
30. Sokolow S, et al. Deleterious effect of butyrylcholinesterase k-variant in donepezil treatment of mild cognitive impairment. J Alzheimers Dis. 2017;56(1):229–37.
31. Hartmann J, et al. Excessive hippocampal acetylcholine levels in acetylcholinesterase-deficient mice are moderated by butyrylcholinesterase activity. J Neurochem. 2007;100(5):1421–9.
32. Jasiecki J, Wasąg B. Butyrylcholinesterase protein ends in the pathogenesis of Alzheimer's disease—could BCHE genotyping be helpful in Alzheimer's therapy? Biomol Ther. 2019;9(10):592.
33. Kanaya K, et al. Changes in cognitive functions of patients with dementia of the Alzheimer type following long-term administration of donepezil hydrochloride: relating to changes attributable to differences in apolipoprotein E phenotype. Geriatr Gerontol Int. 2010;10(1):25–31.
34. Bizzarro A, et al. Apolipoprotein E epsilon4 allele differentiates the clinical response to donepezil in Alzheimer's disease. Dement Geriatr Cogn Disord. 2005;20(4):254–61.
35. Xiao T, et al. Effect of the CYP2D6 and APOE polymorphisms on the efficacy of donepezil in patients with Alzheimer's disease: a systematic review and meta-analysis. CNS Drugs. 2016;30(10):899–907.
36. Lane RM, Darreh-Shori T. Understanding the beneficial and detrimental effects of donepezil and rivastigmine to improve their therapeutic value. J Alzheimers Dis. 2015;44(4):1039–62.
37. Schneider LS, et al. Clinical trials and late-stage drug development for Alzheimer's disease: an appraisal from 1984 to 2014. J Intern Med. 2014;275(3):251–83.
38. Ellis JM. Cholinesterase inhibitors in the treatment of dementia. J Am Osteopath Assoc. 2005;105(3):145–58.
39. Folstein MF, Folstein SE, McHugh PR. "Mini-mental state". A practical method for grading the cognitive state of patients for the clinician. J Psychiatr Res. 1975;12(3):189–98.
40. Rosen WG, Mohs RC, Davis KL. A new rating scale for Alzheimer's disease. Am J Psychiatry. 1984;141(11):1356–64.
41. Gélinas I, et al. Development of a functional measure for persons with Alzheimer's disease: the disability assessment for dementia. Am J Occup Ther. 1999;53(5):471–81.
42. DeJong R, Osterlund OW, Roy GW. Measurement of quality-of-life changes in patients with Alzheimer's disease. Clin Ther. 1989;11(4):545–54.
43. Schneider LS, et al. Validity and reliability of the Alzheimer's disease cooperative study-clinical global impression of change. The Alzheimer's Disease Cooperative Study. Alzheimer Dis Assoc Disord. 1997;11(Suppl 2):S22–32.
44. Bråne G, Gottfries CG, Winblad B. The Gottfries-Bråne-Steen scale: validity, reliability and application in anti-dementia drug trials. Dement Geriatr Cogn Disord. 2001;12(1):1–14.
45. Cummings JL, et al. The Neuropsychiatric Inventory: comprehensive assessment of psychopathology in dementia. Neurology. 1994;44(12):2308–14.
46. Saxton J, Swihart AA. Neuropsychological assessment of the severely impaired elderly patient. Clin Geriatr Med. 1989;5(3):531–43.
47. Schneider LS, et al. Differences in Alzheimer disease clinical trial outcomes based on age of the participants. Neurology. 2015;84(11):1121–7.
48. Laver K, et al. Interventions to delay functional decline in people with dementia: a systematic review of systematic reviews. BMJ Open. 2016;6(4):e010767.
49. Cooper C, et al. Systematic review of the effectiveness of pharmacologic interventions to improve quality of life and well-being in people with dementia. Am J Geriatr Psychiatry. 2013;21(2):173–83.

50. Farlow MR, et al. Effectiveness and tolerability of high-dose (23 mg/d) versus standard-dose (10 mg/d) donepezil in moderate to severe Alzheimer's disease: A 24-week, randomized, double-blind study. Clin Ther. 2010;32(7):1234–51.
51. Homma A, et al. Efficacy and safety of sustained release donepezil high dose versus immediate release donepezil standard dose in japanese patients with severe Alzheimer's disease: a randomized, double-blind trial. J Alzheimers Dis. 2016;52(1):345–57.
52. Schneider LS, et al. Eligibility of Alzheimer's disease clinic patients for clinical trials. J Am Geriatr Soc. 1997;45(8):923–8.
53. Courtney C, et al. Long-term donepezil treatment in 565 patients with Alzheimer's disease (AD2000): randomised double-blind trial. Lancet. 2004;363(9427):2105–15.
54. Loy C, Schneider L. Galantamine for Alzheimer's disease and mild cognitive impairment. Cochrane Database Syst Rev. 2006(1):Cd001747.
55. Brodaty H, et al. Galantamine prolonged-release formulation in the treatment of mild to moderate Alzheimer's disease. Dement Geriatr Cogn Disord. 2005;20(2–3):120–32.
56. Rockwood K, et al. Effects of a flexible galantamine dose in Alzheimer's disease: a randomised, controlled trial. J Neurol Neurosurg Psychiatry. 2001;71(5):589–95.
57. Tariot PN, et al. A 5-month, randomized, placebo-controlled trial of galantamine in AD. The Galantamine USA-10 Study Group. Neurology. 2000;54(12):2269–76.
58. Burns A, et al. Safety and efficacy of galantamine (Reminyl) in severe Alzheimer's disease (the SERAD study): a randomised, placebo-controlled, double-blind trial. Lancet Neurol. 2009;8(1):39–47.
59. Erkinjuntti T, et al. Efficacy of galantamine in probable vascular dementia and Alzheimer's disease combined with cerebrovascular disease: a randomised trial. Lancet. 2002;359(9314):1283–90.
60. Birks JS, Chong LY, Grimley Evans J. Rivastigmine for Alzheimer's disease. Cochrane Database Syst Rev. 2015;9(9):Cd001191.
61. Alva G, et al. Efficacy of rivastigmine transdermal patch on activities of daily living: item responder analyses. Int J Geriatr Psychiatry. 2011;26(4):356–63.
62. Winblad B, Poritis N. Memantine in severe dementia: results of the 9M-Best Study (Benefit and efficacy in severely demented patients during treatment with memantine). Int J Geriatr Psychiatry. 1999;14(2):135–46.
63. McShane R, et al. Memantine for dementia. Cochrane Database Syst Rev. 2019;3(3): Cd003154.
64. Matsunaga S, Kishi T, Iwata N. Memantine monotherapy for Alzheimer's disease: a systematic review and meta-analysis. PLoS One. 2015;10(4):e0123289.
65. Blanco-Silvente L, et al. Predictors of discontinuation, efficacy, and safety of memantine treatment for Alzheimer's disease: meta-analysis and meta-regression of 18 randomized clinical trials involving 5004 patients. BMC Geriatr. 2018;18(1):168.
66. Winblad B, et al. Memantine in moderate to severe Alzheimer's disease: a meta-analysis of randomised clinical trials. Dement Geriatr Cogn Disord. 2007;24(1):20–7.
67. Tan CC, et al. Efficacy and safety of donepezil, galantamine, rivastigmine, and memantine for the treatment of Alzheimer's disease: a systematic review and meta-analysis. J Alzheimers Dis. 2014;41(2):615–31.
68. Jakobsen JC, et al. Thresholds for statistical and clinical significance in systematic reviews with meta-analytic methods. BMC Med Res Methodol. 2014;14:120.
69. Hansen RA, et al. Efficacy and safety of donepezil, galantamine, and rivastigmine for the treatment of Alzheimer's disease: a systematic review and meta-analysis. Clin Interv Aging. 2008;3(2):211–25.
70. Wilcock G, et al. A long-term comparison of galantamine and donepezil in the treatment of Alzheimer's disease. Drugs Aging. 2003;20(10):777–89.
71. Jones RW, et al. A multinational, randomised, 12-week study comparing the effects of donepezil and galantamine in patients with mild to moderate Alzheimer's disease. Int J Geriatr Psychiatry. 2004;19(1):58–67.

72. Wilkinson DG, et al. A multinational, randomised, 12-week, comparative study of donepezil and rivastigmine in patients with mild to moderate Alzheimer's disease. Int J Clin Pract. 2002;56(6):441–6.
73. Bullock R, et al. Rivastigmine and donepezil treatment in moderate to moderately-severe Alzheimer's disease over a 2-year period. Curr Med Res Opin. 2005;21(8):1317–27.
74. Tricco AC, et al. Comparative effectiveness and safety of cognitive enhancers for treating Alzheimer's disease: systematic review and network metaanalysis. J Am Geriatr Soc. 2018;66(1):170–8.
75. Alva G, Cummings JL. Relative tolerability of Alzheimer's disease treatments. Psychiatry (Edgmont). 2008;5(11):27–36.
76. Khoury R, Rajamanickam J, Grossberg GT. An update on the safety of current therapies for Alzheimer's disease: focus on rivastigmine. Ther Adv Drug Saf. 2018;9(3):171–8.
77. Grossberg GT. Cholinesterase inhibitors for the treatment of Alzheimer's disease:: getting on and staying on. Curr Ther Res Clin Exp. 2003;64(4):216–35.
78. Maclean LE, Collins CC, Byrne EJ. Dementia with Lewy bodies treated with rivastigmine: effects on cognition, neuropsychiatric symptoms, and sleep. Int Psychogeriatr. 2001;13(3):277–88.
79. Feldman HH, et al. Analyses of mortality risk in patients with dementia treated with galantamine. Acta Neurol Scand. 2009;119(1):22–31.
80. Mayor S. Regulatory authorities review use of galantamine in mild cognitive impairment. BMJ. 2005;330(7486):276.
81. Park-Wyllie LY, et al. Cholinesterase inhibitors and hospitalization for bradycardia: a population-based study. PLoS Med. 2009;6(9):e1000157.
82. Schneider LS. Open-label extension studies and misinformation. Arch Neurol. 2006;63(7):1036. author reply 1036-7
83. Rountree SD, et al. Persistent treatment with cholinesterase inhibitors and/or memantine slows clinical progression of Alzheimer disease. Alzheimers Res Ther. 2009;1(2):7.
84. Kaushik V, et al. Acetylcholinesterase inhibitors: beneficial effects on comorbidities in patients with Alzheimer's disease. Am J Alzheimers Dis Other Dement. 2018;33(2):73–85.
85. Howes LG. Cardiovascular effects of drugs used to treat Alzheimer's disease. Drug Saf. 2014;37(6):391–5.
86. Monacelli F, Rosa G. Cholinesterase inhibitors: cardioprotection in Alzheimer's disease. J Alzheimers Dis. 2014;42(4):1071–7.
87. Nordström P, et al. The use of cholinesterase inhibitors and the risk of myocardial infarction and death: a nationwide cohort study in subjects with Alzheimer's disease. Eur Heart J. 2013;34(33):2585–91.
88. Rolinski M, et al. Cholinesterase inhibitors for dementia with Lewy bodies, Parkinson's disease dementia and cognitive impairment in Parkinson's disease. Cochrane Database Syst Rev. 2012(3):Cd006504.
89. Aarsland D, et al. Memantine in patients with Parkinson's disease dementia or dementia with Lewy bodies: a double-blind, placebo-controlled, multicentre trial. Lancet Neurol. 2009;8(7):613–8.
90. Emre M, et al. Memantine for patients with Parkinson's disease dementia or dementia with Lewy bodies: a randomised, double-blind, placebo-controlled trial. Lancet Neurol. 2010;9(10):969–77.
91. Menéndez González M, Calatayud M, Blazquez-Menes B. Exacerbation of Lewy bodies dementia due to memantine. J Alzheimers Dis. 2006;8:289–91.
92. Levin OS, et al. Efficacy and safety of memantine in Lewy body dementia. Neurosci Behav Physiol. 2009;39(6):597–604.
93. Van Der Putt R, et al. Effectiveness of acetylcholinesterase inhibitors: diagnosis and severity as predictors of response in routine practice. Int J Geriatr Psychiatry. 2006;21(8):755–60.
94. Malouf R, Birks J. Donepezil for vascular cognitive impairment. Cochrane Database Syst Rev. 2004(1):Cd004395.

95. Birks J, Craig D. Galantamine for vascular cognitive impairment. Cochrane Database Syst Rev. 2006(4):Cd004746.
96. Birks J, McGuinness B, Craig D. Rivastigmine for vascular cognitive impairment. Cochrane Database Syst Rev. 2013(5):Cd004744.
97. McShane R, Areosa Sastre A, Minakaran N. Memantine for dementia. Cochrane Database Syst Rev. 2006(2):Cd003154.
98. Kavirajan H, Schneider LS. Efficacy and adverse effects of cholinesterase inhibitors and memantine in vascular dementia: a meta-analysis of randomised controlled trials. Lancet Neurol. 2007;6(9):782–92.
99. Moretti R, et al. Cholinesterase inhibition as a possible therapy for delirium in vascular dementia: a controlled, open 24-month study of 246 patients. Am J Alzheimers Dis Other Dement. 2004;19(6):333–9.
100. Li Y, et al. Cholinesterase inhibitors for rarer dementias associated with neurological conditions. Cochrane Database Syst Rev. 2015(3):Cd009444.
101. Litvan I, et al. Randomized placebo-controlled trial of donepezil in patients with progressive supranuclear palsy. Neurology. 2001;57(3):467–73.
102. Dichgans M, et al. Donepezil in patients with subcortical vascular cognitive impairment: a randomised double-blind trial in CADASIL. Lancet Neurol. 2008;7(4):310–8.
103. Moretti R, et al. Rivastigmine in frontotemporal dementia: an open-label study. Drugs Aging. 2004;21(14):931–7.
104. Tenovuo O, Alin J, Helenius H. A randomized controlled trial of rivastigmine for chronic sequels of traumatic brain injury-what it showed and taught? Brain Inj. 2009;23(6):548–58.
105. McDermott CL, Gray SL. Cholinesterase inhibitor adjunctive therapy for cognitive impairment and depressive symptoms in older adults with depression. Ann Pharmacother. 2012;46(4):599–605.
106. Reynolds CF III, et al. Maintenance treatment of depression in old age: a randomized, double-blind, placebo-controlled evaluation of the efficacy and safety of donepezil combined with antidepressant pharmacotherapy. Arch Gen Psychiatry. 2011;68(1):51–60.
107. Bauer A, et al. Valuing Alzheimer's disease drugs: a health technology assessment perspective on outcomes. Int J Technol Assess Health Care. 2020:1–7.
108. Wimo A, et al. Quantifying and describing the natural history and costs of Alzheimer's disease and effects of hypothetical interventions. J Alzheimers Dis. 2020;75(3):891–902.
109. Clegg A, et al. Clinical and cost-effectiveness of donepezil, rivastigmine and galantamine for Alzheimer's disease: a rapid and systematic review. Health Technol Assess. 2001;5(1):1–137.
110. Howard R, et al. Donepezil and memantine for moderate-to-severe Alzheimer's disease. N Engl J Med. 2012;366(10):893–903.
111. Howard R, et al. Nursing home placement in the Donepezil and Memantine in Moderate to Severe Alzheimer's Disease (DOMINO-AD) trial: secondary and post-hoc analyses. Lancet Neurol. 2015;14(12):1171–81.
112. Jelic V, Winblad B. Alzheimer disease. Donepezil and nursing home placement--benefits and costs. Nat Rev Neurol. 2016;12(1):11–3.
113. Russ TC, Morling JR. Cholinesterase inhibitors for mild cognitive impairment. Cochrane Database Syst Rev. 2012(9):Cd009132.
114. Petersen RC, et al. Vitamin E and donepezil for the treatment of mild cognitive impairment. N Engl J Med. 2005;352(23):2379–88.
115. Winblad B, et al. Safety and efficacy of galantamine in subjects with mild cognitive impairment. Neurology. 2008;70(22):2024–35.
116. Jessen F, et al. AD dementia risk in late MCI, in early MCI, and in subjective memory impairment. Alzheimers Dement. 2014;10(1):76–83.
117. Jessen F, et al. The characterisation of subjective cognitive decline. Lancet Neurol. 2020;19(3):271–8.
118. Handels RLH, et al. Predicting progression to dementia in persons with mild cognitive impairment using cerebrospinal fluid markers. Alzheimers Dement. 2017;13(8):903–12.

119. Jack CR Jr, et al. Introduction to the recommendations from the National Institute on Aging-Alzheimer's Association workgroups on diagnostic guidelines for Alzheimer's disease. Alzheimers Dement. 2011;7(3):257–62.
120. Dubois B, et al. Preclinical Alzheimer's disease: definition, natural history, and diagnostic criteria. Alzheimers Dement. 2016;12(3):292–323.
121. Frederiksen KS, et al. Biomarker counseling, disclosure of diagnosis and follow-up in patients with mild cognitive impairment: a European survey of EADC centers. Eur J Neurol. 2020;27:105.
122. Bertens D, et al. Use of mild cognitive impairment and prodromal AD/MCI due to AD in clinical care: a European survey. Alzheimers Res Ther. 2019;11(1):74.
123. O'Brien JT, et al. Clinical practice with anti-dementia drugs: a revised (third) consensus statement from the British Association for Psychopharmacology. J Psychopharmacol. 2017;31(2):147–68.
124. Frisoni GB, et al. Strategic roadmap for an early diagnosis of Alzheimer's disease based on biomarkers. Lancet Neurol. 2017;16(8):661–76.
125. Nielsen TR, et al. The process of disclosing a diagnosis of dementia and mild cognitive impairment: a national survey of specialist physicians in Denmark. Dementia (London). 2020;19(3):547–59.
126. Dou KX, et al. Comparative safety and effectiveness of cholinesterase inhibitors and memantine for Alzheimer's disease: a network meta-analysis of 41 randomized controlled trials. Alzheimers Res Ther. 2018;10(1):126.
127. O'Brien JT, Burns A. Clinical practice with anti-dementia drugs: a revised (second) consensus statement from the British Association for Psychopharmacology. J Psychopharmacol. 2011;25(8):997–1019.
128. Ueda K, et al. Efficacy, safety, and tolerability of switching from oral cholinesterase inhibitors to rivastigmine transdermal patch with 1-step titration in patients with mild to moderate Alzheimer's disease: a 24-week, open-label, multicenter study in Japan. Dement Geriatr Cogn Dis Extra. 2019;9(2):302–18.
129. Gill SS, et al. Syncope and its consequences in patients with dementia receiving cholinesterase inhibitors: a population-based cohort study. Arch Intern Med. 2009;169(9):867–73.
130. O'Regan J, et al. Cholinesterase inhibitor discontinuation in patients with Alzheimer's disease: a meta-analysis of randomized controlled trials. J Clin Psychiatry. 2015;76(11):e1424–31.
131. Herrmann N, et al. A randomized placebo-controlled discontinuation study of cholinesterase inhibitors in institutionalized patients with moderate to severe Alzheimer disease. J Am Med Dir Assoc. 2016;17(2):142–7.
132. Renn BN, et al. A systematic review of practice guidelines and recommendations for discontinuation of cholinesterase inhibitors in dementia. Am J Geriatr Psychiatry. 2018;26(2):134–47.
133. Moore A, et al. Fourth Canadian consensus conference on the diagnosis and treatment of dementia: recommendations for family physicians. Can Fam Physician. 2014;60(5):433–8.
134. Bond M, et al. The effectiveness and cost-effectiveness of donepezil, galantamine, rivastigmine and memantine for the treatment of Alzheimer's disease (review of Technology Appraisal No. 111): a systematic review and economic model. Health Technol Assess. 2012;16(21):1–470.
135. Hort J, et al. EFNS guidelines for the diagnosis and management of Alzheimer's disease. Eur J Neurol. 2010;17(10):1236–48.
136. Schmidt R, et al. EFNS-ENS/EAN Guideline on concomitant use of cholinesterase inhibitors and memantine in moderate to severe Alzheimer's disease. Eur J Neurol. 2015;22(6):889–98.
137. Albert MS, et al. The diagnosis of mild cognitive impairment due to Alzheimer's disease: recommendations from the National Institute on Aging-Alzheimer's Association workgroups on diagnostic guidelines for Alzheimer's disease. Alzheimers Dement. 2011;7(3):270–9.
138. Sevigny J, et al. The antibody aducanumab reduces Aβ plaques in Alzheimer's disease. Nature. 2016;537(7618):50–6.
139. Weitz TM, Town T. Amyloid cascade into clarity. Immunity. 2016;45(4):717–8.

140. Sperling RA, et al. Amyloid-related imaging abnormalities in amyloid-modifying therapeutic trials: Recommendations from the Alzheimer's Association Research Roundtable Workgroup. Alzheimers Dement. 2011;7(4):367–85.
141. La Joie R, et al. Prospective longitudinal atrophy in Alzheimer's disease correlates with the intensity and topography of baseline tau-PET. Sci Transl Med. 2020;12(524):eaau5732.
142. Novak P, et al. Safety and immunogenicity of the tau vaccine AADvac1 in patients with Alzheimer's disease: a randomised, double-blind, placebo-controlled, phase 1 trial. Lancet Neurol. 2017;16(2):123–34.
143. Stephenson D, et al. Charting a path toward combination therapy for Alzheimer's disease. Expert Rev Neurother. 2015;15(1):107–13.
144. Jack CR Jr, et al. NIA-AA research framework: toward a biological definition of Alzheimer's disease. Alzheimers Dement. 2018;14(4):535–62.
145. Palop JJ, Mucke L. Epilepsy and cognitive impairments in Alzheimer disease. Arch Neurol. 2009;66(4):435–40.
146. Friedman D, Honig LS, Scarmeas N. Seizures and epilepsy in Alzheimer's disease. CNS Neurosci Ther. 2012;18(4):285–94.
147. Xiao R. Levetiracetam might act as an efficacious drug to attenuate cognitive deficits of Alzheimer's disease. Curr Top Med Chem. 2016;16(5):565–73.

Review of Medication in Patients with Dementia

6

Dorota Religa, Katarzyna Wieczorowska-Tobis, and Björn Johansson

List of Abbreviations

AChEI	Acetylcholinesterase inhibitor
AGS	American Geriatrics Association
ATC	Anatomical Therapeutic Chemical Classification System
BZD	Benzodiazepines
CNS	Central nervous system
eGFR	Estimated glomerular filtration rate
NSAID	Non-steroidal anti-inflammatory drug
PIM	Potentially inappropriate medication
PIP	Potentially inappropriate prescribing
SSRI	Selective serotonin reuptake inhibitor
START	Screening Tool to Alert to Right Treatment
STOPP	Screening Tool of Older Persons' Prescriptions

D. Religa (✉)
Division of Clinical Geriatrics, Department of Neurobiology, Care Sciences and Society, Center for Alzheimer Research, Karolinska Institutet, Huddinge, Sweden

Karolinska University Hospital, Huddinge, Sweden
e-mail: dorota.religa@ki.se

K. Wieczorowska-Tobis
Poznan University of Medical Sciences, Poznan, Poland
e-mail: kwt@tobis.pl

B. Johansson
Karolinska University Hospital, Huddinge, Sweden

Department of Clinical Neuroscience, Karolinska Institutet, Stockholm, Sweden

Department of Molecular Medicine and Surgery, Karolinska Institutet, Stockholm, Sweden
e-mail: bjorn.johansson@ki.se

K. S. Frederiksen, G. Waldemar (eds.), *Management of Patients with Dementia*,
https://doi.org/10.1007/978-3-030-77904-7_6

Introduction

Physicians have access to potent drugs, which represent an important and common form of treatment. Prescribing medication is a longitudinal process that stretches from the initial decision to write a prescription and increasing the dosage to lowering it and making the choice to stop the medication. During this journey many opportunities arise to review the drug therapy in a structured way, e.g. during the work-up for cognitive impairment or dementia.

Many drugs can lower cognitive ability, typically those with anticholinergic effects but also ones that specifically target the central nervous system (CNS), for example antiepileptic drugs may have unwanted effects on cognition. Taking this into account is especially important when investigating older adults who simultaneously take many different drugs and have reduced cognitive reserve.

As a result, acquiring an accurate drug history is important during the work-up for cognitive impairment. In patients with cognitive disorders the history needs to be supplemented by relatives, other caregivers and by reviewing medical records. When addressing compliance, any drugs prescribed must be compared with the medicines that patient is taking. Equally important, non-prescription over-the-counter drugs and nutritional supplements that the patient uses must be considered. Quickly obtaining information about who the person with the most up-to-date knowledge on the patient's medical history is valuable, especially if the patient lives alone. The next imperative step is to ensure that patient consent is provided to obtain information from other sources. When setting up an appointment, it is advisable to ask the patient (or caregiver) in advance to bring a medication list to the appointment and, if possible, the actual packages. Any differences in terms of the actual current drug use can then be discussed during the patient's visit. Often well-received by patients, dose dispensing systems are increasingly available in many countries (Fig. 6.1).

Not only is the type of drug but also dosage important. The most common drug-related problem in older adults is prescribing a dose that is too high, with older

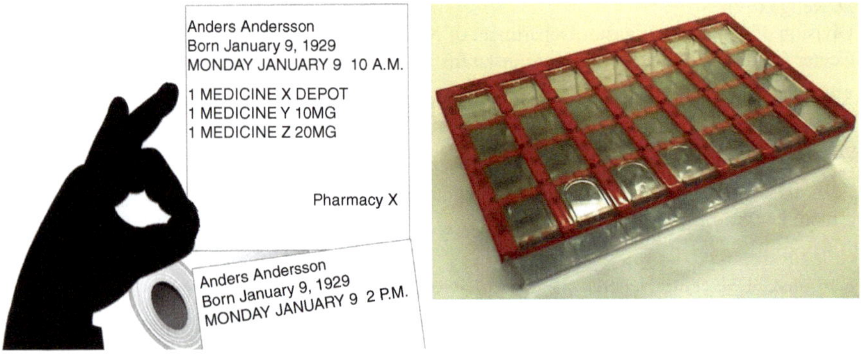

Fig. 6.1 Dose dispensation bags and convenient medicine boxes are often helpful tools for patients with memory problems, especially when compliance is an issue

adults possibly responding with side effects to doses recommended for younger patients.

Since age is the most important risk factor for dementia, it must also be taken into account in terms of problems related to drug treatment. With increasing age, both the body's ability to absorb, distribute, convert and secrete drugs (pharmacokinetics) and its sensitivity to drugs (pharmacodynamics) change.

In the following some of the drug-related problems that need special consideration are described that can occur in patients with cognitive impairment.

Lack of Follow-Up

It is not uncommon that drug treatment is not followed up on in patients with cognitive problems. Patients can experience side effects, or the drug may be ineffective because the dose is not appropriate. Start low, go slow is an essential rule of thumb in older adults when scheduling follow-ups for increasing the dose, but it must be kept in mind that a drug can become ineffective if the patient stays on a lower dose for too long. For instance, a 68-year-old female patient diagnosed with depression and mild cognitive impairment after a memory work-up was prescribed an antidepressant. During the one-year follow-up at a memory clinic, she clearly had mild dementia. Unfortunately, the follow-up on the depression medication was not appropriate because the patient had not visited her primary care doctor enough in between. This example highlights the critical issue that patients with cognitive impairment or dementia may not seek out medical attention on their own but need a pre-scheduled appointment and that medical staff should actively ensure compliance, e.g. telephone consultation with a nurse.

Doing a medication review is essential from a medical perspective. Many countries have enacted legislation regulating regular medication reviews that puts the responsibility for medication (e.g. writing prescriptions) on the physician [1] and, if necessary, in collaboration with other healthcare professionals. Emphasising patient involvement is also important and differs from patient consent. Physicians must familiarise themselves with the patient's current medication and systematically discuss the therapy and therapeutic options with the patient using suitable tools. In Sweden patients 75 years of age or older taking at least five prescription medications must be given a patient medication review at visits to outpatient doctors, during inpatient enrolment, home care visits, when moving to a nursing home and yearly if receiving home care or when living in a nursing home, but also when drug-related problems exist or are suspected [2].

In some countries, pharmacists are available for consultation but are not usually a mandatory part of a medication review. However, in some locations, pharmacists play a crucial role in medication reviews, a practice reflected in the large share of recently published articles on medication reviews written by clinical pharmacists. Regardless, it is important to decide on the division of tasks in a medication review and to conduct the follow-up as early as possible and if feasible, especially when a patient is cognitively impaired.

A systematic review of medicines management issues in dementia [1] identified challenges and solutions to medication management described by people with dementia and their carers. A common issue was a worsening of the ability to plan, organise and execute medicine management tasks. Additional related issues were forgetfulness, confusion and lack of insight. A proposed solution was accepting assistance with medication and transferring responsibility for medicine management to the family carer. However, the review showed that sometimes caregivers can be forgetful themselves, which is why it is also important to assess the ability and resources of the family caregiver before delegating the responsibility. Other solutions for dealing with reduced organisational abilities were visual aids and/or external memory reminders such as diaries, alarms and activity planners. The review also pointed out that risk of medication errors (e.g. under/overdose) was an issue, especially when new medications are introduced. Medicine aids [pill box (Fig. 6.1)] represent a possible solution, just as internal and external memory strategies can be helpful, for instance by linking to the patient's daily routine. Difficulties in maintaining a continuous supply of medicine was another issue, but one that could possibly be solved by sending/faxing prescriptions from the hospital to the pharmacy and the patient's home, using online prescription systems, home delivery of medications and simplifying dosing regimens. The review also pinpointed stress caused by non-professional care responsibilities as an issue for carers, but one that the temporary replacement of the carer could ameliorate. The review indicated that family caregiver communication with healthcare professionals was important and played a role in giving medications safely, recognising side effects and increasing preparedness on how to deal with medication-related emergencies.

Prescribing Cascade

The prescribing (or prescription) cascade is an undesirable sequence of events that begins when the drug is prescribed and a side effect occurs that is misinterpreted as a new medical condition, causing another drug to be prescribed to treat this condition. In the memory clinic setting a very commonly occurring prescribing cascade in the memory clinic setting is antipsychotic → parkinsonism → antiparkinsonian drug therapy. Another common cascade links the initiation of a non-steroidal anti-inflammatory drug to the development of hypertension and subsequent initiation of antihypertensive therapy [2]. A recent study also carefully examined a common cascade that occurs when older adults with hypertension are newly prescribed a calcium channel blocker and then subsequently given a loop diuretic at higher rates than those who began taking other antihypertensive medications [3] due to oedema misinterpreted as a new medical condition. An obvious way to prevent prescription cascades that should be kept in mind during medication review in dementia is alternative treatment strategies such as non-pharmacological treatment, e.g. for pain.

After a dementia diagnosis, newly prescribed acetylcholinesterase inhibitors (AChEIs) can result in sudden worsening of urinary incontinence, a new problem often treated with anticholinergic drugs (e.g. oxybutynin chloride, tolterodine tartrate and flavoxate hydrochloride), resulting in what can be considered a prescribing cascade. A Canadian study showed that older adults with dementia on AChEIs had a 1.55 times higher risk of being subsequently prescribed an anticholinergic drug for urinary incontinence compared to older adults with dementia not on AChEIs [4]. Dementia patients taking donepezil and an anticholinergic drug had worse cognitive outcomes at 2 years, showed a seven-point decline in the Mini-Mental State Examination score compared to a two-point decline in patients taking donepezil only [5]. However, not all studies found that cognition or function worsened with the AChEI-anticholinergic combination [6]. A recent meta-analysis reported that anticholinergic drug use is associated with increased dementia and cognitive decline, but causation has not yet been confirmed [7]. The aforementioned Canadian dataset, with data from 1.8 million older adults, which allowed the identification of a link between use of cholinesterase inhibitor therapy to initiation of urinary anticholinergics [4], also showed a prescription cascade with lithium use and that treatment for parkinsonism began later [8].

The path to reducing **prescribing cascades** should include prevention, detection and reversion. The best strategy for reversion of prescription cascades is to ask what the indication for this drug is, in addition to providing education about de-prescribing and dose-tapering strategies. Other available resources to reduce cascades include detection algorithms, protocols, games [9] and checklists [2]. Case reports also represent a highly illustrative method, e.g. dose reduction to reverse rhinorrhoea after starting AChEI treatment [10].

Polypharmacy

In polypharmacy, defined as the use of multiple [5–10] medications, with >10 known as excessive polypharmacy, the risk of drug side effects increases exponentially. The most important risk factor for side effects is the number of drugs used. The risk of drug interactions also increases exponentially. At the same time, adherence to drug prescriptions diminishes, presenting the risk that patients will neglect the most important drugs.

In a recent analysis with data from 18 countries, the prevalence of polypharmacy in older adults (although mostly without dementia) was 26.3% to 39.9% [11]. A recent Danish study in a dementia population showed that, from 2011 to 2014, the prevalence of polypharmacy decreased negligibly from 69.4% to 68.1% in people with dementia and from 36.1% to 35.2% in people without dementia [12]. Polypharmacy in patients with dementia is associated with an increased risk of visiting the emergency department, hospitalisation and death, as the risk of any or unplanned hospitalisation may increase by 12% in those taking 4–6 medications, with a dose-response relationship between number of medications and adverse health outcomes [13].

Potentially Inappropriate Medications

The American Geriatrics Society (AGS) Beers Criteria® defines potentially inappropriate medications (PIMs) as medications that should generally be avoided in people 65 years or older because they are either ineffective, pose an unnecessarily high risk for older people and a safer alternative is available. One study showed an independent association between PIM use and dementia (odds ratio 1.69) [14], the authors suggesting that identifying inappropriate medication use can help prevent, delay and reduce PIM use and related adverse health outcomes.

De-prescribing

Physicians in a memory clinic setting must be willing to de-prescribe medications that are inappropriate, even if they are not the main prescriber for most of them. The best way to approach de-prescription is in dialogue and agreement with other physicians, though with one of them taking responsibility for initiating the discussion and de-prescription. A crucial issue for hospital-based physicians is to get the general practitioner on board. Other obstacles can be family caregivers and professional caregivers who might be concerned that de-prescription may lead to the re-emergence of symptoms. As a result, shared decision making and setting goals with adequate follow-up, for instance a contact number for the patient or caregiver to use in case of re-emergence of symptoms, may be useful.

Review of Drugs in Patients with Advanced Dementia

Dementia is an age-associated morbidity that ultimately becomes a life-defining illness. As such, when the disease unavoidably progresses, the goal of treatment shifts towards promoting quality of life and reducing the burden of pharmacotherapy to the greatest extent possible. It has been shown that patients with advanced dementia are at greater risk of receiving aggressive pharmacotherapy, which may not align with the proper goals of treatment but, at the same time, these patients may be experiencing physical and psychological symptoms, including agitation, depression, pain and constipation. Hence, they may significantly benefit from appropriate pharmacotherapy at the end of life. As a result, the goal of the treatment at the end of life is to reduce unnecessary pharmacotherapy and introduce other more suitable drugs, i.e. ones that reduce symptoms rather than prevent future illnesses. Examples of the drugs used, which may be referred to as essential in palliative care, are antidepressants, analgesics and laxatives.

Kidney Function

As decreased kidney function is a feature of normal aging, chronic kidney disease is common in older individuals. In all patients with renal abnormalities, the adjustment of drug doses is an essential issue in all those who are treated with nephrotoxic drugs or drugs removed by the kidney. Furthermore, there are drug combinations which may be harmful to the kidney, e.g., they may increase the risk of pre-renal kidney injury: a combination of non-steroidal anti-inflammatory drugs (NSAIDs), diuretics, ACEI or ARB (angiotensin receptor blockers) [15]. In patients treated with any harmful combinations, adding a drug that worsens kidney function may be dangerous. Consequently, to avoid the side effects of drugs that may negatively impact kidney function, it is imperative to calculate the estimated glomerular filtration rate (eGFR) based on creatinine level, bearing in mind that eGFR can easily change when the water balance is altered (e.g. less fluid intake and vomiting). Thus, in patients with an unstable clinical condition, a current eGFR value is needed.

A list of drugs with prescription recommendations for patients with an eGFR below 30 ml/min/1.73 m^2 can be compiled based on updated AGS Beers Criteria® [16] and consensus guidelines for oral dosing of primarily renally cleared medication in older adults [17] and include the following neuropsychotropic drugs:

- duloxetine—avoid
- venlafaxine—reduce dose
- gabapentin—reduce dose
- levetiracetam—reduce dose
- pregabalin—reduce dose
- topiramate—reduce dose
- memantine—reduce dose
- piracetam—reduce dose
- risperidone—reduce dose
- sulpiride—reduce dose

Every drug description included information on how to dose according to kidney function and helpful reminders. Today, the most important step is to integrate the kidney function and electronic advice on dosage. In some countries the prescription module in electronic patient records is integrated with renal status (eGFR), leading to an increase in follow-up on patients and concrete suggestions for drug reduction as renal function/dysfunction may have some merits.

Potentially Inappropriate Prescribing

Potentially inappropriate prescribing (PIP) is defined as the use of medicines that pose more risk than benefits, especially when safer alternatives exist, and mainly involves medications that should generally be avoided in older populations. The risk of PIP varies from patient to patient, though patients with dementia are particularly sensitive to PIP due to the spectrum of drugs used to treat them.

Literature reviews show that the prevalence of PIP in dementia varies significantly between studies due to their high level of clinical heterogeneity [18]. It is safe to assume, however, that PIP occurs in one third of community dwelling individuals (the lowest value identified by a study focusing on individuals with mild dementia only), and in even every other resident in nursing homes/specialised care homes [19].

Two types of PIP in patients with dementia can be distinguished [20]. The first one results from a more frequent application of medicines like benzodiazepines (BZDs), antidepressants, neuroleptics in patients with dementia than in the general population because these medications are used to control various behavioural and psychological symptoms common in dementia (e.g. aggression, wandering and sleep disturbances). They often pose more risk than benefit due to narrow therapeutic indices. The second type of PIP emerges from medications used in the treatment of comorbid medical conditions. As dementia is frequently accompanied by comorbidities, they are often managed with multiple medications that lead straight down a path to polypharmacy, which itself creates the risk of both adverse drug reactions and thus PIP. Based on a literature review, Parsons [21] reported that people with dementia take an average of 5–10 medications, one to two of which are prescribed because of dementia, the remaining ones indicated for treating other comorbid conditions. Although polypharmacy is a significant risk factor of PIP [22], it is not always inappropriate by itself but contributes to the complexity of managing the possible side effects of every medication and the potential consequences of drug interactions.

PIP is always related to adverse drug reactions, which are an unwanted, undesirable effect of a medication that occurs during typical clinical use. Cognitive impairment contributes to the substantially higher prevalence of adverse drug reactions, mainly due to nonadherence. Patients with cognitive impairment may not follow their medication regimen, forgetting to take their medication or taking it inappropriately. Notably, the risk of medication nonadherence increases with a higher number of drugs, further increasing the risk of adverse drug reactions.

Multiple tools are available to help identify PIP, but most of them are designed with older adults in mind and not specifically tailored to dementia. Even though this is the case, the tools contain items that can be applied to the review of medication in patients with dementia. These three tools are used most widely:

- AGS Beers Criteria® for Potentially Inappropriate Medication Use in Older adults [16]
- Screening Tool of Older Persons' Prescriptions (STOPP) and Screening Tool to Alert to Right Treatment (START) [23, 24]
- PRISCUS list [25]

AGS Beers Criteria for Potentially Inappropriate Medication (PIM) Use in Older adults

These criteria, which have been in common use for 30 years worldwide, not only by physicians but also by other professionals [26], provide a list of PIM that should be avoided in older patients in most situations but also certain circumstances and in specific conditions. Many countries have incorporated the list into their electronic medical record systems so that the physician receives a warning when the drug is prescribed for people over the age of 65 or 75 years, for example. Since 2011, AGS has updated the criteria every 3 years. For the last update (2019), a multidisciplinary expert panel examined the evidence published since the previous update (2015) to verify whether new criteria were necessary, or whether existing criteria were still valid or needed changes (in terms of their rationale, level of evidence or strength of recommendations). The current AGS Beers Criteria® is the third update by AGS and the fifth since the original release. The criteria include a list of drugs that are strongly recommended to be avoided in older individuals. Among them are drugs that negatively effect on the CNS:

1. *Anticholinergics*, due to high risk of confusion (quality of evidence: moderate): first-generation antihistamines: brompheniramine, carbinoxamine, chlorpheniramine, clemastine, cyproheptadine, dexbrompheniramine, dexchlorpheniramine, dimenhydrinate, diphenhydramine (oral: use of diphenhydramine in situations such as acute treatment of severe allergic reaction may be appropriate), doxylamine, hydroxyzine, meclizine, promethazine, pyrilamine, triprolidine
2. *Antispasmodics*, as they are highly anticholinergic and their effectiveness is uncertain (quality of evidence: moderate): atropine (excludes ophthalmic), belladonna alkaloids, clidinium-chlordiazepoxide, dicyclomine, homatropine (excludes ophthalmic), hyoscyamine, methscopolamine, propantheline, scopolamine
3. *CNS alpha-agonists*, due to high risk of adverse effects on the CNS (quality of evidence: moderate): clonidine for first-line treatment of hypertension, other CNS alpha-agonists: guanabenz, guanfacine, methyldopa, reserpine (>0.1 mg/day)
4. *CNS antidepressants*, alone or in combination due to their highly anticholinergic effect (quality of evidence: high): amitriptyline, amoxapine, clomipramine, desipramine, doxepin >6 mg/day, imipramine, nortriptyline, paroxetine, protriptyline, trimipramine
5. *Antipsychotics (first (conventional) and second (atypical) generation)*, due to increased risk of cerebrovascular accident (stroke) and a greater rate of cognitive decline and mortality in persons with dementia; should be avoided for behavioural problems in dementia or delirium unless non-pharmacological options (e.g. behavioural interventions) have failed or are not possible and the older adult is threatening substantial harm to self or others (except in schizophrenia or bipolar disorder, or for short-term use as antiemetic during chemotherapy) (quality of evidence: moderate)
6. *Barbiturates*, due to high rate of physical dependence, tolerance to sleep benefits, greater risk of overdose at low dosages (being phased out in many European countries)
7. *BZDs*, all of which increase the risk of cognitive impairment, delirium (may be appropriate for seizure disorders, rapid eye movement sleep behaviour disorder, benzodiazepine withdrawal, ethanol withdrawal, severe generalised anxiety disorder, periprocedural anaesthesia (quality of evidence: moderate): short- and intermediate-acting: alprazolam, estazolam, lorazepam, oxazepam, temazepam, triazolam; long-acting BZDs: chlordiazepoxide (alone or in combination with

amitriptyline or clidinium), clonazepam, clorazepate, diazepam, flurazepam, oxazepam
8. *Meprobamate*, due to high rate of physical dependence and sedating (quality of evidence: moderate)
9. *Nonbenzodiazepine, benzodiazepine receptor agonist hypnotics (i.e. Z-drugs)*, due to their adverse events (e.g. delirium), which are similar to those of BZDs in older adults and include increased emergency room visits/hospitalisations, minimal improvement in sleep latency and duration (quality of evidence: moderate): eszopiclone, zaleplon, zolpidem

The 2019 AGS Beers Criteria® also comprises a list of drugs that are discouraged in certain clinical conditions due to drug–disease or drug–syndrome interactions. Among them there are drugs which may exacerbate:

1. *May exacerbate dementia and cognitive impairment:*
   (a) Anticholinergics (quality of evidence: moderate)
   (b) BZDs (quality of evidence: moderate)
   (c) Nonbenzodiazepine, benzodiazepine receptor agonist hypnotics: eszopiclone, zaleplon, zolpidem (quality of evidence: moderate)
2. *May exacerbate* delirium:
   (a) Anticholinergics (quality of evidence: moderate)
   (b) Antipsychotics (quality of evidence: moderate)
   (c) Benzodiazepine (quality of evidence: moderate)
   (d) Corticosteroids (oral and parenteral) (quality of evidence: moderate)
   (e) H2-receptor antagonists (cimetidine, famotidine, nizatidine, ranitidine, meperidine) (quality of evidence: low)
   (f) Nonbenzodiazepine, benzodiazepine receptor agonist hypnotics: eszopiclone, zaleplon, zolpidem (quality of evidence: moderate)

Note that, due to weak supporting evidence, the most recent AGS Beers Criteria® update removed H2-receptor antagonists from the "avoid" list of drugs that can potentially affect the CNS in patients with dementia or cognitive impairment. This criterion, combined with another one that de-recommends chronic use of proton pump inhibitors without strong indications, could have severely restricted the therapeutic possibilities for older individuals with dementia and gastroesophageal reflux or similar conditions. H2-receptor antagonists remain, however, on the "avoid" list for patients with delirium.

STOPP/START

In 2003, due to the limitations of existing criteria (including the AGS Beers Criteria®, which had some deficiencies, e.g. several listed drugs were not available in Europe or were not contraindicated), a European panel of experts reached a consensus based on a literature review and validation discussions, leading to the publication of the two-part STOPP/START criteria [27]. STOPP lists drugs to be avoided due to their potential inappropriateness in older persons and START lists drugs frequently omitted in prescriptions but that should be considered for older patients where no contraindications exist. The STOPP part also includes drugs that adversely affect older patients at risk of falls, analgesics and duplicate drug class prescriptions (e.g. two angiotensin converting enzyme inhibitors or two proton pump inhibitors). In both tools, drugs were grouped by physiological systems (e.g. the cardiovascular system or CNS), making their use easier.

A group of experts in geriatric medicine, clinical pharmacology, clinical pharmacy, old age psychiatry and primary care subsequently validated the STOPP/START criteria in 2006. These experts were also invited to suggest additional criteria that were not included in the original drafts of STOPP/START. They finally agreed on a list of 65 STOPP and 22 START criteria (STOPP/START version 1).

In 2015, following expansion of the therapeutics evidence base, a thorough literature review was performed to reassess the 2008 criteria and create a new version, in accordance with the same rules as previously (STOPP/START version 2).

The 2015 STOPP list [24] mentions dementia twice, which means that two groups of drugs should be avoided in patients with dementia. Among the central nervous system drugs there are tricyclic antidepressants (due to the risk of worsening cognitive impairment) and among urogenital system drugs—the bladder antimuscarinic drugs (due to the risk of increased confusion and agitation). The previous STOPP lists (2003/2006) contained analgesics, also long-term opioids, due to the risk of exacerbation of cognitive impairment, unless indicated for palliative care or management of moderate/severe chronic pain syndrome. They were removed from the 2015 list as the evidence was weak.

The STOPP criteria also include, however, drugs that should be used with caution in patients with dementia. The reason suggested for avoiding them is related to potentially harmful CNS effects:

- Long-term (>1 month), long-acting BZDs, e.g. chlordiazepoxide, flurazepam, nitrazepam, clorazepate and BZDs with long-acting metabolites, e.g. diazepam (risk of prolonged sedation, confusion)
- Long-term (>1 month) neuroleptics like long-term hypnotics (risk of confusion, hypotension, extrapyramidal side effects)
- Anticholinergics to treat extrapyramidal side effects of neuroleptic medications (risk of anticholinergic toxicity)
- Prolonged use (>1 week) of first-generation antihistamines, e.g. diphenhydramine, chlorpheniramine, cyclizine, promethazine (risk of sedation and anticholinergic side effects)

The START list is limited to the general population of older individuals and does not mention patients with dementia or cognitive impairment.

PRISCUS List

The history of the PRISCUS list is similar to that of the STOPP/START criteria. International recommendations regarding the correct treatment of older patients, particularly those with multimorbidities, were difficult to apply in Germany because they often did not apply to the situation in German because of differences in which drugs are approved, prescribing behaviour and therapeutic guidelines. The project, named PRISCUS, which is Latin for old and frail, was dedicated to PIM for older patients in the German-speaking countries. The PRISCUS list includes drugs whose use in older adults carries an increased risk of adverse drug events. The list was put together after a review of existing lists from other countries and a review of the current literature. This list has not been updated since its inception, but it has the significant advantage that possible therapeutic alternatives are indicated for each PIM.

The PRISCUS list contains 83 PIMs, which includes drugs that can potentially affect the CNS or that should be used with caution in patients with cognitive impairment. The following items only indicate how they act on the CNS:

1. Non-steroidal anti-inflammatory drugs: indomethacin, due to central nervous disturbances; possible alternatives are: paracetamol, weak opioids (tramadol, codeine) and weak NSAIDs (e.g. ibuprofen)
2. Opioid analgesics: pethidine, due to elevated risk of delirium; possible alternatives are: paracetamol, other opioids (with lower risk of delirium, e.g. tilidine/naloxone, morphine, oxycodone, buprenorphine, hydroxymorphone) and weak NSAIDs (e.g. ibuprofen)
3. Antiarrhythmic drugs:
   (a) quinidine, due to CNS side effects; possible alternatives are: beta blockers, verapamil, diltiazem, amiodarone, defibrillator implantation
   (b) flecainide, due to higher rate of adverse effects, CNS effects (e.g. vertigo, cognitive impairment) should be monitored; possible alternatives are: beta blockers, amiodarone
4. Anticholinergic drugs due to impaired cognitive performance:
   (a) Antihistamines: hydroxyzine, clemastine, dimetindene, chlorpheniramine, triprolidine; possible alternatives are: non-sedating, non-anticholinergic antihistamines (e.g. cetirizine, loratadine, desloratadine)
   (b) Urological spasmolytic agents: oxybutynin (non-sustained-release and sustained-release formulations), tolterodine (non-sustained-release), solifenacin; possible alternatives are: trospium, non-pharmacological treatment (e.g. pelvic floor exercises, physical and behavioural therapy)
5. Antidepressants:
   (a) Tricyclic antidepressants (amitriptyline, doxepin, imipramine, clomipramine, maprotiline, trimipramine), due to central anticholinergic side effects (e.g. drowsiness, inner unrest, confusion, other types of delirium) and cognitive deficit; possible alternatives are: Selective serotonin reuptake inhibitors (SSRIs) (e.g. citalopram, sertraline), mirtazapine, non-pharmacological treatments such as behavioural therapy

   (b) Among SSRIs: fluoxetine, due to CNS side effects (e.g. insomnia, dizziness, confusion), hyponatraemia; possible alternatives are: another SSRI (e.g. citalopram, sertraline), trazodone, mirtazapine, non-pharmacological treatments such as behavioural therapy
   (c) Monoamine oxidase inhibitors: tranylcypromine, due to risk of cerebral haemorrhage; possible alternatives are: SSRIs (other than fluoxetine), non-pharmacological treatments such as behavioural therapy
6. Antiemetic drugs: dimenhydrinate, due to anticholinergic side effects; possible alternatives are: domperidone, metoclopramide (beware of extrapyramidal side effects)
7. Antihypertensive agents and other cardiovascular drugs: Clonidine, due to CNS side effects (sedation, cognitive impairment); Alpha blockers (doxazosin, prazosin, terazosin (as an antihypertensive agent), due to CNS side effects (e.g. vertigo, light-headedness, somnolence), increased risk of cerebrovascular disease; Methyldopa, due to sedation; Reserpine due to CNS effects (sedation, depression). Possible alternatives are: other antihypertensive agents, e.g. angiotensin converting enzyme inhibitors, AT1 receptor blockers, thiazide (diuretics), beta blockers, calcium antagonists (long-acting, with peripheral effect)
8. Neuroleptic drugs: Classic neuroleptic drugs: thioridazine, fluphenazine, levomepromazine, perphenazine, haloperidol (>2 mg); Atypical neuroleptic drugs: olanzapine (>10 mg), clozapine. The main concerns are anticholinergic and extrapyramidal side effects, parkinsonism, sedation, falls and increased mortality in patients with dementia; fewer extrapyramidal side effects when atypical neuroleptics are used; possible alternatives are neuroleptics of low potency (e.g. melperone, pipamperone) or atypical neuroleptics with a favourable risk/benefit profile (e.g. risperidone)
9. Muscle relaxants: baclofen, tetrazepam due to CNS effects: amnesia, confusion; possible alternatives for baclofen are: tolperisone, tizanidine, physical therapy; for tetrazepam: short/intermediate-acting BZDs in low doses
10. BZDs, due to psychiatric reactions (sometimes paradoxical, e.g. agitation, irritability, hallucinations, psychosis), cognitive impairment, depression, increased risk of falls (excluding depression for Z-drugs).
    (a) Long-acting BZDs: chlordiazepoxide, diazepam, flurazepam, dipotassium clorazepate, bromazepam, prazepam, clobazam, nitrazepam, flunitrazepam, medazepam
    (b) Short-/intermediate-acting BZDs (alprazolam, temazepam, triazolam, lorazepam (>2 mg/d), oxazepam (>60 mg/d), lormetazepam (>0.5 mg/d), brotizolam (>0.125 mg/d)
    (c) Z-drugs: zolpidem (>5 mg/d), zopiclone (>3.75 mg/d), zaleplon (>5 mg/d)

Possible alternatives for long-acting BZDs are short-/shorter-acting benzodiazepines, Z-drugs (a low dose), opipramol, sedating antidepressants (e.g. mirtazapine), neuroleptic drugs of low potency (e.g. melperone, pipamperone); for short-/intermediate-acting and Z-drugs: valerian, sedating antidepressants (trazodone, mianserin, mirtazapine), opipramol, low-potency neuroleptic drugs (melperone, pipamperone), non-pharmacological treatment of sleep disturbances (sleep hygiene); for short-/intermediate-acting BZDs: zolpidem ($\leq$5 mg/d).

11. Other sedative agents:
    (a) Doxylamine, diphenhydramine due to anticholinergic effects and dizziness; possible alternatives are the same as for short-/intermediate-acting BZDs
    (b) Chloral hydrate due to dizziness

Possible alternatives for both listed above are the same as for short-/intermediate-acting BZDs.

12. Other antiepileptic drugs: phenobarbital, due to sedation and paradoxical excitation; possible alternatives are other antiepileptic drugs: lamotrigine, valproic acid, levetiracetam, gabapentin

Possible Cognitive Side Effects of Major Drug Classes

This section provides a list of the major classes of drugs in the Anatomical Therapeutic Chemical Classification System (ATC) that have cognitive side effects and a brief description of their side effects, with a focus on elderly people with dementia. This list can aid in assessing possible cognitive side effects of a particular drug during a medication review for patients with dementia.

Cognitive effects are seen not only in drug treatment affecting the CNS [28–30] but may also occur in electrolyte balance disorders [29], for example in diuretics treatment. Anticholinergic effects are found in many different drug groups, such as antihistamines, anti-incontinence drugs and tricyclic antidepressants. The degree of anticholinergic effect of the drugs varies and the overall anticholinergic effect should be taken into account rather than the anticholinergic effect of individual substances. Scales are available for estimating a patient's total anticholinergic load that can be of help in the medication review. Drugs less known for their potential anticholinergic activity are digoxin, amantadine, prednisolone, metoprolol, warfarin and morphine

Individual Assessment

Some patients are more sensitive than others to the side effects of drugs, which is why individual assessment is necessary, even if studies do not show impairment or impairment cognitive function

Below is a selected list of drugs with their ACT code and a brief description of how they act. The first level of each code indicates the anatomical main group, of which there are 14, and consists of one letter. The groups listed below include: 'A', which stands for alimentary tract and metabolism; 'G', which stands for genitourinary system and sex hormones; 'M', which stands for musculo-skeletal system; and 'N', which stands for nervous system. The second level comprises two digits and indicates the therapeutic subgroup, while the third level indicates the therapeutic/pharmacological subgroup and comprises one letter

A04 Antiemetics

Serotonin receptor antagonists do not appear to affect cognition in a negative direction, while scopolamine exhibits clear anticholinergic and thus cognitive effects.

A10 Diabetes agents

Most importantly, hypoglycaemia may be an issue with antidiabetics, which may have adverse cognitive effects. Studies have shown that experimentally keeping blood glucose at 4.5 mmol/l in type 2 diabetes had a negative impact on process speed, memory and attention compared to blood glucose at 16 mmol/l [31]. The influence of hyperglycaemia is generally less than for hypoglycaemia [32] but some studies in blood glucose >20 mmol/l showed a potentially negative effect.

The American Diabetes Association has recently added three new recommendations on hypoglycaemia in the elderly, for instance: glycaemic goals can be relaxed in the older population as part of individualised care that focuses on individualised pharmacotherapy with glucose-lowering agents with a low risk of hypoglycaemia and proven cardiovascular safety [33].

Insulin therapy always carries a potential risk of severe hypoglycaemia, which gradually influences the cognitive function and results in the occurrence of diabetic coma. Since severe hypoglycaemia renders the individual unconscious, someone else must intervene to reverse it. Severe hypoglycaemia often refers to a fixed blood sugar level, often 2.8 mmol/L, but other values may occur.

Insulin therapy increases the risk of severe hypoglycaemia. In most studies, patient-reported hypoglycaemia symptoms are most often described and often hypoglycaemia is not verified with the measurement of blood/plasma glucose. In the studies examined, hypoglycaemia was usually confirmed at blood glucose <3.3 mmol/l, sometimes <2.2 mmol/l, the latter blood glucose sometimes considered severe hypoglycaemia. Metformin appears to have a low hypoglycaemia rate, comparable to placebo, in a larger study reported at 4.2% of all participants [34]. The newest drugs used in diabetes, used alone or in combination, have different risk levels in terms of hypoglycaemia.

Recommendation: Ensure that patients with dementia, carers and healthcare staff can monitor glucose level and detect signs of hypoglycaemia.

G04 Urological Agents

An overactive bladder is successfully treated with anticholinergic drugs, but cognitive impact is more likely with increasing age. Darifenacin does not appear to have any impact on cognitive function, which is fortunate considering its high efficacy.

A recent review article asserted that oxybutynin may impair cognition in the elderly. For this age group, darifenacin, trospium, solifenacin and tolterodine are considered to have little risk of CNS side effects, but caution is still warranted in dementia, especially for the last-mentioned compound [35]

Darifenacin 15 mg × 1 (slow release) does not affect cognitive function and is comparable to placebo regarding adverse effects on cognition. Single dose oxybutynin (5 and 10 mg) has been shown to result in impaired cognitive test results in seven out of 15 neuropsychological tests [36]. Slow-release oxybutynin (20 mg) affects cognition, especially memory, in the elderly when compared to placebo and darifenacin (15 mg) [37]. Studies on tolterodine are lacking, though a couple of case histories have been described with memory impairment [38] and confusion [39].

M01A NSAID

In general, single-dose NSAIDs do not appear to affect cognitive function, while both improved and impaired test results may be detected with longer term treatment. It is well known that NSAIDs may have effects on the CNS in overdose [40].

N01 Anaesthetics

A review by Wu et al. [41] showed that the risk of postoperative impairment in cognitive function did not differ between general anaesthesia and regional anaesthesia. The review also showed that especially elderly people were sensitive to postoperative cognitive dysfunction, which could persist for one week postoperatively in 26% of patients, in some cases for up to months.

N02 Analgesics

There are three key issues to be aware of when reviewing analgesics in patients with dementia in terms of cognitive side effects: (1) pain has been shown to affect reaction speed and other cognitive functions, which is why treating it adequately is essential; (2) opioids negatively impact cognitive function, especially upon initiation of the therapy (up to 2 weeks but highly dependent on the individual); and (3) a stable dose of opioids is better than short-term, extra doses. Also note that with morphine, it is important to start with short acting before moving on to long acting.

N03 Antiepileptics

The cognitive side effects of antiepileptics are more common, although less studied, in elderly patients. The cognitive influence of most antiepileptic drugs has been described, but discerning whether it is the effect of the disease or drugs is difficult, as attested to by how results differ considerably among studies. Risk of cognitive side effect differs between various antiepileptics, but valproate, phenytoin, clonazepam, clobazam and gabapentin should be given special attention. Sarkis et al. [42], who did a review of phase-III studies on newer drugs, found adverse reactions in placebo patients (cognitive in 0–10.6%; fatigue in 2.5–37.7%), making the results difficult to interpret. However, dose-response relationships were found for most antiepileptics, except for brivaracetam and zonisamide (for cognitive side effects) and tiagabine, topiramate and zonisamide (for fatigue). Cognitive side effects were present in at least 5% more patients than placebo subjects for eslicarbazepine (high load), perampanel (high load), pregabalin (average and high load), tiagabine (high load), topiramate (average and high load) and vigabatrin (high load). About 3% had cognitive side effects with placebo or low drug load, but 5.8% with average drug load and 8.7% with high drug load. Levetiracetam is reported by some to improve cognition [43] and lamotrigine to relieve depression in patients with cognitive impairment, while phenobarbital and lamotrigine could worsen cognition, and levetiracetam and phenobarbital could worsen mood. Levetiracetam does not appear to reduce cognitive ability but can produce undesirable effects in terms of aggressiveness and impulsivity. Chapter 12 provides detailed information on antiepileptics.

When monitoring antiepileptic treatment in patients with cognitive problems that are known or suspected, it is important to observe cognitive abilities. Patients can be asked whether they experience cognitive problems and cognitive tests can be administered. When a cognitive side effect is suspected, modification of the treatment should be considered.

N04 Anti-Parkinson Drugs

Cognitive function may be affected already in the early stages of the disease. For elderly patients with cognitive impairment it is important to choose medication that does not have a sedative effect (or as little as possible) and that does not contain an anticholinergic component. L-DOPA, also called levodopa, appears to be the best option. Selegiline and tolcapone seem to have the potential to improve cognition, and rasagiline seems to be neutral from a cognitive point of view.

N05A Neuroleptics

Clozapine appears to have less impact on cognitive function than other neuroleptics, but its anticholinergic effects may have significance, at least for elderly patients.

N05C Hypnotics and Sedatives

In some countries, half or more of patients with mild to moderate Alzheimer's disease were prescribed a sedative. Sedative load was associated with the risk of delirium and falls, which is why optimal prescribing is needed in individuals with Alzheimer's disease.

Recent evidence indicates that the use of BZDs and Z-drugs may be strongly associated with the risk of developing dementia [44]. Unfortunately, there is limited evidence to aid in selecting pharmacotherapy for sleeping problems specifically for patients with dementia [45]. Recent studies examining the use of ramelteon and mirtazapine to treat sleep disorders in Alzheimer's disease showed they had no significant therapeutic effects. BZDs, the most common drugs for insomnia, may have significant side effects in older patients. The orexin receptor antagonist suvorexant was recently reported to be beneficial in insomnia in Alzheimer's disease [46]. Although melatonin is widely used because it has no side effects in people with dementia, studies on melatonin are very limited for this patient group.

Some hypnotics provide considerable effects on cognitive function measured using various neuropsychological tests. More long-acting hypnotics are found among BZDs, where nitrazepam, lorazepam, oxazepam and flunitrazepam have been studied.

N06A Antidepressants

Depression is a condition that requires special consideration in dementia (see Chap. 7). In one study, more than 20% of patients reported subjective cognitive symptoms in long-term treatment with SSRIs [47]. Tricyclic antidepressants initially have an impact on cognitive function, while paroxetine has some negative impact on it. Other antidepressants have varying degrees of influence and tolerance development, except venlafaxine and reboxetine, which seem to have no impact on cognitive function. SSRIs in dementia may be preferable, but depression itself may impair cognitive function.

Other Medicines and Electroconvulsive Therapy

A meta-analysis has shown that it is not possible to show impaired cognition in the long term measured with psychometric tests, but some patients experience a memory disorder long after electroconvulsive therapy. Cancer treatments such as radiation therapy and chemotherapy can also affect cognitive function. Moreover, subjective experiences of cognitive problems are common after chemotherapy, radiation treatment and other pharmacological treatments for cancer. Nootropics are an example of substances that claim to improve cognition, which is why asking patients about them is also relevant.

Other Issues

Non-cardiac drugs with proarrhythmic potential include antihistamines, selective serotonin reuptake inhibitors and AChEIs for dementia. Prolonged QT intervals (from the beginning of the QRS complex to the end of the T wave) can lead to life-threatening heart arrhythmias such as torsades de pointes. In recent years, donepezil and memantine have been known to increase the QT interval, resulting in sudden cardiac death. Drug interactions can also lead to a cumulative effect on the QT interval [48]. To identify and prevent long QT intervals, calculating the QT interval has been suggested when elderly patients are treated for dementia [49]. Electronic resources, e.g. CredibleMeds®, are available to help avoid QT intervals that are too long.

Box 6.1 and 6.2 provide tips on doing the two main types of medication review; Table 6.1 is an example patient case.

Box 6.1 Patient Medication Review

Depending on how the clinic is organised, a physician, pharmacist or nurse speaks with the patient to secure a complete and accurate medication list. Checking with caregivers is important to know exactly which medications are used. Keep an eye out for pharmaceutical drugs with an unfavourable cognitive profile. Both cognition and other bodily functions should be optimised. Conducting a medication review in dementia often includes contacting physicians in other areas of medicine, e.g. urologists. Follow-up is always essential.

Electronic resources are often available for drug–drug interactions. For example, it is important to look for medications that prolong the QT interval of the electrocardiogram.

Based on documentation and the patient's own data identify:

- Drugs prescribed and why
- Strength and dose prescribed versus what is actually taken
- Non-prescription medicines, including over-the-counter drugs, herbal medicines and nutritional supplements
- If there are practical problems with the medicines and compliance

The physician will assess the effectiveness and safety of the drug treatment. Drug-related problems that can be readily solved should be addressed and, if a major drug-related problem is suspected, an in-depth medication review should be provided.

After the review:

- Update the drugs being used in the patient file
- Note the drug-related problems detected, measures taken, and follow-up planned
- Provide patient with individually tailored information on drug treatment and any actions taken
- Give the patient an updated list of medicines
- Give the patient a complete drug report once the patient is enrolled in inpatient care

Source: Modified based on Bergqvist M. and Segander, M. (2020) [50]

Box 6.2 Clinical Medication Review

An in-depth clinical medication review is based on:

- Updated list of medicines and other documentation from the patient medication review
- Estimation of symptoms, e.g. PHASE-20 1
- Test results, e.g. haemoglobin, sodium, potassium, creatinine, depending on the diagnoses and medicines
- Blood pressure (orthostatic if necessary), heart rate and weight
- Estimated glomerular filtration rate
- Interaction control, SFINX 2
- Declaration of any falls

A main goal of the clinical medication review is to identify potentially inappropriate drugs. Renal function and interactions are important. For each medicine:

- Check that there is an indication
- Evaluate the treatment effect based on treatment objectives
- Assess appropriateness of medication based on diagnoses, age, kidney function and other medicines
- Assess whether the dose is correct based on diagnoses, age, kidney function and other medicines
- Evaluate whether the drug's benefit is greater than its side effects or risk thereof
- Assess whether non-pharmacological alternatives or complement are available

For the drug treatment in its entirety:

- Check whether it follows current recommendations
- Assess whether the patient has problems taking action or understanding information
- Assess whether the patient can manage the drug treatment or has sufficient support to do so
- Assess whether undertreatment is present
- Check for clinically relevant interactions

After or during the clinical medication review:

- Update the patient file

- Note which medicines the patient uses
- Note the objectives of the drug treatment
- Indicate which drug-related problems have come to light and how to remedy them
- Note how and when to follow up, clearly indicating which healthcare provider/care unit is responsible for doing so
- Provide the patient with individually tailored information on measures taken and why; when and how to follow up; which healthcare provider/care unit is responsible for follow-up; and who participated in the review
- Give the patient an updated list of medicines

Source: Modified based on Bergqvist M. and Segander, M. (2020) [50]

Table 6.1 Patient case

Patient's story	Physician's view
Retired 67-year-old male who worked in sales in various countries; non-smoker, moderate alcohol intake. Uses a walker, pain problems starting from the right hip; surgery is planned. Lives alone but is in regular contact with sons and sister. Receives home care every morning and gets help once a week with his medicine box. Otherwise functions independently. Recently prescribed levodopa and benserazide for investigative reasons but says he does not feel any tangible effects from the drug. Although prescribed propiomazine at night he says today that he only takes one every 3 months. Has previously been informed of the risk of hangovers. Comments that he has accidentally taken a propiomazine instead of ibuprofen at one of the test sessions during his examination and believes this may have worsened his results. Seen in 2017 in a memory clinic for diagnostic evaluation. Neuropsychological testing showed impairments in various cognitive domains. Interpreting the findings was difficult due to a recent period of confusion caused by an orthopaedic injury. Dementia markers in the cerebrospinal fluid were all in the normal range. A component of neurodegeneration such as Alzheimer's, however, could not be excluded. Information about these conclusions given to relatives who seem to understand the content.	The physician notes that the patient has been drinking alcohol for years, a combination of wine and strong spirits. Intake estimated to be at least three bottles of wine weekly for several years, with a similar intake of whisky. The only break in alcohol consumption occurred after an accident and while patient admitted to a geriatric ward. Sleeps satisfactorily at night, has no depressive symptoms and maintains weight. Neurological status: rigidity, mostly on the right side; hypomimia; normal eye movements, no vertical gaze paresis; Romberg unremarkable; balance difficulties, uses a walker (due to hip problems). Referred to neurological specialist. Hand tremor of the parkinsonian type visible at later visit to the doctor's office, albeit weak; patient tries to downplay it. Cognition appears improved after initiation of anti-Parkinson drug.

Conclusion

Medication reviews are a method for mapping all of the drugs prescribed to and used by a patient and ensure an accurate and up-to-date list of medicines. The method also makes it possible to analyse, retest and follow up on a patient's entire medication use in order to detect, address and prevent drug-related problems.

References

1. Lim RH, Sharmeen T. Medicines management issues in dementia and coping strategies used by people living with dementia and family carers: a systematic review. Int J Geriatr Psychiatry. 2018;33(12):1562–81.
2. Brath H, Mehta N, Savage RD, Gill SS, Wu W, Bronskill SE, et al. What is known about preventing, detecting, and reversing prescribing cascades: a scoping review. J Am Geriatr Soc. 2018;66(11):2079–85.
3. Savage RD, Visentin JD, Bronskill SE, Wang X, Gruneir A, Giannakeas V, et al. Evaluation of a common prescribing cascade of calcium channel blockers and diuretics in older adults with hypertension. JAMA Intern Med. 2020;180(5):643–51.
4. Gill SS, Mamdani M, Naglie G, Streiner DL, Bronskill SE, Kopp A, et al. A prescribing cascade involving cholinesterase inhibitors and anticholinergic drugs. Arch Intern Med. 2005;165(7):808–13.
5. Lopez-Gongora M, Martinez-Domeno A, Garcia C, Escartin A. Effect of levetiracetam on cognitive functions and quality of life: a one-year follow-up study. Epileptic Disord. 2008;10(4):297–305.
6. Triantafylidis LK, Clemons JS, Peron EP, Roefaro J, Zimmerman KM. Brain over bladder: a systematic review of dual cholinesterase inhibitor and urinary anticholinergic use. Drugs Aging. 2018;35(1):27–41.
7. Pieper NT, Grossi CM, Chan WY, Loke YK, Savva GM, Haroulis C, et al. Anticholinergic drugs and incident dementia, mild cognitive impairment and cognitive decline: a meta-analysis. Age Ageing. 2020;49(6):939–47.
8. Marras C, Herrmann N, Fischer HD, Fung K, Gruneir A, Rochon PA, et al. Lithium use in older adults is associated with increased prescribing of parkinson medications. Am J Geriatr Psychiatry. 2016;24(4):301–9.
9. Testman JA. The prescribing cascade game: Applying geriatric pharmacotherapy principles in the classroom. Curr Pharm Teach Learn. 2014;6(5):646–51.
10. Vouri SM, Chung JM, Binder EF. Successful intervention to mitigate an acetylcholinesterase inhibitor-induced rhinorrhea prescribing cascade: a case report. J Clin Pharm Ther. 2017;42(3):370–1.
11. Midao L, Giardini A, Menditto E, Kardas P, Costa E. Polypharmacy prevalence among older adults based on the survey of health, ageing and retirement in Europe. Arch Gerontol Geriatr. 2018;78:213–20.
12. Kristensen RU, Norgaard A, Jensen-Dahm C, Gasse C, Wimberley T, Waldemar G. Changes in the prevalence of polypharmacy in people with and without dementia from 2000 to 2014: a nationwide study. J Alzheimers Dis. 2019;67(3):949–60.
13. Mueller C, Molokhia M, Perera G, Veronese N, Stubbs B, Shetty H, et al. Polypharmacy in people with dementia: associations with adverse health outcomes. Exp Gerontol. 2018;106:240–5.
14. Kucukdagli P, Bahat G, Bay I, Kilic C, Oren MM, Turkmen BO, et al. The relationship between common geriatric syndromes and potentially inappropriate medication use among older adults. Aging Clin Exp Res. 2020;32(4):681–7.
15. Rivosecchi RM, Kellum JA, Dasta JF, Armahizer MJ, Bolesta S, Buckley MS, et al. Drug class combination-associated acute kidney injury. Ann Pharmacother. 2016;50(11):953–72.

16. By the American Geriatrics Society Beers Criteria Update Expert P. American Geriatrics Society 2019 updated AGS Beers Criteria(R) for potentially inappropriate medication use in older adults. J Am Geriatr Soc. 2019;67(4):674–94.
17. Hanlon JT, Aspinall SL, Semla TP, Weisbord SD, Fried LF, Good CB, et al. Consensus guidelines for oral dosing of primarily renally cleared medications in older adults. J Am Geriatr Soc. 2009;57(2):335–40.
18. Patel T, Slonim K, Lee L. Use of potentially inappropriate medications among ambulatory home-dwelling elderly patients with dementia: A review of the literature. Can Pharm J (Ott). 2017;150(3):169–83.
19. Hukins D, Macleod U, Boland JW. Identifying potentially inappropriate prescribing in older people with dementia: a systematic review. Eur J Clin Pharmacol. 2019;75(4):467–81.
20. Delgado J, Bowman K, Clare L. Potentially inappropriate prescribing in dementia: a state-of-the-art review since 2007. BMJ Open. 2020;10(1):e029172.
21. Parsons C. Polypharmacy and inappropriate medication use in patients with dementia: an underresearched problem. Ther Adv Drug Saf. 2017;8(1):31–46.
22. Barry HE, Cooper JA, Ryan C, Passmore AP, Robinson AL, Molloy GJ, et al. Potentially inappropriate prescribing among people with dementia in primary care: a retrospective cross-sectional study using the enhanced prescribing database. J Alzheimers Dis. 2016;52(4):1503–13.
23. O'Mahony D. STOPP/START criteria for potentially inappropriate medications/potential prescribing omissions in older people: origin and progress. Expert Rev Clin Pharmacol. 2020;13(1):15–22.
24. Mahony DO, Sullivan DO, Byrne S, Connor MNO, Ryan C, Gallagher P. Corrigendum: STOPP/START criteria for potentially inappropriate prescribing in older people: version 2. Age Ageing. 2018;47(3):489.
25. Holt S, Schmiedl S, Thurmann PA. Potentially inappropriate medications in the elderly: the PRISCUS list. Dtsch Arztebl Int. 2010;107(31–32):543–51.
26. Beers MH. Explicit criteria for determining potentially inappropriate medication use by the elderly. Arch Intern Med. 1997;157(14):1531.
27. Armitage S. STOPP (Screening Tool of Older Person's Prescriptions) and START (Screening Tool to Alert doctors to Right Treatment) as a pharmacy service. Eur J Hosp Pharm. 2012;19(2):221.1.
28. Low LF, Anstey KJ, Sachdev P. Use of medications with anticholinergic properties and cognitive function in a young-old community sample. Int J Geriatr Psychiatry. 2009;24(6):578–84.
29. Carnahan RM, Lund BC, Perry PJ, Pollock BG, Culp KR. The Anticholinergic Drug Scale as a measure of drug-related anticholinergic burden: associations with serum anticholinergic activity. J Clin Pharmacol. 2006;46(12):1481–6.
30. Ancelin ML, Artero S, Portet F, Dupuy AM, Touchon J, Ritchie K. Non-degenerative mild cognitive impairment in elderly people and use of anticholinergic drugs: longitudinal cohort study. BMJ. 2006;332(7539):455–9.
31. Sommerfield AJ, Deary IJ, Frier BM. Acute hyperglycemia alters mood state and impairs cognitive performance in people with type 2 diabetes. Diabetes Care. 2004;27(10):2335–40.
32. Holmes CS, Hayford JT, Gonzalez JL, Weydert JA. A survey of cognitive functioning at difference glucose levels in diabetic persons. Diabetes Care. 1983;6(2):180–5.
33. Freeman J. Management of hypoglycemia in older adults with type 2 diabetes. Postgrad Med. 2019;131(4):241–50.
34. Bolen S, Feldman L, Vassy J, Wilson L, Yeh HC, Marinopoulos S, et al. Systematic review: comparative effectiveness and safety of oral medications for type 2 diabetes mellitus. Ann Intern Med. 2007;147(6):386–99.
35. Pagoria D, O'Connor RC, Guralnick ML. Antimuscarinic drugs: review of the cognitive impact when used to treat overactive bladder in elderly patients. Curr Urol Rep. 2011;12(5):351–7.
36. Katz IR, Sands LP, Bilker W, DiFilippo S, Boyce A, D'Angelo K. Identification of medications that cause cognitive impairment in older people: the case of oxybutynin chloride. J Am Geriatr Soc. 1998;46(1):8–13.

37. Kay G, Crook T, Rekeda L, Lima R, Ebinger U, Arguinzoniz M, et al. Differential effects of the antimuscarinic agents darifenacin and oxybutynin ER on memory in older subjects. Eur Urol. 2006;50(2):317–26.
38. Womack KB, Heilman KM. Tolterodine and memory: dry but forgetful. Arch Neurol. 2003;60(5):771–3.
39. Salvatore S, Serati M, Cardozo L, Uccella S, Bolis P. Cognitive dysfunction with tolterodine use. Am J Obstet Gynecol. 2007;197(2):e8.
40. Auriel E, Regev K, Korczyn AD. Chapter 38 - Nonsteroidal anti-inflammatory drugs exposure and the central nervous system. In: Biller J, Ferro JM, editors. Handbook of clinical neurology, vol. 119. Elsevier; 2014. p. 577–84.
41. Wu CL, Hsu W, Richman JM, Raja SN. Postoperative cognitive function as an outcome of regional anesthesia and analgesia. Reg Anesth Pain Med. 2004;29(3):257–68.
42. Sarkis RA, Goksen Y, Mu Y, Rosner B, Lee JW. Cognitive and fatigue side effects of anti-epileptic drugs: an analysis of phase III add-on trials. J Neurol. 2018;265(9):2137–42.
43. Ciesielski AS, Samson S, Steinhoff BJ. Neuropsychological and psychiatric impact of add-on titration of pregabalin versus levetiracetam: a comparative short-term study. Epilepsy Behav. 2006;9(3):424–31.
44. Tseng LY, Huang ST, Peng LN, Chen LK, Hsiao FY. Benzodiazepines, z-hypnotics, and risk of dementia: special considerations of half-lives and concomitant use. Neurotherapeutics. 2020;17(1):156–64.
45. McCleery J, Sharpley AL. Pharmacotherapies for sleep disturbances in dementia. Cochrane Database Syst Rev. 2020;11(11):CD009178.
46. Ferini-Strambi L, Galbiati A, Casoni F, Salsone M. Therapy for insomnia and circadian rhythm disorder in Alzheimer disease. Curr Treat Options Neurol. 2020;22(2):4.
47. Popovic D, Vieta E, Fornaro M, Perugi G. Cognitive tolerability following successful long term treatment of major depression and anxiety disorders with SSRi antidepressants. J Affect Disord. 2015;173:211–5.
48. Jackson EG, Stowe S. Lesson of the month 1: prolonged QT syndrome due to donepezil: a reversible cause of falls? Clin Med (Lond). 2019;19(1):80–1.
49. Leitch A, McGinness P, Wallbridge D. Calculate the QT interval in patients taking drugs for dementia. BMJ. 2007;335(7619):557.
50. Bergqvist M, Segander M. Läkemedelsgenomgångar. Vårdhandboken; 2020.

Management Approaches for Behavioural and Psychological Symptoms of Dementia

7

Maarten J. A. Van Den Bossche and Mathieu Vandenbulcke

Abbreviations

AChI	Acetylcholinesterase inhibitors
AD	Alzheimer's disease
BPSD	Behavioural and psychological symptoms of dementia
ECT	Electroconvulsive therapy
FTD	frontotemporal dementia
LBD	Lewy body dementia
NPI	Neuropsychiatric Inventory
SSRI	Selective serotonin reuptake inhibitor
PD	Parkinson's dementia

Introduction

Dementia is characterised by a loss of cognitive functioning in, e.g. memory, language and judgement. However, behavioural and psychological symptoms of dementia (BPSD), also known as neuropsychiatric symptoms of dementia, are as clinically relevant as cognitive symptoms. In recent years the term BPSD has

M. J. A. Van Den Bossche (✉) · M. Vandenbulcke
Department of Geriatric Psychiatry, University Psychiatric Center KU Leuven, Leuven, Belgium

Department of Neurosciences, Research Group Psychiatry, Center for Neuropsychiatry, Leuven Brain Institute, KU Leuven, Leuven, Belgium
e-mail: maarten.vandenbossche@upckuleuven.be; mathieu.vandenbulcke@uzleuven.be

K. S. Frederiksen, G. Waldemar (eds.), *Management of Patients with Dementia*,
https://doi.org/10.1007/978-3-030-77904-7_7

become somewhat contentious but is still widely used in the literature as a better substitute has yet to emerge. The International Psychogeriatric Association defines BPSD as “symptoms of disturbed perception, thought content, mood or behaviour that frequently occur in patients with dementia” [1]. The symptoms can be further divided into behavioural symptoms (e.g. aggression), usually identified by observation of a patient, and psychological symptoms (e.g. delusions), usually assessed based on interviews with patients and relatives. BPSD encompasses highly diverse symptoms ranging from agitation, aggression, wandering, screaming, cursing and sexual disinhibition to anxiety, depressive mood, hallucinations and delusions.

Prevalent in every type of dementia (e.g. Alzheimer’s disease (AD), frontotemporal dementia (FTD), Lewy body dementia (LBD), Parkinson’s dementia (PD) and vascular dementia) BPSD develops in almost everyone with dementia over the course of the disease [2]. Even in the early stages of neurodegenerative diseases, neuropsychiatric symptoms are already frequently present, with an estimated 35–85% of patients with mild cognitive impairment experiencing neuropsychiatric symptoms [3]. The 5-year prevalence of neuropsychiatric symptoms in patients with dementia was 97% in the Cache County Study of Memory in Aging [2].

Associated with faster cognitive decline, faster progression of dementia [4, 5], lower quality of life of patients [6, 7] and a substantial increase in caregiver burden [8, 9], BPSD is the most important reason for institutionalisation, even more so than cognitive decline alone [10, 11]. By increasing caregiver burden and earlier institutionalisation, BPSD also leads to increased healthcare and economic costs. An estimated 30% of all care costs for patients with AD living in a community dwelling are due to BPSD [12]; this is even higher in institutionalised patients. According to a large study in almost 2000 patients in eight European countries, agitation alone was responsible for a mean total extra cost per person per month of €445 in home care and €561 in institutional long-term care [13].

The many potential causes or triggers for BPSD (Fig. 7.1) range from medical problems like pain and infection to an environment that is either over- or under-stimulating. Interactional and communication issues between patients and formal or informal caregivers can also cause or worsen BPSD. These underlying causes and modifiers of BPSD are highly variable from patient to patient and can also vary within one patient over time. Consequently, a thorough assessment and personalised treatment plan are warranted in individual patients, especially when the physician is confronted with particularly challenging behaviour.

Assessment

Every treatment of BPSD should start with a careful, detailed assessment of the symptoms, the patient and the context. This implies obtaining a full medical and psychiatric history of the patient, conducting a physical exam, reviewing medication and analysing the characteristics of the behavioural and psychological problems and any relevant information on the context of the patient and the BPSD. This assessment is crucial as often this will quickly provide the physician with clues on how to treat BPSD.

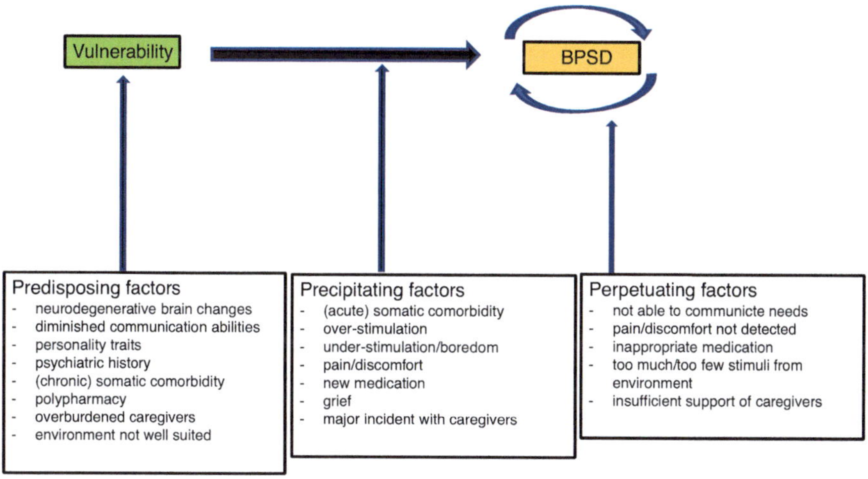

Fig. 7.1 Overview of some of the possible underlying factors for BPSD. Predisposing factors create a vulnerability for the development of BPSD. Precipitating factors can then result in clinical symptoms of BPSD. Perpetuating factors can result in chronic symptoms

A full history should include details on underlying dementia, the current cognitive deficits and substance use, but also on any other past or current medical problems. Since patients may often have difficulties with memory and in expressing themselves, obtaining information from caregivers, relatives and other medical providers is also essential. The medical history and physical exam may point to medical problems that play a significant role in the behavioural problems, such as infection, obstipation or pain.

A medication review is mandatory as numerous drugs can cause or worsen BPSD. Recent drug changes should be thoroughly inspected, especially when new behavioural or psychological symptoms occur or when symptoms have recently worsened.

BPSD must be analysed in detail because the symptoms are highly diverse, ranging from apathy to agitation to hallucinations. It is vital to establish which symptoms are present and which of the symptoms are most important to focus on in a specific patient. Also, symptoms are sometimes only intermittently present or even gradually disappear. Failure to take into account the exact nature of the symptoms in an individual patient with dementia will have negative implications for choosing the right treatment and evaluating it [14]. Several questions should be asked: What type of symptoms do we specifically observe? When did they start? What elicits them, makes them worse or improves them? Do they occur at specific times during the day or in connection with specific activities? How severe are the problems, and how often do the problematic symptoms occur? Careful analysis will determine the focus of treatment, enable evaluation of the treatment effect and help determine treatment goals. For example in a patient with highly intrusive, seemingly therapy-resistant screaming, reducing the frequency of the behaviour by half may be considered a success. These treatment goals are preferably set at the beginning of treatment.

It is best to involve caregivers and, if possible, patients in determining these treatment objectives.

Taking into account the context of the BPSD is also crucial. What is the environment the patient is living in? Is it possible to make changes to this environment? What environmental factors have a beneficial or worsening effect on the behaviour? For example wandering may not be a problem in the setting of a specialist care unit specifically designed to deal with patients with dementia, but it is a reason for concern in a community dwelling patient living alone. The same is true for "internal" contextual factors, like the beliefs and values of the patient. What matters to this patient? Are there life events the patient has gone through that have an effect on the current behaviour?

In recent years several models for structured assessment of patients with BPSD have been proposed that chiefly provide ways to do careful assessments but also to establish treatment plans and to evaluate treatment progression.

- The DICE (describe, investigate, create, evaluate) approach, developed by a national expert panel in the USA in 2014 [15], comprises four steps: (1) describing the symptoms and context in which they occur, including antecedents and triggers for the behaviour and which behaviours the patient and caregivers see as the most problematic; (2) investigating possible causes of the behaviour; (3) creating a treatment plan, which can include all kinds of treatments and modifications to the environment; and (4) evaluating the outcome of the treatment plan. The approach is the basis for a web-based tool called WeCareAdvisor™, which can be used to assess, manage and track BPSD [16].
- The Wisconsin STAR method maps five factors (medical, medication, social, personal and behavioural) that can contribute to BPSD into a single graphical interface, a five-pointed star. The visual representation takes into account the various factors simultaneously and aids in identifying missing data [17].
- Dynamic system analysis, a method developed in the Netherlands, assesses patients based on six dimensions, each assigned a colour: somatic, cognitive, personality, experience, communication and social. After observation and assessment, the problems identified in the analysis can be used to develop a treatment plan and establish treatment goals [18].

Scales exist for assessing BPSD in general and in terms of specific symptoms. Likely used most for general symptoms, the Neuropsychiatric Inventory (NPI) [19] comprises 12 domains with 7–9 items each. Per domain, frequency and severity over the past month are rated. A brief NPI questionnaire (NPI-Q) [20] is also available for use in routine clinical practice, and the nursing home version (NPI-NH) for use in extended care settings where professional caregivers provide the information [21]. The Behavioural Pathology in Alzheimer's Disease Rating Scale (BEHAVE-AD), also based on a caregiver interview, consists of 26 items [22] and is geared somewhat more to psychotic disorders [23]. Specific rating scales for various symptom domains are also available, for example the Cohen Mansfield Agitation Inventory [24], the Apathy Evaluation Scale [25], the Apathy Scale [26], the Apathy

Inventory [27], the Lille Apathy Rating Scale [28] and the Cornell Scale for Depression in Dementia [29].

Note that completing a full assessment of BPSD takes a considerable amount of time. In acute situations, it may be necessary to first address urgent symptom control, for example when violent behaviour is present. However, once the situation is safer, further careful assessment of BPSD should be undertaken.

Addressing Causative Problems of BPSD

After careful assessment, it is important to first look at modifiable causes of the behavioural and psychological symptoms. We will discuss some of the most frequent causes: medical problems, medication, caregiver approach and environmental factors.

Medical Problems

Virtually all medical problems may result in triggering or worsening BPSD. An acute onset of BPSD should cause suspicion of delirium. There is considerable overlap in symptoms between dementia, BPSD and delirium [30], and most patients with both dementia and delirium will manifest with some degree of BPSD. However, only a minority of patients with dementia and BPSD will also have comorbid delirium.

Of the possible medical problems that can cause BPSD, some of the most frequent are infection, pain, urinary retention, constipation, vision or hearing problems, electrolyte imbalances or metabolic disorders. As a result, a work-up of a patient with new or worsened BPSD should also include a full physical exam, blood analysis (blood count, c-reactive protein, serum electrolytes, serum glucose, kidney and liver function, thyroid-stimulating hormone and thiamine) and urine analysis (urinalysis with microscopy and urine culture). When necessary, other tests such as a chest X-ray or head CT scan should be ordered.

People with dementia are especially vulnerable to developing infections, e.g. urinary tract infections and pneumonia. Asymptomatic bacteriuria is often present in seniors, and most guidelines advise against treating it [31]. However, treatment of the bacteriuria in cases without typical symptoms of a urinary tract infection (dysuria, urgency, frequency and urethral purulence) but with an acute onset or worsening of BPSD may result in rapid improvement of BPSD. If possible, obtain a urine culture before starting antibiotic treatment [32].

Pain is especially prevalent in patients with dementia, with studies suggesting that undiagnosed and untreated pain may be present in more than 30% of community dwelling patients with dementia and 54–78% of patients with dementia in nursing homes [33]. As patients with dementia are less able to report, describe or deal with their pain (for instance, by changing posture), pain may manifest as BPSD-like agitation, depression and resistance to care. It is important to detect and remediate possible causes for pain, such as inadequate posture and ergonomic measures that cause the patient pain. If a painful condition is suspected and specific therapy directed at the underlying cause is not possible or is insufficient, it is recommended to start pain treatment with paracetamol (3 × 1000 mg daily) [34] in patients without a history of hepatic disease. When paracetamol proves insufficient, a stepwise approach for further pain treatment is advised; however, caution must be exercised when using other pain medication like non-steroidal anti-inflammatory drugs, tramadol and opioids, which can cause severe side effects in the elderly. Currently, routinely treating behavioural problems (without specific pain complaints) with mild analgesics is not recommended as this could neglect the identification of underlying causes [35]. Chapter 9 discusses the management of pain further.

Fairly innocent somatic problems, like constipation or cerumen, can give rise to severe behavioural problems and should be ruled out and regularly reassessed before moving to other forms of treatment for BPSD.

Medication

Various medications can also provoke or worsen BPSD. As polypharmacy is even more frequent in elderly people with dementia compared to people without dementia [36], medication or medication interactions may likely play a role in BPSD. Chapter 6 provides a full discussion and review of medication in patients with dementia. Medication with anticholinergic effects, in particular, are potentially harmful and can cause cognitive, emotional and behavioural problems [37]. Reducing the anticholinergic burden decreases the frequency and severity of BPSD among elderly people with dementia [38]. Sedatives are another class of drugs that can cause or worsen BPSD, for instance, benzodiazepines, which are frequently associated with delirium or apathy. Before considering additional drugs, conducting a thorough review of the medication list in patients with BSPD is advised. When a new medication is introduced, or an increased dose coincides with worsening of BPSD, it should, of course, be looked at more closely.

Caregiver Approach

Symptoms like agitation or depression can be triggered or worsened when formal or informal caregivers have a misunderstanding of or lack of familiarity with them. (Psycho)education on BPSD can thus often be effective in reducing the burden of these symptoms for both patients and caregivers [39].

Because the dementia process affects language and communication, it is important for caregivers to adjust their communication. Speaking clearly and slowly, offering step-by-step instructions, along with giving the person with dementia sufficient time to respond, are vital to avoiding frustration and agitation in a patient with moderate to severe dementia. On the other hand, since communication skills are not invariably impaired in dementia, making assumptions simply because of a dementia diagnosis should be avoided [40, 41].

The person-centred care approach, also known as patient-centred care, takes into account the individuality of the patient in relation to surrounding attitudes and care practices [42]. Evidence shows that training professional caregivers in person-centred care methods and skills reduces agitation and helps prevent emergent agitation [43].

Psychoeducation of informal caregivers can lead to better understanding of the neuropsychiatric symptoms of dementia. Explaining that for example agitation and aggressive behaviour are part of dementia and almost always not intentional can be helpful to family members. This can reduce the behavioural problems but also increase confidence and reduce stress in caregivers [44].

Environment

Information on the environment is important to determine further management of BPSD. For example confined spaces may more easily trigger agitation or even aggression. Adjusting the environment to reduce BPSD may be possible, with quite simple adaptations available, like creating more space to wander, removing unsafe objects, smartly using colours or camouflaging doors that trigger unrest. Some institutions have dementia-friendly gardens as green spaces and proximity to natural elements have a favourable impact on the wellbeing of people with dementia [45]. A sufficient influx of daylight is advisable to provide cues about the time of day and reduce circadian rhythm problems. Similarly, assorted options exist to adapt new architecture to people with dementia. This of course cannot always be changed in the short term but should be taken into account when building facilities to provide care for patients with dementia.

Non-pharmacological Treatment of BPSD

After careful assessment of the neuropsychiatric symptoms and after dealing with direct causes, the need for further treatment should be evaluated. When there are no symptoms associated with immediate danger to the patient (e.g. severe self-harm) or to others (such as severe physical aggression), non-pharmacological treatments should be considered first, not so much because these interventions are more evidence-based than medication—in general, they are not—but because they have less adverse effects compared to medication, especially in a population with already considerable frailty and polypharmacy. This does not mean that non-pharmacological interventions have no side effects at all. For example increased agitation has been described in cognitive or emotion-focused interventions, music therapy, massage and aromatherapy [46]. Like with most pharmacological treatments, the evidence in terms of the efficacy of various non-pharmacological treatments is rather limited.

The effects of various therapies can also vary significantly between individuals with dementia. Managing BPSD often requires taking a trial-and-error approach.

Specific Psychotherapeutic Interventions

There is a moderate amount of quality evidence that psychotherapeutic interventions like cognitive behavioural therapy can reduce depressive symptoms in people with dementia and limited evidence that they reduce anxiety [47]. For other symptoms like agitation or aggression, studies on systematic psychotherapy are lacking. Reminiscence therapy involves the discussion of past activities, events and experiences, usually aided by objects like photographs or familiar items from the past. There is some evidence that reminiscence therapy can improve mood and possibly behaviour in dementia [48].

Daily Routine and Activities

Keeping a daily routine provides structure, which helps the patient and caregivers by giving them something to navigate by. A tailored activity programme can be used to train caregivers in customised activity based on the person with dementia's current and previous interests and cognitive and physical abilities [46]. Reality orientation therapy uses repeated and meaningful stimulation of orientation in daily life to people, time or surroundings [49]. This can have beneficial effects on BPSD, mainly in combination with other interventions [50]. Occupational therapy attempts to find a fit between occupation, a person's capabilities and the physical and social environment in which they live in order to optimise participation in valued activities, roles and relationships. Occupational therapy in dementia tries to identify activities that are meaningful to the patient, taking into account the individual's capabilities and the physical and social environment in which they live [51, 52]. Occupational therapy was shown to have a positive effect on overall BPSD, the quality of life of both patients and carers, and on carer distress, but no significant effects were apparent in terms of depression or anxiety in patients [52]. Gardening can also help reduce BPSD [53], especially in patients who already have a history of gardening [54].

Exercise Therapy

Physical exercise can be defined as planned, structured, repetitive and purposeful physical activity. Exercise training seems to have a small beneficial effect in reducing depression in people with dementia [55]. There are also promising results for aberrant motor behaviour, agitation, apathy and eating disorders. There may also be a positive effect on sleep [55]. Another study found that physical exercise can inhibit or delay the emergence of more severe BPSD with dementia progression [56]. The positive effect of exercise may be due to psychological mechanisms like stress reduction, but also because it stimulates neuroplasticity or has an anti-inflammatory effect [55, 57]. The best type of exercise or duration has yet to be determined, although walking at least 30 min several times a week appears to be beneficial [58]. The effect of exercise on BPSD varies between individuals depending on the underlying mechanisms. For example structured exercise training may to some degree alleviate purposeless wandering due to psychomotor agitation, whereas wandering because of disorientation and feeling lost may not improve with exercise [58].

Sensory-Based Interventions

Both under- and overstimulation of the senses can result in BPSD-like agitation and hallucinations.

Moreover, age and dementia impact all sensory systems: vision, hearing, smell and taste, as well as proprioception and vestibular senses [54]. Progressive neuronal loss in major neurocognitive disorders may also lead to impaired processing of sensory stimuli, rendering normal stimuli confusing and thus resulting in BPSD [59].

Aromatherapy

Aromatherapy using aromatic oils is an olfactory stimulation intervention that is thought to have potential psychological effects based on an association between a pleasant smell and positive emotions, which involves limbic connections between the olfactory bulb and the amygdala. As many patients with dementia have at least partial anosmia caused by neurodegeneration, processing olfactory stimuli and the benefits of aromatherapy may differ considerably between subjects [60]. The terpenes used in aromatherapy may also have pharmacological effects that could affect GABA augmentation or acetylcholine receptors [61]. Existing studies exhibit significant differences in the use of aromatic oils (direct inhalation, oil directly on the skin, applying oil to a pillow and ingestion of oil), scents (lavender, lemon, thyme and rosemary) and duration of the intervention (2–4 weeks on average) [54]. A Cochrane Review [62] showing that there is a lack of large studies only included seven studies, two of which had useable data but inconclusive evidence. Side effects like nausea, diarrhoea and drowsiness have been reported [63].

Massage Therapy

Massage or touch therapy is a form of tactile sensory stimulation. Touch can have an immediate calming, reassuring effect, possibly by stimulating the production of hormones like oxytocin. Touch also represents a way of communicating meaningfully with others when verbal communication is hampered, a way of literally "staying in touch" [64]. The areas of the body involved (back, shoulders, back of the neck, hands, arms, feet and legs) vary between studies, just as the type of stroking or style of touching, the duration of the intervention (1–30 min), number of sessions (10–50) and the provider (nursing staff, therapist, family members) [64]. A 2012 review [65] found only one study of good methodological quality, and that study showed that massage had a good effect on agitated behaviours with no documented negative side effects [66].

Multisensory Stimulation, Snoezelen and Virtual Reality

Snoezelen rooms derive their name from a blend of the Dutch word *snuffelen* (to sniff) and *doezelen* (to doze), the former referring to the more active aspects of the intervention and the latter to the more passive elements. Snoezelen is a therapy that takes place in a specially designed room filled with diverse soothing, multisensory stimulation, which usually includes aromatherapy, lighting effects, colour, water columns, sandboxes and music. It involves one-to-one attention, a nondirective approach encouraging patients to engage with sensory stimuli of their choice, and does not require any cognitive processing [67]. Although evidence is limited, Snoezelen rooms appear to have some positive effects on BPSD like agitation [59].

Other controlled multisensory environments include sensory gardens designed for people with dementia in mind in several hospitals across the globe. Fragrant (and edible) plants, water and art installations are examples of the assorted elements that can be incorporated [68]. Simulation of an external sensory world using virtual reality is also a therapeutic option that makes virtually visiting the beach, forest or a cathedral possible. Emerging evidence indicates that this can help improve mood and reduce aggression. Virtual reality can also be used as an aid in reminiscence therapy [69]. Newer virtual reality applications no longer require practice beforehand, as was previously the case. For example immersive virtual reality uses head-mounted displays to achieve immersion by excluding external visual input and updating the simulated visual environment in relation to head movements [70]. These applications can also be built into rooms, or interactive virtual environments can be projected onto a table [71].

Arts-Based Interventions

Humour Therapy and Elder Clowns

Humour therapy involves using comedy to elicit laughter and induce a feeling of happiness. Elderly clowns engage with each patient on a personal level. They usually work with information obtained from caregivers about each individual's history, abilities and interests. They combine this information with their own experience and intuition to create tailored interactions with the patient with dementia. The clown often uses techniques like stimulating questions to engage in conversation, acting foolish to provide patients with the opportunity to tell the clown what to do, but also magic, singing, musical instruments and dance [72]. A large Australian study involving 35 nursing homes showed a reduction in agitation after 9–12 weekly humour therapy sessions with elderly clowns, augmented by resident engagement involving staff trained as laughter bosses (healthcare practitioners trained to assist elder clowns in introducing humour in care practices and to continue the humour intervention between elder clown visits) [73, 74]. A smaller Canadian study also found a reduction in overall BPSD and particularly agitation [74].

Music Therapy

Even as people with dementia lose the ability to speak or understand language, they may still be able to hum or play along with the music. Music-based therapeutic interventions can be receptive (listening to music played or selected by the therapist), active (actively involved in making the music) or a combination of the two. Most studies used an intervention with both receptive and active elements [75]. There is some evidence that suggests that receptive music therapy is better than active in reducing BPSD [76]. Music therapy seems to be mainly effective for depressive symptoms [75] and apathy [77]. Effects on symptoms like agitation and aggression are less clear [75], although beneficial effects have been reported [78].

Art Therapy

There is some anecdotal evidence that participating in an art class [79] or individualised art therapy [80] can reduce symptoms like agitation.

Bright Light Therapy

Improving the lighting in residential care to whole-day bright light could possibly have a positive effect on mood and agitation [81, 82]. One randomised controlled trial found an effect on agitation, though only in combination with melatonin [81]. Effects may be better in patients with milder dementia due to a more intact suprachiasmatic nucleus [83], and effects may be larger in winter months [82]. Overall the evidence is mixed and not very convincing [84, 85].

Pharmacological Treatment of BPSD

When non-pharmacological treatment fails, in the case of an emergency or when BPSD poses a threat to the patient with dementia or others, pharmacological treatment may be warranted. It must be noted, however, that virtually no drugs are officially approved for the treatment of BPSD, with only risperidone approved in some parts of the world [44]. Physicians should carefully weigh the benefits versus the risks. We provide an overview of the different medication classes that can be

Table 7.1 Pharmacological and neuromodulation treatments to consider for various neuropsychiatric symptoms of dementia when biological treatment is deemed necessary

Symptom	Consider	When treatment-resistant also consider	Specific circumstances
Agitation	SSRI, atypical antipsychotics, AChI	Trazodone	In FTD consider trazodone as first-choice pharmacological treatment
Aggression	Atypical antipsychotics	AChI, benzodiazepines, trazodone	When rapid, short-term sedation is necessary, consider benzodiazepines
Apathy	AChI	Methylphenidate	
Depression	SSRI (except paroxetine)	SNRI, ECT	With severe concomitant loss of appetite or sleeping problems, consider mirtazapine
Anxiety	SSRI (except paroxetine)		When quick relief of severe anxiety is necessary, consider benzodiazepines
Hallucinations/delusions	Atypical antipsychotics, AChI		In LBD/PD, preferably use quetiapine, rivastigmine or clozapine
Sexually inappropriate behaviour	SSRI (except paroxetine)	Atypical antipsychotics	In very severe hypersexuality, consider consulting an endocrinologist to discuss anti-androgens and gonadotrophin-releasing hormone analogues

AChI acetylcholinesterase inhibitor, *ECT* electroconvulsive therapy, *FTD* frontotemporal dementia, *LBD* Lewy body dementia, *PD* Parkinson's dementia, *SNRI* serotonin-norepinephrine reuptake inhibitor, *SSRI* selective serotonin reuptake inhibitor

considered for the treatment of BPSD, with Table 7.1 containing a synopsis of which drugs to consider for specific symptoms.

Cognitive Enhancers

Acetylcholinesterase inhibitors (AChI), like rivastigmine, donepezil and galantamine, are generally used for the treatment of cognitive symptoms of dementia but can be used for some BPSD as well. Probably the strongest evidence for AChI exists for the treatment of apathy. Donepezil, rivastigmine and galantamine have all shown to be beneficial to patients with apathy, in several types of dementia, probably with the exception of FTD [86]. AChI, like rivastigmine, can have good effects on hallucinations, especially in LBD [87]. AChI may also have some beneficial effects on agitation and aggression, although results are inconsistent [88, 89]. A 2017 study found significant effects of the rivastigmine patch on non-aggressive agitated behaviours [90]; however, there is currently insufficient evidence to recommend one AChI over another. Common side effects of AChI include bradycardia (Special caution is warranted in patients with pre-existing cardiovascular disorders), gastrointestinal side effects (e.g. nausea, anorexia, diarrhoea, etc.), headache and dizziness.

Memantine, an *N*-Methyl-D-aspartate receptor antagonist, may have some beneficial effects on mood and behaviour, especially in moderate to severe Alzheimer's dementia and in vascular dementia [91]. Smaller studies also suggest some improvement of mood and behaviour in PD, LBD and FTD [91]. In patients with moderate to severe AD not selected for agitation at baseline, the proportion reporting agitation at follow-up is reduced by memantine [91]. However, memantine is not effective for treating agitation in dementia and may even worsen agitation [91]. Common side effects include headache, dizziness, obstipation, confusion and hallucinations.

A combination of AChI and memantine results in better outcomes on mood and behaviour when compared to memantine in monotherapy. However, patients on memantine monotherapy probably develop less agitation than patients receiving placebo or memantine plus an AChI. Further studies are needed to determine the efficacy of AChI and memantine in the treatment of BPSD [91].

Antidepressants

Antidepressants are often used for the treatment of BPSD, mainly because they are well tolerated and have less side effects compared to other pharmacological interventions.

Antidepressants are the first choice in the treatment of depression in dementia. However, there is actually little evidence of their efficacy in depression in dementia [92]. There is insufficient evidence to recommend one antidepressant over another, but antidepressants with high anticholinergic activity like tricyclic antidepressants and paroxetine should be avoided because of side effects. On the other hand, other selective serotonin reuptake inhibitors (SSRIs) like sertraline and (es)citalopram are generally well tolerated. Although not proven effective specifically in the treatment of depression in dementia, other antidepressants could be considered in specific circumstances or treatment-resistant depression. Serotonin-norepinephrine reuptake inhibitors like venlafaxine and duloxetine could be considered when depression responds insufficiently to SSRIs and could be especially useful in patients with comorbid chronic (neuropathic) pain. Mirtazapine could be considered when there is a severe concomitant loss of appetite or sleeping problems [93]. Almost all antidepressants can cause hyponatremia, which is why checking the plasma sodium level at baseline and at follow-up is recommended [94].

For the treatment of agitation, there is evidence for the beneficial effect of citalopram. However, the Citalopram for Agitation in Alzheimer Disease (CitAD) trial [95] showed this beneficial effect at a dose of 30 mg, a dose that also resulted in mild cognitive adverse effects and, more worrisome, in QT interval prolongation. Risk of QT prolongation may be somewhat lower with escitalopram [96], although when citalopram is not utilised based on risk factors for torsades de pointes, use of escitalopram is probably not the safest alternative [97]. Doses higher than 20 mg of citalopram or 10 mg of escitalopram in the elderly are not recommended. Sertraline, which has also shown effects on agitation in dementia [98], has a more favourable cardiac side effect profile [97]. Trazodone could have minor effects on agitation, although the effect in two studies was not significant [99, 100]. A small study in patients with FTD showed beneficial effects of trazodone 150–300 mg on eating disorders, irritability, agitation and depressive symptoms [101, 102]. We recommend starting with low doses of trazodone (e.g. 25 mg) and titrate slowly (cave risk of orthostatic hypotension and falls).

There have been no trials specifically involving the use of antidepressants for anxiety in dementia [103], but based on their effects in other patients groups, starting SSRIs for anxiety disorders in dementia appears to be reasonable.

A specific symptom in which antidepressants can be useful is sexually inappropriate behaviours in dementia, probably because of their anti-obsessional and anti-libidinal effects. An SSRI (sertraline and (es)citalopram) or trazodone should be considered first [104].

Finally, antidepressants can be used to treat pseudobulbar affect [105].

Antipsychotics

Antipsychotics are very frequently used in the management of BPSD, especially in the treatment of agitation and aggression. However, for many years, there have been safety concerns regarding antipsychotics in dementia, as highlighted by the US Food and Drug Administration's 2005 black box warning and by the European Medicines Agency's safety warnings in 2004 and 2009 [106]. These warnings cover both typical and atypical antipsychotics. Meta-analyses of clinical trials have demonstrated 1.5–1.7 times increased risk of mortality. Atypical antipsychotics are also linked to a 2–3 times higher risk of cerebrovascular events. The absolute risk difference for death is estimated to be around 1%, at least for treatment for 8–12 weeks [107, 108]. The actual risk may be as high as 4–5%, depending on the drug [107]. It is unclear whether this risk further increases with treatment beyond 8–12 weeks [107], but it is very likely that the elevated risk of death and morbidity is present even with short durations of treatment. Conventional antipsychotics, like haloperidol, have a similar, if not higher, risk of death than atypical agents [109]. Other adverse effects include extrapyramidal symptoms, cardiovascular and metabolic effects, cognitive worsening, infections and falls [110]. This is all reason for concern, and the prescription of antipsychotics to patients with dementia should not be taken lightly. On the other hand, antipsychotics can have a good effect on patients with severe agitation, aggression and psychosis. Expert consensus suggests that the use of an antipsychotic medication in individuals with dementia can be appropriate, particularly in individuals with dangerous agitation or psychosis, and can lower the risk of violence, reduce patient distress, improve patient quality of life and reduce caregiver burden [111]. However, in clinical trials, the benefits of antipsychotic medications are at best small and have not been shown to be effective beyond 3 months [111].

As also advised by the American Psychiatric Association [111], their use should be reserved for symptoms that are severe, dangerous and/or cause significant distress to the patient. In a non-urgent context, non-pharmacological interventions should be considered first, and of course, other causes for BPSD (e.g. pain and other medication) should be considered, as described above. Patients should be started on a low dose that is titrated slowly to the minimum effective dose [111]. In general, long-acting injectable antipsychotic medication is not recommended (unless otherwise indicated for a co-occurring chronic psychotic disorder) [111]. In general, in patients with LBD and PD, antipsychotics should be avoided, as severe neuroleptic sensitivity reactions are possible [112]. Before initiation of antipsychotics, it is advised to perform electrocardiography. Evidence on the metabolic effects of antipsychotics is not as strong in individuals with dementia as in younger adults, and specific recommendations about the timing of laboratory monitoring have not been developed for individuals with dementia. Based on recommendations for individuals with psychotic disorders like schizophrenia, it can be recommended to assess the blood pressure, weight, body mass index, waist circumference, fasting glucose, fasting lipid profile and personal/family history of patients with dementia. These assessments should be repeated regularly as long as patients are on an antipsychotic [111, 113].

When looking at specific antipsychotics in detail, randomised placebo-controlled trials seem to suggest efficacy for risperidone in treating psychosis and for risperidone, olanzapine and aripiprazole in treating agitation. Insufficient evidence exists on which atypical antipsychotic is both safest and most beneficial [114, 115]. Risperidone is the only drug licenced for the treatment of severe BPSD in some parts of the world. Quetiapine, which shows somewhat mixed evidence, likely requires doses of 100–200 mg, resulting in more side effects [44, 111, 114, 115]. In LBD and PD, quetiapine and clozapine are the antipsychotic medications of choice because of fewer extrapyramidal side effects [116]. However, close follow-up is mandatory in those conditions, given the risk of sedation for both drugs and the risk of agranulocytosis for clozapine.

Given the similar, or even higher, risk of death when using conventional antipsychotics [109, 111], it is generally advisable to avoid using them in patients with dementia, with the exception of the treatment of delirium with haloperidol.

A 2018 Cochrane Review [117] concluded that discontinuation of antipsychotics after patients had taken them for at least 3 months probably has little or no effect on BPSD. In light of the possible negative effects of antipsychotics, tapering and stopping the antipsychotics after 8–12 weeks of treatment for BPSD should be considered. However, according to the same review, it remains unclear whether there are any positive effects on cognitive functioning, quality of life or mortality when the antipsychotic agent is withdrawn [117]. Two studies suggest there may be a benefit from continuing antipsychotic treatment in patients with severe neuropsychiatric symptoms at baseline (NPI score > 14) [118, 119].

Mood Stabilisers

Carbamazepine has shown efficacy for the treatment of global BPSD and the symptoms of aggression, hostility and (possibly) agitation [120]. However, the high risk of drug-drug interactions and serious adverse effects like Stevens-Johnson syndrome limit its use considerably. Evidence for antipsychotics in BPSD is more robust. Carbamazepine could be considered for patients who are sensitive or unresponsive to antipsychotics, have significant cardiovascular risk factors and are aggressive or hostile, but not delusional [120]. There is no evidence of the beneficial effects of valproate on agitation, and serious adverse effects are possible [121]. There is not enough evidence to currently recommend other anti-epileptic drugs or lithium for BPSD [120].

Benzodiazepines

There is only limited data on the efficacy of the use of benzodiazepines for the treatment of BPSD [122]. However, they can have severe adverse effects, especially in the elderly, like drowsiness, increased risk of falls and fractures [122] and negative effects on cognition [123]. In general, it is not advisable to use benzodiazepines in the treatment of BPSD, but there are specific situations where benzodiazepines may be useful. For example, when other psychotropic medications are deemed unsafe or not tolerated by the patient (e.g. for cardiovascular reasons or in severe PD or LBD) or in emergency use where sedation or fast relief of severe anxiety is wanted [122]. Generally, lorazepam and oxazepam are preferred, as they require no oxidative metabolism in the liver and have no active metabolites [122, 124]. Occasionally, the ultra-brief-acting midazolam could be considered in acute (response) agitation [125, 126].

Other Drugs

Methylphenidate has been proposed for the treatment of apathy in dementia, although evidence is currently of low quality [127]. Methylphenidate and dextroamphetamine could also have a positive effect on risk taking and disinhibition, and apathy, respectively, in FTD [102]. However, methylphenidate is contraindicated in agitation and can have side effects like hypertension [127, 128].

Dextromethorphan with quinidine showed promise for the treatment of agitation in one randomised controlled trial, but the effects were small [129]. More research is needed to confirm these findings.

Melatonin may have some beneficial effects on sundowning, but the evidence is mixed. Care should be taken not to advance the sleep-wake cycle, just as an effort should be made to align exogenous melatonin administration with estimated endogenous secretion [130].

Neuromodulation

Electroconvulsive therapy (ECT) involves the delivery of direct electrical current to the patient under general anaesthesia to induce a generalised seizure for therapeutic purposes. ECT is a safe and remarkably effective therapy for depression in the elderly, including in patients with dementia [131]. ECT may also be a safe, effective treatment for severe and treatment-refractory agitation and aggression in dementia. A systematic review found a clinically significant improvement in 88% of 122 patients treated with ECT. Adverse effects from ECT were most commonly mild and transient [131]. Although the cumulated anecdotal evidence favours the use of ECT in treatment-resistant severe symptoms of agitation and aggression, a randomised clinical trial to support its efficacy is currently lacking [132].

There is emerging evidence that repetitive transcranial magnetic stimulation, which uses a magnetic field to stimulate the (dorsolateral prefrontal) cortex, might have a positive effect on BPSD, but larger trials are needed to confirm these findings [133]. Transcranial direct current stimulation delivers mild electric currents to the scalp but does not seem to result so far in substantial effects on BPSD [133].

Conclusion

BPSD is very prevalent in dementia, the symptoms debilitating to both the patient with dementia and the patient's environment. By increasing caregiver burden and earlier institutionalisation, BPSD is also strongly associated with increased healthcare and economic costs.

Every treatment of BPSD should start with careful assessment of the symptoms, the patient and the context. After this assessment, it is important to identify modifiable underlying causes of the BPSD, like medical problems, medication, caregiver approach and environmental factors. After careful assessment of the neuropsychiatric symptoms, and after dealing with direct causes, the need for further treatment should be evaluated. When there are no symptoms associated with immediate danger to the patient or others, non-pharmacological treatments should be considered first. When non-pharmacological treatment fails, in the case of an emergency or when BPSD poses a threat to the individual with dementia or others, pharmacological treatment may be warranted.

However, few of the non-pharmacological or pharmacological treatment interventions for BPSD have shown convincing efficacy so far. In clinical practice, treatment strategies that work well in one patient may result in no effect or even have an adverse outcome in others. This is related to the diverse nature of these symptoms and their varying pathogenesis between individuals with dementia. For example one intervention may be useful for hallucinations but not for delusions. Similarly, one person with dementia may be agitated because of under-stimulation due to boredom and a lack of personal contact, whereas another subject may be agitated because of overstimulation. For the first person, interventions with extra stimuli may of course be helpful but not in the latter subject, resulting in a lack of overall efficacy in the context of a clinical trial. Moreover, in many studies, patients with the most severe BPSD are likely to be underrepresented. There is thus a clear need for more detailed studies focusing on subgroups of patients, and with a careful description of the symptoms, variables and outcomes, to develop more personalised treatment strategies.

Just as important, some of these patients with very severe BPSD and sometimes multiple comorbidities will require a multifaceted approach and much creativity on the part of the physicians caring for them.

References

1. Finkel SI, Burns A. BPSD consensus statement. International Psychogeriatric Association. Northfield, IL, United States; 1999.
2. Steinberg M, Shao H, Zandi P, Lyketsos CG, Welsh-Bohmer KA, Norton MC, et al. Point and 5-year period prevalence of neuropsychiatric symptoms in dementia: the Cache County Study. Int J Geriatr Psychiatry. 2008;23(2):170–7. https://doi.org/10.1002/gps.1858.
3. Monastero R, Mangialasche F, Camarda C, Ercolani S, Camarda R. A systematic review of neuropsychiatric symptoms in mild cognitive impairment. J Alzheimers Dis. 2009;18(1):11–30. https://doi.org/10.3233/JAD-2009-1120.
4. Ismail Z, Smith EE, Geda Y, Sultzer D, Brodaty H, Smith G, et al. Neuropsychiatric symptoms as early manifestations of emergent dementia: provisional diagnostic criteria for mild behavioral impairment. Alzheimers Dement. 2016;12(2):195–202. https://doi.org/10.1016/j.jalz.2015.05.017.
5. Canevelli M, Adali N, Cantet C, Andrieu S, Bruno G, Cesari M, et al. Impact of behavioral subsyndromes on cognitive decline in Alzheimer's disease: data from the ICTUS study. J Neurol. 2013;260(7):1859–65. https://doi.org/10.1007/s00415-013-6893-3.
6. Tatsumi H, Nakaaki S, Torii K, Shinagawa Y, Watanabe N, Murata Y, et al. Neuropsychiatric symptoms predict change in quality of life of Alzheimer disease patients: a two-year follow-up study. Psychiatry Clin Neurosci. 2009;63(3):374–84. https://doi.org/10.1111/j.1440-1819.2009.01955.x.
7. Karttunen K, Karppi P, Hiltunen A, Vanhanen M, Valimaki T, Martikainen J, et al. Neuropsychiatric symptoms and quality of life in patients with very mild and mild Alzheimer's disease. Int J Geriatr Psychiatry. 2011;26(5):473–82. https://doi.org/10.1002/gps.2550.
8. Ryu SH, Ha JH, Park DH, Yu J, Livingston G. Persistence of neuropsychiatric symptoms over six months in mild cognitive impairment in community-dwelling Korean elderly. Int Psychogeriatr. 2011;23(2):214–20. https://doi.org/10.1017/S1041610210001766.
9. Chen P, Guarino PD, Dysken MW, Pallaki M, Asthana S, Llorente MD, et al. Neuropsychiatric symptoms and caregiver burden in individuals with Alzheimer's disease: the TEAM-AD VA cooperative study. J Geriatr Psychiatry Neurol. 2018;31(4):177–85. https://doi.org/10.1177/0891988718783897.
10. Schoenmakers B, Buntinx F, Devroey D, Van Casteren V, DeLepeleire J. The process of definitive institutionalization of community dwelling demented vs non demented elderly: data obtained from a network of sentinel general practitioners. Int J Geriatr Psychiatry. 2009;24(5):523–31. https://doi.org/10.1002/gps.2147.
11. Gaugler JE, Wall MM, Kane RL, Menk JS, Sarsour K, Johnston JA, et al. The effects of incident and persistent behavioral problems on change in caregiver burden and nursing home admission of persons with dementia. Med Care. 2010;48(10):875–83. https://doi.org/10.1097/MLR.0b013e3181ec557b.
12. Beeri MS, Werner P, Davidson M, Noy S. The cost of behavioral and psychological symptoms of dementia (BPSD) in community dwelling Alzheimer's disease patients. Int J Geriatr Psychiatry. 2002;17(5):403–8. https://doi.org/10.1002/gps.490.
13. Costa N, Wubker A, De Mauleon A, Zwakhalen SMG, Challis D, Leino-Kilpi H, et al. Costs of care of agitation associated with dementia in 8 European countries: results from the RightTimePlaceCare study. J Am Med Dir Assoc. 2018;19(1):95.e1–e10. https://doi.org/10.1016/j.jamda.2017.10.013.
14. Maust DT, Kales HC. Bringing precision medicine to the management of BPSD. Am J Geriatr Psychiatry. 2017;25(5):469–70. https://doi.org/10.1016/j.jagp.2017.02.010.

15. Kales HC, Gitlin LN, Lyketsos CG, Detroit Expert Panel on Assessment and Management of Neuropsychiatric Symptoms of Dementia. Management of neuropsychiatric symptoms of dementia in clinical settings: recommendations from a multidisciplinary expert panel. J Am Geriatr Soc. 2014;62(4):762–9. https://doi.org/10.1111/jgs.12730.
16. Kales HC, Gitlin LN, Stanislawski B, Myra Kim H, Marx K, Turnwald M, et al. Effect of the WeCareAdvisor on family caregiver outcomes in dementia: a pilot randomized controlled trial. BMC Geriatr. 2018;18(1):113. https://doi.org/10.1186/s12877-018-0801-8.
17. Howell T. The Wisconsin Star Method: understanding and addressing complexity in geriatrics. In: Malone M, Capezuti E, Palmer R, editors. Geriatric models of care: bringing 'best practice' to an aging America. Cham: Springer International; 2015. p. 87–94.
18. van Helden M. Kleur bekennen in de psychogeriatrie—DSA in zakformaat. Maarssen: Elsevier gezondheidszorg; 2004.
19. Cummings JL. The neuropsychiatric inventory: assessing psychopathology in dementia patients. Neurology. 1997;48(5 Suppl 6):S10–6. https://doi.org/10.1212/wnl.48.5_suppl_6.10s.
20. Kaufer DI, Cummings JL, Ketchel P, Smith V, MacMillan A, Shelley T, et al. Validation of the NPI-Q, a brief clinical form of the neuropsychiatric inventory. J Neuropsychiatry Clin Neurosci. 2000;12(2):233–9. https://doi.org/10.1176/jnp.12.2.233.
21. Wood S, Cummings JL, Hsu MA, Barclay T, Wheatley MV, Yarema KT, et al. The use of the neuropsychiatric inventory in nursing home residents. Characterization and measurement. Am J Geriatr Psychiatry. 2000;8(1):75–83. https://doi.org/10.1097/00019442-200002000-00010.
22. Reisberg B, Auer SR, Monteiro IM. Behavioral pathology in Alzheimer's disease (BEHAVE-AD) rating scale. Int Psychogeriatr. 1996;8(Suppl 3):301–8.; discussion 51-4. https://doi.org/10.1097/00019442-199911001-00147.
23. David R, Mulin E, Mallea P, Robert PH. Measurement of neuropsychiatric symptoms in clinical trials targeting Alzheimer's disease and related disorders. Pharmaceuticals (Basel). 2010;3(8):2387–97. https://doi.org/10.3390/ph3082387.
24. Cohen-Mansfield J. Conceptualization of agitation: results based on the Cohen-Mansfield agitation inventory and the agitation behavior mapping instrument. Int Psychogeriatr. 1996;8(Suppl 3):309–15.; discussion 51-4. https://doi.org/10.1017/s1041610297003530.
25. Marin RS, Biedrzycki RC, Firinciogullari S. Reliability and validity of the apathy evaluation scale. Psychiatry Res. 1991;38(2):143–62. https://doi.org/10.1016/0165-1781(91)90040-v.
26. Starkstein SE, Mayberg HS, Preziosi TJ, Andrezejewski P, Leiguarda R, Robinson RG. Reliability, validity, and clinical correlates of apathy in Parkinson's disease. J Neuropsychiatry Clin Neurosci. 1992;4(2):134–9. https://doi.org/10.1176/jnp.4.2.134.
27. Robert PH, Clairet S, Benoit M, Koutaich J, Bertogliati C, Tible O, et al. The apathy inventory: assessment of apathy and awareness in Alzheimer's disease, Parkinson's disease and mild cognitive impairment. Int J Geriatr Psychiatry. 2002;17(12):1099–105. https://doi.org/10.1002/gps.755.
28. Sockeel P, Dujardin K, Devos D, Deneve C, Destee A, Defebvre L. The Lille apathy rating scale (LARS), a new instrument for detecting and quantifying apathy: validation in Parkinson's disease. J Neurol Neurosurg Psychiatry. 2006;77(5):579–84. https://doi.org/10.1136/jnnp.2005.075929.
29. Alexopoulos GS, Abrams RC, Young RC, Shamoian CA. Cornell scale for depression in dementia. Biol Psychiatry. 1988;23(3):271–84. https://doi.org/10.1016/0006-3223(88)90038-8.
30. Holtta E, Laakkonen ML, Laurila JV, Strandberg TE, Tilvis R, Kautiainen H, et al. The overlap of delirium with neuropsychiatric symptoms among patients with dementia. Am J Geriatr Psychiatry. 2011;19(12):1034–41. https://doi.org/10.1097/JGP.0b013e31820dcbb6.
31. Nicolle LE, Gupta K, Bradley SF, Colgan R, DeMuri GP, Drekonja D, et al. Clinical practice guideline for the management of asymptomatic bacteriuria: 2019 update by the Infectious Diseases Society of America. Clin Infect Dis. 2019;68(10):e83–e110. https://doi.org/10.1093/cid/ciy1121.
32. Miller J. To treat or not to treat: managing bacteriuria in elderly people. CMAJ. 2001;164(5):619–20.

33. Husebo BS, Strand LI, Moe-Nilssen R, Borgehusebo S, Aarsland D, Ljunggren AE. Who suffers most? Dementia and pain in nursing home patients: a cross-sectional study. J Am Med Dir Assoc. 2008;9(6):427–33. https://doi.org/10.1016/j.jamda.2008.03.001.
34. Husebo BS, Achterberg W, Flo E. Identifying and managing pain in people with Alzheimer's disease and other types of dementia: a systematic review. CNS Drugs. 2016;30(6):481–97. https://doi.org/10.1007/s40263-016-0342-7.
35. Frederiksen KS, Cooper C, Frisoni GB, Frolich L, Georges J, Kramberger MG, et al. A European Academy of Neurology guideline on medical management issues in dementia. Eur J Neurol. 2020; https://doi.org/10.1111/ene.14412.
36. Kristensen RU, Norgaard A, Jensen-Dahm C, Gasse C, Wimberley T, Waldemar G. Polypharmacy and potentially inappropriate medication in people with dementia: a nationwide study. J Alzheimers Dis. 2018;63(1):383–94. https://doi.org/10.3233/JAD-170905.
37. Pinto T, Lanctot KL, Herrmann N. Revisiting the cholinergic hypothesis of behavioral and psychological symptoms in dementia of the Alzheimer's type. Ageing Res Rev. 2011;10(4):404–12. https://doi.org/10.1016/j.arr.2011.01.003.
38. Jaidi Y, Nonnonhou V, Kanagaratnam L, Bertholon LA, Badr S, Noel V, et al. Reduction of the anticholinergic burden makes it possible to decrease behavioral and psychological symptoms of dementia. Am J Geriatr Psychiatry. 2018;26(3):280–8. https://doi.org/10.1016/j.jagp.2017.08.005.
39. Livingston G, Sommerlad A, Orgeta V, Costafreda SG, Huntley J, Ames D, et al. Dementia prevention, intervention, and care. Lancet. 2017;390(10113):2673–734. https://doi.org/10.1016/S0140-6736(17)31363-6.
40. Banovic S, Zunic LJ, Sinanovic O. Communication difficulties as a result of dementia. Mater Sociomed. 2018;30(3):221–4. https://doi.org/10.5455/msm.2018.30.221-224.
41. Alzheimer's Association. Communication and Alzheimer's. https://www.alz.org/help-support/caregiving/daily-care/communications. Accessed 2 Dec 2020.
42. Kim SK, Park M. Effectiveness of person-centered care on people with dementia: a systematic review and meta-analysis. Clin Interv Aging. 2017;12:381–97. https://doi.org/10.2147/CIA.S117637.
43. Livingston G, Kelly L, Lewis-Holmes E, Baio G, Morris S, Patel N, et al. A systematic review of the clinical effectiveness and cost-effectiveness of sensory, psychological and behavioural interventions for managing agitation in older adults with dementia. Health Technol Assess. 2014;18(39):1–226, v–vi. https://doi.org/10.3310/hta18390.
44. Bessey LJ, Walaszek A. Management of behavioral and psychological symptoms of dementia. Curr Psychiatry Rep. 2019;21(8):66. https://doi.org/10.1007/s11920-019-1049-5.
45. Liao ML, Ou SJ, Heng Hsieh C, Li Z, Ko CC. Effects of garden visits on people with dementia: a pilot study. Dementia (London). 2020;19(4):1009–28. https://doi.org/10.1177/1471301218793319.
46. Kales HC, Gitlin LN, Lyketsos CG. Assessment and management of behavioral and psychological symptoms of dementia. BMJ. 2015;350:h369. https://doi.org/10.1136/bmj.h369.
47. Orgeta V, Qazi A, Spector A, Orrell M. Psychological treatments for depression and anxiety in dementia and mild cognitive impairment: systematic review and meta-analysis. Br J Psychiatry. 2015;207(4):293–8. https://doi.org/10.1192/bjp.bp.114.148130.
48. Woods B, Spector A, Jones C, Orrell M, Davies S. Reminiscence therapy for dementia. Cochrane Database Syst Rev. 2005;2:CD001120. https://doi.org/10.1002/14651858.CD001120.pub2.
49. Chiu HY, Chen PY, Chen YT, Huang HC. Reality orientation therapy benefits cognition in older people with dementia: a meta-analysis. Int J Nurs Stud. 2018;86:20–8. https://doi.org/10.1016/j.ijnurstu.2018.06.008.
50. Tible OP, Riese F, Savaskan E, von Gunten A. Best practice in the management of behavioural and psychological symptoms of dementia. Ther Adv Neurol Disord. 2017;10(8):297–309. https://doi.org/10.1177/1756285617712979.
51. Law M, Cooper B, Strong S, Stewart D, Rigby P, Letts L, et al. Can J Occup Ther. 1996;63(1):9–23. https://doi.org/10.1177/000841749606300103.

52. Bennett S, Laver K, Voigt-Radloff S, Letts L, Clemson L, Graff M, et al. Occupational therapy for people with dementia and their family carers provided at home: a systematic review and meta-analysis. BMJ Open. 2019;9(11):e026308. https://doi.org/10.1136/bmjopen-2018-026308.
53. Pedrinolla A, Tamburin S, Brasioli A, Sollima A, Fonte C, Muti E, et al. An indoor therapeutic garden for behavioral symptoms in Alzheimer's disease: a randomized controlled trial. J Alzheimers Dis. 2019;71(3):813–23. https://doi.org/10.3233/JAD-190394.
54. Smith BC, D'Amico M. Sensory-based interventions for adults with dementia and Alzheimer's disease: a scoping review. Occup Ther Health Care. 2020;34(3):171–201. https://doi.org/10.1080/07380577.2019.1608488.
55. Barreto Pde S, Demougeot L, Pillard F, Lapeyre-Mestre M, Rolland Y. Exercise training for managing behavioral and psychological symptoms in people with dementia: a systematic review and meta-analysis. Ageing Res Rev. 2015;24(Pt B):274–85. https://doi.org/10.1016/j.arr.2015.09.001.
56. Hoffmann K, Sobol NA, Frederiksen KS, Beyer N, Vogel A, Vestergaard K, et al. Moderate-to-high intensity physical exercise in patients with Alzheimer's disease: a randomized controlled trial. J Alzheimers Dis. 2016;50(2):443–53. https://doi.org/10.3233/JAD-150817.
57. Matura S, Carvalho AF, Alves GS, Pantel J. Physical exercise for the treatment of neuropsychiatric disturbances in Alzheimer's dementia: possible mechanisms, current evidence and future directions. Curr Alzheimer Res. 2016;13(10):1112–23. https://doi.org/10.2174/1567205013666160502123428.
58. Thune-Boyle IC, Iliffe S, Cerga-Pashoja A, Lowery D, Warner J. The effect of exercise on behavioral and psychological symptoms of dementia: towards a research agenda. Int Psychogeriatr. 2012;24(7):1046–57. https://doi.org/10.1017/S1041610211002365.
59. Cheng C, Baker GB, Dursun SM. Use of multisensory stimulation interventions in the treatment of major neurocognitive disorders. Psychiatr Clin Psychopharmacol. 2019;29(4):916–21. https://doi.org/10.1080/24750573.2019.1699738.
60. Holmes C, Ballard C. Aromatherapy in dementia. Adv Psychiatr Treat. 2004;10(4):296–300. https://doi.org/10.1192/apt.10.4.296.
61. Nguyen QA, Paton C. The use of aromatherapy to treat behavioural problems in dementia. Int J Geriatr Psychiatry. 2008;23(4):337–46. https://doi.org/10.1002/gps.1886.
62. Forrester LT, Maayan N, Orrell M, Spector AE, Buchan LD, Soares-Weiser K. Aromatherapy for dementia. Cochrane Database Syst Rev. 2014;2:CD003150. https://doi.org/10.1002/14651858.CD003150.pub2.
63. Fung JK, Tsang HW, Chung RC. A systematic review of the use of aromatherapy in treatment of behavioral problems in dementia. Geriatr Gerontol Int. 2012;12(3):372–82. https://doi.org/10.1111/j.1447-0594.2012.00849.x.
64. Viggo Hansen N, Jorgensen T, Ortenblad L. Massage and touch for dementia. Cochrane Database Syst Rev. 2006;4:CD004989. https://doi.org/10.1002/14651858.CD004989.pub2.
65. Moyle W, Murfield JE, O'Dwyer S, Van Wyk S. The effect of massage on agitated behaviours in older people with dementia: a literature review. J Clin Nurs. 2013;22(5–6):601–10. https://doi.org/10.1111/j.1365-2702.2012.04234.x.
66. Holliday-Welsh DM, Gessert CE, Renier CM. Massage in the management of agitation in nursing home residents with cognitive impairment. Geriatr Nurs. 2009;30(2):108–17. https://doi.org/10.1016/j.gerinurse.2008.06.016.
67. Lancioni GE, Cuvo AJ, O'Reilly MF. Snoezelen: an overview of research with people with developmental disabilities and dementia. Disabil Rehabil. 2002;24(4):175–84. https://doi.org/10.1080/09638280110074911.
68. Prolo P, Sassi E. A sensory garden in dementia care: from design to practice. Balerna Diurnal Therapeutic Centre. Alzheimers Dement Cogn Neurol. 2017;1(3):1–5. https://doi.org/10.15761/ADCN.1000116.
69. Tabbaa L, Ang CS, Rose V, Siriaraya P, Stewart I, Jenkins KG, et al. Bring the outside in: providing accessible experiences through VR for people with dementia in locked psychiatric

hospitals. Proceedings of the 2019 CHI Conference on Human Factors in Computing Systems. 2019. p. 1–15.
70. Clay F, Howett D, FitzGerald J, Fletcher P, Chan D, Price A. Use of immersive virtual reality in the assessment and treatment of Alzheimer's disease: a systematic review. J Alzheimers Dis. 2020;75(1):23–43. https://doi.org/10.3233/JAD-191218.
71. Bruil L, Adriaansen MJM, Groothuis JWM, Bossema ER. [Quality of life of nursing home residents with dementia before, during and after playing with a magic table]. Tijdschr Gerontol Geriatr 2018;49(2):72–80. https://doi.org/10.1007/s12439-017-0243-3.
72. Warren B, Spitzer P. Laughing to longevity—the work of elder clowns. Lancet. 2011;378(9791):562–3. https://doi.org/10.1016/s0140-6736(11)61280-4.
73. Low LF, Brodaty H, Goodenough B, Spitzer P, Bell JP, Fleming R, et al. The Sydney Multisite Intervention of LaughterBosses and ElderClowns (SMILE) study: cluster randomised trial of humour therapy in nursing homes. BMJ Open. 2013;3(1) https://doi.org/10.1136/bmjopen-2012-002072.
74. Kontos P, Miller KL, Colobong R, Palma Lazgare LI, Binns M, Low LF, et al. Elder-clowning in long-term dementia care: results of a pilot study. J Am Geriatr Soc. 2016;64(2):347–53. https://doi.org/10.1111/jgs.13941.
75. van der Steen JT, Smaling HJ, van der Wouden JC, Bruinsma MS, Scholten RJ, Vink AC. Music-based therapeutic interventions for people with dementia. Cochrane Database Syst Rev. 2018;7:CD003477. https://doi.org/10.1002/14651858.CD003477.pub4.
76. Tsoi KKF, Chan JYC, Ng YM, Lee MMY, Kwok TCY, Wong SYS. Receptive music therapy is more effective than interactive music therapy to relieve behavioral and psychological symptoms of dementia: a systematic review and meta-analysis. J Am Med Dir Assoc. 2018;19(7):568–76.e3. https://doi.org/10.1016/j.jamda.2017.12.009.
77. Holmes C, Knights A, Dean C, Hodkinson S, Hopkins V. Keep music live: music and the alleviation of apathy in dementia subjects. Int Psychogeriatr. 2006;18(4):623–30. https://doi.org/10.1017/S1041610206003887.
78. Raglio A, Bellelli G, Traficante D, Gianotti M, Ubezio MC, Villani D, et al. Efficacy of music therapy in the treatment of behavioral and psychiatric symptoms of dementia. Alzheimer Dis Assoc Disord. 2008;22(2):158–62. https://doi.org/10.1097/WAD.0b013e3181630b6f.
79. McLean J, Woodhouse A, Goldie I, Chylarova E, Williamson T. An evidence review of the impact of participatory arts on older people. Mental Health Foundation, Edinburgh, Scotland; 2011.
80. Peisah C, Lawrence G, Reutens S. Creative solutions for severe dementia with BPSD: a case of art therapy used in an inpatient and residential care setting. Int Psychogeriatr. 2011;23(6):1011–3. https://doi.org/10.1017/S1041610211000457.
81. Riemersma-van der Lek RF, Swaab DF, Twisk J, Hol EM, Hoogendijk WJ, Van Someren EJ. Effect of bright light and melatonin on cognitive and noncognitive function in elderly residents of group care facilities: a randomized controlled trial. JAMA. 2008;299(22):2642–55. https://doi.org/10.1001/jama.299.22.2642.
82. Burns A, Allen H, Tomenson B, Duignan D, Byrne J. Bright light therapy for agitation in dementia: a randomized controlled trial. Int Psychogeriatr. 2009;21(4):711–21. https://doi.org/10.1017/S1041610209008886.
83. Ancoli-Israel S, Martin JL, Gehrman P, Shochat T, Corey-Bloom J, Marler M, et al. Effect of light on agitation in institutionalized patients with severe Alzheimer disease. Am J Geriatr Psychiatry. 2003;11(2):194–203.
84. Livingston G, Kelly L, Lewis-Holmes E, Baio G, Morris S, Patel N, et al. Non-pharmacological interventions for agitation in dementia: systematic review of randomised controlled trials. Br J Psychiatry. 2014;205(6):436–42. https://doi.org/10.1192/bjp.bp.113.141119.
85. Cibeira N, Maseda A, Lorenzo-Lopez L, Rodriguez-Villamil JL, Lopez-Lopez R, Millan-Calenti JC. Application of light therapy in older adults with cognitive impairment: a systematic review. Geriatr Nurs. 2020; https://doi.org/10.1016/j.gerinurse.2020.07.005.
86. Berman K, Brodaty H, Withall A, Seeher K. Pharmacologic treatment of apathy in dementia. Am J Geriatr Psychiatry. 2012;20(2):104–22. https://doi.org/10.1097/JGP.0b013e31822001a6.

87. McKeith I, Del Ser T, Spano P, Emre M, Wesnes K, Anand R, et al. Efficacy of rivastigmine in dementia with Lewy bodies: a randomised, double-blind, placebo-controlled international study. Lancet. 2000;356(9247):2031–6. https://doi.org/10.1016/S0140-6736(00)03399-7.
88. Wang J, Yu JT, Wang HF, Meng XF, Wang C, Tan CC, et al. Pharmacological treatment of neuropsychiatric symptoms in Alzheimer's disease: a systematic review and meta-analysis. J Neurol Neurosurg Psychiatry. 2015;86(1):101–9. https://doi.org/10.1136/jnnp-2014-308112.
89. Cumbo E, Ligori LD. Differential effects of current specific treatments on behavioral and psychological symptoms in patients with Alzheimer's disease: a 12-month, randomized, open-label trial. J Alzheimers Dis. 2014;39(3):477–85. https://doi.org/10.3233/JAD-131190.
90. Yoon SJ, Choi SH, Na HR, Park KW, Kim EJ, Han HJ, et al. Effects on agitation with rivastigmine patch monotherapy and combination therapy with memantine in mild to moderate Alzheimer's disease: a multicenter 24-week prospective randomized open-label study (the Korean EXelon Patch and combination with mEmantine Comparative Trial study). Geriatr Gerontol Int. 2017;17(3):494–9. https://doi.org/10.1111/ggi.12754.
91. McShane R, Westby MJ, Roberts E, Minakaran N, Schneider L, Farrimond LE, et al. Memantine for dementia. Cochrane Database Syst Rev. 2019;3:CD003154. https://doi.org/10.1002/14651858.CD003154.pub6.
92. Dudas R, Malouf R, McCleery J, Dening T. Antidepressants for treating depression in dementia. Cochrane Database Syst Rev. 2018;8:CD003944. https://doi.org/10.1002/14651858.CD003944.pub2.
93. Espinoza RT, Unützer J. Diagnosis and management of late-life unipolar depression. 2020. Waltham, MA: Wolters Kluwer. Accessed Sept 2020.
94. Viramontes TS, Truong H, Linnebur SA. Antidepressant-induced hyponatremia in older adults. Consult Pharm. 2016;31(3):139–50. https://doi.org/10.4140/TCP.n.2016.139.
95. Porsteinsson AP, Drye LT, Pollock BG, Devanand DP, Frangakis C, Ismail Z, et al. Effect of citalopram on agitation in Alzheimer disease: the CitAD randomized clinical trial. JAMA. 2014;311(7):682–91. https://doi.org/10.1001/jama.2014.93.
96. Beach SR, Celano CM, Noseworthy PA, Januzzi JL, Huffman JC. QTc prolongation, torsades de pointes, and psychotropic medications. Psychosomatics. 2013;54(1):1–13. https://doi.org/10.1016/j.psym.2012.11.001.
97. Funk KA, Bostwick JR. A comparison of the risk of QT prolongation among SSRIs. Ann Pharmacother. 2013;47(10):1330–41. https://doi.org/10.1177/1060028013501994.
98. Seitz DP, Adunuri N, Gill SS, Gruneir A, Herrmann N, Rochon P. Antidepressants for agitation and psychosis in dementia. Cochrane Database Syst Rev. 2011;2:CD008191. https://doi.org/10.1002/14651858.CD008191.pub2.
99. Sultzer DL, Gray KF, Gunay I, Berisford MA, Mahler ME. A double-blind comparison of trazodone and haloperidol for treatment of agitation in patients with dementia. Am J Geriatr Psychiatry. 1997;5(1):60–9.
100. Teri L, Logsdon RG, Peskind E, Raskind M, Weiner MF, Tractenberg RE, et al. Treatment of agitation in AD: a randomized, placebo-controlled clinical trial. Neurology. 2000;55(9):1271–8. https://doi.org/10.1212/wnl.55.9.1271.
101. Lebert F, Stekke W, Hasenbroekx C, Pasquier F. Frontotemporal dementia: a randomised, controlled trial with trazodone. Dement Geriatr Cogn Disord. 2004;17(4):355–9. https://doi.org/10.1159/000077171.
102. Nardell M, Tampi RR. Pharmacological treatments for frontotemporal dementias: a systematic review of randomized controlled trials. Am J Alzheimers Dis Other Dement. 2014;29(2):123–32. https://doi.org/10.1177/1533317513507375.
103. Kwak YT, Yang Y, Koo MS. Anxiety in dementia. Dement Neurocogn Disord. 2017;16(2):33–9. https://doi.org/10.12779/dnd.2017.16.2.33.
104. Black B, Muralee S, Tampi RR. Inappropriate sexual behaviors in dementia. J Geriatr Psychiatry Neurol. 2005;18(3):155–62. https://doi.org/10.1177/0891988705277541.
105. Chen JJ. Pharmacotherapeutic management of pseudobulbar affect. Am J Manag Care. 2017;23(18 Suppl):S345–S50.

106. Sultana J, Leal I, de Ridder M, Sturkenboom M, Trifiro G. Antipsychotic use in dementia patients in a general practice setting: a Dutch population-based study. Epidemiol Psychiatr Sci. 2016;25(4):403–6. https://doi.org/10.1017/S2045796016000111.
107. Schneider LS, Dagerman KS, Insel P. Risk of death with atypical antipsychotic drug treatment for dementia: meta-analysis of randomized placebo-controlled trials. JAMA. 2005;294(15):1934–43. https://doi.org/10.1001/jama.294.15.1934.
108. Jeste DV, Blazer D, Casey D, Meeks T, Salzman C, Schneider L, et al. ACNP White Paper: update on use of antipsychotic drugs in elderly persons with dementia. Neuropsychopharmacology. 2008;33(5):957–70. https://doi.org/10.1038/sj.npp.1301492.
109. Trifiro G, Spina E, Gambassi G. Use of antipsychotics in elderly patients with dementia: do atypical and conventional agents have a similar safety profile? Pharmacol Res. 2009;59(1):1–12. https://doi.org/10.1016/j.phrs.2008.09.017.
110. Steinberg M, Lyketsos CG. Atypical antipsychotic use in patients with dementia: managing safety concerns. Am J Psychiatry. 2012;169(9):900–6. https://doi.org/10.1176/appi.ajp.2012.12030342.
111. Reus VI, Fochtmann LJ, Eyler AE, Hilty DM, Horvitz-Lennon M, Jibson MD, et al. The American Psychiatric Association practice guideline on the use of antipsychotics to treat agitation or psychosis in patients with dementia. Am J Psychiatry. 2016;173(5):543–6.
112. Aarsland D, Perry R, Larsen JP, McKeith IG, O'Brien JT, Perry EK, et al. Neuroleptic sensitivity in Parkinson's disease and parkinsonian dementias. J Clin Psychiatry. 2005;66(5):633–7.
113. De Hert M, Detraux J, van Winkel R, Yu W, Correll CU. Metabolic and cardiovascular adverse effects associated with antipsychotic drugs. Nat Rev Endocrinol. 2011;8(2):114–26. https://doi.org/10.1038/nrendo.2011.156.
114. Maglione M, Maher AR, Hu J, Wang Z, Shanman R, Shekelle PG, et al. Off-Label Use of Atypical Antipsychotics: An Update. Comparative Effectiveness Review No. 43. (Prepared by the Southern California Evidence-based Practice Center under Contract No. HHSA290-2007-10062-1.) Rockville, MD: Agency for Healthcare Research and Quality. September 2011. Available at: www.effectivehealthcare.ahrq.gov/reports/final.cfm.
115. Yunusa I, Alsumali A, Garba AE, Regestein QR, Eguale T. Assessment of reported comparative effectiveness and safety of atypical antipsychotics in the treatment of behavioral and psychological symptoms of dementia: a network meta-analysis. JAMA Netw Open. 2019;2(3):e190828. https://doi.org/10.1001/jamanetworkopen.2019.0828.
116. Fernandez HH, Trieschmann ME, Burke MA, Friedman JH. Quetiapine for psychosis in Parkinson's disease versus dementia with Lewy bodies. J Clin Psychiatry. 2002;63(6):513–5. https://doi.org/10.4088/jcp.v63n0608.
117. Van Leeuwen E, Petrovic M, van Driel ML, De Sutter AI, Vander Stichele R, Declercq T, et al. Withdrawal versus continuation of long-term antipsychotic drug use for behavioural and psychological symptoms in older people with dementia. Cochrane Database Syst Rev. 2018;3:CD007726. https://doi.org/10.1002/14651858.CD007726.pub3.
118. Ballard CG, Thomas A, Fossey J, Lee L, Jacoby R, Lana MM, et al. A 3-month, randomized, placebo-controlled, neuroleptic discontinuation study in 100 people with dementia: the neuropsychiatric inventory median cutoff is a predictor of clinical outcome. J Clin Psychiatry. 2004;65(1):114–9. https://doi.org/10.4088/jcp.v65n0120.
119. Ballard C, Hanney ML, Theodoulou M, Douglas S, McShane R, Kossakowski K, et al. The dementia antipsychotic withdrawal trial (DART-AD): long-term follow-up of a randomised placebo-controlled trial. Lancet Neurol. 2009;8(2):151–7. https://doi.org/10.1016/S1474-4422(08)70295-3.
120. Yeh YC, Ouyang WC. Mood stabilizers for the treatment of behavioral and psychological symptoms of dementia: an update review. Kaohsiung J Med Sci. 2012;28(4):185–93. https://doi.org/10.1016/j.kjms.2011.10.025.
121. Baillon SF, Narayana U, Luxenberg JS, Clifton AV. Valproate preparations for agitation in dementia. Cochrane Database Syst Rev. 2018;10:CD003945. https://doi.org/10.1002/14651858.CD003945.pub4.

122. Tampi RR, Tampi DJ. Efficacy and tolerability of benzodiazepines for the treatment of behavioral and psychological symptoms of dementia: a systematic review of randomized controlled trials. Am J Alzheimers Dis Other Dement. 2014;29(7):565–74. https://doi.org/10.1177/1533317514524813.
123. Barker MJ, Greenwood KM, Jackson M, Crowe SF. Cognitive effects of long-term benzodiazepine use: a meta-analysis. CNS Drugs. 2004;18(1):37–48. https://doi.org/10.2165/00023210-200418010-00004.
124. Rabins PV, McIntyre JS, American Psychiatric Association. Practice Guideline for the Treatment of Patients with Alzheimer's Disease and Other Dementias. 2nd ed. Arlington, VA: American Psychiatric Publishing; 2010.
125. Passmore MJ, Sheldon L, Lax S, Wilkins-Ho M, Illing M. Oral midazolam for dementia-related response agitation. J Am Geriatr Soc. 2009;57(3):561–2. https://doi.org/10.1111/j.1532-5415.2009.02162.x.
126. Bloch F, Karoui I, Boutalha S, Defouilloy C, Dubaele JM. Tolerability of Midazolam to treat acute agitation in elderly demented patients: a systematic review. J Clin Pharm Ther. 2019;44(2):143–7. https://doi.org/10.1111/jcpt.12785.
127. Ruthirakuhan MT, Herrmann N, Abraham EH, Chan S, Lanctot KL. Pharmacological interventions for apathy in Alzheimer's disease. Cochrane Database Syst Rev. 2018;5:CD012197. https://doi.org/10.1002/14651858.CD012197.pub2.
128. Padala PR, Padala KP, Lensing SY, Ramirez D, Monga V, Bopp MM, et al. Methylphenidate for apathy in community-dwelling older veterans with mild Alzheimer's disease: a double-blind, randomized, placebo-controlled trial. Am J Psychiatry. 2018;175(2):159–68. https://doi.org/10.1176/appi.ajp.2017.17030316.
129. Cummings JL, Lyketsos CG, Peskind ER, Porsteinsson AP, Mintzer JE, Scharre DW, et al. Effect of dextromethorphan-quinidine on agitation in patients with Alzheimer disease dementia: a randomized clinical trial. JAMA. 2015;314(12):1242–54. https://doi.org/10.1001/jama.2015.10214.
130. Blais J, Zolezzi M, Sadowski CA. Treatment options for sundowning in patients with dementia. Mental Health Clin. 2014;4(4):189–95. https://doi.org/10.9740/mhc.n204525.
131. van den Berg JF, Kruithof HC, Kok RM, Verwijk E, Spaans HP. Electroconvulsive therapy for agitation and aggression in dementia: a systematic review. Am J Geriatr Psychiatry. 2018;26(4):419–34. https://doi.org/10.1016/j.jagp.2017.09.023.
132. Kaster TS, Blumberger DM. Palliating severe refractory neuropsychiatric symptoms of dementia: is there a role for electroconvulsive therapy? Am J Geriatr Psychiatry. 2018;26(4):435–7. https://doi.org/10.1016/j.jagp.2018.01.002.
133. Wang X, Mao Z, Yu X. The role of noninvasive brain stimulation for behavioral and psychological symptoms of dementia: a systematic review and meta-analysis. Neurol Sci. 2020;41(5):1063–74. https://doi.org/10.1007/s10072-020-04245-4.

Management of Vascular Risk Factors in Dementia

8

Ana Verdelho and Manuel Gonçalves Pereira

Abbreviations

CI Confidence Interval
CT Computerized tomography
GP General practitioner
MCI Mild cognitive impairment
TIA Transient ischemic attack

Introduction

Vascular risk factors (e.g., hypertension, diabetes, smoking) play an important role in cognitive decline and dementia [1, 2]. This applies not only to vascular dementia, but also to dementia due to Alzheimer's disease, endorsing the emerging concept of a mixed etiology. In fact, Alzheimer's disease and vascular dementia share both protective and risk factors, namely these vascular risk factors, which are potentially modifiable. Prevention is better than cure [1] and vascular risk factors' management has been suggested as one of the best ways of preventing dementia in the next decades [1–3]. In fact, the 2017 Lancet Commission on

A. Verdelho (✉)
Faculdade de Medicina, Department of Neurosciences and Mental Health, CHULN-Hospital de Santa Maria, Instituto de Medicina Molecular – IMM e Instituto de Saúde Ambiental – ISAMB, University of Lisbon, Lisbon, Portugal
e-mail: averdelho@medicina.ulisboa.pt

M. G. Pereira
Comprehensive Health Research Centre (CHRC), CEDOC, NOVA Medical School/Faculdade de Ciências Médicas, Universidade Nova de Lisboa, Lisbon, Portugal
e-mail: gpereira@nms.unl.pt

K. S. Frederiksen, G. Waldemar (eds.), *Management of Patients with Dementia*,
https://doi.org/10.1007/978-3-030-77904-7_8

dementia prevention, intervention, and care suggested that around 35% of dementia was attributable to a combination of modifiable risk factors including midlife hypertension and obesity, diabetes, smoking and inactivity, among other factors of non-vascular nature—less education, hearing impairment, depression, and low social contact [1]. Recently, alcohol consumption, traumatic brain injury and air pollution were added to the list. The 2020 update consists of a 12 risk factor life course model of dementia prevention: 12 modifiable risk factors account for around 40% of worldwide dementias that could theoretically be prevented or delayed [4].

Not all dementia prediction models developed in high-income countries can be simply extrapolated worldwide [5]. However, it was recently estimated, after adjusting for non-independence of risk factors, that 24.4%, to 40.1% of dementia cases could be related to seven potentially modifiable risk factors in Mozambique, Brazil, and Portugal [6]. In this study, the risk factors selected for estimate calculations included low education and depression, but mostly vascular risk factors. Reducing the prevalence of each risk factor by 20% per decade could, by 2050, potentially reduce the prevalence of dementia in Mozambique, Brazil, and Portugal by 12.9%, 16.2%, and 19.5%, respectively [6].

Notwithstanding, studies investigating cognitive benefits from treatment of vascular risk factors sometimes led to conflicting results. Hence, evidence is still too sparse to support clear recommendations concerning the beneficial impact on cognition of specific treatments for vascular risk factors. This is so regarding not only the prevention of incident cognitive decline but also the progression of cognitive deficits in the presence of diagnosed dementia. On the other hand, despite that vascular risk factors and dementia are both frequent, and frequently co-exist, they are seldom managed altogether in effective ways. In fact, clinicians tend to target primarily either vascular risk factors or cognitive decline. Unfortunately, combined approaches are often neglected in daily practice.

In this chapter, the authors present the bulk of current knowledge concerning vascular risk factors and dementia, the impact of managing vascular risk factors in dementia, and the influence of living with dementia in the treatment of vascular risk factors, including in adherence. A few clinical dilemmas will be discussed, inspired by two vignettes introducing examples of the complex situations surrounding this topic. The authors do not intend to conduct yet another exhaustive review. Recognizing that much is still controversial or inconsistent, they aim to provide instead a critical appraisal based on the best evidence available and discuss some practical implications. Systematic reviews and meta-analyses are easily accessible, as acknowledged throughout the chapter, and are recommended for further reading.

Clinical Case A: Why Should Doctors Focus on Vascular Factors?

Teresa is a recently widowed 78-years-old woman, who worked as a primary school teacher for many years.

During the past year or so, she had daily support from a payed caregiver, who helped her in the difficult task of caring for her severely ill husband, and also in household chores.

Teresa has hypertension and diabetes, and she always took care of her own medication. Her daughter recently realised that Teresa is increasingly forgetful for 1 or 2 years now, and there were even some lapses with her medication. Nevertheless, she always seemed able to carry out her duties as usual. After her husband's passing, Teresa started to socially withdraw, preferring to stay alone at home. She often forgets messages and things she planned to do. Her thinking and even movements seem much slower. The daughter took her to the general practitioner (GP), suspecting of 'depression'. Surprisingly for the daughter, the GP was more concerned about vascular risk factors' control. Teresa was remarkably hypertensive at the GP's office, with a systolic blood pressure of 187 mmHg and a diastolic of 110 mmHg. Glycaemia was also high, and she had lost weight, comparing to an appointment 6 months earlier.

Over the clinical interview, Teresa seemed confused and had difficulties in identifying the correct date and recalling the exact day of her husband's death. The GP asked for a computerized tomography (CT) that showed severe cerebral small vessel disease. A neuropsychological evaluation was compatible with multi-domain cognitive impairment (with major problems in attention and executive functions, mental and motor processing speed, and working memory). These findings were clearly interfering with the patient's autonomy and vascular dementia (subcortical type) was diagnosed after consulting with a dementia specialist in regular liaison with the primary care team. Despite the daughter's begging for a 'brain supplement', the GP mainly insisted on a better control of vascular risk factors and recommended that Teresa should keep the caregiver with her, for continuous support.

The Importance of Vascular Risk Factors in Cognitive Decline and Incident Dementia

So far, the study of vascular risk factors in the context of cognitive disorders has focused on their role as determinants of incident cognitive impairment, including dementia, and not exactly of further complications when dementia is already established. Overall, there are caveats regarding the study of risk factors in producing a clinical outcome (e.g., a disease). A first issue is to contrast the impact of a single risk factor with the impact of a cluster of risk factors. In the latter approach, the different associations considered are also relevant in themselves, and in the case of vascular risk factors (Table 8.1), associations are highly diverse indeed. It is not difficult to sustain that the impact of a certain factor is not independent from the co-existence of other, concomitant factors [7], or from genetic, environmental, sociocultural, and economic factors which may further interfere. A second issue regards the consideration of the age of starting, frequency, length, and severity of the exposure to risk factors. Aging is a dynamic process and it may moderate or even change the direction of the effect.

Table 8.1 Main vascular risk factors

Cognitive decline: Vascular risk factors
Midlife hypertension
Midlife hyperlipidemias
Midlife obesity
Diabetes Stroke
Excessive alcohol consumption
Smoking
Low physical activity/sedentarism

The traditional approach in the context of dementia was to consider the role of vascular risk factors in separate [6], trying to make inferences about their individual impact in cognitive decline, over the lifetime. Relevant information can be retrieved from those studies and the following sections describe these "individual" approaches, but multiple risk factors' models will also be discussed afterwards. For an important example of the exploration of communality of risk factors, along with a thorough discussion of limitations in estimating population attributable fractions, refer to Livingston et al. [1].

Hypertension, Hypercholesterolemia, and Obesity

Vascular risk factors probably have a different impact according to the age of manifestation. This is somehow clear concerning hypertension, hypercholesterolemia, and obesity [7, 8].

Starting with hypertension, midlife, and late-onset hypertension do not seem to represent the same level of risk regarding late cognitive decline. Midlife hypertension has been consistently associated with the risk of cognitive decline and incident dementia [8–12], not only of the vascular type but also of dementia due to Alzheimer's disease [13, 14]. A higher risk is associated with non-treated midlife hypertension [10, 11]. In accordance, midlife hypertension was also implicated in brain atrophy [15]. Notwithstanding, in the Honolulu Asia Aging study, there was an increased risk of later hippocampal atrophy for those men who had never been treated for hypertension in midlife, compared to those who had been treated [16]. Although vascular mechanisms could explain the association between hypertension and hippocampal atrophy, there is also evidence that hypertension may be implicated in amyloid deposition. This effect seems to be independent of age but depending on the presence of the Apolipoprotein E epsilon 4 genotype in cognitively intact subjects of middle and older ages [17].

The relationship between late-onset hypertension and cognitive decline and incident dementia has been a subject of controversy over the last decades. Recently, Arvanitakis et al. [18], in a clinicopathological study, found that late-life hypertension was associated with a higher risk of vascular pathology and with a higher number of tangles in the brain, but not of amyloid plaques [18]. Some studies even suggested an increased risk of cognitive decline due to low blood pressure or to a decline in values of blood pressure in old age [19–22]. Of note, late-life hypotension was not found to decrease the risk of dementia [19].

Despite encouraging results concerning the potential effect of antihypertensive medication in Alzheimer's neuropathology [23] and in reducing dementia risk in older people [24], the main randomized controlled studies using antihypertensive medication to prevent dementia showed no consistent protective effect [25–31]. Only one study showed a modest effect [29] and one other a protective effect in post-stroke dementia only [30]. Recently, a phase III investigator-driven clinical trial tested a calcium channel blocker (nilvadipine) that had been associated with reduction of amyloid production and anti-tau activity in pre-clinical studies. Unfortunately, the drug failed to reduce cognitive decline in patients with mild to moderate Alzheimer's disease [32]. The ONTARGET and TRANSCEND studies also failed to reduce incidence of dementia by lowering blood pressure [33]. In the HOPE-3 study, treating high blood pressure and lipidemia over 5.7 years did not reduce the progression in cognitive decline and, namely the incidence of dementia [34]. In a substudy of the SPRINT project, intensive blood pressure control failed to significantly lower the risk of probable dementia [35]. Notwithstanding, the authors found a reduction of incident mild cognitive impairment (MCI) [35].

A recent meta-analysis that included broad neurocognitive outcomes (not only dementia) found promising results regarding the effect of lowering blood pressure. These effects were mostly found in subgroups of patients with more severe hypertension [35, 36] and when clinical assessments and not necessarily cognitive test scores were considered as outcomes [36].

Studies conducted among patients with small vessel disease (who could most likely benefit from intervention) generated contradicting results [37–39].

In summary, blood pressure control should be implemented at any life stage, starting very early, severe hypertension should be it is effective in preventing recurrent vascular events [40], and general recommendations should be followed over the entire lifespan in order to prevent cognitive decline [41, 42]. The maximization of brain protection may be jeopardized by poor awareness regarding the control of hypertension and its consequences in drug adherence, especially among younger persons as compared to middle age or older adults [43, 44]. In fact, the so-called health optimism hinders the early prevention of late cognitive problems, a potential that may be underestimated by younger people.

A few additional comments on hypercholesterolemia and obesity are needed, when considering them as isolated risk factors. Evidence is stronger for both as risk factors of Alzheimer's disease when they are present in midlife [7, 19, 45, 46]. However, evidence about the benefits of treatment with statins to prevent cognitive impairment is low [31, 47–49]. One of the reasons may be, again, a possible modulatory effect of age [50]. Higher body mass index at midlife was independently associated with deposition of amyloid more than 25 years after [8]. Overall, obesity seems to be a risk factor for cognitive decline and dementia in midlife [51] but not in old age [52].

Diabetes

The high number of publications under the topic of diabetes and dementia broadly reflects a growing knowledge about the links between both conditions, along with the investment being made to change the associated risk profile. Diabetes is a clearly identified risk factor for cognitive impairment and dementia of all causes, including vascular dementia and Alzheimer's disease [53–56]. The risk of dementia seems to double in diabetics, comparing to non-diabetics [53], and it is higher in non-treated compared to treated diabetics [57]. Even among old age people without dementia, diabetes was implicated in worse cognitive performance in several cognitive domains [58–60].

The strong link between diabetes and dementia, with specific metabolic changes and cognitive, structural, and functional profiles, recently led to the suggestion of a phenomenon coined as "diabetes-related dementia." This condition, specifically linked to diabetes, is not necessarily mediated through amyloid (in fact, it is more likely Tau-dependent) nor vascular links [61, 62]. In any case, diabetes, either type 1 [63, 64] or type 2 [65, 66], and independently of the age of onset, is an established risk factor for dementia.

Mechanisms linking diabetes and dementia include vascular disease, inflammation, mitochondrial dysfunction, and impaired insulin signaling [67–69]. Ultimately, metabolic changes can alter the production of both amyloid and tau protein deposits, promoting neuronal degeneration [70, 71]. Alzheimer-disease-related biomarkers have been investigated to clarify underlying pathways [72]. Different interactions were described that worsen the cognitive decline in diabetes. These include poor glycemic control and hypoglycemic episodes, but also metabolic syndrome, insulin resistance, and a genetic linkage [73–75]. Probably the direction of research should move towards identifying individual risk profiles, which can be highly relevant to anticipate complications among diabetics [76]. Despite all the evidence linking diabetes with the incidence of cognitive problems and dementia, specific evidence supporting the efficacy of diabetes treatment in dementia risk reduction is still lacking [53, 77].

Stroke

Stroke and dementia share the same vascular risk factors. Furthermore, there is a bidirectional relationship between them: stroke doubles the risk of dementia, and patients with dementia have a higher risk of stroke [78–83]. The risk is increased for all-cause dementia, i.e., not only for vascular dementia but also for Alzheimer's disease. It is not only stroke but also transient ischemic attack (TIA) [82, 84] and silent infarcts [85] that are implicated in higher risk of cognitive decline. This reflects the considerable risk of cognitive impairment in the presence of cerebrovascular disease, regardless of the heterogeneity of vascular etiologies.

Risk of dementia after stroke depends on multiple factors, including: higher age, lower educational level and cognitive reserve, previous cognitive impairment, vascular risk factors (e.g., hypertension, diabetes, atrial fibrillation, coronary disease, tobacco and alcohol consumption, stroke characteristics—recurrence, severity, functional impairment, and complications), and concomitant neurodegenerative and vascular changes, namely small vessel disease changes (as white matter changes, microbleeds, or lacunes), global and medial temporal lobe atrophy, and Alzheimer's disease pathology [81, 82, 86–90].

Stroke prevention and early treatment, together with interventions in long-term care are essential for dementia prevention or management [91]. Special considerations will be done, later in this chapter, considering reperfusion treatments in stroke patients with a previous diagnosis of dementia, together with other aspects of managing vascular risk factors in those patients. However, a few related ideas are worth noting already at this stage.

In patients with dementia who suffered a stroke, current guidelines apply as there is no evidence to proceed otherwise [91, 92]. It remains a matter of debate whether specific treatments can reduce the likelihood of dementia, per se, or indirectly by preventing stroke, e.g., by treating atrial fibrillation [93, 94]. Patients with dementia should be prescribed antiplatelets and anticoagulants, following the usual guidelines for primary and secondary stroke prevention [95, 96]. However, the emphasis should always be on a personalized approach, namely in the presence of microbleeds or other manifestations of particular conditions (as is the case of amyloid angiopathy). This should obviously take into consideration factors like stage of dementia and treatment adherence. Of note, there is no evidence that antiplatelets improve cognition or should be recommended without a specific indication such as cardiovascular disease or previous stroke/TIA.

There is a long-standing debate concerning the nature of interactions between vascular pathology and Alzheimer's pathology. It may be that vascular disease is itself (either through stroke or through chronic injuries translated into small vessel disease) directly involved in higher amyloid production. Alternatively, it may increase the brain vascular burden, with an "add-on" effect regarding Alzheimer's pathology [97]. A third hypothesis could be that vascular disease triggers the manifestations of ongoing degenerative processes (of the amyloid line), with combined effects. Overall, the co-existence of vascular and Alzheimer's disease has been acknowledged for decades [98, 99], with difficulties distinguishing the contribution of each pathology and ascertaining the exact relation between them, but there is no doubt that their combination will double the risk of dementia, as compared to the risk associated with Alzheimer pathology alone [100]. Nevertheless, stroke does change the trajectories of subjects previously diagnosed with Alzheimer's disease and vice versa. Moreover, stroke can cause dementia even without amyloid deposition [101]: remote astrogliosis phenomena are a possible explanation [83, 102, 103], or else the expression of small vessel disease and vascular burden may be determinant [104, 105].

Alcohol Consumption and Smoking

Alcohol consumption and smoking may influence many clinical outcomes, especially because excessive consumption, harmful use, or dependence are prevalent conditions. Most of the evidence relating alcohol and tobacco consumption with cognition is driven from observational studies, which means that the effect of confounders may limit the interpretation of results, including the fact that habits may change due to concomitant health conditions. It would be unfeasible to implement appropriate randomized and controlled studies on the impact of drinking or smoking in cognitive status and dementia, namely among never drinkers or never smokers. One must remind the current knowledge of potential risks for general health due to smoking and alcohol, the potential neurotoxicity of the latter, and the addictive properties of both. It has been suggested that the use of metabolites or components of both may be a way to go in further studies aiming to understand the impact of those substances in cognition and in dementia risk [106, 107].

Relationships between alcohol consumption and incident dementia are controversial. Many factors undermine the interpretation of these studies, namely operational definitions of mild, moderate, or excessive intake (taking into consideration frequency, type of exposure, and amount by exposure), variations in individuals' tolerance, or that they do not include participants who never drank or that stopped drinking due to health reasons. Excessive alcohol consumption has been systematically associated with brain atrophy [108–111], including hippocampal atrophy [112], worse vascular risk control [108], and higher risk of dementia [108, 113–115]. Clinically, we sometimes observe cognitive impairment reverting upon alcohol abstinence. It is also known that alcohol effects are age-dependent, as metabolism, distribution, and elimination of ethanol decrease with age, leading to increased effects of alcohol in persons of old age [116]. On the contrary, some beneficial effects of alcohol may be mediated through cardiovascular effects, and, for instance, resveratrol [106] was recently investigated in this context. A recent meta-analysis [108] found an optimal range of alcohol consumption associated with a lower risk of dementia (<12.5 g/day). However, this is not enough to make a recommendation to drink moderately to prevent dementia, namely among never drinkers or patients with alcohol intolerance.

In summary, excessive drinking and binge drinking stand as risk factors for dementia. Alcohol-related disorders, either as harmful use or dependence, should be managed whenever identified. Among usual drinkers, mild consumption should be aimed for. No recommendation should be done for non-usual drinkers to start drinking alcohol, and individual tolerance must also always be taken into consideration.

Nicotine is an exogenous agonist of nicotinic acetylcholine receptors [117], thereby with a potentially beneficial effect in cognition [118]. Theoretically, exploring some of its pharmacologically active metabolites may be a clue for interventional studies [107]. Nevertheless, in observational studies, smoking was associated with an increased risk of dementia [119], whereas stopping smoking was associated with a decreased risk in the long term [119, 120].

Associations Between Risk Factors

In the last two decades, more consideration has been given to the role of interactions among risk factors in increasing the risk of cognitive decline and dementia. It would be expected that the simultaneous impact of different risk factors on cognition might differ from the effect of single risk factors by themselves. A recent meta-analysis found that the risk of dementia increased with the number of risk factors involved, suggesting a dose-related response [121]. Despite that the type of risk factors was not coincident in the different studies included, the authors found a risk ratio of 1.2 (95% Confidence Interval (CI) 1.0–1.4) for one risk factor, a combined risk ratio of 1.7 (95% CI 1.4–1.9) for two risk factors, and a combined risk ratio of 2.2 (95% CI 1.8–2.7) for three risk factors, hence meaning that three risk factors roughly doubled the risk of dementia comparing to no risk factor.

This effect was not circumscribed to midlife vascular risk factors and unhealthy behavior [45, 46, 122–124] but was also described in late life [125, 126], including in very old people [127]. Notwithstanding, the impact can be observed since early age: cumulative exposure of several risk factors in early adult (18–30 years) was associated with worse cognitive performance in neuropsychological evaluation 25 years later (in midlife) even without dementia, underlining the need to early and effectively address the vascular risk factors.

Recently, Suri et al. analyzed a subsample of the Whitehall II Imaging Substudy cohort. They found that subjects with vascular risk factors and without dementia in midlife had lower perfusion in gray matter areas at older ages (25 years after) [128]. Accordingly, in the ARIC study [129], an increased number of midlife vascular risk factors was significantly associated with a higher risk of positivity using the amyloid tracer florbetapir later in life [129].

An established example of clustering of vascular risk factors is the metabolic syndrome [130]. This umbrella term refers to a combination of vascular risk factors, including raised fasting glucose (>100 mg/dL), raised blood pressure (systolic ≥130 and/or diastolic ≥85 mm Hg), dyslipidemia defined as high level of triglycerides (>150 mg/dL) and low level of high-density lipoprotein cholesterol (<40 mg/dL in males and <50 mg/dL in females), and central obesity (elevated waist circumference), with three out of the five being necessary to diagnose the condition [130].

The analysis of relationships between metabolic syndrome and risk of incident dementia has yielded controversial results: a meta-analysis including studies between 2000 and 2018 pooled nine studies and was unable to find a relation between metabolic syndrome and increased incident dementia, including Alzheimer's disease. However, an effect was found in the increased risk of pure vascular dementia and of progression from MCI into dementia [131]. Metabolic syndrome was also associated with incident dementia in a large observational study [132], as previously reported by others [133, 134]. The normalization of metabolic syndrome (although within a relatively small range of 2 years) was also associated with a lower risk of dementia; among all metabolic syndrome components, controlling fasting glucose and blood pressure were the most strongly associated with lowering dementia risk [132], especially so in the younger group as compared to the older group. In the same study, metabolic syndrome increased the risk of both Alzheimer's disease and vascular dementia, with a stronger association with vascular dementia.

In the last decade, some epidemiological studies suggested a stabilization or even declining prevalence or incidence of dementia in a few countries [135, 136]. Despite no single risk factor change that could fully explain these findings, one of the possible contributors could be better vascular risk control at earlier stages in life. On the contrary, discrepancies and non-stabilization in some other countries could also be partially explained by lack of control in cardiovascular risk factors [137], namely diseases associated with sedentarism, as diabetes and obesity. Overall, the debate on secular trends regarding the epidemiology of dementia continues. Prince et al. suggested that the age-specific prevalence of dementia is unlikely to change significantly in the coming years, even if incidence falls in high-income countries because of improvements in public health [137]. Perhaps there are mixed effects and opposite influences in dementia risk, in what concerns the particular trends in vascular risk factors.

Despite promising data from recent trials [138], the evidence concerning combined approaches to prevent dementia remains quite limited. Early in this chapter, important studies were cited estimating the potential magnitude of dementia prevalence decrease attributable to better control of vascular risk, among other factors amenable to intervention [1, 4, 6]. Obviously, however, those were not field trials.

In a population-based cohort, healthy lifestyle (defined as a combination of physical activity according to usual recommendations, non-smoking, light to moderate alcohol consumption, Mediterranean-type diet, and involvement in cognitive activities) was associated with lower risk of dementia of the Alzheimer type [139]. In the FINGER trial, a combination of diet, exercise, cognitive training, and vascular risk monitoring led to encouraging results, with stabilization or improvement in cognitive function. However, the selective impact of vascular risk monitoring was not entirely clear [140]. Furthermore, among high-risk vascular patients, and particularly in stroke patients (where interventions would be more prone to produce beneficial results), previous studies using multiple lifestyle interventions have not globally changed outcomes [141–143].

It is likely that published studies might have been too short in time to produce useful evidence. Their targets may be difficult to capture with fully quantitative measures (as opposed to, e.g., cognitive clinical end-points, the clinical impression of decline), or they could have started too late in life to be able to prevent degenerative consequences. Moreover, long-standing interventions designed to capture the effects of preventive therapies may be difficult to conduct and maintain over time without high attrition rates and other limitations (e.g., comorbidities as confounders).

Evidence is quite low concerning the risk of cognitive deterioration due to vascular risk in patients already diagnosed with MCI or dementia and the impact of specifically controlling vascular risk factors in order to reduce the progression of cognitive decline among patients with any of these established diagnoses.

In a recent study, the presence of modifiable risk factors was specifically associated with an increased risk of non-reversion from a diagnosis of MCI (versus reversion from MCI) [144], while in another study, subjects with MCI and vascular risk vascular factors converted faster and declined faster, compared to subjects without vascular risk factors [145] Concerning patients with established dementia, there is a dearth of studies specifically designed to study the impact of controlling vascular risk factors, and specific recommendations are limited [95]. However, and following common sense, there is no reason to believe that patients with dementia will not profit from regular vascular risk control, as it happens with any person in general. The few data available (namely from observational studies) suggest that controlling several vascular risk factors altogether could be more effective to prevent cognitive decline among subjects with an established diagnosis of cognitive impairment than a single risk factor control approach [145]. In a retrospective study, treatment of one or more vascular risk factors in subjects with dementia was associated with less decline in Mini Mental State Examination scores comparing to no treatment [146]. This suggests that vascular risk factors' control can contribute by itself to slow down cognitive decline.

Dementia and Control of Vascular Risk Factors

Dementia is associated with increased mortality [147, 148], including the risk of death during hospitalization [149]. Among patients with dementia, the presence of vascular risk factors and cardiovascular diseases is associated with an additional risk of death [148]. Despite this growing evidence that the control of vascular risk factors is effective in preventing—if not cognitive decline—at least further medical complications and death, patients with dementia may be undertreated regarding their general health, and this is specifically so in what concerns vascular risk factors. Several reasons may contribute. First, these patients tend to have less insight regarding their medical symptoms and health conditions. They also usually depend on others in order to receive appropriate care. Additionally, clinicians may withhold a prescription decision or be afraid to reach therapeutic dose ranges due to concerns about medication risks or side effects, including the risk of compromising adherence.

In fact, inappropriate drug use seems to be more frequent among patients with dementia [150]. A study conducted in the UK analyzed the quality of care for vascular conditions and risk factors in people with dementia in primary care services. The authors found that the level of care received by people with dementia was significantly lower compared with those without dementia [151]. Other studies suggested that patients with dementia may receive inappropriate prescriptions due to lack of evidence on expected benefits or fear of secondary effects. For instance, patients with cardiovascular diseases were not treated according to the evidence-base if they had a diagnosis of dementia in different samples from different countries [152, 153]. One may also speculate about the role of dementia-related stigma in this regard.

Now let us go back to Teresa and see how a few complications were effectively managed:

Teresa underwent adequate correction of her vascular risk factors and for some time she steadily improved in mental speed, becoming more prone to undertake activities beyond her strict routine. She accepted to participate in a few leisure activities, and although her medication was broadly supervised, Teresa took a greater role in remembering names, times and dosages of her own pills.

Then, after 2 years of clinical stabilization, Teresa's condition deteriorated rapidly. In a few weeks she became lethargic, drowsy and refusing to cooperate and engage in any activities. Once more, she did not want to go out even for a short walk.

Her daughter brought her again to the GP. She was bradycardic, and a atrioventricular block became apparent, with intermittent changes into a 3rd degree blockage. She was under mild doses of β-blockers that were then stopped. Teresa had allergic rhinitis and antihistamine drugs were also stopped. As she was in better shape and glucose levels were lower, antidiabetic medication was reduced. Teresa returned to her previous condition in several weeks and another stabilization period ensued, her general health status being closely monitored by her GP.

In a population-based study on MCI and conversion to dementia that considered vascular risk factors, having an appropriate drug prescription was more frequent among the group of stable MCI and reverters (into the normal cognitive state) and not in the converters into dementia [154]. This supports the idea that vascular risk management can be efficient, at least regarding cognitive stabilization.

In summary, although there is no evidence that systematic follow-up with the implementation of strict vascular risk factor control can prevent cognitive decline in patients with dementia, there is no reason to assume that these patients do not benefit from the same level of care than patients without dementia [95]. A final message should be taken from cases like the one above, and not only in primary care. The efficient management of chronic diseases in old age may be compromised by the still prevailing but unrealistic views that multiple health problems can be effectively managed independently (by separate national strategies for diabetes and dementia, for instance) [155]. There is now a strong emphasis from the World Health Organization in promoting more comprehensive, integrated care for old age people at the community level and relying on primary care-based interventions [156].

Clinical Case B: Reperfusion Therapies in Dementia

John, an 83-year-old man, was diagnosed with Alzheimer's disease 3 years ago. He forgets plain things he has to do, and most messages given to him. John is quite happy during family meetings and enjoys a chat with his grandchildren, although he keeps repeating the same questions over and over. By the end of the afternoon he usually becomes more confused and sometimes starts wandering, trying to leave home as he does not recognise the place as his own. John's relatives are now pretty used to these behaviours and are able to deal with them very well, reducing his activities over the afternoon and redirecting John to simple but purposeful tasks.

One day after having had lunch and rested for half an hour, John awaked aphasic and with right hemiparesis to his family surprise. Astonishingly, he was completely well 1 h before. They brought him to the emergency room, where the diagnosis was not difficult. John had suffered a stroke, with mean cerebral artery occlusion, probably due to new onset atrial fibrillation. A CT scan showed leukoaraiosis. Thrombectomy after thrombolysis was conducted at once. John recovered partially, with mild aphasia, and slowly improving right paresis.

As stated above, dementia and stroke share several risk factors, and stroke is more frequent in patients with dementia.

Thrombolysis and thrombectomy are both approved treatments for acute stroke, but there is no study specifically addressing the benefits of thrombolysis or thrombectomy in acute stroke patients with a previous diagnosis of dementia. Patients with dementia are less likely admitted to a stroke unit or submitted to thrombolysis [157, 158], and most previous studies conducted on reperfusion therapies tend to have an unrepresentative number of patients with dementia.

In principle, a diagnosis of dementia should not preclude any acute stroke treatment from being considered. Overall, the risks of hemorrhage and death associated with thrombolysis in acute stroke are not increased in patients with dementia compared to those without dementia [158, 159]. This said, a personalized approach is needed, namely in those highly dependent patients who will probably have worse outcomes after thrombolysis [160–162]. Patients in whom an aggressive intervention will likely not promote significant clinical improvement (due, for instance, to the extension of the lesion or because they were already bedridden and highly dependent before stroke) should also be cautiously approached. A thorough evaluation of any potential complications is also necessary.

A few additional points are pertinent to this discussion. First, patients with dementia more frequently have small vessel disease (expressed through leukoaraiosis, lacunes, and microbleeds) and cerebral amyloid angiopathy. Microbleeds may be a hemorrhagic expression of small vessel disease [161] and are highly associated with hypertension, where they are seen mainly in subcortical locations (deep grey and white matter). Otherwise, they may be the expression of concomitant cerebral amyloid angiopathy, in which case they would have a preferential lobar localization in subcortical-cortical junctions and would rather be associated with cortical superficial siderosis. Leukoaraiosis, another expression of small vessel disease, potentially increases intracerebral hemorrhages after intravenous thrombolysis [162]. Controversial data concerning improvement in outcome after thrombolysis sustain, at least, the consideration of its use in patients with leukoaraiosis [161–163]. Increased risk of symptomatic intracerebral hemorrhage after thrombolysis in stroke patients with cerebral microbleeds [164, 165] should not exclude those patients, as the risk of ischemic stroke is nonetheless higher than the risk of hemorrhagic stroke [166]. Nevertheless, special attention should be paid to those with a higher number of microbleeds (>10) and with cortical superficial siderosis (another expression of cerebral amyloid angiopathy) [167, 168]. In these patients, the relative hazard ratio for intracerebral hemorrhages is higher than ischemic stroke [166].

In summary, thrombolysis and thrombectomy should be considered in all acute stroke patients, despite cognitive status. That is why current recommendations for thrombolysis do not exclude patients with dementia [161, 165].

Concluding Remarks

Vascular risk factors increase the risk of cognitive decline and dementia over time, as well as the risk of death among patients with an established diagnosis of dementia. As an aide-mémoire for the busy clinician, a few take-home messages are summarized in Table 8.2. Notably, these messages are not fully evidence-based but are mainly inspired by the authors' clinical experience. In the forthcoming years (even months), they will hopefully have to be confronted with new research data.

Table 8.2 Vascular risk factors management in patients with the diagnosis of dementia: practical suggestions

Vascular risk factor	Suggestion	Special remarks
Hypertension	Treat according to usual guidelines[a] Regular measurements of blood pressure should be recommended at home[b] In case of general health or cognitive instability, increase surveillance Side effects such as hypotension should be avoided	Blood pressure measurements should be part of any medical appointment
Diabetes	Treat according to usual guidelines[a] and vascular risk Severity of diabetes should determine type of monitoring (could be prescribed at home, if necessary-BM test) In case of general health or cognitive instability, increase surveillance Hypoglycemia is not the aim	Blood tests should follow usual guidelines
Stroke	Treat according to usual guidelines[a] Antiplatelets and anticoagulants should be considered for secondary prevention reperfusion treatment should be considered in acute stroke patients with previous dementia	Particular decisions are based on risk of hemorrhagic events, previous functional status, and expectable benefits
Hypercholesterolemia	Treatment according to usual guidelines[a]	Diet counseling should be offered, trying to follow patient preferences, whenever clinically reasonable
Smoking	Should be avoided in patients with high vascular risk	
Excessive alcohol intake	Should be avoided	Mild alcohol intake may be accepted
Obesity, sedentarism, and physical activity	Promote physical activity to reduce sedentarism and control weight	Screen for depression Check if altered dietary intake reflects a behavior problem

[a]See main text for appropriate guidelines references
[b]Frequency should depend on the level and stability of usual blood pressure

Among all vascular risk factors, hypertension, hypercholesterolemia, and excessive weight should be especially addressed since early life in order to prevent later cognitive deterioration. Diabetes and stroke should also be prevented and treated following current guidelines. Patients with dementia should be regularly monitored concerning vascular risk factors and should never be denied the possibility of receiving appropriate treatments, including antiplatelets, anticoagulants, or reperfusion therapies, provided a thorough clinical evaluation is conducted.

References

1. Livingston G, Sommerlad A, Orgeta V, et al. Dementia prevention, intervention, and care. Lancet. 2017;390:2673–734.
2. METACOHORTS Consortium. METACOHORTS for the study of vascular disease and its contribution to cognitive decline and neurodegeneration: an initiative of the Joint Programme for Neurodegenerative Disease Research. Alzheimers Dement. 2016;12:1235–49.
3. Smith D, Yaffe K. Dementia (including Alzheimer's disease) can be prevented: statement supported by International Experts. J Alzheimers Dis. 2014;38:699–703.
4. Livingston G, Huntley J, Sommerlad A, Ames D, Ballard C, Banerjee S, Brayne C, Burns A, Cohen-Mansfield J, Cooper C, Costafreda SG, Dias A, Fox N, Gitlin LN, Howard R, Kales HC, Kivimäki M, Larson EB, Ogunniyi A, Orgeta V, Ritchie K, Rockwood K, Sampson EL, Samus Q, Schneider LS, Selbæk G, Teri L, Mukadam N. Dementia prevention, intervention, and care: 2020 report of the Lancet Commission. Lancet. 2020;396(10248):413–46.
5. Stephan BCM, Pakpahan E, Siervo M, et al. Prediction of dementia risk in low-income and middle-income countries (the 10/66 Study): an independent external validation of existing models. Lancet Glob Health. 2020;8(4):e524–35.
6. Oliveira D, Jun Otuyama L, Mabunda D, et al. Reducing the number of people with dementia through primary prevention in Mozambique, Brazil, and Portugal: an analysis of population-based data. J Alzheimers Dis. 2019;70(s1):S283–91.
7. Yaffe K, Vittinghoff E, Pletcher MJ, et al. Early adult to midlife cardiovascular risk factors and cognitive function. Circulation. 2014;129:1560–7.
8. Gottesman RF, Albert MS, Alonso A, et al. Associations between midlife vascular risk factors and 25-year incident dementia in the atherosclerosis risk in communities (ARIC) cohort. JAMA Neurol. 2017;74(10):1246–54.
9. Verdelho A. Role of cerebrovascular disease in cognitive decline. In: Galimberti D, Scarpini E, editors. Neurodegeneration: clinical aspects, molecular genetics and biomarkers for early diagnosis and treatment. Cham: Springer; 2014.
10. Muller M, Sigurdsson S, Kjartansson O, Aspelund T, Lopez OL, Jonnson PV, et al. Joint effect of mid- and late-life blood pressure on the brain: the AGES-Reykjavik Study. Neurology. 2014;82:2187–95.
11. Gottesman RF, Schneider AL, Albert M, Alonso A, Bandeen-Roche K, Coker L, Coresh J, Knopman D, Power MC, Rawlings A, Sharrett AR, Wruck LM, Mosley TH. Midlife hypertension and 20-year cognitive change: the atherosclerosis risk in communities neurocognitive study. JAMA Neurol. 2014;71:1218–27.
12. Iadecola C, Gottesman RF. Neurovascular and cognitive dysfunction in hypertension. Circ Res. 2019;124(7):1025–44.
13. Kivipelto M, Helkala EL, Laakso MP, Hänninen T, Hallikainen M, Alhainen K, et al. Midlife vascular risk factors and Alzheimer's disease in later life: longitudinal, population based study. BMJ. 2001;322:1447–51.
14. Launer LJ, Ross GW, Petrovitch H, Masaki K, Foley D, White LR, Havlik RJ. Midlife blood pressure and dementia: the Honolulu-Asia aging study. Neurobiol Aging. 2000;21:49–55.

15. Power MC, Schneider ALC, Wruck L, Griswold M, Coker LH, Alonso A, Jack CR Jr, Knopman D, Mosley TH, Gottesman RF. Life-course blood pressure in relation to brain volumes. Alzheimers Dement. 2016;12:890–9.
16. Korf ES, White LR, Scheltens P, Launer LJ. Midlife blood pressure and the risk of hippocampal atrophy: the Honolulu Asia Aging Study. Hypertension. 2004;44(1):29–34.
17. Rodrigue KM, Rieck JR, Kennedy KM, Devous MD Sr, Diaz-Arrastia R, Park DC. Risk factors for β-amyloid deposition in healthy aging: vascular and genetic effects. JAMA Neurol. 2013;70:600–6.
18. Arvanitakis Z, Capuano AW, Lamar M, et al. Late-life blood pressure association with cerebrovascular and Alzheimer disease pathology. Neurology. 2018;91(6):e517–25.
19. Walker KA, Sharrett AR, Wu A, et al. Association of midlife to late-life blood pressure patterns with incident dementia. JAMA. 2019;322(6):535–45.
20. Qiu C, Winblad B, Fratiglioni L. Low diastolic pressure and risk of dementia in very old people: a longitudinal study. Dement Geriatr Cogn Disord. 2009;28:213–9.
21. Razay G, Williams J, King E, Smith AD, Wilcock G. Blood pressure, dementia and Alzheimer's disease: the OPTIMA longitudinal study. Dement Geriatr Cogn Disord. 2009;28:70–4.
22. Stewart R, Xue QL, Masaki K, Petrovitch H, Ross GW, White LR, Launer LJ. Change in blood pressure and incident dementia: a 32-year prospective study. Hypertension. 2009;54:233–40.
23. Hoffman LB, Schmeidler J, Lesser GT, Beeri MS, Purohit DP, Grossman HT, Haroutunian V. Less Alzheimer disease neuropathology in medicated hypertensive than nonhypertensive persons. Neurology. 2009;72:1720–6.
24. van Middelaar T, van Vught LA, van Charante EPM, et al. Lower dementia risk with different classes of antihypertensive medication in older patients. J Hypertens. 2017;35(10):2095–101.
25. SHEP Cooperative Research Group. Prevention of stroke by antihypertensive drug treatment in older persons with isolated systolic hypertension. Final results of the Systolic Hypertension in the Elderly Program (SHEP). JAMA. 1991;265:3255–64.
26. Lithell H, Hansson L, Skoog I, Elmfeldt D, Hofman A, Olofsson B, et al. The Study on Cognition and Prognosis in the Elderly (SCOPE): principal results of a randomized double-blind intervention trial. J Hypertens. 2003;21:875–86.
27. Peters R, Beckett N, Forette F, Tuomilehto J, Clarke R, Ritchie C, et al. Incident dementia and blood pressure lowering in the Hypertension in the Very Elderly Trial cognitive function assessment (HYVET-COG): a double-blind, placebo controlled trial. Lancet Neurol. 2008;7:683–9.
28. Yusuf S, Diener HC, Sacco RL, Cotton D, Ounpuu S, Lawton WA, et al. Telmisartan to prevent recurrent stroke and cardiovascular events. N Engl J Med. 2008;359:1225–37.
29. Forette F, Seux ML, Staessen JA, Thijs L, Birkenhager WH, Babarskiene MR, et al. Prevention of dementia in randomised double-blind placebocontrolled Systolic Hypertension in Europe (Syst-Eur) trial. Lancet. 1998;352:1347–51.
30. Tzourio C, Anderson C, Chapman N, Woodward M, Neal B, MacMahon S, et al. Effects of blood pressure lowering with perindopril and indapamide therapy on dementia and cognitive decline in patients with cerebrovascular disease. Arch Intern Med. 2003;163:1069–75.
31. Larsson SC, Markus HS. Does treating vascular risk factors prevent dementia and Alzheimer's disease? A systematic review and meta-analysis. J Alzheimers Dis. 2018;64(2):657–68.
32. Lawlor B, Segurado R, Kennelly S, et al. Nilvadipine in mild to moderate Alzheimer disease: a randomised controlled trial. PLoS Med. 2018;15(9):e1002660. https://doi.org/10.1371/journal.pmed.1002660.
33. Anderson C, Teo K, Gao P, et al. Renin-angiotensin system blockade and cognitive function in patients at high risk of cardiovascular disease: analysis of data from the ONTARGET and TRANSCEND studies. Lancet Neurol. 2011;10(1):43–53.
34. Bosch J, O'Donnell M, Swaminathan B, et al. Effects of blood pressure and lipid lowering on cognition: results from the HOPE-3 study. Neurology. 2019;92(13):e1435–46.
35. Williamson JD, Pajewski NM, et al. SPRINT MIND investigators for the SPRINT research group, effect of intensive vs standard blood pressure control on probable dementia: a randomized clinical trial. JAMA. 2019;321(6):553–61.

36. Hughes D, Judge C, Murphy R, et al. Association of blood pressure lowering with incident dementia or cognitive impairment: a systematic review and meta-analysis. JAMA. 2020;323(19):1934–44. https://doi.org/10.1001/jama.2020.4249.
37. Dufouil C, Chalmers J, Coskun O, Besançon V, Bousser MG, Guillon P, MacMahon S, Mazoyer B, Neal B, Woodward M, TzourioMazoyer N, Tzourio C, PROGRESS MRI Substudy Investigators. Effects of blood pressure lowering on cerebral white matter hyperintensities in patients with stroke: the PROGRESS (perindopril protection against recurrent stroke study) magnetic resonance imaging substudy. Circulation. 2005;112:1644–50. https://doi.org/10.1161/CIRCULATIONAHA.104.501163.
38. Weber R, Weimar C, Blatchford J, Hermansson K, Wanke I, MöllerHartmann C, Gizewski ER, Forsting M, Demchuk AM, Sacco RL, Saver JL, Warach S, Diener HC, Diehl A, PRoFESS Imaging Substudy Group. Telmisartan on top of antihypertensive treatment does not prevent progression of cerebral white matter lesions in the Prevention Regimen for Effectively Avoiding Second Strokes (PRoFESS) MRI substudy. Stroke. 2012;43(9):2336–42.
39. Smith EE, Markus HS. New treatment approaches to modify the course of cerebral small vessel diseases. Stroke. 2020;51(1):38–46.
40. Zonneveld TP, Richard E, Vergouwen MD, et al. Blood pressure-lowering treatment for preventing recurrent stroke, major vascular events, and dementia in patients with a history of stroke or transient ischaemic attack. Cochrane Database Syst Rev. 2018;7(7):CD007858.
41. Williams B, Mancia G, Spiering W, Agabiti Rosei E, Azizi M, Burnier M, et al. 2018 ESC/ESH guidelines for the management of arterial hypertension: the task force for the management of arterial hypertension of the European Society of Cardiology and the European Society of hypertension: the task force for the management of arterial hypertension of the European Society of Cardiology and the European Society of Hypertension. J Hypertens. 2018;36:1953–2041.
42. Iadecola C, Yaffe K, Biller J, Bratzke LC, Faraci FM, Gorelick PB, Gulati M, Kamel H, Knopman DS, Launer LJ, Saczynski JS, Seshadri S, Zeki Al Hazzouri A, American Heart Association Council on Hypertension, Council on Clinical Cardiology, Council on Cardiovascular Disease in the Young, Council on Cardiovascular and Stroke Nursing, Council on Quality of Care and Outcomes Research, Stroke Council. Impact of hypertension on cognitive function: a scientific statement from the American Heart Association. Hypertension. 2016;68:e67–94.
43. Zhang Y, Moran AE. Trends in the prevalence, awareness, treatment, and control of hypertension among young adults in the United States, 1999 to 2014. Hypertension. 2017;70(4):736–42. https://doi.org/10.1161/HYPERTENSIONAHA.117.09801.
44. Burnier M, Polychronopoulou E, Wuerzner G. Hypertension and drug adherence in the elderly. Front Cardiovasc Med. 2020;7:49. https://doi.org/10.3389/fcvm.2020.00049.
45. Anstey KJ, Sargent-Cox K, Garde E, et al. Cognitive development over 8 years in midlife and its association with cardiovascular risk factors. Neuropsychology. 2014;28:653–65.
46. Knopman DS, Gottesman RF, Sharrett AR, et al. Midlife vascular risk factors and midlife cognitive status in relation to prevalence of mild cognitive impairment and dementia in later life: the Atherosclerosis Risk in Communities Study. Alzheimers Dement. 2018;14(11):1406–15.
47. Wong WB, Lin VW, Boudreau D, Devine EB. Statins in the prevention of dementia and Alzheimer's disease: a meta-analysis of observational studies and an assessment of confounding. Pharmacoepidemiol Drug Saf. 2013;22(4):345–58.
48. Chang CF, Liou YS, Lin TK, et al. High exposure to statins decrease the risk of new-onset dementia: a nationwide population-based longitudinal cohort study. Medicine (Baltimore). 2019;98(34):e16931.
49. Power MC, Weuve J, Sharrett AR, Blacker D, Gottesman RF. Statins, cognition, and dementia—systematic review and methodological commentary. Nat Rev Neurol. 2015;11(4):220–9.
50. Alsehli AM, Olivo G, Clemensson LE, Williams MJ, Schiöth HB. The cognitive effects of statins are modified by age. Sci Rep. 2020;10(1):6187.
51. Dye L, Boyle NB, Champ C, Lawton C. The relationship between obesity and cognitive health and decline. Proc Nutr Soc. 2017;76(4):443–54.

52. Pedditzi E, Peters R, Beckett N. The risk of overweight/obesity in mid-life and late life for the development of dementia: a systematic review and meta-analysis of longitudinal studies [published correction appears in Age Ageing. 2016 Sep;45(5):740]. Age Ageing. 2016;45(1):14–21.
53. Xue M, Xu W, Ou YN, et al. Diabetes mellitus and risks of cognitive impairment and dementia: a systematic review and meta-analysis of 144 prospective studies. Ageing Res Rev. 2019;55:100944.
54. Bello-Chavolla OY, Antonio-Villa NE, Vargas-Vázquez A, Ávila-Funes JA, Aguilar-Salinas CA. Pathophysiological mechanisms linking type 2 diabetes and dementia: review of evidence from clinical, translational and epidemiological research. Curr Diabetes Rev. 2019;15(6):456–70.
55. Huang CC, Chung CM, Leu HB, et al. Diabetes mellitus and the risk of Alzheimer's disease: a nationwide population-based study. PLoS One. 2014;9(1):e87095. https://doi.org/10.1371/journal.pone.0087095.
56. Cheng G, Huang C, Deng H, Wang H. Diabetes as a risk factor for dementia and mild cognitive impairment: a meta-analysis of longitudinal studies. Intern Med J. 2012;42(5):484–91. https://doi.org/10.1111/j.1445-5994.2012.02758.x.
57. Buchmann N, Fink A, Tegeler C, Demuth I, Doblhammer G, Steinhagen-Thiessen E. Different treatment forms of type II diabetes and the risk of dementia in German health claims data. Acta Diabetol. 2019;56(9):995–1003.
58. Verdelho A, Madureira S, Moleiro C, Ferro JM, Santos CO, Erkinjuntti T, et al. White matter changes and diabetes predict cognitive decline in the elderly: the ladis study. Neurology. 2010;75:160–7.
59. Verdelho A, Madureira S, Ferro JM, Basile AM, Chabriat H, Erkinjuntti T, et al. Differential impact of cerebral white matter changes, diabetes, hypertension and stroke on cognitive performance among non-disabled elderly. The ladis study. J Neurol Neurosurg Psychiatry. 2007;78:1325–30.
60. Teixeira MM, Passos VMA, Barreto SM, et al. Association between diabetes and cognitive function at baseline in the Brazilian Longitudinal Study of Adult Health (ELSA—Brasil). Sci Rep. 2020;10(1):1596.
61. Hanyu H. Diabetes-related dementia. Adv Exp Med Biol. 2019;1128:147–60. https://doi.org/10.1007/978-981-13-3540-2_8.
62. Hanyu H, Hirose D, Fukasawa R, Hatanaka H, Namioka N, Sakurai H. Guidelines for the clinical diagnosis of diabetes mellitus-related dementia. J Am Geriatr Soc. 2015;63:1721–2.
63. Takenoshita N, Fukasawa R, Ogawa Y, et al. Amyloid and tau positron emission tomography in suggested diabetes related dementia. Curr Alzheimer Res. 2018;15(11):1062–9.
64. Li W, Huang E, Gao S. Type 1 diabetes mellitus and cognitive impairments: a systematic review. J Alzheimers Dis. 2017;57(1):29–36. https://doi.org/10.3233/JAD-161250.
65. Biessels GJ, Despa F. Cognitive decline and dementia in diabetes mellitus: mechanisms and clinical implications. Nat Rev Endocrinol. 2018;14(10):591–604. https://doi.org/10.1038/s41574-018-0048-7.
66. Vázquez A, Ávila-Funes JA, Aguilar-Salinas CA. Pathophysiological mechanisms linking type 2 diabetes and dementia: review of evidence from clinical, translational and epidemiological research. Curr Diabetes Rev. 2019;15(6):456–70.
67. Kimura N. Diabetes mellitus induces Alzheimer's disease pathology: histopathological evidence from animal models. Int J Mol Sci. 2016;17(4):503. https://doi.org/10.3390/ijms17040503.
68. Wijesekara N, Gonçalves RA, De Felice FG, Fraser PE. Impaired peripheral glucose homeostasis and Alzheimer's disease. Neuropharmacology. 2018;136(Pt B):172–81.
69. Vieira MNN, Lima-Filho RAS, De Felice FG. Connecting Alzheimer's disease to diabetes: underlying mechanisms and potential therapeutic targets. Neuropharmacology. 2018;136(Pt B):160–71.

70. Morsi M, Maher A, Metwally A, Abo-Elmagd O, Johar D, Bernstein L. A shared comparison of diabetes mellitus and neurodegenerative disorders. J Cell Biochem. 2017;120(9):14318–25. https://doi.org/10.1002/jcb.26261.
71. Folch J, Pedrós I, Patraca I, Martínez N, Sureda F, Camins A. Metabolic basis of sporadic Alzheimer's disease. Role of hormones related to energy metabolism. Curr Pharm Des. 2013;19(38):6739–48.
72. Movassat J, Delangre E, Liu J, Gu Y, Janel N. Hypothesis and theory: circulating Alzheimer's-related biomarkers in type 2 diabetes. Insight from the Goto-Kakizaki Rat. Front Neurol. 2019;10:649. https://doi.org/10.3389/fneur.2019.00649.
73. Santiago JA, Bottero V, Potashkin JA. Transcriptomic and network analysis highlight the association of diabetes at different stages of Alzheimer's disease. Front Neurosci. 2019;13:1273. https://doi.org/10.3389/fnins.2019.01273.
74. Mirza Z, Kamal MA, Abuzenadah AM, Al-Qahtani MH, Karim S. Establishing genomic/transcriptomic links between Alzheimer's disease and type II diabetes mellitus by meta-analysis approach. CNS Neurol Disord Drug Targets. 2014;13:501–16.
75. Abdul-Rahman O, Sasvari-Szekely M, Ver A, Rosta K, Szasz BK, Kereszturi E, Keszler G. Altered gene expression profiles in the hippocampus and prefrontal cortex of type 2 diabetic rats. BMC Genomics. 2012;13:81.
76. Stephan BCM, Minett T, Muniz-Terrera G, Harrison SL, Matthews FE, Brayne C. Neuropsychological profiles of vascular disease and risk of dementia: implications for defining vascular cognitive impairment no dementia (VCI-ND). Age Ageing. 2017;46(5):755–60.
77. Moran C, Callisaya ML, Srikanth V, Arvanitakis Z. Diabetes therapies for dementia. Curr Neurol Neurosci Rep. 2019;19(8):58. https://doi.org/10.1007/s11910-019-0973-4.
78. Rostamian S, Mahinrad S, Stijnen T, et al. Cognitive impairment and risk of stroke: a systematic review and meta-analysis of prospective cohort studies. Stroke. 2014;45:1342–134.
79. Lee M, Saver JL, Hong KS, et al. Cognitive impairment and risk of future stroke: a systematic review and meta-analysis. CMAJ. 2014;186(14):E536–46.
80. Heshmatollah A, Mutlu U, Koudstaal PJ, Ikram MA, Ikram MK. Cognitive and physical impairment and the risk of stroke—a prospective cohort study. Sci Rep. 2020;10(1):6274.
81. Pendlebury ST, Rothwell PM. Prevalence, incidence, and factors associated with pre-stroke and post-stroke dementia: a systematic review and meta-analysis. Lancet Neurol. 2009;8(11):1006–18.
82. Pendlebury S, Rothwell P, Study OV. Incidence and prevalence of dementia associated with transient ischaemic attack and stroke: analysis of the population-based oxford vascular study. Lancet Neurol. 2019;18:248–58.
83. Hachinski V, Einhäupl K, Ganten D, et al. Preventing dementia by preventing stroke: the Berlin manifesto. Alzheimers Dement. 2019;15(7):961–84.
84. Mok VCT, Lam BYK, Wang Z, et al. Delayed-onset dementia after stroke or transient ischemic attack. Alzheimers Dement. 2016;12(11):1167–76.
85. Lei C, Deng Q, Li H, Zhong L. Association between silent brain infarcts and cognitive function: a systematic review and meta-analysis. J Stroke Cerebrovasc Dis. 2019;28(9):2376–87.
86. Yang J, Wong A, Wang Z, et al. Risk factors for incident dementia after stroke and transient ischemic attack. Alzheimers Dement. 2015;11(1):16–23.
87. Surawan J, Areemit S, Tiamkao S, Sirithanawuthichai T, Saensak S. Risk factors associated with post-stroke dementia: a systematic review and meta-analysis. Neurol Int. 2017;9(3):7216.
88. Mijajlović MD, Pavlović A, Brainin M, et al. Post-stroke dementia—a comprehensive review. BMC Med. 2017;15(1):11.
89. Casolla B, Caparros F, Cordonnier C, et al. Biological and imaging predictors of cognitive impairment after stroke: a systematic review. J Neurol. 2018;266(11):2593–604.
90. Puy L, Barbay M, Roussel M, et al. Neuroimaging determinants of poststroke cognitive performance. Stroke. 2018;49:2666–73.

91. Kernan WN, Ovbiagele B, Black HR, et al. Guidelines for the prevention of stroke in patients with stroke and transient ischemic attack: a guideline for healthcare professionals from the American Heart Association/American Stroke Association. Stroke. 2014;45:2160–236.
92. Powers WJ, Rabinstein AA, Ackerson T, et al. Guidelines for the early management of patients with acute ischemic stroke: 2019 update to the 2018 guidelines for the early management of acute ischemic stroke: a guideline for healthcare professionals from the American Heart Association/American Stroke Association. Stroke. 2019;50:e344–418.
93. Friberg L, Rosenqvist M. Less dementia with oral anticoagulation in atrial fibrillation. Eur Heart J. 2018;39(6):453–60.
94. Mongkhon P, Fanning L, Lau WCY, et al. Oral anticoagulant and reduced risk of dementia in patients with atrial fibrillation: a population-based cohort study. Heart Rhythm. 2020;17(5 Pt A):706–13.
95. Frederiksen KS, Cooper C, Frisoni GB, et al. European Academy of Neurology guideline on medical management issues in dementia. Eur J Neurol. 2020;27:1805–20.
96. Subic A, Cermakova P, Religa D, et al. Treatment of atrial fibrillation in patients with dementia: a cohort study from the Swedish Dementia Registry. J Alzheimers Dis. 2018;61(3):1119–28. https://doi.org/10.3233/JAD-170575.
97. Rabin JS, Schultz AP, Hedden T, et al. Interactive associations of vascular risk and β-amyloid burden with cognitive decline in clinically normal elderly individuals: findings from the Harvard Aging Brain Study. JAMA Neurol. 2018;75(9):1124–31.
98. Attems J, Jellinger KA. The overlap between vascular disease and Alzheimer's disease--lessons from pathology. BMC Med. 2014;12:206.
99. Iadecola C, Gottesman RF. Cerebrovascular alterations in Alzheimer disease. Circ Res. 2018;123(4):406–8.
100. Azarpazhooh MR, Avan A, Cipriano LE, Munoz DG, Sposato LA, Hachinski V. Concomitant vascular and neurodegenerative pathologies double the risk of dementia. Alzheimers Dement. 2018;14(2):148–56.
101. Hagberg G, Ihle-Hansen H, Fure B, et al. No evidence for amyloid pathology as a key mediator of neurodegeneration post-stroke—a seven-year follow-up study. BMC Neurol. 2020;20(1):174.
102. Wollenweber FA, Därr S, Müller C, Duering M, Buerger K, Zietemann V, Malik R, Brendel M, Ertl-Wagner B, Bartenstein P, Rominger A, Dichgans M. Prevalence of amyloid positron emission tomographic positivity in poststroke mild cognitive impairment. Stroke. 2016;47:2645–8.
103. Schmidt A, Diederich K, Strecker JK, Geng B, Hoppen M, Duning T, Schäbitz WR, Minnerup J. Progressive cognitive deficits in a mouse model of recurrent photothrombotic stroke. Stroke. 2015;46:1127–31.
104. Mok VC, Lam BY, Wong A, Ko H, Markus HS, Wong LK. Early-onset and delayed-onset poststroke dementia—revisiting the mechanisms. Nat Rev Neurol. 2017;13(3):148–59.
105. Banerjee G, Chan E, Ambler G, et al. Effect of small-vessel disease on cognitive trajectory after atrial fibrillation-related ischaemic stroke or TIA. J Neurol. 2019;266(5):1250–9.
106. Cicero AFG, Ruscica M, Banach M. Resveratrol and cognitive decline: a clinician perspective. Arch Med Sci. 2019;15(4):936–43. https://doi.org/10.5114/aoms.2019.85463.
107. Majdi A, Kamari F, Sadigh-Eteghad S, Gjedde A. Molecular insights into memory-enhancing metabolites of nicotine in brain: a systematic review. Front Neurosci. 2019;12:1002.
108. Xu W, Wang H, Wan Y, et al. Alcohol consumption and dementia risk: a dose-response meta-analysis of prospective studies. Eur J Epidemiol. 2017;32(1):31–42.
109. Kim JW, Lee DY, Lee BC, et al. Alcohol and cognition in the elderly: a review. Psychiatry Investig. 2012;9(1):8–16.
110. Verbaten MN. Chronic effects of low to moderate alcohol consumption on structural and functional properties of the brain: beneficial or not? Hum Psychopharmacol. 2009;24:199–205.
111. Neiman J. Alcohol as a risk factor for brain damage: neurologic aspects. Alcohol Clin Exp Res. 1998;22:346S–51S.

112. Mechtcheriakov S, Brenneis C, Egger K, Koppelstaetter F, Schocke M, Marksteiner J. A widespread distinct pattern of cerebral atrophy in patients with alcohol addiction revealed by voxel-based morphometry. J Neurol Neurosurg Psychiatry. 2007;78(6):610–4.
113. Handing EP, Andel R, Kadlecova P, Gatz M, Pedersen NL. Midlife alcohol consumption and risk of dementia over 43 years of follow-up: a population-based study from the Swedish Twin Registry. J Gerontol Ser A Biol Sci Med Sci. 2015;70(10):1248–54.
114. Langballe EM, Ask H, Holmen J, et al. Alcohol consumption and risk of dementia up to 27 years later in a large, population-based sample: the HUNT study, Norway. Eur J Epidemiol. 2015;30(9):1049–56.
115. Weyerer S, Schaufele M, Wiese B, et al. Current alcohol consumption and its relationship to incident dementia: results from a 3-year follow-up study among primary care attenders aged75 years and older. Age Ageing. 2011;40(4):456–63. https://doi.org/10.1093/ageing/afr007.
116. Meier P, Seitz HK. Age, alcohol metabolism and liver disease. Curr Opin Clin Nutr Metab Care. 2008;11(1):21–6.
117. Majdi A, Kamari F, Vafaee MS, Sadigh-Eteghad S. Revisiting nicotine's role in the ageing brain and cognitive impairment. Rev Neurosci. 2017;28(7):767–81.
118. Newhouse P, Kellar K, Aisen P, White H, Wesnes K, Coderre E, et al. Nicotine treatment of mild cognitive impairment: a 6-month double-blind pilot clinical trial. Neurology. 2012;78:91–101.
119. Zhong G, Wang Y, Zhang Y, Guo JJ, Zhao Y. Smoking is associated with an increased risk of dementia: a meta-analysis of prospective cohort studies with investigation of potential effect modifiers. PLoS One. 2015;10(4):e0126169.
120. Choi D, Choi S, Park SM. Effect of smoking cessation on the risk of dementia: a longitudinal study. Ann Clin Transl Neurol. 2018;5(10):1192–9.
121. Peters R, Booth A, Rockwood K, Peters J, D'Este C, Anstey KJ. Combining modifiable risk factors and risk of dementia: a systematic review and meta-analysis. BMJ Open. 2019;9(1):e022846. https://doi.org/10.1136/bmjopen-2018-022846.
122. Virta JJ, Heikkilä K, Perola M, Koskenvuo M, Räihä I, Rinne JO, Kaprio J. Midlife cardiovascular risk factors and late cognitive impairment. Eur J Epidemiol. 2013;28:405–16.
123. Kesse-Guyot E, Andreeva VA, Lassale C, Hercberg S, Galan P. Clustering of midlife lifestyle behaviors and subsequent cognitive function: a longitudinal study. Am J Public Health. 2014;104(11):e170–7. https://doi.org/10.2105/AJPH.2014.302121.
124. Kivipelto M, Ngandu T, Laatikainen T, Winblad B, Soininen H, Tuomilehto J. Risk score for the prediction of dementia risk in 20 years among middle aged people: a longitudinal, population-based study. Lancet Neurol. 2006;5(9):735–41.
125. Gardener H, Wright CB, Dong C, et al. Ideal cardiovascular health and cognitive aging in the Northern Manhattan Study. J Am Heart Assoc. 2016;5:e002731.
126. Norton MC, Dew J, Smith H, et al. Lifestyle behavior pattern is associated with different levels of risk for incident dementia and Alzheimer's disease : the cache county study. J Am Geriatr Soc. 2012;60:405–12.
127. Qiu C, Xu W, Winblad B, et al. Vascular risk profiles for dementia and Alzheimer's disease in very old people: a population-based longitudinal study. J Alzheimers Dis. 2010;20:293–300.
128. Suri S, Topiwala A, Chappell MA, et al. Association of midlife cardiovascular risk profiles with cerebral perfusion at older ages. JAMA Netw Open. 2019;2(6):e195776.
129. Gottesman RF, Schneider AL, Zhou Y, Coresh J, Green E, Gupta N, et al. Association between midlife vascular risk factors and estimated brain amyloid deposition. JAMA. 2017;317(14):1443–50.
130. Alberti KG, Eckel RH, Grundy SM, Zimmet PZ, Cleeman JI, Donato KA, Fruchart JC, James WP, Loria CM, Smith SC Jr, International Diabetes Federation Task Force on Epidemiology and Prevention, National Heart, Lung, and Blood Institute, American Heart Association, World Heart Federation, International Atherosclerosis Society, International Association for the Study of Obesity. Harmonizing the metabolic syndrome: a joint interim statement of the International Diabetes Federation Task Force on Epidemiology and Prevention; National Heart, Lung, and Blood Institute; American Heart Association; World Heart Federation; International

Atherosclerosis Society; and International Association for the Study of Obesity. Circulation. 2009;120(16):1640–5. https://doi.org/10.1161/CIRCULATIONAHA.109.192644.
131. Atti AR, Valente S, Iodice A, et al. Metabolic syndrome, mild cognitive impairment, and dementia: a meta-analysis of longitudinal studies. Am J Geriatr Psychiatry. 2019;27(6):625–37. https://doi.org/10.1016/j.jagp.2019.01.214.
132. Lee JE, Shin DW, Han K, et al. Changes in metabolic syndrome status and risk of dementia. J Clin Med. 2020;9(1):122. https://doi.org/10.3390/jcm9010122.
133. Ng TP, Feng L, Nyunt MSZ, Feng L, Gao Q, Lim ML. Metabolic syndrome and the risk of mild cognitive impairment and progression to dementia: follow-up of the Singapore Longitudinal Ageing Study Cohort. JAMA Neurol. 2016;73:456–63.
134. Akbaraly TN, Kivimaki M, Shipley MJ, Tabak AG, Jokela M, Virtanen M. Metabolic syndrome over 10 years and cognitive functioning in late midlife: the Whitehall II study. Diabetes Care. 2010;33:84–9.
135. Wu YT, Beiser AS, Breteler MMB, et al. The changing prevalence and incidence of dementia over time—current evidence. Nat Rev Neurol. 2017;13(6):327–39.
136. Wu YT, Fratiglioni L, Matthews FE, et al. Dementia in western Europe: epidemiological evidence and implications for policy making [published correction appears in Lancet Neurol. 2016 Feb;15(2):135]. Lancet Neurol. 2016;15(1):116–24.
137. Prince M, Ali GC, Guerchet M, Prina AM, Albanese E, Wu YT. Recent global trends in the prevalence and incidence of dementia, and survival with dementia. Alzheimers Res Ther. 2016;8(1):23.
138. Kivipelto M, Mangialasche F, Ngandu T. Lifestyle interventions to prevent cognitive impairment, dementia and Alzheimer disease. Nat Rev Neurol. 2018;14(11):653–66.
139. Dhana K, Evans DA, Rajan KB, Bennett DA, Morris MC. Healthy lifestyle and the risk of Alzheimer dementia: findings from 2 longitudinal studies. Neurology. 2020;95(4):e374–83. https://doi.org/10.1212/WNL.0000000000009816.
140. Ngandu T, Lehtisalo J, Solomon A, et al. A 2 year multidomain intervention of diet, exercise, cognitive training, and vascular risk monitoring versus control to prevent cognitive decline in at-risk elderly people (FINGER): a randomised controlled trial. Lancet. 2015;385(9984):2255–63.
141. Teuschl Y, Ihle-Hansen H, Matz K, et al. Multidomain intervention for the prevention of cognitive decline after stroke—a pooled patient-level data analysis. Eur J Neurol. 2018;25:1182–8.
142. Teuschl Y, Matz K, Firlinger B, et al. Preventive effects of multiple domain interventions on lifestyle and risk factor changes in stroke survivors: evidence from a two-year randomized trial. Int J Stroke. 2017;12:976–84.
143. Dalen V, Willem J, Moll EP, et al. Effect of long-term vascular care on progression of cerebrovascular lesions: magnetic resonance imaging substudy of the PreDIVA trial (prevention of dementia by intensive vascular care). Stroke. 2017;48:1842–8.
144. Katayama O, Lee S, Bae S, et al. Modifiable risk factor possession patterns of dementia in elderly with MCI: a 4-year repeated measures study. J Clin Med. 2020;9(4):1076. https://doi.org/10.3390/jcm9041076.
145. Li J, Wang YJ, Zhang M, et al. Vascular risk factors promote conversion from mild cognitive impairment to Alzheimer disease. Neurology. 2011;76(17):1485–91.
146. Deschaintre Y, Richard F, Leys D, Pasquier F. Treatment of vascular risk factors is associated with slower decline in Alzheimer disease. Neurology. 2009;73(9):674–80.
147. Alzheimer's Association. 2016 Alzheimer's disease facts and figures. Alzheimers Dement. 2016;12(4):459–509. https://doi.org/10.1016/j.jalz.2016.03.001.
148. van de Vorst IE, Koek HL, de Vries R, Bots ML, Reitsma JB, Vaartjes I. Effect of vascular risk factors and diseases on mortality in individuals with dementia: a systematic review and meta-analysis. J Am Geriatr Soc. 2016;64(1):37–46. https://doi.org/10.1111/jgs.13835.
149. Golüke NMS, van de Vorst IE, Vaartjes IH, et al. Risk factors for in-hospital mortality in patients with dementia. Maturitas. 2019;129:57–61. https://doi.org/10.1016/j.maturitas.2019.08.0071.

150. Johnell K. Inappropriate drug use in people with cognitive impairment and dementia: a systematic review. Curr Clin Pharmacol. 2015;10(3):178–84. https://doi.org/10.2174/1574884710666150609154741).
151. Connolly A, Campbell S, Gaehl E, et al. Under-provision of medical care for vascular diseases for people with dementia in primary care: a cross-sectional review. Br J Gen Pract. 2013;63(607):e88–96. https://doi.org/10.3399/bjgp13X663046.
152. Rattinger GB, Dutcher SK, Chhabra PT, et al. The effect of dementia on medication use and adherence among Medicare beneficiaries with chronic heart failure. Am J Geriatr Pharmacother. 2012;10(1):69–80. https://doi.org/10.1016/j.amjopharm.2011.11.003.
153. Lopponen M, Raiha I, Isoaho R, Vahlberg T, Puolijoki H, Kivela SL. Dementia associates with undermedication of cardiovascular diseases in the elderly: a population-based study. Dement Geriatr Cogn Disord. 2006;22(2):132–41.
154. Ganguli M, Jia Y, Hughes TF, et al. Mild cognitive impairment that does not progress to dementia: a population-based Study. J Am Geriatr Soc. 2019;67(2):232–8.
155. Balsinha C, Gonçalves-Pereira M, Iliffe S, Freitas JA, Grave J. Healthcare delivery for older people with dementia in primary care. In: de Mendonça-Lima C, Ivbijaro G, editors. Primary care mental health for older people. Cham: Springer; 2019. p. 311–29. https://doi.org/10.1007/978-3-030-10814-4_23. isbn:978-3-030-10812-0 (Print) 978-3-030-10814-4.
156. World Health Organization. Integrated care for older people: guidelines on community-level interventions to manage declines in intrinsic capacity. 2017. isbn:978-92-4-155010-9. https://www.who.int/ageing/publications/guidelines-icope/en/
157. Saposnik G, Cote R, Rochon PA, Mamdani M, Liu Y, Raptis S, Kapral MK, Black SE. Care and outcomes in patients with ischemic stroke with and without preexisting dementia. Neurology. 2011;77(18):1664–73. https://doi.org/10.1212/WNL.0b013e31823648f1.
158. Alshekhlee A, Li CC, Chuang SY, et al. Does dementia increase risk of thrombolysis? A case-control study. Neurology. 2011;76(18):1575–80. https://doi.org/10.1212/WNL.0b013e3182190d37.
159. Zupanic E, von Euler M, Kåreholt I, et al. Thrombolysis in acute ischemic stroke in patients with dementia: a Swedish registry study. Neurology. 2017;89(18):1860–8.
160. Gensicke H, Strbian D, Zinkstok SM, Scheitz JF, Bill O, Hametner C, Moulin S, Zini A, Kägi G, Pezzini A, Padjen V, Béjot Y, Corbiere S, Zonneveld TP, Seiffge DJ, Roos YB, Traenka C, Putaala J, Peters N, Bonati LH, Curtze S, Erdur H, Sibolt G, Koch P, Vandelli L, Ringleb P, Leys D, Cordonnier C, Michel P, Nolte CH, Lyrer PA, Tatlisumak T, Nederkoorn PJ, Engelter ST, Thrombolysis in Stroke Patients (TriSP) Collaborators. Intravenous thrombolysis in patients dependent on the daily help of others before stroke. Stroke. 2016;47:450–6.
161. Paciaroni M, Pantoni L. Thrombolysis in dementia patients with acute stroke: is it justified? Neurol Sci. 2017;38(1):27–31. https://doi.org/10.1007/s10072-016-2725-4.
162. Charidimou A, Pasi M, Fiorelli M, et al. Leukoaraiosis, cerebral hemorrhage, and outcome after intravenous thrombolysis for acute ischemic stroke: a meta-analysis (v1) [published correction appears in Stroke. 2016 Oct;47(10):e244]. Stroke. 2016;47(9):2364–72.
163. Demchuk AM, Khan F, Hill MD, et al. Importance of leukoaraiosis on CT for tissue plasminogen activator decision making: evaluation of the NINDS rt-PA Stroke Study. Cerebrovasc Dis. 2008;26(2):120–5.
164. Charidimou A, Kakar P, Fox Z, Werring DJ. Cerebral microbleeds and the risk of intracerebral haemorrhage after thrombolysis for acute ischaemic stroke: systematic review and meta-analysis. J Neurol Neurosurg Psychiatry. 2013;84:277–80.
165. Demaerschalk BM, Kleindorfer DO, Adeoye OM, Demchuk AM, Fugate JE, Grotta JC, Khalessi AA, Levy EI, Palesch YY, Prabhakaran S, Saposnik G, Saver JL, Smith EE. American Heart Association Stroke Council and Council on Epidemiology and Prevention Scientific rationale for the inclusion and exclusion criteria for intravenous alteplase in acute ischemic stroke: a statement for healthcare professionals from the American Heart Association/American Stroke Association. Stroke. 2016;47(2):581–641.

166. Wilson D, Ambler G, Lee KJ, et al. Cerebral microbleeds and stroke risk after ischaemic stroke or transient ischaemic attack: a pooled analysis of individual patient data from cohort studies [published correction appears in Lancet Neurol. 2019 Sep;18(9):e8] [published correction appears in Lancet Neurol. 2020 Feb;19(2):e2]. Lancet Neurol. 2019;18(7):653–65.
167. Charidimou A, Boulouis G, Greenberg SM, Viswanathan A. Cortical superficial siderosis and bleeding risk in cerebral amyloid angiopathy: a meta-analysis. Neurology. 2019;93:e2192–202.
168. Wollenweber FA, Opherk C, Zedde M, et al. Prognostic relevance of cortical superficial siderosis in cerebral amyloid Angiopathy. Neurology. 2019;92:e792–801.

9 Assessment and Management of Pain in Patients with Dementia

Christina Jensen-Dahm

Abbreviations

AD	Alzheimer's disease
CNS	Central nervous system
DLB	Dementia with Lewy Bodies
FTD	Frontotemporal Dementia
MMSE	Minimental state examination
NSAID	Non-steroidal anti-inflammatory drug
PACSLAC	Pain Assessment Checklist for Seniors with Limited Ability to Communicate
PAINAD	Pain in Advanced Dementia
WHO	World Health Organization

Introduction

Pain is defined by the International Association for Study of Pain as "an unpleasant sensory and emotional experience associated with actual or potential tissue damage or described in terms of such damage" [1]. It is classified as acute—associated with trauma or injury—or chronic (lasting longer than 3 months). Pain perception is a subjective and complex experience, which involves sensory-discriminative components (i.e., location, intensity, duration), affective-motivational (e.g., unpleasantness of the noxious stimuli), and cognitive components. The prevalence of pain rises with increasing age [2, 3], and likewise does the incidence of dementia. Thus, it

C. Jensen-Dahm (✉)
Danish Dementia Research Centre, Rigshospitalet, University of Copenhagen, Copenhagen, Denmark
e-mail: christina.jensen-dahm@regionh.dk

K. S. Frederiksen, G. Waldemar (eds.), *Management of Patients with Dementia*,
https://doi.org/10.1007/978-3-030-77904-7_9

must be expected that a considerable number of patients experience both pain and dementia.

Any cognitive disorder, in which deficits in memory and reasoning are cardinal symptoms, could be expected to have a profound effect on an individual's appraisal of the pain experience and its future implications. In judging pain severity, we rely on previous experiences and knowledge of pain, underpinned by episodic memory and semantic memory. Memory problems may lead to patients forgetting that they experienced pain recently and therefore not communicating they were in pain. Likewise, aphasia could lead to problems expressing pain. Lack of insight may also mean that patients with dementia fail to report pain when consulting a physician. In terms of pain assessment dementia is a double-edged sword. Pain affects cognitive function [4], and cognitive function also affects pain assessment as patient's report still is the primary mean for pain assessment [5, 6].

Pain in the Elderly

The prevalence of pain in the elderly population in general is difficult to estimate and has varied from 0 to 93% depending on the population and definition of pain [7]. The prevalence of pain rises with increasing age, though some studies have found that it reaches a plateau after age 65 [7, 8]. The prevalence of chronic pain is estimated to be 20–25% in men over the age of 65 and 30–35% in women over the age of 65 [9, 10]. The most frequent causes of pain in the elderly are related to osteoarthritis, especially in the back and neck, which is present in up to 65% of elderly with chronic pain. Other frequent causes are musculoskeletal problems (40%), neuropathic pain (35%), and chronic joint pain (15–25%) [8]. Elderly patients with musculoskeletal pain often have pain from several regions. Likewise, the elderly with chronic pain often have different pain-causing conditions. Older people with dementia have worse overall oral health than older people without dementia, including coronal caries, root caries, and retained roots [11]. Orofacial pain and its potential causes were frequently present in elderly with dementia [11, 12] and more so than in elderly without dementia [11]. Furthermore, one study found a correlation between the severity of cognitive impairment and potential painful oral conditions [12].

Epidemiology of Pain in Dementia

Knowledge about the epidemiology of pain in patients with dementia is to a large extent, based on studies of nursing home residents. A review of studies published between 1999 and 2009 found that pain prevalence among nursing home residents varied between 3.7 and 79.5% depending on the method used [13]. In a large study of almost 10,000 nursing home residents, a negative association between dementia and pain was observed [14]. This was supported by a study that observed that increasing degree of cognitive impairment leads to lower frequencies of observed pain among nursing home residents [15]. However, both studies were based on observer ratings (minimum dataset), and one may speculate whether the lower frequency of pain was due to communication problems, leading to undiagnosed pain. An alternative explanation may be that patients with and without dementia were admitted to a nursing home for different reasons, i.e., patients with dementia were living in a nursing home due to cognitive impairment, whereas the cognitively intact were living at nursing homes due to severe illness or disability and therefore were more likely to suffer from pain.

Few studies have investigated prevalence of pain in community-dwelling patients with dementia. A Finnish population-based study of elderly over 75 years found that the prevalence of pain was significantly lower in patients with dementia. This was irrespective of whether they evaluated pain during the preceding month, presence of daily pain, pain interfering with routine activities, or daily pain at rest. The findings did not seem to depend on the degree of dementia, though patients were mainly suffering from mild to moderate dementia [16]. In contrast, results from the "Swedish National Study of Aging and Care—Kungsholmen" found a similar prevalence of pain in home-living patients with dementia compared to those without dementia [17]. Thirty-five percent of nursing home residents without dementia were reporting pain in contrast to 8.6% of nursing home residents with dementia. However, 48.9% of nursing home residents with dementia were unable to answer the question, and this may point toward one obvious mechanism behind the epidemiological finding of a lower prevalence of pain in patients with dementia, i.e., problems with communicating pain.

The majority of studies have not distinguished between different types of dementia when assessing pain prevalence or pain report. The studies that have focused on subtypes of dementia have mainly focused on Alzheimer's disease, and a few have focused on vascular dementia and/or mixed dementia. At present, there is limited evidence about pain prevalence in dementia with Lewy bodies and frontotemporal dementia [18].

Alzheimer's Disease

In 1997 Fisher-Morris and Gellatly published a report of two patients with Alzheimer's disease (AD), where they had observed a marked decrease in pain responses. The first case was a 90-year-old woman with a fungating carcinoma of the breast, which ulcerated through the skin and destroyed the breast and chest wall. During the 18 month the patient lived in a nursing home, her response to the lesions was gradually diminished, and she did not complain of pain. The second case was a 70-year-old man with AD, who sustained a femur fracture, but still walked around without complaining of pain, which lead the authors to speculate if AD leads to a change in pain perception [19].

A reduced report of pain is supported by a study comparing pain intensity ratings in cognitively intact elderly and patients with early and moderate AD matched for painful conditions, which showed that cognitively intact peers rated pain significantly higher than patients with AD. The study also found a correlation between pain intensity and stage of AD, as patients with early AD rated pain higher than patients with moderate AD [20]. In a similar study, the same authors were able to show that patients with early AD reported lower pain scores on a visual analog scale and lower affective distress associated with pain compared to the cognitively intact [21]. The same authors found that the patients experienced less pain during activities of daily living, and pain had a lower impact on daily life than controls. Similar in a study examining patient's and proxy's ratings of pain in 321 patients with early AD using part of a self-rated health scale (EQ-5D), it was found that 32.9% of the patients reported pain, whereas 51.4% of their caregivers judged the patients to experience pain. The authors compared the finding to EQ-5D norms for the elderly Danish population, in which approximately 50% reported pain, which was considerably higher than in patients with early AD [22]. In a recent study of pain complaints in outpatient memory clinic patients, it was found that elderly with AD complained significantly less than elderly with subjective cognitive impairment [23]. The exact prevalence of pain varies considerably from study to study depending on the sample and what is measured (any pain, daily pain, chronic pain, etc.). A systematic recent review found that the pain sample-weighted pain prevalence was 45.8% (95% CI: 33.4–58.5%) for AD [18].

Other Types of Dementia

To date, there have been no studies examining the prevalence of pain in frontotemporal dementia (FTD). There is very limited evidence about dementia with Lewy bodies (DLB). In Parkinson's disease pain is frequent and is a frequent pre-motor symptom [24], but if this the case in DLB is not known. Studies have shown that nursing home patients with "possible" or "probable" vascular dementia were more likely to self-report pain [25], more likely to suffer from chronic pain [26], and reported higher pain intensity than nursing home residents without dementia [27]. Furthermore, more pain locations were observed in patients with vascular dementia and mixed dementia compared to AD [28]. A recent study found a positive relationship between white matter hyperintensities and self-reported pain intensity in older patients with and without dementia [29]. However, a recent systematic review found no differences in pain prevalence among dementia subtypes, although limited data about vascular dementia [18].

Pathophysiology of Pain in Dementia

Supraspinal Mechanism of Pain

Pain is the psychophysiological result of an unpleasant internal or external stimulus, which activates a group of receptors called nociceptors. Nociceptors are located in the skin, and other tissues (first-order neurons) and information is projected to the dorsal horn of the spinal cord (second-order neurons) [30]. From the spinal cord, the information is transmitted via the spinoreticular, spinomesencephalic, and spinothalamic tract to the brain stem and thalamus. Areas of the brain stem such as the periaqueductal gray, rostral ventromedial medulla, and locus coeruleus are important sites for pain modulating systems and constitute part of a descending modulatory pain system [30]. From the brain stem information is transmitted to the spinal cord and the central nervous system (CNS) (third-order neurons). The thalamus, located within the diencephalon, is the major relay station for sensory information projected to the CNS.

Pain perception is a complex experience, which involves sensory-discriminative components (i.e., location, intensity, duration), affective-motivational (e.g., unpleasantness of the noxious stimuli), and cognitive components. It has been suggested that the sensory-discriminative and affective-motivational components of pain are largely represented by separate pathways that target lateral and medial nuclei of the dorsal thalamus [30–33].

The spinothalamic tracts have their main targets in the lateral thalamic nuclei (ventral posterolateral, ventral posteromedial and ventral posterior inferior nuclei), which project to the contralateral primary sensory cortex, secondary somatosensory cortex, parietal operculum, and the mid- and posterior part of the insula also referred to as the lateral pain pathway. The lateral pain pathway encodes sensory-discriminative aspects of pain, i.e., spatial localization and intensity of painful stimuli [30, 31]. This is supported by the clinical finding that patients with lesions in the primary and secondary sensory cortices have deficits in pain sensations and disturbed ability to localize pain [34]. However, lesions at different levels of the somatosensory pathway can lead to central pain, which can occur in stroke patients [35].

The medial thalamic nuclei (central median nucleus and intralaminar complex) projects to structures of the limbic system (anterior cingulate cortex, amygdala, hippocampus, insula, and prefrontal cortex) and is thought to process the affective-motivational and cognitive components of pain [36, 37], also referred to as the medial pathway [30–33]. The anterior cingulate cortex has been shown to be important for the affective-motivational and cognitive aspects of pain [33, 38]. Connections between the anterior cingulate cortex, prefrontal cortex, and periaqueductal gray and connections between insula, amygdala, and periaqueductal gray constitutes part of the descending pain modulatory pathways [30, 37].

Pathological Changes in Alzheimer's and Pain Processing

The pathological changes in AD patients develop over decades. Coinciding with the diagnosis of AD, the patients have widespread changes of the limbic system with interruption of connections between components of the limbic system, and its influence on the prefrontal cortex is markedly reduced (equivalent to Braak stage IV–V) [39, 40]. At stage V, there are widespread changes of the neocortex, but the primary motor and sensory cortex remain largely unaffected until the severe stages of AD (stage VI). The pathological changes in AD have a wide impact on the limbic system, which plays an important role in processing the "affective-motivational" component of pain. Furthermore, patients with AD have pathological changes in the intralaminar and medical nuclei of the thalamus, which are progressively affected by the disease, with severe changes in pathological stages equivalent to clinical AD [41]. The relative sparing of the sensory cortex and the impact on the limbic system and medial thalamic nuclei led Scherder et al. to conclude that the pathological changes in AD have a wide impact on the medial pain system [42], but the lateral system (sensory-discriminative aspects) are largely unaffected. However, at severe stages of AD amyloid plaques have been found in almost all thalamic nuclei [43].

Pathological alterations have also been found in areas of the brain stem, with evidence of neuronal loss in the locus coeruleus [44], parabrachial region [41, 45] and in the periaqueductal gray matter [46], which are important for modulating pain. Thus, AD pathology affects several areas of the brain important for processing and modulating pain.

Pathological Changes in Other Types of Dementia

Vascular dementia is a heterogenous disorder, and because infarctions of the brain can occur at many locations, all areas involved in pain processing can potentially be affected. Disruption of connections in the cortex and between the cortex and subcortex by white matter lesions may theoretically increase the experience of pain in vascular dementia [42], and white matter hyperintensities have also been associated with increased self-reported pain in patients with dementia [29]. Furthermore, there is an increased risk of post-stroke central pain [35]. In frontotemporal dementia, there can be atrophy of part of the medial pain system such as the prefrontal gyrus, the insula, and the anterior cingulate cortex. Thus, theoretically patients with FTD may have a change in pain perception [42, 47], but clinical date about pain in FTD is missing making it difficult to judge potential effects of neuropathology. In Parkinson's disease, there is Lewy body pathology in areas of the brainstem important for pain processing such periaqueductal gray and locus coeruleus [24], but this have not been specifically assessed in dementia with Lewy bodies.

Evidence from Experimental Pain Studies

A number of experimental studies have investigated the effect that dementia have on pain processing. To date, the majority of studies have focused on AD or mixed groups of patients.

Experimental studies have investigated the hypothesis that AD leads to a change in pain processing and thus, in pain experience. The sensory-discriminative aspects of pain can be studied by investigating the pain threshold. Consistent with the neuropathological finding that the sensory cortex remains intact until late in the disease, the majority of studies have found that the pain threshold (a measure of the sensory-discriminative component of pain) was intact [48–54]. The affective-emotional aspect of pain can be studied by investigating pain tolerance, where results have been differing [49], but with the majority pointing toward a decrease in pain tolerance in mild to moderate AD [51, 52].

A few studies have assessed motor, facial, and brain responses to experimentally induced pain. Here, the picture tends to look more consistent with most findings pointing to a somewhat augmented processing of nociceptive information in patients with AD. More precisely, it was found that patients with dementia showed increased facial responses to pain compared to healthy individuals [53, 55, 56]. Importantly, this increase was not accompanied by an overall increase in facial responsiveness (e.g., unspecific grimacing) but was solely due to an augmentation of pain-specific facial expressions. Regarding brain responses, supraspinal processing of nociceptive inputs in patients with AD has only been investigated in a few studies. Despite the hypothesis of impaired pain pathway in AD patients, functional brain imaging studies (fMRI) show that brain activity in response to noxious stimulation is preserved and even elevated in both the medial and lateral pathways [57, 58]. Interestingly, these studies also observed prolonged activation in the pain pathways and increased activity in cognitive regions, such as the dorsolateral prefrontal cortex. This suggests that cognitive integration of pain may be altered in elderly with AD and could also suggest that they experience greater distress than those without dementia. Thus, taken together, the lower frequency of self-reported pain in AD cannot be explained by impaired processing due to selective impairment of the affective-motivational or cognitive component of pain, suggesting that pain is not less frequent and intense even if no longer reported.

Observation and Assessment of Pain in Dementia

General Assessment of Pain in the Elderly

Assessment of pain requires a comprehensive assessment across all populations and should include a detailed investigation of a patient's pain and medical history, a physical examination, and diagnostic testing if needed. A pain history should include characterization of the current complaint, including associated features or secondary signs and symptoms. The present pain complaint should be described in terms of intensity, quality, location(s) (including radiation), pattern (including onset, duration, and frequency), and aggravating and relieving factors and consequences [7, 8, 59–61]. Nonverbal cues (e.g., guarding, grimacing, and restricted movement) should be noted, particularly if the older person is unable to provide a description of the pain, and furthermore, in circumstances where self-report is unobtainable, gathering information and history from other sources, such as the primary caregiver, can be helpful [60, 62–64]. One of the main purposes of the history and physical exam is to identify a cause of pain. Older adults typically present with multiple pain etiologies. Indeed, a comprehensive assessment is even more critical in this population, in order to gather complete information on all of the locations of pain and the types of conditions that may be causing pain.

Mild to Moderate Dementia

Assessment of pain gets increasingly difficult with the increasing severity of dementia. Studies investigating the capacity of patients with dementia to self-report pain have shown that this ability declines across the course of dementia [20, 21, 65–67]. One study examined the ability of elderly with dementia to understand and use four standard pain assessment scales in different stages of dementia ((1) Horizontal visual analog scale, which consists of a 10-cm line anchored by two extremes of pain: no pain and extreme pain; (2) Vertical visual analog scale is similar to the prior scale but is presented vertically; (3) The faces pain scale consists of a drawing of seven faces that express increasing pain; (4) The 6-point verbal rating scale consists of a list of adjectives which describe different levels of pain) [65]. The study found that in patient with mild dementia 97% were able to understand and use at least one scale and 80% understood all four scales. In patients with moderate dementia 90% understood at least one scale and 59% understood all four scales. There was a high-reliability and correlation between scales. Patients with dementia had the most difficulty using the Faces Pain Scale. Thus, according to published guidelines self-reporting of pain is the standard gold method for identifying pain in those with mild to moderate cognitive impairment [7, 63, 68]. It is recommended to use the numerical rating scale or verbal descriptors with categories of a degree of pain (such as "no pain," "mild pain," "moderate pain," "severe pain," and "worst pain imaginable"). If using a visual analog scale, it is recommended to use a vertical visual analog scale and preferably a colored visual analog scale. The Faces Pain Scale has been shown to be the most difficult to use and is not recommended [20, 65, 66]. People with moderate to severe communication problems should be offered additional assistance with self-report, and the health care provider may need to try different measures.

Severe Dementia

Assessment of pain poses the greatest challenges in cases of severe dementia. The ability to self-report pain has been examined in elderly with severe dementia. In a study of the ability to use and comprehend standard pain assessment scales (Horizontal visual analog scale, Verbal rating scale, and Faces Pain Scale, see previously for description) in patients with severe dementia, it was found that 60% were able to understand at least one of the three scales and even in those with an mini-mental state examination (MMSE) below 6 50% demonstrated comprehension of at least one scale [66]. In patients who demonstrated good comprehension, the reliability of the three self-assessment scales was good. Thus, when people with severe cognitive impairment can self-report pain, these reports are valid [68]. It is important to try to achieve a self-report of pain from all patients, even if the patient can only confirm that they are in pain, as self-report is the gold-standard [64] and the only way to be certain that the patient has pain. If a patient answer "yes" to the question it is important to check that the individual understood the question and does not reply "yes" to every question asked. In patients with moderate to severe communication problems additional assistance needs to be provided and different measures used to achieve self-report [60, 63, 68].

In cases with severe communication difficulties and in situations where a procedure can cause pain, an observational assessment of pain behavior is additionally required and is a valid approach [60, 63]. Patients with dementia, who have difficulty communicating, may express pain by a change in behavior. The American Geriatric Society has defined a number of common behaviors that may indicate pain [63], please see Table 9.1. Some behaviors are common and typically considered to be pain related (e.g., facial grimacing, moaning, groaning, rubbing a body part), but others are less obvious (e.g., agitation, restlessness, irritability, confusion, combativeness particularly with care, changes in appetite or

Table 9.1 Observational changes associated with pain and alternative explanations

Type	Symptoms	Alternative explanations
Autonomic changes	Pale, sweating, tachypnea, change in breathing, increase in pulse and/or blood pressure	Infection, worsening of chronic obstructive pulmonary disorder, pulmonary edema, heart disease
Facial expression	Slight frown; sad, frightened face Grimacing, wrinkled forehead, closed, or tightened eyes Any distorted expression Rapid blinking	Distress associated with the situation Psychosocial circumstances, for instance, problematic social relations at the nursing home
Body movements	Rigid, tense body posture, guarding Fidgeting Increased pacing, rocking Restricted movement Gait or mobility changes	Neuropsychiatric symptoms. Parkinsonism Side effect to antipsychotic Bad fitting shoes
Verbalizations/ vocalizations	Sighing, moaning, groaning Grunting, chanting, calling out Noisy breathing Asking for help Verbally abusive	Neuropsychiatric symptoms Psychosocial circumstances, for instance, problematic social relations at the nursing home Lung disease
Changes in interpersonal interactions	Aggressive, combative, resisting care Decreased social interactions Socially inappropriate, disruptive Withdrawn	Psychosocial circumstances, for instance, problematic social relations at the nursing home Depression Neuropsychiatric symptoms
Changes in activity patterns	Refusing food, appetite change Increase in rest periods Sleep, rest pattern changes Sudden cessation of common routines Increased wandering	Psychosocial circumstances, for instance, problematic social relations at the nursing home Depression Infection
Mental status changes	Crying or tears Increased confusion Distress or irritability	Psychosocial circumstances, for instance, problematic social relations at the nursing home Depression Medication side effects Neuropsychiatric symptoms

Reproduced with permission of American Geriatrics Society. AGS Panel on Persistent Pain in Older Persons. The Management of Persistent Pain in Older Persons. J Am Geriatr Soc 2002;50(Suppl.):S205–S224 usual activities) [64]. Typical pain behaviors may not be present, and more subtle indicators may be the only indicator of unrecognized pain. Unusual behavior in a patient with severe dementia should trigger assessment for pain as a potential cause. Furthermore, if pain is suspected, it is important to investigate the cause of pain as it may be due to serious underlying disease. Pain behaviors are not specific reflections of pain and can be caused many underlying causes of which pain is one, but also other sources of distress, such as physiologic or emotional distress [62, 64, 69]. Pain behaviors differ between individuals, so assessment should include insights from familiar caregivers and family members to interpret the meaning of their behaviors. Box 9.1 shows an algorithm for assessment of pain in patients with dementia [60–64, 68, 70].

Box 9.1 Algorithm for Assessment of Pain in Elderly with Dementia

1. *Is the patient able to communicate sufficiently?*
   (a) If no, continue to 2.
   (b) If yes, ask the patient if he/she is in pain. Use alternate words such as sore, ache, discomfort, or agony. Try to get a detailed pain history. Treat the cause of pain or the pain.
2. *Use observations from caregivers or relatives familiar with the patient.*
3. *Observe for potential pain indicators, assess changes in the following*:
   (a) Autonomic changes
   (b) Facials expression
   (c) Body movement/language
   (d) Verbalizations
   (e) Changes in interpersonal interactions
   (f) Change in activity patterns
   (g) Mental status changes
4. *If potential "pain indicators" are observed ask the following questions to examine what the behavior means*:
   (a) Are basic need fulfilled, i.e., thirst, hunger, need for visiting the toilet, hearing or visual aid?
      (i) If not, correct this. If it does not help, continue the search.
   (b) Are behavior present during movement/transfer?
      (i) If yes, consider strategies to prevent movements that induce pain, provide reassurance and/or consider premedication before provocative movements.
   (c) Are there evidence of morbidity which may cause pain?
      (i) Examine for the potential disease which may cause pain such as pressure ulcers, constipation, or infection among others.
5. *Consider analgesic trial. Monitor response carefully and plan for close follow-up.*
6. *If behavior persist, search for alternative causes by involving caregivers or relatives familiars with the patient*

Pain Assessment Scales

Pain assessment scales can be used to recognize behavior, which may indicate pain and can be used as a proxy for the presence of pain. Most of the instruments are based on the assumption and recommendations of the American Geriatrics Society Panel that pain can be expressed by changes in facial expression (e.g., frowning), vocalization and verbalization (e.g., groaning, mumbling), and body movements [59, 63]. A large number of scales have been developed and aim to make a systematic approach to observe pain behavior in the elderly with dementia [64]. In 2014 28 different scales had been developed to assess pain in different situations and groups of patients. For all 28 scales, there is limited evidence about their reliability, validity, and clinical utility [71]. The interpretation of many of these behaviors is complex when applied to dementia due to considerable overlap with other common behavioral symptoms or cognitive deficits which may confound an assessment, manifesting from boredom, hunger, anxiety, depression, or disorientation [72]. This increases the complexity of identifying the presence of pain accurately in patients with dementia. Generally, none of the scales are specific for pain and measure other sources of distress as well. Importantly, most scales are validated for ascertaining the presence of pain, but not the pain intensity. In most scales, we do not know if scoring a higher number of behavioral items also means more pain [72]. It is important that the pain assessment is not the sole measure but are used to identify patients who may have pain as a part of a comprehensive pain assessment [7, 60, 62, 64, 72].

In the British Geriatric Societies guideline from 2018, they highlight three pain scales: (1) Pain in Advanced Dementia (PAINAD), (2) Doloplus-2 and (3) Pain Assessment Checklist for Seniors with Limited Ability to Communicate (PACSLAC). PAINAD assesses five domains (breathing, negative vocalization, facial expression, body language, and consolability) from 0 to 2 points (max score of 10). It is a sensitive tool for detecting pain in adults with dementia, but does have a high false-positive rate [73]. The scale has not been evaluated in adults with mild to moderate dementia. PAINAD has a high sensitivity (92%) but low specificity for pain (62%). It is easy and simple to use [74]. Doloplus-2 assesses somatic reactions (5 domains), psychomotor reactions (2 domains), and psychosocial reaction (3 domains), which are graded from 0 to 3, yielding a max score of 30 [66, 75, 76]. Doloplus-2 has been translated into many languages, including English, for use across Europe. The PACSLAC consists of four subscales: facial expression, activity/body movement, social/personality mood, and others. Each sub-scale is scored, and a total score is generated. The PACSLAC scale has good inter-rater reliability [77–79], but does need a short form and more testing in larger scale studies.

Treatment of Pain in Dementia

General Principles of Pain Treatment

Treatment of pain in elderly with dementia follows the same guidelines as for elderly without dementia, and for an extensive review we refer to designated texts [7, 8, 59, 80–85].

With age, a number of physiological changes occur, which affect the ability to handle drugs, and these changes need to be kept in mind [59, 86, 87], see Table 9.2 for a summary. Physiological changes in older people increase the sensitivity to some analgesic drugs, resulting in them being more susceptible to side effects and sometimes requiring lower doses. Thus, in choosing analgesics, comorbidity and interactions with other medication need to be taken into account in order to reduce the chance of drug–disease and drug–drug interactions [7, 59, 80]. Especially in frail, multimorbid patients, it is important to preserve function and avoid treatment-related morbidities such as falls, confusion, and delirium [82].

Only one drug should be initiated at a time using a low dose, and this should be followed by slow dose titration, using the principle "start low and go slow." Sufficiently long intervals between introducing drugs should be allowed to assess the effect. Analgesics should, however, always be titrated to response or alternatively discontinued because of side effects and insufficient effect. The least invasive route of administration should be preferred, and subcutaneous formulations reserved for patients with dysphagia [84]. Timing of medication administration is important. Severe, episodic pain requires treatment with medicines with a rapid onset of action and short duration. However, if a patient is experiencing continuous pain, regular analgesics are the most effective, possibly using modified release formulations. Treatment should be constantly monitored and adjusted if required to improve

Table 9.2 Pharmacological changes with aging

Pharmacological function	Change with normal aging	Common effect of disease
Gastrointestinal absorption and function	Increased gastrointestinal transit time may increase the risk of opioid-related obstipation	Change in gastric PH may alter the absorption of drugs
Transdermal absorption	Usually no age-related changes	Increase in body temperature may increase absorption from patches
Distribution	Increased fat/muscle ratio may increase volume for distribution of fat-soluble drugs	Aging and obesity may increase the distribution of fat-soluble drugs, which result in longer effective drug half-life
Liver metabolism	Pre-, intra, and post-hepatic age-related changes may lead to a decrease in conjugation, metabolism, and clearance of drugs. The exact effect can be difficult to predict	Cirrhosis may change metabolism and clearance of drugs
Renal excretion	Glomerular filtration rates decreased with advancing age which leads to a decrease in clearance and excretion of drugs and metabolites, leading to the prolonged half-life of drugs	Chronic kidney disease may predispose to renal toxicity and accumulation of drugs leading to systemic toxicity
Anticholinergic side effects	Increased confusion, constipation, incontinence, and movement disorders	Enhanced by neurological disease

efficacy and limit adverse events. Combination therapy using drugs with complementary mechanisms of action may have synergistic effects to provide greater pain relief with fewer side effects than higher doses of a single drug [7, 59, 80]. However, in patients receiving polypharmacy, this may decrease compliance. Treatment of pain should follow a step-wise approach following the World Health Organization (WHO) analgesic ladder [88]. When starting an analgesic, a plan for follow-up with evaluation of effect and side effects should be made. At every follow-up, discontinuation of analgesics should be considered [89].

Paracetamol

Paracetamol is first-choice due to a favorable side effect profile [7, 8, 47, 80, 90]. It is effective towards musculoskeletal pain. Paracetamol is relatively safe and without significant side effects. It is important that the dose is not increased beyond the maximum dose of 4 g/day. In malnourished patients (weight below 50 kg), acute liver failure secondary to maximum dose oral paracetamol has been reported, and in this population, a dose reduction (max 2 g/day) is recommended [91].

Non-steroidal Anti-inflammatory Drugs

Non-steroidal anti-inflammatory drugs (NSAIDs) are more effective for persistent inflammatory pain than paracetamol [7, 59]. Despite good efficacy, NSAIDs must be used with caution in older people because of a high risk of potentially serious and life-threatening side effects [7]. Caution must be made in patients with low creatinine clearance, gastropathy, cardiovascular disease, or congestive heart failure. A study found that NSAIDs was implicated in up to a quarter (23.5%) of hospital admissions due to adverse drug reactions in older people [92]. NSAIDs may be considered as a treatment option when paracetamol or topical NSAID are ineffective or insufficient to treat osteoarthritis [93] and low back pain [94], considering the individual risk of side effects.

Opioider

Nonpharmacologic therapy and nonopioid pharmacologic therapy are preferred for chronic pain [59, 81, 83, 85]. In carefully selected and monitored patients, opioids can be used as part of a multimodal pain treatment also in patients with dementia. Clinicians should consider opioid therapy only if expected benefits for both pain and function are anticipated to outweigh risks to the patient [81, 83, 85]. Due to reduced renal function and medication clearance even in the absence of renal disease, patients aged ≥65 years might have increased susceptibility to accumulation of opioids and a smaller therapeutic window between safe dosages and dosages associated with respiratory depression and overdose [81]. Thus, clinicians should use additional caution and increased monitoring to minimize the risks of opioids prescribed for patients aged ≥65 years [81]. Age is a significant predictor in opioid-related harm with patients over 60 having a two to eightfold increased risk of respiratory depression, falls, and fracture [95], hospitalization and death [82, 96, 97]. For safety reasons, long-acting opioids should not be introduced before short-acting opioids.

Due to changes in gastrointestinal motility, elderly have an increased risk of suffering constipation when treated with an opioid and a laxative should be co-prescribed. Special caution should be made in patients with reduced renal function in whom treatment with tramadol, morphine, oxycodone, and fentanyl as these opioids are cleared by the kidneys, and there is a risk of reduced clearance of the drugs and increased susceptibility to accumulation of opioids and side effect. Buprenorphine is not cleared by the kidney and can be used in patients with reduced renal function.

There have been very few studies examining the effect and side effect of opioids in patients with dementia. At double-blinded trial of buprenorphine in people with advanced dementia found a high risk of adverse events, and the adverse symptoms that were described overlapped with common behavioral symptoms in dementia such as changes in personality, confusion, sedation or somnolence [98]. Opioids central side effects such as sedation, confusion, and dizziness pose a special concern in elderly with dementia as they, due to their brain diseases, are more susceptible to the central side effects. Furthermore, a considerable proportion of elderly with dementia receives another centrally acting drug such as a benzodiazepine or an antipsychotic drug [99, 100]. Sedative drugs such as antipsychotics, benzodiazepines, anxiolytics, hypnotics, antihistamines, tricyclic antidepressant all increase the risk of sedation and dizziness, and one should be especially cautious when initiating opioid treatment in a patient receiving either of these drugs. Recently, the US Federal Drug Administration issued their strongest warning against combining opioids and benzodiazepines due to the risk of serious adverse events and death [101]. Elderly with dementia are more susceptible to central side effects related to opioids and can experience a cognitive decline and loss of function when treated with an opioid. A recently published European Academy of Neurology guideline on medical management issues in dementia state that it is good clinical practice to consider discontinuation of opioids in patients for whom there are no complaints of pain and no clear indication, where mild analgesics have not been tried and in patients in whom there is suspicion of side effects, such as rapid cognitive decline, sedation, falls, respiratory problems, constipation, nausea, or reduced appetite [89].

Use of Analgesics in Elderly with Dementia

A common belief has been that elderly with dementia were being undertreated for pain due to a number of older studies showing that they were less likely to receive analgesics compared to cognitively intact elderly [16, 21, 102, 103]. However, over the past 15–20 year there have been increased prescribing of analgesics in elderly with dementia internationally [104–106]. Several more recent cohorts have shown that elderly with dementia are prescribed analgesics more often than cognitively intact elderly [17, 107]. The largest study to date examining the use of opioids in elderly with and without dementia in the entire elderly Danish population found that among home-living elderly 27.5% of elderly with dementia prescribed an opioid and 16.9% of those without dementia. Among nursing home resident, use of opioids were higher and 37.8% of nursing home residents diagnosed with dementia and 43% of elderly not diagnosed with dementia received an opioid [107]. Elderly with dementia received longer use than elderly without dementia. Transdermal formulations were used by 2% of home-living without dementia, 11% of home-living elderly, and 19% of nursing home resident with and without dementia [107]. Furthermore, significant geographical variation in the use of opioids among elderly with dementia has been demonstrated [108], which was not explained by differences in age, sex, and comorbidity, suggesting different approaches towards either pain assessment and/or pain treatment in primary care.

Several factors may have influenced increases in opioid prescriptions. Clinicians are more cautious about NSAIDS and may prescribe opioids as an alternative. A Finnish study saw a reduction in NSAID use in nursing home facilities from 13.0% in 2003 to 2.6% in 2011 [109] as did a Norwegian study (6.8% in 2000 to 3.2% in 2011), alongside increases in opioids and acetaminophen [106]. Concerns have been expressed that opioids are used for their sedative effect, not just pain [104, 107, 109], especially since the increase in opioids has occurred concurrently with a decrease in the use of antipsychotics [104].

Dilemmas in Treating Pain in Dementia

Treating pain in the elderly with dementia is complex and challenging. The first challenge relates to identifying whether the patient is in pain. In patients with severe communication difficulties, pain assessment relies on observation. It can be difficult to judge whether a behavior is due to pain or not. The problems relating to assessment make it ethically challenging to start a treatment with potentially severe side effects if the indication for treatment is doubtful and the patient is unable to consent to treatment. The assessment of pain also poses a problem in relation to monitoring the effect and side effects of medication.

A second challenge relates to treatment. It is very much a balancing act between treating pain sufficiently and avoiding loss of function due to sedation and cognitive side effect, and in some cases, both will not be obtainable. Furthermore, there has been very limited research examining the effect and side effects of analgesics in the elderly with dementia.

Conclusion

Elderly with dementia report pain less frequently than cognitively intact elderly, but there is no evidence that they experience less pain. Assessment of pain gets increasingly difficult with an increasing degree of cognitive impairment.

Self-reporting of pain is the standard gold method for identifying pain in those with mild to moderate cognitive impairment. In the older person with severe cognitive impairment, observational assessment of behavior becomes essential for assessing the presence of pain and should follow a systematic approach to investigate the reason for the change in behavior. Treatment of pain follow the same guidelines as for elderly without dementia, but special caution should be made as elderly with dementia are more sensitive to the adverse effects associated with opioids.

Case 1

Mrs. P is an 80-year-old woman who was diagnosed with Alzheimer's disease 4 years ago and lives at a nursing home. She is a widow and moved to the nursing home 6 month prior. She suffers from osteoporosis, hypertension, and cataract, but is otherwise in good health. She suffers from moderate dementia, is apathic, and spends most of the time resting in an armchair.

She has been to a family birthday for 3 hours during the day. In the evening, she gets agitated and irritable. She paces around and does not sleep during the night. She is unable to express what is going on, but her behavior is very unusual. The staff initially thinks she has been overstimulated due to the family event. The following day she is still agitated and unable to find rest. The staff calls her primary care physician, and an examination of her urine is made, which shows traces of blood. On suspicion of a urinary tract infection, she is started on antibiotics. Over the next days she continues to be agitated. After 2 days she starts vomiting and develops a fever. She is admitted to the Hospital. On clinical examination, she is found to have a fever (38.9 °C), low blood pressure (98/60), is sweating and vomiting, and is restless. When her abdomen is examined, she is clearly tender in the right flank, which she expresses by frowning her face and saying "av." An X-ray shows obstruction of the right ureter, and she is diagnosed with kidney stones and acute pyelonephritis. She is treated with extracorporeal shock-wave lithotripsy to remove the kidney stone and iv antibiotics and iv fluids due to sepsis. After removal of the kidney stone, the agitation subsides.

Note: When elderly with dementia develop new behavioral symptoms, a physical cause should always be suspected, and a thorough examination of the patient should be made. In this case, the patient was not able to express what is going on but express pain by developing agitation, restlessness, and disrupted sleep. When a thorough examination was made, she is able to say that it hurts but also expresses pain by facial expressions, when the doctor examines her right flank.

Case 2

Mrs. E is an 85-year-old woman, who was diagnosed with Alzheimer's disease 5 years ago. She suffered a stroke 1 year ago, which left her with a right-sided hemiparesis and aphasia. She is unable to walk and spends the day either in a well-chair or in bed. She also suffers from osteoporosis and is treated with paracetamol 1 g × 4 daily due to pain. Due to spasticity in the right side she receives baclofen 10 mg × 3 daily but has been unable to tolerate higher doses due to sedation. The family physician visits the nursing home and notices that Mrs. E. is screaming. The staff informs him that over the past 2–3 weeks, she has been screaming a lot and been very aggressive and uncooperative during care. The staff think she may be in pain. A systematic evaluation of the patient is made. Due to her not being able to communicate, an observational scale is used (in this case PAINAD), where she scores 4/10 (2 points on vocalization due to "repeated troubling calling out," 1 point on body language due to being tense and 1 point on consolability due to intermittently being distracted by calming talking to her). She is transferred to her bed, and a new assessment is made in order to investigate if this is related to movement. The score increases to 6 due to facial grimacing. A thorough clinical examination is made, which shows a small sacral pressure ulcer. There was also tenderness of the vertebrae at L3 and L4. When moving her right-sided extremities, there was the stiffness of the right arm and upcoming contracture. During the examination mrs E. reacted with restlessness, resistance, and vocalization. It was suspected that pain was the cause of the vocalization and resistance to care as she was unable to express that she was in pain.

Mrs. E. had several reasons for experiencing pain, i.e., a new pressure ulcer, chronic pain due to osteoporosis and developing a contracture. Several non-pharmacological measures were instituted, such as physiotherapy for the contracture, an air madras in her bed, and special pillow in her wheelchair. Furthermore, the staff was made aware that the care and transfer caused pain and found alternate ways. An analgesic trial with morphine 10 mg × 3 daily was instituted as the patient already received paracetamol, and a follow-up 4 days later was arranged. When the physician consulted her 4 days later, he found that she was calmer but also sedated by morphine and spend most of the day sleeping. The dose of morphine was reduced to 5 mg half an hour before care twice daily, which she was able to tolerate without being sedated. A follow-up 1 week later was arranged. At the next consultation, the sacral pressure wound had almost heeled. The patient reacted with less resistance to care, but still had some calling out and had decreased to a 3/10 on PAINAD on transfer. A follow-up 3 weeks later was arranged, where the pressure ulcer was completely healed, and the contracture in the right arm improved. It was possible to discontinue the morphine. Mrs. E. still had episodes of calling out but did not resist care.

Note: in this case, the patient is unable to communicate, and an observational assessment of pain is made. The patient is found to have multiple potential causes of pain aside from potential chronic pain due to osteoporosis. She is also treated with baclofen due to spasticity, and due to the combined sedative load, she is only able to tolerate a small dose of morphine. When starting an analgesic, it is always important to arrange for a follow-up, where effect and side effects are evaluated, and a plan for discontinuation is made. It is also important to be aware of other centrally acting medication, such as antipsychotics, benzodiazepines, hypnotics, etc., which can increase sedation and make side effects unwarranted due to potential loss of function.

References

1. IASP, ed. Task Force on Taxonomy of the International Association for the Study of Pain. Classification of chronic pain—description of chronic pain syndromes and definitions of pain terms. Seattle: IASP Press; 1994.
2. Elliott AM, et al. The epidemiology of chronic pain in the community. Lancet. 1999;354(9186):1248–52.
3. Eriksen J, et al. Epidemiology of chronic non-malignant pain in Denmark. Pain. 2003;106(3):221–8.
4. Berryman C, et al. Evidence for working memory deficits in chronic pain: a systematic review and meta-analysis. Pain. 2013;154(8):1181–96.
5. Borsook D. Neurological diseases and pain. Brain. 2012;135(Pt 2):320–44.
6. Lautenbacher S. Pain assessment in special patient groups such as those with dementia: at the finishing line or just starting from scratch? Pain. 2014;155(8):1419–20.
7. Abdulla A, et al. Guidance on the management of pain in older people. Age Ageing. 2013;42(Suppl 1):i1–57.
8. Savvas SM, Gibson SJ. Overview of pain management in older adults. Clin Geriatr Med. 2016;32(4):635–50.
9. Blyth FM, et al. Chronic pain in Australia: a prevalence study. Pain. 2001;89(2–3):127–34.
10. Sjogren P, et al. Epidemiology of chronic pain in Denmark: an update. Eur J Pain. 2009;13(3):287–92.
11. Delwel S, et al. Oral health and orofacial pain in older people with dementia: a systematic review with focus on dental hard tissues. Clin Oral Investig. 2017;21(1):17–32.
12. Delwel S, et al. Orofacial pain and its potential oral causes in older people with mild cognitive impairment or dementia. J Oral Rehabil. 2019;46(1):23–32.
13. Takai Y, et al. Literature review of pain prevalence among older residents of nursing homes. Pain Manag Nurs. 2010;11(4):209–23.
14. Achterberg WP, et al. Pain in European long-term care facilities: cross-national study in Finland, Italy and The Netherlands. Pain. 2010;148(1):70–4.
15. Reynolds KS, et al. Disparities in pain management between cognitively intact and cognitively impaired nursing home residents. J Pain Symptom Manag. 2008;35(4):388–96.
16. Mantyselka P, et al. Effects of dementia on perceived daily pain in home-dwelling elderly people: a population-based study. Age Ageing. 2004;33(5):496–9.
17. Haasum Y, et al. Pain treatment in elderly persons with and without dementia: a population-based study of institutionalized and home-dwelling elderly. Drugs Aging. 2011;28(4):283–93.
18. van Kooten J, et al. A review of pain prevalence in Alzheimer's, vascular, frontotemporal and Lewy body dementias. Dement Geriatr Cogn Disord. 2016;41(3–4):220–32.
19. Fisher-Morris M, Gellatly A. The experience and expression of pain in Alzheimer patients. Age Ageing. 1997;26(6):497–500.
20. Scherder EJ, Bouma A. Visual analogue scales for pain assessment in Alzheimer's disease. Gerontology. 2000;46(1):47–53.
21. Scherder E, et al. Alzheimer patients report less pain intensity and pain affect than non-demented elderly. Psychiatry. 1999;62(3):265–72.
22. Jensen-Dahm C, et al. Discrepancy between self- and proxy-rated pain in Alzheimer's disease: results from the Danish Alzheimer Intervention Study. J Am Geriatr Soc. 2012;60(7):1274–8.
23. Binnekade TT, et al. Pain in patients with different dementia subtypes, mild cognitive impairment, and subjective cognitive impairment. Pain Med. 2018;19(5):920–7.
24. Blanchet PJ, Brefel-Courbon C. Chronic pain and pain processing in Parkinson's disease. Prog Neuropsychopharmacol Biol Psychiatry. 2018;87(Pt B):200–6.
25. van Kooten J, et al. Prevalence of pain in nursing home residents: the role of dementia stage and dementia subtypes. J Am Med Dir Assoc. 2017;18(6):522–7.
26. Scherder EJ, et al. Chronic pain in "probable" vascular dementia: preliminary findings. Pain Med. 2015;16(3):442–50.

27. Scherder EJ, et al. Pain assessment in patients with possible vascular dementia. Psychiatry. 2003;66(2):133–45.
28. Husebo BS, et al. Who suffers most? Dementia and pain in nursing home patients: a cross-sectional study. J Am Med Dir Assoc. 2008;9(6):427–33.
29. Binnekade TT, et al. White matter hyperintensities are related to pain intensity in an outpatient memory clinic population: preliminary findings. J Pain Res. 2019;12:1621–9.
30. Koltzenburg M. Wall & Melzack's textbook of pain. 6th ed. Philadelphia: Elsevier Health Sciences; 2013.
31. Apkarian AV, et al. Human brain mechanisms of pain perception and regulation in health and disease. Eur J Pain. 2005;9(4):463–84.
32. Treede RD, et al. The cortical representation of pain. Pain. 1999;79(2–3):105–11.
33. Tracey I. Nociceptive processing in the human brain. Curr Opin Neurobiol. 2005;15(4):478–87.
34. Ploner M, Freund HJ, Schnitzler A. Pain affect without pain sensation in a patient with a postcentral lesion. Pain. 1999;81(1–2):211–4.
35. Klit H, Finnerup NB, Jensen TS. Central post-stroke pain: clinical characteristics, pathophysiology, and management. Lancet Neurol. 2009;8(9):857–68.
36. Sewards TV, Sewards MA. The medial pain system: neural representations of the motivational aspect of pain. Brain Res Bull. 2002;59(3):163–80.
37. Wiech K. Deconstructing the sensation of pain: the influence of cognitive processes on pain perception. Science. 2016;354(6312):584–7.
38. Rainville P, et al. Pain affect encoded in human anterior cingulate but not somatosensory cortex. Science. 1997;277(5328):968–71.
39. Braak E, et al. Neuropathology of Alzheimer's disease: what is new since A. Alzheimer? Eur Arch Psychiatry Clin Neurosci. 1999;249(Suppl 3):14–22.
40. Nelson PT, Braak H, Markesbery WR. Neuropathology and cognitive impairment in Alzheimer disease: a complex but coherent relationship. J Neuropathol Exp Neurol. 2009;68(1):1–14.
41. Rub U, et al. The autonomic higher order processing nuclei of the lower brain stem are among the early targets of the Alzheimer's disease-related cytoskeletal pathology. Acta Neuropathol. 2001;101(6):555–64.
42. Scherder EJ, Sergeant JA, Swaab DF. Pain processing in dementia and its relation to neuropathology. Lancet Neurol. 2003;2(11):677–86.
43. Braak H, Braak E. Alzheimer's disease affects limbic nuclei of the thalamus. Acta Neuropathol. 1991;81(3):261–8.
44. Zarow C, et al. Neuronal loss is greater in the locus coeruleus than nucleus basalis and substantia nigra in Alzheimer and Parkinson diseases. Arch Neurol. 2003;60(3):337–41.
45. Parvizi J, Van Hoesen GW, Damasio A. Severe pathological changes of parabrachial nucleus in Alzheimer's disease. Neuroreport. 1998;9(18):4151–4.
46. Parvizi J, Van Hoesen GW, Damasio A. Selective pathological changes of the periaqueductal gray matter in Alzheimer's disease. Ann Neurol. 2000;48(3):344–53.
47. Achterberg W, et al. Pain in dementia. Pain Rep. 2020;5(1):e803.
48. Benedetti F, et al. Pain reactivity in Alzheimer patients with different degrees of cognitive impairment and brain electrical activity deterioration. Pain. 2004;111(1–2):22–9.
49. Benedetti F, et al. Pain threshold and tolerance in Alzheimer's disease. Pain. 1999;80(1–2):377–82.
50. Gibson SJ, et al. An examination of pain perception and cerebral event-related potentials following carbon dioxide laser stimulation in patients with Alzheimer's disease and age-matched control volunteers. Pain Res Manag. 2001;6(3):126–32.
51. Jensen-Dahm C, et al. Quantitative sensory testing and pain tolerance in patients with mild to moderate Alzheimer disease compared to healthy control subjects. Pain. 2014;155(8):1439–45.
52. Jensen-Dahm C, et al. Discrepancy between stimulus response and tolerance of pain in Alzheimer disease. Neurology. 2015;84(15):1575–81.
53. Kunz M, et al. Influence of dementia on multiple components of pain. Eur J Pain. 2009;13(3):317–25.

54. Lints-Martindale AC, et al. A psychophysical investigation of the facial action coding system as an index of pain variability among older adults with and without Alzheimer's disease. Pain Med. 2007;8(8):678–89.
55. Hadjistavropoulos T, et al. Using facial expressions to assess musculoskeletal pain in older persons. Eur J Pain. 2002;6(3):179–87.
56. Kunz M, et al. The facial expression of pain in patients with dementia. Pain. 2007;133(1–3):221–8.
57. Cole LJ, et al. Pain sensitivity and fMRI pain-related brain activity in Alzheimer's disease. Brain. 2006;129(Pt 11):2957–65.
58. Cole LJ, et al. The impact of Alzheimer's disease on the functional connectivity between brain regions underlying pain perception. Eur J Pain. 2011;15(6):568.e1–11.
59. American Geriatrics Society Panel on Pharmacological Management of Persistent Pain in Older Person. Pharmacological management of persistent pain in older persons. J Am Geriatr Soc. 2009;57(8):1331–46.
60. Schofield P. The assessment of pain in older people: UK national guidelines. Age Ageing. 2018;47(suppl_1):i1–i22.
61. Herr K. Pain assessment strategies in older patients. J Pain. 2011;12(3 Suppl 1):S3–S13.
62. Herr K, et al. Pain assessment in the nonverbal patient: position statement with clinical practice recommendations. Pain Manag Nurs. 2006;7(2):44–52.
63. AGS Panel on Persistent Pain in Older Persons. The management of persistent pain in older persons. J Am Geriatr Soc. 2002;50(6 Suppl):S205–24.
64. Herr K, et al. Pain assessment in the patient unable to self-report: position statement with clinical practice recommendations. Pain Manag Nurs. 2011;12(4):230–50.
65. Pautex S, et al. Feasibility and reliability of four pain self-assessment scales and correlation with an observational rating scale in hospitalized elderly demented patients. J Gerontol A Biol Sci Med Sci. 2005;60(4):524–9.
66. Pautex S, et al. Pain in severe dementia: self-assessment or observational scales? J Am Geriatr Soc. 2006;54(7):1040–5.
67. Porter FL, et al. Dementia and response to pain in the elderly. Pain. 1996;68(2–3):413–21.
68. British Geriatrics Society and British Pain Society. The assessment of pain in older people. 2007.
69. Hadjistavropoulos T, et al. Pain assessment in elderly adults with dementia. Lancet Neurol. 2014;13(12):1216–27.
70. Royal College of Physicians, British Pain Society, B.G.S. The assessment of pain in older people—National Guidelines. Concise guidance to good practice—a series of evidence-based guidelines for clinical management. 2007.
71. Lichtner V, et al. Pain assessment for people with dementia: a systematic review of systematic reviews of pain assessment tools. BMC Geriatr. 2014;14:138.
72. Husebo BS, Achterberg W, Flo E. Identifying and managing pain in people with Alzheimer's disease and other types of dementia: a systematic review. CNS Drugs. 2016;30(6):481–97.
73. Warden V, Hurley AC, Volicer L. Development and psychometric evaluation of the Pain Assessment in Advanced Dementia (PAINAD) scale. J Am Med Dir Assoc. 2003;4(1):9–15.
74. Jordan A, et al. The utility of PAINAD in assessing pain in a UK population with severe dementia. Int J Geriatr Psychiatry. 2011;26(2):118–26.
75. Holen JC, et al. Doloplus-2, a valid tool for behavioural pain assessment? BMC Geriatr. 2007;7:29.
76. Pickering G, et al. Reliability study in five languages of the translation of the pain behavioural scale Doloplus. Eur J Pain. 2010;14(5):545.e1–10.
77. Cheung G, Choi P. The use of the Pain Assessment Checklist for Seniors with Limited Ability to Communicate (PACSLAC) by caregivers in dementia care. N Z Med J. 2008;121(1286):21–9.
78. Fuchs-Lacelle S, Hadjistavropoulos T. Development and preliminary validation of the pain assessment checklist for seniors with limited ability to communicate (PACSLAC). Pain Manag Nurs. 2004;5(1):37–49.

79. Zwakhalen SM, van't Hof CE, Hamers JP. Systematic pain assessment using an observational scale in nursing home residents with dementia: exploring feasibility and applied interventions. J Clin Nurs. 2012;21(21–22):3009–17.
80. Reisner L. Pharmacological management of persistent pain in older persons. J Pain. 2011;12(3 Suppl 1):S21–9.
81. Dowell D, Haegerich TM, Chou R. CDC guideline for prescribing opioids for chronic pain--United States, 2016. JAMA. 2016;315(15):1624–45.
82. McLachlan AJ, et al. Clinical pharmacology of analgesic medicines in older people: impact of frailty and cognitive impairment. Br J Clin Pharmacol. 2011;71(3):351–64.
83. Busse J. The 2017 Canadian guideline for opioids for chronic non-cancer pain. 2017. National Pain Center.
84. National Institute for Health and Care Excellence. NICE guideline: palliative care for adults: strong opioids for pain relief. 2016. NICE.
85. Danish National Board of Health. Opioid behandling af kronisk ikke-maligne smerter [danish]; Opioid treatment for chronic non-malignant pain. 2018.
86. Klotz U. Pharmacokinetics and drug metabolism in the elderly. Drug Metab Rev. 2009;41(2):67–76.
87. Shi S, Klotz U. Age-related changes in pharmacokinetics. Curr Drug Metab. 2011;12(7):601–10.
88. World Health Organization. WHO's cancer pain ladder for adults. Available from: https://www.who.int/cancer/palliative/painladder/en/
89. Frederiksen KS, et al. A European Academy of Neurology guideline on medical management issues in dementia. Eur J Neurol. 2020;27:1805–20.
90. Achterberg WP, et al. Pain management in patients with dementia. Clin Interv Aging. 2013;8:1471–82.
91. Claridge LC, et al. Acute liver failure after administration of paracetamol at the maximum recommended daily dose in adults. BMJ. 2010;341:c6764.
92. Franceschi M, et al. Prevalence, clinical features and avoidability of adverse drug reactions as cause of admission to a geriatric unit: a prospective study of 1756 patients. Drug Saf. 2008;31(6):545–56.
93. National Institute for Health and Care Excellence. NICE guidance: osteoarthritis: care and management. 2014. NICE.
94. National Institute for Health and Care Excellence. NICE guidance: low back pain and sciatica in over 16s: assessment and management. 2016.
95. Daoust R, et al. Recent opioid use and fall-related injury among older patients with trauma. CMAJ. 2018;190(16):E500–6.
96. Hoffman EM, et al. Association of Long-term Opioid Therapy with Functional Status, adverse outcomes, and mortality among patients with polyneuropathy. JAMA Neurol. 2017;74(7):773–9.
97. Miller M, Barber CW, Leatherman S. Prescription opioid duration of action and the risk of unintentional overdose-reply. JAMA Intern Med. 2015;175(9):1583.
98. Erdal A, et al. Tolerability of buprenorphine transdermal system in nursing home patients with advanced dementia: a randomized, placebo-controlled trial (DEP.PAIN.DEM). Clin Interv Aging. 2018;13:935–46.
99. Norgaard A, et al. Psychotropic polypharmacy in patients with dementia: prevalence and predictors. J Alzheimers Dis. 2017;56(2):707–16.
100. Norgaard A, et al. Time trends in antipsychotic drug use in patients with dementia: a nationwide study. J Alzheimers Dis. 2016;49(1):211–20.
101. F. D. Administration, FDA Drug Safety Communication. FDA warns about serious risks and death when combining opioid pain or cough medicines with benzodiazepines; requires its strongest warning, F.D. Administration, Editor. 2017.
102. Closs SJ, Barr B, Briggs M. Cognitive status and analgesic provision in nursing home residents. Br J Gen Pract. 2004;54(509):919–21.
103. Scherder E, et al. Pain in dementia. Pain. 2009;145(3):276–8.

104. Jensen-Dahm C, et al. The use of opioids and antipsychotics in elderly with dementia—have opioids replaced antipsychotics in treating behavioral symptoms in dementia? J Alzheimers Dis. 2020;73(1):259–67.
105. La Frenais FL, et al. Temporal trends in analgesic use in long-term care facilities: a systematic review of international prescribing. J Am Geriatr Soc. 2018;66(2):376–82.
106. Sandvik R, et al. Analgesic prescribing patterns in Norwegian nursing homes from 2000 to 2011: trend analyses of four data samples. Age Ageing. 2016;45(1):54–60.
107. Jensen-Dahm C, et al. Frequent use of opioids in patients with dementia and nursing home residents: a study of the entire elderly population of Denmark. Alzheimers Dement. 2015;11(6):691–9.
108. Jensen-Dahm C, et al. Geographical variation in opioid use in elderly patients with dementia: a nationwide study. J Alzheimers Dis. 2019;70(4):1209–16.
109. Pitkala KH, et al. Eight-year trends in the use of opioids, other analgesics, and psychotropic medications among institutionalized older people in Finland. J Am Med Dir Assoc. 2015;16(11):973–8.

Management of Motor Symptoms in Dementia Disorders

10

Zeynep Tufekcioglu, Basar Bilgic, Hasmet Hanagasi, and Murat Emre

List of Abbreviations

AD	Alzheimer's disease
bvFTD	Behavioural variant FTD
CBD	Corticobasal degeneration
CBS	Corticobasal syndrome
DLB	Dementia with Lewy Bodies
EMA	European Medicines Agency
FDA	Food and Drug Administration
FTD	Frontotemporal dementia
HD	Huntington's disease
JHD	Juvenile Huntington's disease
MND	Motor neuron disease
MSA	Multisystem atrophy
PD	Parkinson's disease
PDD	PD dementia
PPA	Primary progressive aphasia
PSP	Progressive supranuclear palsy
svPPA	Semantic variant PPA
UPDRS	Unified Parkinson's Disease Rating Scale
VCI	Vascular cognitive impairment
VaD	Vascular dementia
VaP	Vascular parkinsonism

Z. Tufekcioglu (✉)
Faculty of Medicine, Department of Neurology, Istanbul Aydin University, Istanbul, Turkey

B. Bilgic · H. Hanagasi · M. Emre
Istanbul Faculty of Medicine, Department of Neurology, Movement Disorders and Behavioural Neurology Unit, Istanbul University, Istanbul, Turkey

K. S. Frederiksen, G. Waldemar (eds.), *Management of Patients with Dementia*,
https://doi.org/10.1007/978-3-030-77904-7_10

Introduction

Movement and cognition are the core functions of the nervous system, they are intricately integrated through large-scale networks. As a consequence, co-occurrence of motor and cognitive symptoms are common, encountered in many neurological diseases. Neurodegenerative disorders are slowly progressive entities, typically starting from a distinct area of the central nervous system and spreading to adjacent or inter-connected areas. Depending on the site of origin, motor symptoms can accompany cognitive impairment already at the onset of the disease or emerge as a result of progression of pathology in many neurodegenerative diseases.

Dementia disorders are among the leading causes of disability, especially in the elderly. One of the challenges in the management of dementia is the co-occurrence of cognitive impairment and motor symptoms (Table 10.1), which lead to increased disability and consequent institutionalization. Successful management of motor symptoms is critical to reduce disability and socioeconomic burden of dementias.

There are a variety of motor symptoms which may be seen during the course of the disease in different types of dementias (Table 10.2). These include both hypo- and hyper-kinetic symptoms such as parkinsonism, tremor, dystonia, chorea, myoclonus, and various gait disorders. In this chapter, we will review pharmacological

Table 10.1 Motor symptoms which may be associated with dementia

Motor symptom	Definition
Tremor	Oscillatory, typically rhythmic, and regular movement that affects one or more body parts
Bradykinesia	Slowness of movement unrelated to weakness or spasticity
Akinesia	Loss of movement unrelated to weakness or spasticity
Rigidity	Increased muscle tone to passive motion which is present equally in all directions of the movement
Postural instability	Difficulty righting himself or herself after being pulled off balance
Dystonia	Movements that tend to be sustained at the peak of the movement are usually twisting and frequently repetitive, and often progress to prolonged abnormal postures
Paratonia	Resistance to passive movement of the limb
Myoclonus	Sudden, brief, shock-like involuntary movements caused by muscular contractions (positive myoclonus) or inhibitions (negative myoclonus)
Chorea	Involuntary, irregular, purposeless, non-rhythmic, abrupt, rapid, un-sustained movements
Ataxia	Decomposition of movement flow due to breakdown of normal coordinated execution of a voluntary movement
Hemiparesis	Weakness or inability to move one side of the body
Apraxia	a higher-order motor deficit in executing or planning motor acts that cannot be explained by weakness, spasticity, rigidity, akinesia or sensory loss.
Alien limb	Involuntary movements of an arm or leg which spontaneously moves to adopt odd postures beyond the control or understanding of the patient

Adapted from Fahn et al. [1]

Table 10.2 Dementia disorders associated with motor symptoms

Alzheimer's disease
Dementia with Lewy bodies
Parkinson's disease dementia
Vascular dementia
Normal pressure hydrocephalus
Frontotemporal dementia
Corticobasal degeneration
Progressive supranuclear palsy
Huntington disease
Multisystem atrophy

and non-pharmacological modalities used to treat such motor symptoms. In general, there is a lack of randomized controlled trials on the treatment of motor symptoms associated with dementia, in particular on non-pharmacological treatments.

Management of Motor Symptoms in Alzheimer's Disease

Alzheimer's disease (AD) is the most common form of neurodegenerative disorders. The proto-typical form of AD begins with gradually progressive worsening of memory. As the disease progresses, other cognitive symptoms and non-cognitive features including behavioural, autonomic, and motor symptoms emerge. There are also other initial presentation forms of the disease defined as "atypical AD", including presentations by visual-spatial, aphasic, behavioural, or apraxic symptoms. Although very rare, AD may begin with motor symptoms such as cerebellar ataxia or hemiparesis. Corticobasal syndrome (CBS) may constitute another presentation form of AD presenting with an asymmetrical akinetic-rigid syndrome and limb apraxia; dystonia, myoclonus, and alien limb may be seen in the course of the disease [2, 3]. In contrast to more subtle and later emerging motor symptoms associated with the typical amnestic form, CBS due to AD pathology is associated with substantial motor symptoms, including limb apraxia (90%), myoclonus (81%), and gait disorders (70%) [3].

In the typical, amnestic form of AD, gait disorders, and other movement disorders emerge usually in the later stages of the disease. Motor symptoms in AD are significant and independent predictors of increased cost of care [4]. In a multi-centre study including 533 patients with AD at early stages, the presence of postural-gait impairment was associated with increased risk for institutionalization and mortality whereas the presence of tremor and bradykinesia was linked to increased risk for cognitive and functional decline [5].

There has been some confusion on defining the type of extrapyramidal symptoms seen in AD, in particular features of parkinsonism. Parkinsonian type rigidity has not been discriminated from paratonia in many studies. Unified Parkinson's Disease Rating Scale (UPDRS), which has been used in many studies, may not be ideal for distinguishing parkinsonism from signs that may be mistaken for it such as "gegenhalten", and its use may lead to inaccurate results. The discrepancy in definitions and methodology gave rise to highly variable rates of parkinsonism seen in AD patients ranging from 20 to 100% [6]. On average parkinsonism develops in approximately 1/3 of AD patients and is associated with more severe functional impairment. Most common parkinsonian features are rigidity, bradykinesia, and postural instability, resting tremor is relatively rare. Progression of parkinsonian signs except for tremor is twice as rapid in AD compared to Parkinson's disease (PD) patients [7].

AD patients have an increased rate of falls ranging from 60 to 80%, twice as much as compared to their age-matched cognitively healthy peers. Risk factors for falls include severity of dementia, balance and gait problems, loss of vision, presence of depressive and autonomic symptoms, and use of medications including neuroleptics, hypnotics, and anxiolytics [8]. Falls may lead to serious medical consequences such as death, fractures, and hospitalization. Their aetiology should be evaluated carefully and necessary precautions should be taken.

Myoclonus is another movement disorder seen in AD patients. Its frequency increases gradually over time, younger-onset AD patients are more likely to develop myoclonus. In late-onset AD patients, myoclonus is a late feature; however, it may occur early in younger-onset patients, especially those carrying presenilin 1 (PSEN1) mutations. Along with a variety of drugs used for the symptomatic treatment of AD, both acetylcholine esterase inhibitors and memantine may induce myoclonic jerks in AD patients.

Paratonia, also named "gegenhalten", is a common motor phenomenon in late-stage AD patients. It is characterized by resistance to passive movement of the limb. Unlike rigidity, where there is a constant resistance to passive movement, the speed of movement increases the amount of resistance in paratonia. It is not specific for AD and may be seen in other types of dementia, the presence of paratonia has been associated with a more rapid decline [9]. Since the treatment strategies differ, it is important to differentiate paratonia from rigidity.

The neuropathological substrate of gait disorder and extrapyramidal symptoms in AD is not well established. In a pathological study, it was suggested that neuronal loss in substantia nigra due to tau pathology may be the underlying cause of extrapyramidal symptoms [10]. Another study revealed that alpha-synuclein aggregation and hyperphosphorylated tau accumulation in substantia nigra were associated with extrapyramidal signs observed in AD [11].

Pharmacological Treatment of Parkinsonism in AD

Although parkinsonism is a common feature in the course of the disease, there have been no randomized controlled clinical trials on pharmacological treatment of parkinsonism in AD. Levodopa may provide some benefits, although this needs to be confirmed and it has the potential to induce or worsen behavioural symptoms such as hallucinations. Dopamine agonists and anticholinergics carry a high risk to induce hallucinations and worsen cognitive functions, they should be avoided in AD patients. A small study with galantamine, an acetylcholinesterase inhibitor used in the treatment of cognitive and behavioural symptoms of AD patients, suggested that it may also improve gait [12]. Donepezil was also reported to improve gait in early-stage AD patients in a small phase II trial [13]. Memantine, which is indicated for symptomatic treatment of AD, is an uncompetitive antagonist of *N*-methyl-D-aspartate receptor, also acts as a dopamine D2 receptor agonist. In a small study, improvement in stride time was observed in AD patients receiving memantine (20 mg/day) compared to patients receiving no treatment [14]. All these findings have been in small studies and need confirmation before these drugs can be considered for treatment of motor symptoms in AD.

Non-pharmacological Treatment of Parkinsonism in AD

There has been an increasing interest in the relationship between exercise and cognitive functions in AD. A systematic review, including six randomized clinical trials, showed a positive effect of exercise on the rate of cognitive decline in AD [15]. There are few studies on the effect of exercise and physical therapy on motor signs in AD. A systematic review revealed a moderate effect of exercise on both activities of daily living and physical function, including gait, balance, agility, and strength in AD patients [16]. Home-based exercise programs using computerized game councils have also been reported to show improvements in balance [17].

Treatment of Falls

The aetiology of falls in AD patients is heterogeneous, and treatment should target the underlying etiologic factors. In case falls are mainly related to parkinsonism, levodopa may be initiated empirically although evidence for its efficacy is lacking. In case autonomic dysfunction is the underlying factor, medications that may cause orthostatic hypotension such as antihypertensives, neuroleptics, anxiolytics, and drugs to treat prostate hypertrophy should be discontinued or their dose should be reduced. General principles to avoid orthostatic hypotension including increased intake of fluids and salt (provided there are no contraindications such as renal failure), sleeping with elevated head, abdominal compression and wearing anti-embolic stockings may be useful. In case these measures are not sufficient drugs such as midodrine, fludrocortisone, and pyridostigmine may be considered to increase standing blood pressure, but supine hypertension should be monitored.

Treatment of Myoclonus

Myoclonus in AD is thought to be of cortical origin. Hence, anti-myoclonus drugs known to be effective against cortical myoclonus are first-line treatments. These drugs, however, may be associated with significant adverse events, including cognitive worsening. Therefore, drug treatment should be considered only when myoclonic jerks lead to severe disability or discomfort. Clonazepam, levetiracetam, and valproic acid are the most commonly used medications in AD patients; however, there are no controlled studies with these drugs in this population. Clonazepam should be initiated at low doses (0.5 mg) and gradually titrated up at 5–7 days intervals if needed; doses up to 3 mg/day may be required [18]. The most common side effect is drowsiness, patients may fall because of its sedative effect. Levetiracetam, an anti-epileptic drug, should also be initiated at low doses (500 mg/day) and can be titrated up to 3000 mg/day as necessary. Drowsiness and behavioural changes may occur and should be monitored. Valproic acid is another option, the initial dose should be 250 mg/day, doses around 1000 mg/day are usually needed for sufficient response. Drug-induced parkinsonism and tremor should be monitored in this particularly vulnerable population. It is contraindicated in patients with hepatic failure, and it has the potential to interact with warfarin.

Treatment of Paratonia in AD

No evidence-based treatment is available for managing paratonia in dementia patients. In a small study, botulinum toxin injections showed some beneficial effects, such as increasing the range of motion and reducing caregiver burden [19]. No data is available on the effect of benzodiazepines and baclofen, which are frequently used to treat spasticity and dystonia, other conditions associated with increased muscle tone. A 4-week randomized clinical study, including 101 dementia patients, assessed the effect of passive movement therapy for paratonia and found no benefit [20]. A small study reported that patients might benefit from supporting cushions [21].

Treatment of Motor Symptoms in Parkinson's Disease Dementia and Dementia with Lewy Bodies

In contrast to AD, motor symptoms are initial symptoms and always present in patients with PD dementia (PDD) and they occur in the vast majority of patients with Dementia with Lewy Bodies (DLB), either at the onset or during the course of the disease. There are substantial similarities in the pathological and clinical features of the two diseases, "one-year rule" has been proposed to differentiate these two conditions from each other: in case motor symptoms occur concomitantly with symptoms of dementia or ensue within 1 year of their onset the condition should be defined as DLB whereas it should be defined as PDD in case symptoms of dementia occur at least 1 year after the onset of motor symptoms.

In PDD patients, motor symptoms are generally more symmetrical with a predominance of bradykinesia, rigidity, and postural instability compared to non-demented PD patients. Tremor is less frequent or may disappear as dementia develops in those who initially had tremor [22]. Similar to PDD, an akinetic-rigid phenotype predominates also in patients with DLB, with bradykinesia, rigidity and postural instability as core features. Tremor is less frequent, symptoms tend to be more symmetrical from the onset and during the course of the disease in contrast to the usual asymmetrical presentation of PD. Falls are frequent in both DLB and PDD, they may be the most disabling symptom in some patients leading to severe injuries and institutionalization, recurrent falls is also a supportive diagnostic feature for DLB. Major risk factors associated with falls in DLB and PDD patients are the severity of parkinsonism and dementia and the presence of autonomic symptoms, especially orthostatic hypotension. Medications administered to treat psychotic symptoms and REM sleep behaviour disorder such as neuroleptics and benzodiazepines may exacerbate orthostatic hypotension and can lead to falls. Approximately one-third of DLB patients develop myoclonus [23]. Myoclonus is usually located in the upper extremities and triggered by movement of the limbs or while maintaining a posture.

Pharmacological Treatment of Parkinsonism in DLB and PDD

Half of patients with DLB might show a clinical response to antiparkinsonian drugs [24]. Levodopa is the drug of choice, it should be started at low doses and slowly titrated to the effective and tolerated doses. Levodopa may induce or aggravate hallucinations and excessive daytime sleepiness which may be dose-limiting adverse effects and may render it difficult to attain effective doses. The magnitude of response to levodopa may differ across DLB patients. In a small study, Goldman et al. found a motor benefit (defined as >10% improvement over baseline in UPDRS Part III score) only in 1/3 of treated patients [25]. In another study including 24 DLB patients, positive response to levodopa challenge test was observed in approximately half of the patients. Initial response to levodopa was similar to that seen in PD patients; response to treatment, however, significantly decreased in the first year of treatment [26]. All together the results suggested that half of DLB patients may respond reasonably well to levodopa for a limited time period. The gradual loss of response to levodopa may be due to the predominance of axial symptoms in the later stages, which are usually non-levodopa responsive. The magnitude of motor response to levodopa also seems diminish with time in patients with PDD. In a study investigating response to levodopa in late-stage PD, Fabbri et al. included patients with advanced PD where 70% of patients had also dementia. They found a weak response to a supra-maximal dose of levodopa [27]. Dopamine agonists, monoamine oxidase inhibitors and in particular anticholinergics carry a high risk to induce or worsen behavioural and cognitive symptoms; they should be avoided in patients with PDD or DLB. A Phase II study of zonisamide, a drug approved for treatment of PD in Japan, showed benefits on motor symptoms of DLB patients when combined with levodopa [28].

There is no data on the management of dyskinesias in PDD and DLB. Amantadine, a drug commonly used to treat dyskinesias in PD patients, has the potential to induce or worsen hallucinations and should be used with caution. Clozapine, an atypical antipsychotic which also has some anti-dyskinetic properties, may be considered in patients with both psychosis and severe dyskinesias. It may cause sedation and needs regular blood tests to monitor neutropenia and agranulocytosis which may be life-threatening.

Cholinesterase inhibitors are commonly used in the treatment of PDD and DLB. Donepezil is approved for treatment of DLB in Japan, whereas rivastigmine is world-wide registered for treatment of mild-to-moderate PDD. In a meta-analysis, both medications were found to have no significant effects on motor symptoms of DLB or PDD, rivastigmine may have a potential to worsen tremor in PDD patients [29].

Non-pharmacological Treatment of Parkinsonism in DLB and PDD

There is limited data on the effects of physical exercise in DLB patients. In a case report, stationary cycling (3 sessions/week for 8 weeks) resulted in an improvement of gait speed in a DLB patient [30]. In a small study, auditory rhythmical cueing was shown to improve gait in PD patients with cognitive impairment [31]. Evidence from studies conducted in PD patients suggests short- and long-term benefits of exercise. Hence, it seems reasonable to recommend exercise and physiotherapy to patients who have both dementia and parkinsonism including those with DLB and PDD.

Treatment of Falls in DLB and PDD

The aetiology of falls in this patient population is heterogeneous, it is important to reveal the underlying cause in any given patient with repeated falls. A classification of falls in PD was proposed as follows: (a) transitional (involves a basic transition from one posture to another, e.g., sitting on a sofa), (b) combined (involves everyday walking activities including stair climbing or combined movements, e.g., carrying heavy objects), (c) advanced (involves a complex, high-risk motor activity, e.g., hill walking) [32]. This classification is useful to identify the nature of falls in order to recommend appropriate strategies and exercises (e.g., strength or balance training in "transitional" type, neurocognitive strategies for "combined" type). It is important to recognize orthostatic hypotension as a cause of falls as opposed to those due to symptoms of parkinsonism since the treatment approaches differ. There is substantial data supporting the benefits of physiotherapy, exercise, and dance in reducing the risk of falls and increasing mobility in PD patients [33]. It is, however, not established if these beneficial effects persist in PD patients with dementia or those with DLB. Limited benefits of cognitive strategies such as dual-task, motor task, and complex motor task training to reduce risk of falling have been shown in cognitively healthy subjects and PD patients. However, none of these studies included DLB or PDD patients [34–37]. Although there is no evidence base, individualized exercise and physiotherapy programs fitted to the general, physical and mental status of the patient can be recommended as good clinical practice.

Treatment of Myoclonus in DLB and PDD

Myoclonic jerks seen in patients with DLB are similar to those observed in AD, and strategies for their pharmacological treatment are similar. A caveat is the potential risk for worsening of parkinsonism with valproate in patients with DLB and PDD, treatment with levetiracetam or clonazepam should be preferred in this patient population.

Treatment of Motor Symptoms in Vascular Dementia

Vascular dementia (VaD) is a common form of dementia in which, vascular pathology of various origins is responsible for cognitive, motor, and autonomic symptoms. VaD is not a single disease, it spans a group of syndromes due to varying vascular mechanisms. As an umbrella term, vascular cognitive impairment (VCI) refers to the entire spectrum of cognitive disorders associated with vascular pathology.

In contrast to AD, motor symptoms are usually present in the early stages of VCI. As is the case for the definition of VCI, "vascular parkinsonism" is also a broad term that encompasses motor features of VCI, such as gait disorders, lower body predominant rigidity and bradykinesia, postural instability, freezing of gait, and pyramidal signs. Apart from usually symmetrical lower body parkinsonism, PSP-like syndrome or unilateral parkinsonism may rarely be seen in patients with VCI.

Recently, definition and classification of vascular parkinsonism (VaP) have been proposed by a panel of experts [38]. Acute or subacute presentation of parkinsonism due to vascular pathologies in brainstem or nigrostriatal pathways are defined as "acute/subacute post-stroke VaP" which is usually asymmetric and responsive to dopaminergic drugs. The "insidious onset VaP" is the most common subtype presenting with progressive parkinsonism together with pyramidal, cerebellar, pseudobulbar, cognitive, and urinary symptoms. Response to dopaminergic treatment in the insidious onset VaP subtype is usually poor. The "mixed type VaP" is defined as a clinical syndrome when cerebrovascular disease overlaps with neurodegenerative parkinsonism.

Neuroimaging is essential to demonstrate vascular changes to support the diagnosis of VaP. However, it should be kept in mind that concomitant vascular changes are frequent also in many neurodegenerative diseases, including Parkinson's disease. Severity of white-matter lesions in MRI was shown to be associated with higher UPDRS scores in VaP patients. In some instances, functional imaging with dopamine transporter ligands may help to differentiate VaP from PD by showing normal dopaminergic activity in the basal ganglia of VaD patients provided that vascular lesions do not directly involve the striatum.

Neuropathology of VaP due to small-vessel disease involves perivascular pallor, gliosis, hyaline thickening, and widening of perivascular spaces in the subcortical white-matter, basal ganglia, and brainstem [39].

Pharmacological Treatment of Vascular Parkinsonism

The first step should be to identify and reduce the risk for further vascular damage in order to avoid progression of motor impairment; hence all vascular risk factors should be controlled as much as possible. Changes in lifestyle with pharmacological treatment of hypertension, diabetes mellitus, hyperlipidemia, and following the general guidelines for management of cerebrovascular disease have the potential to reduce the rate of progression of motor symptoms as well as dementia. Nevertheless, there have been no clinical trials that investigate effects of primary or secondary prevention strategies on the severity and progression of motor symptoms of VaD.

For symptomatic treatment, there is limited evidence to support the use of dopaminergic drugs. Levodopa has been reported to be the most beneficial dopaminergic agent in the treatment of motor symptoms of VaP. A study investigating the effect of levodopa in 17 pathologically confirmed vascular parkinsonism cases, a good response to levodopa was observed in 12 patients [39]. On contrary, many other studies showed limited response to levodopa in VaP patients. In a meta-analysis including 17 studies, rate of response to levodopa was 0.304 (95% CI of 0.230–0.388), indicating a low response rate [40]. In four of the studies included in the meta-analysis, UPDRS was used to measure the effect of levodopa on motor symptoms, the reduction in motor score ranged from 5.8 to 22.25% [41–44]. Two studies compared levodopa response in VaP versus PD patients and found a relatively low reduction in the UPDRS scores in VaP patients (5.9–18.7%) as opposed to substantial improvement in PD patients (31.6–64.65%) [42, 43]. There is evidence to suggest that VaP patients with nigrostriatal lesions are more likely to respond to levodopa compared to VaP patients without nigrostriatal lesions. In clinical practice, patients with vascular parkinsonism should receive levodopa in sufficiently high doses, and the treatment should be continued for a sufficient period of time to observe the response; higher doses as compared to those used in PD patients may be required. No data is available on the efficacy of dopamine agonists and monoamine oxidase inhibitors on the treatment of motor symptoms in VaP. An open-label study including 94 VaP and 92 PD patients suggested that vitamin D may have potential to decrease the rate of falls in patients with VaP by increasing muscle strength; no change in symptoms of parkinsonism was observed [45]. In a trial with 40 patients, drainage of cerebrospinal fluid was associated with improvement of gait in 15 patients with a mean duration of 2.4 ± 1.2 months [46]. In a small study, 5 Hz rTMS treatment was associated with a decrease in UPDRS motor scores [47]; a study with 25 Hz stimulation of supplementary motor cortex in VaP patients is in progress.

There are no controlled studies evaluating the effect of non-pharmacological approaches including rehabilitation or physiotherapy. Empirically, gait may benefit from conventional rehabilitation, and behavioural therapy may alleviate the fear of falling, these may be recommended as good clinical practice. Vascular dementia patients usually have primary motor symptoms such as hemiparesis, dysarthria or dysphagia which may benefit from stroke rehabilitation. Gastrostomy and enteral feeding should be considered in patients with severe dysphagia.

Management of Motor Symptoms in Frontotemporal Dementia

Frontotemporal dementia (FTD) is a syndrome characterized by progressive behavioural changes, executive dysfunction, and impairment in language functions, due to neuronal loss in frontal and temporal cortices and striatum, caused by various neurodegenerative disorders [48]. It is the leading cause of dementia before the age of 65 with an overall prevalence ranging from 3 to 26% [49]. Although the majority of cases are sporadic, a family history of dementia, motor neuron disease (MND) or parkinsonism are reported in up to 40% of cases; a clear autosomal dominant history accounts for 10% of cases [50]. Hexanucleotide (GGGGCC) expansions (>30 repeats) in the C9orf72 gene on chromosome 9, mutations in microtubule-associated protein tau, and progranulin genes are the most common (about 60% of all cases) genetic causes of familial FTD and may be associated with parkinsonism or MND [51, 52].

Based on the leading clinical features, three main subtypes have been defined including behavioural variant FTD, and two forms of primary progressive aphasia (PPA), i.e. semantic and non-fluent variants [53]. Behavioural variant FTD (bvFTD), the most common phenotype, manifests with progressive behavioural problems, inappropriate social conduct and executive dysfunction [54]. Semantic variant PPA (svPPA) is characterized by gradual loss of semantic knowledge impairing word comprehension. Non-fluent/agrammatic variant PPA presents with inability to plan and programme the motor aspects of speech and sentence construction [55].

A number of motor symptoms may accompany FTD, occurring usually in the later stages of the disease. These include hypokinetic movement disorders such as parkinsonism, impairment of eye movements, features of CBS as well as hyperkinetic movement disorders such as motor and vocal stereotypies, dystonia, chorea, orofacial dyskinesias, and myoclonus [56]. Although presynaptic dopaminergic dysfunction is involved in the development of parkinsonism, evidence suggests that postsynaptic dopaminergic dysfunction in the striatum may also play a role in the pathogenesis [57, 58].

MND or atypical parkinsonism may accompany both familial and sporadic forms of the disease [59–61]. Mild features of motor neuron disease can occur in up to 40% of FTD patients, 12.5% of patients with bvFTD develop MND with typical signs including upper and lower motor neuron symptoms, dysarthria, dysphagia, and pseudobulbar affect [62]. Epidemiological studies suggest that parkinsonism occurs in up to 50% of FTD patients, predominantly in bvFTD, rarely in svPPA, it may also be associated with MND [54, 63–65]. Parkinsonism may be an initial feature of FTD, it can also emerge during the course of the disease [60, 61]. Atypical parkinsonism with symmetrical, axial akinetic-rigid syndrome, absence of tremor, and poor response to levodopa (including progressive supranuclear palsy phenotype) are the common features in several types of FTD, whereas asymmetrical parkinsonism and dystonia are the leading features in CBS phenotype [61, 66]. The most common hyperkinetic movement disorders in FTD are motor and vocal stereotypies, which have been observed in up to 78% of patients with autopsy-proven FTD. Chorea, orofacial dyskinesias, myoclonus, and dystonia are other hyperkinetic movements observed in some patients with FTD.

There are no randomized clinical trials on the efficacy of dopaminergic treatment for parkinsonism in FTD. Empirically a trial of levodopa up to 1000 mg/day can be given. Adverse effects such as nausea, hypotension, and psychosis may limit dose escalation. Typical neuroleptics should be avoided for the management of behavioural symptoms such as psychosis, quetiapine or clozapine may be considered with appropriate monitoring. Selective serotonin reuptake inhibitors may be considered for the management of stereotypies. In an open-label study fluvoxamine showed improvement in stereotypical behaviour in bvFTD and PPA patients [67]. Tetrabenazine (75 mg/day) has also been used in the management of stereotypies with some improvement [68]. Clonazepam may be used for the treatment of myoclonus [69]. Riluzole (100 mg/day) the only Food and Drug Administration (FDA) and European Medicines Agency (EMA)-approved treatment for MND [70] can be prescribed in FTD patients with motor neuron disease. Physical therapy with gait and balance training might be used to prevent falls and to decrease mortality [71]. Dysphagia is a common *symptom* of MND. Initial management approach should be modification of food and fluid consistency in patients with mild dysphagia. Liquids can be thickened and solid foods may be pureed, diced, or chopped. Gastrostomy and enteral tube feeding should be considered in more advanced patients to reduce the risk of aspiration pneumonia. There is, however, limited data to suggest that PEG placement is associated with prolonged survival [72].

Management of Motor Symptoms in Corticobasal Degeneration

Corticobasal Degeneration (CBD) is a neurodegenerative disease associated with abnormal aggregates of 4-repeat tau (4R-tau) protein. It is characterized by generally asymmetric movement disorders (levodopa non-responsive parkinsonism, dystonia, abnormal gait, and myoclonus) combined with partly lateralized symptoms of higher cortical dysfunction such as apraxia, alien limb phenomenon, cortical sensory loss, cognitive impairment, behavioural changes, and aphasia [73, 74].

Pathology confirmed studies have revealed that diverse clinical presentations are associated with CBD [73]. Conversely, different pathologies such as AD, FTD, progressive supranuclear palsy (PSP), DLB, and Creutzfeldt- Jakob disease might lead to clinical features of classical CBD which is termed as corticobasal syndrome (CBS) [75]. It is estimated that 50% of CBS cases have CBD pathology [76].

There is currently no medication approved for the treatment of CBD. Drugs used for treatment are based on experience in other disorders or on non-randomized historical controls, case series, or expert opinions.

Clinicopathological series revealed that limb rigidity and bradykinesia were the most common motor findings in CBD [73]. Although levodopa response in parkinsonism is considered to be insufficient and excellent/sustained response is an exclusion criterium, it should be tried especially for bradykinesia and rigidity. Where present, benefits are often mild to moderate and transient [73]. Kompoliti et al. reviewed 147 CBS patients (7 were autopsy proven) and found clinical improvement with dopaminergic drugs in 24% of cases, 71% had no improvement [77]. Levodopa was introduced in 87% of all cases and 26% demonstrated modest response (median daily dosage 300 mg, range 100–2000 mg). Bradykinesia and rigidity were the best improved symptoms with levodopa. Dopamine agonists, selegiline, and amantadine were tried in limited number of cases (6–13%) and the response was worse than levodopa. Five percent of the patients experienced drug-associated worsening of parkinsonian features, dystonia, myoclonus, or gait dysfunction. Anticholinergics and benzodiazepines have been tried and found to be usually ineffective. Dyskinesias did not occur with dopaminergic drugs in this series, there are, however, few pathologically confirmed CBD cases who developed levodopa induced dyskinesias [78, 79].

Although dystonia was reported in up to 83% in clinical series and considered as one of the classical features of CBS, pathologically confirmed studies revealed that it was present only in 38% of CBD cases [80]. In the majority of cases presented with a corticobasal syndrome, dystonia occurred earlier (in the first 2 years from disease onset), mostly affecting the upper limb. In other phenotypes with cognitive presentations, dystonia tended to appear later and to affect the cervical region and face [80]. In the PSP phenotype blepharospasm and axial dystonia were the most frequent presentations. Generalized dystonia or hemidystonia may occur during the course of the disease [81, 82]. Dopaminergic agents, amantadine, anticholinergics, benzodiazepines, muscle relaxants (e.g., baclofen), and intramuscular botulinum toxin injections have been tried for the management of dystonia in CBD. Except for botulinum toxin injections, these medications were rarely effective [77, 80, 83]. Botulinum toxin can be useful for pain and hygiene problems due to contractures associated with dystonia. Deep brain stimulation is not recommended for patients with CBD [84].

Myoclonus is one of the common symptoms of CBD. The frequency in pathological series is 27–52% [73, 80]. Myoclonus is usually focal and considered to be of cortical origin. It can present as cortical reflex myoclonus, stimulus-sensitive myoclonus or action myoclonus. It is usually localized in the upper extremities, but can also be present in the face [79, 85, 86]. Low-amplitude action myoclonus may resemble tremor. A clinicopathological study revealed that myoclonus is more common in CBD-mimics [87]. Benzodiazepines (particularly clonazepam), antiepileptics (levetiracetam, gabapentin, valproic acid), piracetam, and neuroleptics have been tried with variable results [77].

The role of exercise in CBD is not well studied. Nevertheless, regular exercise and appropriate physiotherapy may be recommended as good clinical practice in CBD patients with parkinsonism or gait problems [88, 89].

Management of Motor Symptoms in Progressive Supranuclear Palsy

PSP is a tauopathy characterized by parkinsonism, vertical gaze palsy, early postural instability with falls, dysarthria, dysphagia, and a dysexecutive type dementia [90, 91]. The phenotype of parkinsonism is usually a symmetrical, akinetic-rigid form with prominent postural imbalance; tremor is rare. Unprovoked falls are the most significant problem and the main cause of disability, prominent dysphagia, and dysarthria develop in almost all patients.

For treatment of parkinsonism, levodopa is the first drug of choice. While excellent or sustained response to levodopa has previously been a mandatory exclusion criterion, a subtype of PSP defined as PSP-Parkinson has been recognized, such patients may have clear benefit from levodopa, substantially more so as compared to other phenotypes of PSP [92], hence a clear response to levodopa is no longer an exclusion criterion for PSP. Although the evidence base for benefits of levodopa treatment is weak, due to lack of better options up to 1500 mg daily doses are commonly administered [83, 93–96]. There are a few uncontrolled studies which assessed the efficacy of dopamine agonists and which found no or limited benefits [83, 93, 94, 95, 97]. Monoamine oxidase B inhibitors have also failed to show any beneficial effect [83, 93, 95]. The *N*-methyl-D-aspartate-antagonist amantadine up to 600 mg/day has been reported to be of variable benefit in retrospective series [83, 95]. Botulinum toxin injections can be used for focal dystonias including apraxia of eyelid opening with variable success [96]. A study which assessed effects of deep brain stimulation in the pedunculopontine nucleus in eight PSP-RS patients did not show any benefits, there was no difference between on-stimulation and off- stimulation at 6 and 12-month follow-up [98].

Drugs used for the treatment of motor symptoms may lead to various adverse effects. Cognitive and behavioural symptoms may be exacerbated by medication used to treat movement disorders and other symptoms of PSP. Levodopa can cause orthostatic hypotension, hallucinations, delusions, gastrointestinal complaints, and dizziness, amantadine can lead to insomnia, confusion, hallucinations, postural hypotension, anxiety, anorexia, and livedo reticularis [99].

The effect of physiotherapy on motor symptoms has been investigated in a few studies. A randomized controlled study showed that physical exercise may improve balance and gait and reduce falls, the magnitude and duration of effects were, however, limited [100]. Effects of structured physical exercises in patients with advanced PSP are not known. In a systematic review, weight-supported treadmill training, music-cued movement rehabilitation, and robotic-assisted gait training were reported to be beneficial in early PSP [101]. Eyeglasses with bifocal or prismatic lenses may help to look downwards without moving eyes in patients with downward gaze palsy [102]. As pharmacological treatments are of limited benefit in most patients, supportive measures including gait and balance exercises as well as measures to improve dysphagia are important.

Management of Motor Symptoms in Huntington's Disease

Huntington's disease (HD) is an autosomal dominant neurodegenerative disorder caused by an expanded cytosine-adenine-guanine trinucleotide repeat in the huntingtin gene on chromosome 4 which encodes the huntingtin protein. Although medium spiny neurons of the striatum are particularly vulnerable to mutant huntingtin induced pathology, the disease affects the whole brain and body [103]. Clinically, Huntington's disease is characterized by motor symptoms, cognitive impairment, and psychiatric disturbances [103, 104]. Manifest HD is diagnosed in genetically confirmed or at-risk individuals with "unequivocal presence of an otherwise unexplained extrapyramidal movement disorder such as chorea, bradykinesia or rigidity" that indicates 99% diagnostic confidence for HD [105, 106]. Slow saccades and cognitive dysfunction are usually supportive findings for HD [103].

Two main components of motor disorder in HD are involuntary movements (chorea) and impaired voluntary movements (bradykinesia and incoordination). While chorea is common in adult-onset cases, bradykinesia is more common in juvenile onset patients in earlier phases of the disease [107, 108]. Bradykinesia, dystonia, and parkinsonism are more prominent features in Juvenile HD (JHD), and chorea may not be seen during the whole course of the disease. Myoclonus and epileptic seizures are also reported in half of the JHD patients. In adult-onset HD, chorea often decreases during the course of the disease whereas bradykinesia, dystonia, and rigidity begin to predominate and predict functional disability [103, 109, 110]. Dysarthria and dysphagia usually appear at the later stages of the disease.

Chorea is thought to be a result of imbalance between glutamate and dopamine activity in basal ganglia. Treatment for chorea is based on dopamine depletion or dopamine receptor blockade [111, 112]. Tetrabenazine, a synaptic vesicular amine transporter inhibitor 2 (VMAT2) depletes dopamine and has been licensed by the US FDA for the treatment of chorea in HD. The initial dose is 12.5 mg/day, titration should be done slowly by weekly intervals of 12.5 mg/day to identify dose that reduces chorea and is tolerated, maximum dose is 100 mg/day. The main and dose-limiting adverse events have been reported to be sedation, akathisia, parkinsonism, depression, and suicide attempt [113]. However, recent studies reported that use of Tetrabenazine is not associated with increased risk of suicide [114, 115]. Deutetrabenazine, recently approved by FDA, is a novel Vesicular Amine Transporter Inhibitor 2 inhibitor with prolonged active metabolite half-lives and has a favourable tolerability profile with lower adverse effect rates than tetrabenazine [116, 117]. The most common adverse events with deutetrabenazine include somnolence, insomnia, headache, diarrhoea, and akathisia which are usually mild to moderate [118].

Chorea is also treated with typical or atypical neuroleptics (dopamine receptor blockers). These are, however, associated with potentially serious adverse effects such as parkinsonism, imbalance, akathisia, neuroleptic malignant syndrome, acute dystonic reactions, tardive dyskinesia, blunting of affect, and generalized apathy. Since parkinsonism dominates in the later stages of the adult-onset disease, use of neuroleptics requires caution. Neuroleptic drugs may be preferred in the treatment of chorea when accompanied with psychiatric symptoms. Tiapride (in Europe), olanzapine, and risperidone are preferred as the first-line treatment of chorea, in addition to Vesicular Amine Transporter Inhibitor 2 inhibitors [119]. Considering the glutamate arm of chorea pathophysiology, inhibitors of glutamate transmission (riluzole 200 mg/day, amantadine 400 mg/day) have also been tried. Although they are recommended in the 2011 AAN evidence-based guidelines, their use is controversial [120, 121].

Dopaminergic drugs, such as levodopa and dopamine agonists can be used to treat rigidity and bradykinesia [122]. They may be used in selected cases of JHD or in the late stages of the adult-onset disease, where hypokinetic symptoms are more prominent. They should be avoided in early stages of adult forms or late stages of JHD where chorea is more prominent. Based on limited data, non-invasive stimulation with transcranial magnetic stimulation to supplementary motor and primary motor area may be effective for chorea, depression, and cognitive functions; these effects, however, need to be confirmed in larger studies [123–125]. Deep brain stimulation of pallidum may be effective in the treatment of medically resistant chorea. It does not, however, seem to improve daily living activities, current data are limited, there are challenges such as severe pallidal atrophy, clinical variety in different stages of the disease and coexisting problems [125]. Baclofen, benzodiazepines, and botulinum toxin injections can be used to treat dystonia.

Physiotherapy should be part of the management of motor symptoms, recommendations have been published to guide physical therapy [126]. Aerobic exercise, resistance training, and supervised gait training are recommended to improve fitness, motor function, and gait with grade A evidence. It has been suggested that these approaches also improve balance although they do not reduce the frequency of falls. Inspiratory and expiratory training may be beneficial to improve respiratory functions. Educating caregivers on the value of these exercises may lead to a higher rate of engagement in training and integrating these into daily life.

Treatment of Motor Symptoms in Multisystem Atrophy

Multisystem atrophy (MSA) is a neurodegenerative disease associated with abnormal aggregates of fibrillary α-synuclein protein in both glia and neurons [127, 128]. Depending on the predominant clinical features, the disease is sub-classified as MSA-parkinsonism and MSA-cerebellar. Dementia was considered as a non-supporting feature of MSA clinical criteria, however, emerging evidence demonstrated that approximately 30% of patients with MSA develop mild cognitive impairment. Cognitive decline sufficient to justify a diagnosis of dementia may be found in some patients with advanced stages of MSA [129, 130].

Response of parkinsonism to levodopa is variable and limited. In pathologically confirmed series, 30–70% of patients with MSA had an initial good response to levodopa [131–135]. In order to fully evaluate therapeutic response patients should be given up to a maximum dose of 1.5 g per day for at least 3 months [136]. One should be cautioned that levodopa may induce psychotic symptoms and worsening of orthostatic hypotension in the absence of any motor benefit. In a minority of patients with levodopa responsiveness, dyskinesia can develop, mostly at the craniocervical region and even after short-term use [137]. There are no controlled studies on the efficacy of dopamine agonists in MSA, in a retrospective study only 10% of patients had benefit with dopamine agonists [133]. Dopamine agonists also have a higher rate of side effects, especially worsening of orthostatic hypotension [138, 139], they are not recommended as first-line treatment. A retrospective case study revealed good response to amantadine in 15% of patients. A small, placebo-controlled study, however, failed to demonstrate any efficacy of amantadine in patients with MSA [140]. There is no evidence supporting the benefits of entacapone and Monoamine oxidase inhibitors in MSA [141, 142]. Because of limited experience suggesting poor outcome, and the possibility of harmful effects, DBS is not recommended in patients with MSA [143–145].

Although there are no randomized controlled studies, available data suggests that medical rehabilitation may improve balance, motor impairment, functional capacity, and reduce falls [146, 147].

Case Presentation

A 74-year-old female was referred to Memory Clinic for gradually progressive forgetfulness during the past 3 years with a rapid worsening in the last 3 months. Her memory problems included repeating questions, inability to recall new events, and recent conversations. She had trouble finding her way in familiar environments which had developed over the last 1 year, she became more apathetic and had increasingly more difficulty understanding complex sentences. Her movements became slower and resting tremor emerged on the right hand in the past few years. Her cognitive and motor performance fluctuated within the day as well as from today. Her past medical history was conspicuous for paranoid delusions for more than 30 years without hallucinations. There was no history of REM sleep behaviour or autonomic dysfunction. On admission she was receiving rivastigmine patch 4.6 mg/day, pimozide 4 mg/day for delusions, and trihexyphenidyl 4 mg/day as prophylaxis against extrapyramidal side effects. Her neurological examination revealed a right-sided resting tremor, mild-to-moderate rigidity, and bradykinesia, her gait was slow with short stride length and stooped posture. Mini mental state examination score was 19/30, her neuropsychological exam revealed deficits in memory (both encoding and retrieval), attention, executive, and visuo-spatial functions. Cranial MRI revealed mild bilateral hippocampal and parietal atrophy. Differential diagnosis included Dementia with Lewy Bodies versus Alzheimer disease with secondary parkinsonism due to pimozide and aggravated cognitive impairment due to adverse effects of anticholinergic medication. Pimozide and trihexyphenidyl were discontinued, rivastigmine patch was increased to 9.6 mg/day. Her motor and cognitive symptoms improved within a month, mini-mental state examination score increased to 24/30, both gait and bradykinesia improved, but a slight resting tremor on the right hand as well as mild bradykinesia-rigidity remained. A treatment with L-dopa 300 mg/day was initiated upon which her tremor and bradykinesia further improved. Our final diagnosis was Alzheimer disease with concomitant Lewy-body pathology as well as drug-induced worsening of motor and cognitive symptoms.

References

1. Fahn S, Jankovic J, Hallett M. Clinical overview and phenomenology of movement disorders. In: Principles and practice of movement disorders. 2nd ed. Philadelphia: Elsevier Health Sciences; 2011. p. 1–35. isbn:10:1437723691.
2. Alladi S, Xuereb J, Bak T, Nestor P, Knibb J, Patterson K, Hodges JR. Focal cortical presentations of Alzheimer's disease. Brain. 2007;130(Pt 10):2636–45. https://doi.org/10.1093/brain/awm213.
3. Sakae N, Josephs KA, Litvan I, Murray ME, Duara R, Uitti RJ, Wszolek ZK, van Gerpen J, Graff-Radford NR, Dickson DW. Clinicopathologic subtype of Alzheimer's disease presenting as corticobasal syndrome. Alzheimers Dement. 2019;15(9):1218–1228. https://doi.org/10.1016/j.jalz.2019.04.011.
4. Murman DL, Kuo SB, Powell MC, Colenda CC. The impact of parkinsonism on costs of care in patients with AD and dementia with Lewy bodies. Neurology. 2003;61(7):944–9. https://doi.org/10.1212/wnl.61.7.944.
5. Scarmeas N, Albert M, Brandt J, Blacker D, Hadjigeorgiou G, Papadimitriou A, Dubois B, Sarazin M, Wegesin D, Marder K, Bell K, Honig L, Stern Y. Motor signs predict poor outcomes in Alzheimer disease. Neurology. 2005;64(10):1696–703. https://doi.org/10.1212/01.WNL.0000162054.15428.E9.
6. Kurlan R, Richard IH, Papka M, Marshall F. Movement disorders in Alzheimer's disease: more rigidity of definitions is needed. Mov Disord. 2000;15(1):24–9. https://doi.org/10.1002/1531-8257(200001)15:1<24::aid-mds1006>3.0.co;2-x.
7. Wilson RS, Bennett DA, Gilley DW, Beckett LA, Schneider JA, Evans DA. Progression of parkinsonian signs in Alzheimer's disease. Neurology. 2000;54(6):1284–9. https://doi.org/10.1212/wnl.54.6.1284.
8. Fernando E, Fraser M, Hendriksen J, Kim CH, Muir-Hunter SW. Risk factors associated with falls in older adults with dementia: a systematic review. Physiother Can. 2017;69(2):161–70. https://doi.org/10.3138/ptc.2016-14.
9. Gladstone DJ, Black SE. The neurological examination in aging, dementia and cerebrovascular disease. Part 2: motor examination. Geriatr Aging. 2002;5:44–9.
10. Attems J, Quass M, Jellinger KA. Tau and alpha-synuclein brainstem pathology in Alzheimer disease: relation with extrapyramidal signs. Acta Neuropathol. 2007;113(1):53–62. https://doi.org/10.1007/s00401-006-0146-9.
11. Burns JM, Galvin JE, Roe CM, Morris JC, McKeel DW. The pathology of the substantia nigra in Alzheimer disease with extrapyramidal signs. Neurology. 2005;64(8):1397–403. https://doi.org/10.1212/01.WNL.0000158423.05224.7F.

12. Assal F, Allali G, Kressig RW, Herrmann FR, Beauchet O. Galantamine improves gait performance in patients with Alzheimer's disease. J Am Geriatr Soc. 2008;56(5):946–7. https://doi.org/10.1111/j.1532-5415.2008.01657.x.
13. Montero-Odasso M, Muir-Hunter SW, Oteng-Amoako A, Gopaul K, Islam A, Borrie M, Wells J, Speechley M. Donepezil improves gait performance in older adults with mild Alzheimer's disease: a phase II clinical trial. J Alzheimers Dis. 2015;43(1):193–9. https://doi.org/10.3233/JAD-140759.
14. Beauchet O, Allali G, Launay C, Fantino B, Annweiler C. Does memantine improve the gait of individuals with Alzheimer's disease? J Am Geriatr Soc. 2011;59(11):2181–2. https://doi.org/10.1111/j.1532-5415.2011.03648.x. Erratum in: J Am Geriatr Soc. 2012; 60(10):2001
15. Farina N, Rusted J, Tabet N. The effect of exercise interventions on cognitive outcome in Alzheimer's disease: a systematic review. Int Psychogeriatr. 2014;26(1):9–18. https://doi.org/10.1017/S1041610213001385.
16. Rao AK, Chou A, Bursley B, Smulofsky J, Jezequel J. Systematic review of the effects of exercise on activities of daily living in people with Alzheimer's disease. Am J Occup Ther. 2014;68(1):50–6. https://doi.org/10.5014/ajot.2014.009035.
17. Padala KP, Padala PR, Lensing SY, Dennis RA, Bopp MM, Roberson PK, Sullivan DH. Home-based exercise program improves balance and fear of falling in community-dwelling older adults with mild Alzheimer's disease: a pilot study. J Alzheimers Dis. 2017;59(2):565–74. https://doi.org/10.3233/JAD-170120.
18. Caviness JN. Treatment of myoclonus in degenerative disorders. Curr Clin Neurol. 2019:277–80. https://doi.org/10.1007/978-3-319-97897-0_63.
19. Kleiner-Fisman G, Khoo E, Moncrieffe N, Forbell T, Gryfe P, Fisman D. A randomized, placebo controlled pilot trial of botulinum toxin for paratonic rigidity in people with advanced cognitive impairment. PLoS One. 2014;9(12):e114733. https://doi.org/10.1371/journal.pone.0114733.
20. Hobbelen JH, Tan FE, Verhey FR, Koopmans RT, de Bie RA. Passive movement therapy in severe paratonia: a multicenter randomized clinical trial. Int Psychogeriatr. 2012;24(5):834–44. https://doi.org/10.1017/S1041610211002468.
21. Van Deun B, Van Den Noortgate N, Van Bladel A, De Weerdt K, Cambier D. Managing Paratonia in Persons With Dementia: Short-term Effects of Supporting Cushions and Harmonic Techniques. J Am Med Dir Assoc. 2019;20(12):1521–1528. https://doi.org/10.1016/j.jamda.2019.04.031.
22. Alves G, Larsen JP, Emre M, Wentzel-Larsen T, Aarsland D. Changes in motor subtype and risk for incident dementia in Parkinson's disease. Mov Disord. 2006;21(8):1123–30. https://doi.org/10.1002/mds.20897.
23. Tartaglia MC, Johnson DY, Thai JN, Cattaruzza T, Wong K, Garcia P, Dearmond SJ, Miller BL, Geschwind MD. Clinical overlap between Jakob-Creutzfeldt disease and Lewy body disease. Can J Neurol Sci. 2012;39(3):304–10. https://doi.org/10.1017/s0317167100013421.
24. Farina E, Baglio F, Caffarra P, Magnani G, Scarpini E, Appollonio I, Bascelli C, Cheldi A, Nemni R, Franceschi M; Italian Group for Lewy Body Dementia and Dementias Associated to Parkinsonism, Messa G, Mantovani F, Bellotti M, Olivotto F, Alberoni M, Isella V, Regazzoni R, Schiatti E, Vismara C, Falautano M, Barbieri A, Restelli I, Fetoni V, Donato M, Zuffi M, Castiglioni S. Frequency and clinical features of Lewy body dementia in Italian memory clinics. Acta Biomed. 2009;80(1):57–64. PMID: 19705622.
25. Goldman JG, Goetz CG, Brandabur M, Sanfilippo M, Stebbins GT. Effects of dopaminergic medications on psychosis and motor function in dementia with Lewy bodies. Mov Disord. 2008;23(15):2248–50. https://doi.org/10.1002/mds.22322.
26. Lucetti C, Logi C, Del Dotto P, Berti C, Ceravolo R, Baldacci F, Dolciotti C, Gambaccini G, Rossi G, Bonuccelli U. Levodopa response in dementia with lewy bodies: a 1-year follow-up study. Parkinsonism Relat Disord. 2010;16(8):522–6. https://doi.org/10.1016/j.parkreldis.2010.06.004.

27. Fabbri M, Coelho M, Abreu D, Guedes LC, Rosa MM, Costa N, Antonini A, Ferreira JJ. Do patients with late-stage Parkinson's disease still respond to levodopa? Parkinsonism Relat Disord. 2016;26:10–6. https://doi.org/10.1016/j.parkreldis.2016.02.021.
28. Murata M, Odawara T, Hasegawa K, Iiyama S, Nakamura M, Tagawa M, Kosaka K. Adjunct zonisamide to levodopa for DLB parkinsonism: a randomized double-blind phase 2 study. Neurology. 2018;90(8):e664–72. https://doi.org/10.1212/WNL.0000000000005010.
29. Stinton C, McKeith I, Taylor JP, Lafortune L, Mioshi E, Mak E, Cambridge V, Mason J, Thomas A, O'Brien JT. Pharmacological Management of Lewy Body Dementia: A Systematic Review and Meta-Analysis. Am J Psychiatry. 2015;172(8):731–42. https://doi.org/10.1176/appi.ajp.2015.14121582.
30. Tabak R, Aquije G, Fisher BE. Aerobic exercise to improve executive function in Parkinson disease: a case series. J Neurol Phys Ther. 2013;37(2):58–64. https://doi.org/10.1097/NPT.0b013e31829219bc.
31. Rochester L, Burn DJ, Woods G, Godwin J, Nieuwboer A. Does auditory rhythmical cueing improve gait in people with Parkinson's disease and cognitive impairment? A feasibility study. Mov Disord. 2009;24(6):839–45. https://doi.org/10.1002/mds.22400.
32. Ross A, Yarnall AJ, Rochester L, Lord S. A novel approach to falls classification in Parkinson's disease: development of the Fall-Related Activity Classification (FRAC). Physiotherapy. 2017;103(4):459–64. https://doi.org/10.1016/j.physio.2016.08.002.
33. Joza S, Camicioli R, Ba F. Falls in Synucleinopathies. Can J Neurol Sci. 2019;27:1–14. https://doi.org/10.1017/cjn.2019.287.
34. Mirelman A, Maidan I, Herman T, Deutsch JE, Giladi N, Hausdorff JM. Virtual reality for gait training: can it induce motor learning to enhance complex walking and reduce fall risk in patients with Parkinson's disease? J Gerontol A Biol Sci Med Sci. 2011;66(2):234–40. https://doi.org/10.1093/gerona/glq201.
35. You JH, Shetty A, Jones T, Shields K, Belay Y, Brown D. Effects of dual-task cognitive-gait intervention on memory and gait dynamics in older adults with a history of falls: a preliminary investigation. NeuroRehabilitation. 2009;24(2):193–8. https://doi.org/10.3233/NRE-2009-0468.
36. Verghese J, Mahoney J, Ambrose AF, Wang C, Holtzer R. Effect of cognitive remediation on gait in sedentary seniors. J Gerontol A Biol Sci Med Sci. 2010;65(12):1338–43. https://doi.org/10.1093/gerona/glq127.
37. Silsupadol P, Shumway-Cook A, Lugade V, van Donkelaar P, Chou LS, Mayr U, Woollacott MH. Effects of single-task versus dual-task training on balance performance in older adults: a double-blind, randomized controlled trial. Arch Phys Med Rehabil. 2009;90(3):381–7. https://doi.org/10.1016/j.apmr.2008.09.559.
38. Rektor I, Bohnen NI, Korczyn AD, Gryb V, Kumar H, Kramberger MG, de Leeuw FE, Pirtošek Z, Rektorová I, Schlesinger I, Slawek J, Valkovič P, Veselý B. An updated diagnostic approach to subtype definition of vascular parkinsonism—recommendations from an expert working group. Parkinsonism Relat Disord. 2018;49:9–16. https://doi.org/10.1016/j.parkreldis.2017.12.030.
39. Zijlmans JC, Katzenschlager R, Daniel SE, Lees AJ. The L-dopa response in vascular parkinsonism. J Neurol Neurosurg Psychiatry. 2004;75(4):545–7. https://doi.org/10.1136/jnnp.2003.018309.
40. Miguel-Puga A, Villafuerte G, Salas-Pacheco J, Arias-Carrión O. Therapeutic interventions for vascular parkinsonism: a systematic review and meta-analysis. Front Neurol. 2017;8:481. https://doi.org/10.3389/fneur.2017.00481.
41. Zijlmans J, Evans A, Fontes F, Katzenschlager R, Gacinovic S, Lees AJ, Costa D. [123I] FP-CIT spect study in vascular parkinsonism and Parkinson's disease. Mov Disord. 2007;22(9):1278–85. https://doi.org/10.1002/mds.21479.
42. Gago MF, Fernandes V, Ferreira J, Silva H, Rodrigues ML, Rocha L, Bicho E, Sousa N. The effect of levodopa on postural stability evaluated by wearable inertial measurement units for idiopathic and vascular Parkinson's disease. Gait Posture. 2015;41(2):459–64. https://doi.org/10.1016/j.gaitpost.2014.11.008.

43. Vale TC, Caramelli P, Cardoso F. Vascular parkinsonism: a case series of 17 patients. Arq Neuropsiquiatr. 2013;71(10):757–62. https://doi.org/10.1590/0004-282X20130117.
44. Vale TC, Caramelli P, Cardoso F. Clinicoradiological comparison between vascular parkinsonism and Parkinson's disease. J Neurol Neurosurg Psychiatry. 2015;86(5):547–53. https://doi.org/10.1136/jnnp-2014-307867.
45. Sato Y, Iwamoto J, Honda Y, Amano N. Vitamin D reduces falls and hip fractures in vascular Parkinsonism but not in Parkinson's disease. Ther Clin Risk Manag. 2013;9:171–6. https://doi.org/10.2147/TCRM.S43811.
46. Ondo WG, Chan LL, Levy JK. Vascular parkinsonism: clinical correlates predicting motor improvement after lumbar puncture. Mov Disord. 2002;17(1):91–7. https://doi.org/10.1002/mds.1270.
47. Yip CW, Cheong PW, Green A, Prakash PK, Fook-Cheong SK, Tan EK, Lo YL. A prospective pilot study of repetitive transcranial magnetic stimulation for gait dysfunction in vascular parkinsonism. Clin Neurol Neurosurg. 2013;115(7):887–91. https://doi.org/10.1016/j.clineuro.2012.08.032.
48. Bang J, Spina S, Miller BL. Frontotemporal dementia. Lancet. 2015;386(10004):1672–82. https://doi.org/10.1016/S0140-6736(15)00461-4.
49. Vieira RT, Caixeta L, Machado S, Silva AC, Nardi AE, Arias-Carrión O, Carta MG. Epidemiology of early-onset dementia: a review of the literature. Clin Pract Epidemiol Ment Health. 2013;9:88–95. https://doi.org/10.2174/1745017901309010088.
50. Rohrer JD, Guerreiro R, Vandrovcova J, Uphill J, Reiman D, Beck J, Isaacs AM, Authier A, Ferrari R, Fox NC, Mackenzie IR, Warren JD, de Silva R, Holton J, Revesz T, Hardy J, Mead S, Rossor MN. The heritability and genetics of frontotemporal lobar degeneration. Neurology. 2009;73(18):1451–6. https://doi.org/10.1212/WNL.0b013e3181bf997a.
51. Le Ber I. Genetics of frontotemporal lobar degeneration: an up-date and diagnosis algorithm. Rev Neurol (Paris). 2013;169(10):811–9. https://doi.org/10.1016/j.neurol.2013.07.014.
52. Renton AE, Majounie E, Waite A, Simón-Sánchez J, Rollinson S, Gibbs JR, et al. A hexanucleotide repeat expansion in C9ORF72 is the cause of chromosome 9p21-linked ALS-FTD. Neuron. 2011;72(2):257–68. https://doi.org/10.1016/j.neuron.2011.09.010.
53. Woollacott IO, Rohrer JD. The clinical spectrum of sporadic and familial forms of frontotemporal dementia. J Neurochem. 2016;138(Suppl 1):6–31. https://doi.org/10.1111/jnc.13654.
54. Rascovsky K, Hodges JR, Knopman D, Mendez MF, Kramer JH, Neuhaus J, van Swieten JC, Seelaar H, Dopper EG, Onyike CU, Hillis AE, Josephs KA, Boeve BF, Kertesz A, Seeley WW, Rankin KP, Johnson JK, Gorno-Tempini ML, Rosen H, Prioleau-Latham CE, Lee A, Kipps CM, Lillo P, Piguet O, Rohrer JD, Rossor MN, Warren JD, Fox NC, Galasko D, Salmon DP, Black SE, Mesulam M, Weintraub S, Dickerson BC, Diehl-Schmid J, Pasquier F, Deramecourt V, Lebert F, Pijnenburg Y, Chow TW, Manes F, Grafman J, Cappa SF, Freedman M, Grossman M, Miller BL. Sensitivity of revised diagnostic criteria for the behavioural variant of frontotemporal dementia. Brain. 2011;134(Pt 9):2456–77. https://doi.org/10.1093/brain/awr179.
55. Gorno-Tempini ML, Hillis AE, Weintraub S, Kertesz A, Mendez M, Cappa SF, Ogar JM, Rohrer JD, Black S, Boeve BF, Manes F, Dronkers NF, Vandenberghe R, Rascovsky K, Patterson K, Miller BL, Knopman DS, Hodges JR, Mesulam MM, Grossman M. Classification of primary progressive aphasia and its variants. Neurology. 2011;76(11):1006–14. https://doi.org/10.1212/WNL.0b013e31821103e6.
56. Baizabal-Carvallo JF, Jankovic J. Parkinsonism, movement disorders and genetics in frontotemporal dementia. Nat Rev Neurol. 2016;12(3):175–85. https://doi.org/10.1038/nrneurol.2016.14.
57. Pal PK, Wszolek ZK, Kishore A, de la Fuente-Fernandez R, Sossi V, Uitti RJ, Dobko T, Stoessl AJ. Positron emission tomography in pallido-ponto-nigral degeneration (PPND) family (frontotemporal dementia with parkinsonism linked to chromosome 17 and point mutation in tau gene). Parkinsonism Relat Disord. 2001;7(2):81–8. https://doi.org/10.1016/s1353-8020(00)00026-2.

58. Rinne JO, Laine M, Kaasinen V, Norvasuo-Heilä MK, Någren K, Helenius H. Striatal dopamine transporter and extrapyramidal symptoms in frontotemporal dementia. Neurology. 2002;58(10):1489–93. https://doi.org/10.1212/wnl.58.10.1489.
59. Espay AJ, Litvan I. Parkinsonism and frontotemporal dementia: the clinical overlap. J Mol Neurosci. 2011;45(3):343–9. https://doi.org/10.1007/s12031-011-9632-1.
60. Kertesz A, McMonagle P, Jesso S. Extrapyramidal syndromes in frontotemporal degeneration. J Mol Neurosci. 2011;45(3):336–42. https://doi.org/10.1007/s12031-011-9616-1.
61. Park HK, Chung SJ. New perspective on parkinsonism in frontotemporal lobar degeneration. J Mov Disord. 2013;6(1):1–8. https://doi.org/10.14802/jmd.13001.
62. Burrell JR, Kiernan MC, Vucic S, Hodges JR. Motor neuron dysfunction in frontotemporal dementia. Brain. 2011;134(Pt 9):2582–94. https://doi.org/10.1093/brain/awr195.
63. Coon EA, Sorenson EJ, Whitwell JL, Knopman DS, Josephs KA. Predicting survival in frontotemporal dementia with motor neuron disease. Neurology. 2011;76(22):1886–93. https://doi.org/10.1212/WNL.0b013e31821d767b.
64. Coyle-Gilchrist IT, Dick KM, Patterson K, Vázquez Rodríquez P, Wehmann E, Wilcox A, Lansdall CJ, Dawson KE, Wiggins J, Mead S, Brayne C, Rowe JB. Prevalence, characteristics, and survival of frontotemporal lobar degeneration syndromes. Neurology. 2016;86(18):1736–43. https://doi.org/10.1212/WNL.0000000000002638.
65. Irwin DJ, Brettschneider J, McMillan CT, Cooper F, Olm C, Arnold SE, Van Deerlin VM, Seeley WW, Miller BL, Lee EB, Lee VM, Grossman M, Trojanowski JQ. Deep clinical and neuropathological phenotyping of pick disease. Ann Neurol. 2016;79(2):272–87. https://doi.org/10.1002/ana.24559.
66. Rowe JB. Parkinsonism in frontotemporal dementias. Int Rev Neurobiol. 2019;149:249–75. https://doi.org/10.1016/bs.irn.2019.10.012.
67. Ikeda M, Shigenobu K, Fukuhara R, Hokoishi K, Maki N, Nebu A, Komori K, Tanabe H. Efficacy of fluvoxamine as a treatment for behavioral symptoms in frontotemporal lobar degeneration patients. Dement Geriatr Cogn Disord. 2004;17(3):117–21. https://doi.org/10.1159/000076343.
68. Ondo WG. Tetrabenazine treatment for stereotypies and tics associated with dementia. J Neuropsychiatry Clin Neurosci. 2012;24(2):208–14. https://doi.org/10.1176/appi.neuropsych.11030077.
69. Pail M, Matej R, Husarova I, Rektorova I. Generalized myoclonus as a prominent symptom in a patient with FTLD-TDP. J Neurol. 2013;260(6):1681–3. https://doi.org/10.1007/s00415-013-6942-y.
70. Bensimon G, Lacomblez L, Meininger V. A controlled trial of riluzole in amyotrophic lateral sclerosis. ALS/Riluzole Study Group. N Engl J Med. 1994;330(9):585–91. https://doi.org/10.1056/NEJM199403033300901.
71. Tsai RM, Boxer AL. Treatment of frontotemporal dementia. Curr Treat Options Neurol. 2014;16(11):319. https://doi.org/10.1007/s11940-014-0319-0.
72. Janssens AI, Ruytings M, Al-Chalabi A, Chio A, Hardiman O, Mcdermott CJ, et al. A mapping review of international guidance on the management and care of amyotrophic lateral sclerosis (ALS). Amyotroph Lateral Scler Frontotemporal Degener. 2016;17(5–6):325–36. https://doi.org/10.3109/21678421.2016.1167911.
73. Armstrong MJ, Litvan I, Lang AE, Bak TH, Bhatia KP, Borroni B, Boxer AL, Dickson DW, Grossman M, Hallett M, Josephs KA, Kertesz A, Lee SE, Miller BL, Reich SG, Riley DE, Tolosa E, Tröster AI, Vidailhet M, Weiner WJ. Criteria for the diagnosis of corticobasal degeneration. Neurology. 2013;80(5):496–503. https://doi.org/10.1212/WNL.0b013e31827f0fd1.
74. Kovacs GG, Murrell JR, Horvath S, Haraszti L, Majtenyi K, Molnar MJ, Budka H, Ghetti B, Spina S. TARDBP variation associated with frontotemporal dementia, supranuclear gaze palsy, and chorea. Mov Disord. 2009;24(12):1843–7. https://doi.org/10.1002/mds.22697.
75. Hassan A, Whitwell JL, Josephs KA. The corticobasal syndrome-Alzheimer's disease conundrum. Expert Rev Neurother. 2011;11(11):1569–78. https://doi.org/10.1586/ern.11.153.

76. Boeve BF. Links between frontotemporal lobar degeneration, corticobasal degeneration, progressive supranuclear palsy, and amyotrophic lateral sclerosis. Alzheimer Dis Assoc Disord. 2007;21(4):S31–8.
77. Kompoliti K, Goetz CG, Boeve BF, Maraganore DM, Ahlskog JE, Marsden CD, Bhatia KP, Greene PE, Przedborski S, Seal EC, Burns RS, Hauser RA, Gauger LL, Factor SA, Molho ES, Riley DE. Clinical presentation and pharmacological therapy in corticobasal degeneration. Arch Neurol. 1998a;55(7):957–61.
78. Frucht S, Fahn S, Chin S, Dhawan V, Eidelberg D. Levodopa-induced dyskinesias in autopsy-proven cortical-basal ganglionic degeneration. Mov Disord. 2000;15:340–3. https://doi.org/10.1002/1531-8257(200003)15:2<340::aid-mds1025>3.0.co;2-o.
79. Ling H, O'Sullivan SS, Holton JL, Revesz T, Massey LA, Williams DR, Paviour DC, Lees AJ. Does corticobasal degeneration exist? A clinicopathological re-evaluation. Brain. 2010;133(Pt 7):2045–57. https://doi.org/10.1093/brain/awq123.
80. Stamelou M, Alonso-Canovas A, Bhatia KP. Dystonia in corticobasal degeneration: a review of the literature on 404 pathologically proven cases. Mov Disord. 2012;27(6):696–702. https://doi.org/10.1002/mds.24992.
81. Mastrolilli F, Benvenga A, Di Biase L, Giambattistelli F, Trotta L, Salomone G, Quintiliani L, Landi D, Melgari JM, Vernieri F. An unusual cause of dementia: essential diagnostic elements of corticobasal degeneration-a case report and review of the literature. Int J Alzheimers Dis. 2011;2011:536141. https://doi.org/10.4061/2011/536141.
82. Rinne JO, Lee MS, Thompson PD, Marsden CD. Corticobasal degeneration. A clinical study of 36 cases. Brain. 1994;117(Pt 5):1183–96.
83. Kompoliti K, Goetz CG, Litvan I, Jellinger K, Verny M. Pharmacological therapy in progressive supranuclear palsy. Arch Neurol. 1998b;55(8):1099–102.
84. Shih LC, Tarsy D. Deep brain stimulation for the treatment of atypical parkinsonism. Mov Disord. 2007;22(15):2149–55.
85. Grimes DA, Lang AE, Bergeron CB. Dementia as the most common presentation of cortical-basal ganglionic degeneration. Neurology. 1999;53(9):1969–74.
86. Wenning GK, Litvan I, Jankovic J, Granata R, Mangone CA, McKee A, Poewe W, Jellinger K, Ray Chaudhuri K, D'Olhaberriague L, Pearce RK. Natural history and survival of 14 patients with corticobasal degeneration confirmed at postmortem examination. J Neurol Neurosurg Psychiatry. 1998;64(2):184–9.
87. Alexander SK, Rittman T, Xuereb JH, Bak TH, Hodges JR, Rowe JB. Validation of the new consensus criteria for the diagnosis of corticobasal degeneration. J Neurol Neurosurg Psychiatry. 2014;85(8):925–9. https://doi.org/10.1136/jnnp-2013-307035.
88. Capecci M, Pournajaf S, Galafate D, Sale P, Le Pera D, Goffredo M, De Pandis MF, Andrenelli E, Pennacchioni M, Ceravolo MG, Franceschini M. Clinical effects of robot-assisted gait training and treadmill training for Parkinson's disease. A randomized controlled trial. Ann Phys Rehabil Med. 2019;62(5):303–12. https://doi.org/10.1016/j.rehab.2019.06.016.
89. Schenkman M, Moore CG, Kohrt WM, Hall DA, Delitto A, Comella CL, Josbeno DA, Christiansen CL, Berman BD, Kluger BM, Melanson EL, Jain S, Robichaud JA, Poon C, Corcos DM. Effect of high-intensity treadmill exercise on motor symptoms in patients with de novo Parkinson disease: a phase 2 randomized clinical trial. JAMA Neurol. 2018;75(2):219–26. https://doi.org/10.1001/jamaneurol.2017.3517.
90. Kovacs GG. Invited review: neuropathology of tauopathies: principles and practice. Neuropathol Appl Neurobiol. 2015;41(1):3–23. https://doi.org/10.1111/nan.12208.
91. Litvan I, Mangone CA, McKee A, et al. Natural history of progressive supranuclear palsy (Steele-Richardson-Olszewski syndrome) and clinical predictors of survival: a clinicopathological study. J Neurol Neurosurg Psychiatry. 1996;60:615–20.
92. Williams DR, de Silva R, Paviour DC, Pittman A, Watt HC, Kilford L, et al. Characteristics of two distinct clinical phenotypes in pathologically proven progressive supranuclear palsy: Richardson's syndrome and PSP- parkinsonism. Brain. 2005;128(Pt 6):1247–58.

93. Birdi S, Rajput AH, Fenton M, Donat JR, Rozdilsky B, Robinson C, Macaulay R, George D. Progressive supranuclear palsy diagnosis and confounding features: report on 16 autopsied cases. Mov Disord. 2002;17(6):1255–64.
94. Jackson JA, Jankovic J, Ford J. Progressive supranuclear palsy: clinical features and response to treatment in 16 patients. Ann Neurol. 1983;13(3):273–8.
95. Nieforth KA, Golbe LI. Retrospective study of drug response in 87 patients with progressive supranuclear palsy. Clin Neuropharmacol. 1993;16(4):338–46.
96. Stamelou M, Höglinger G. A review of treatment options for progressive supranuclear palsy. CNS Drugs. 2016;30(7):629–36. https://doi.org/10.1007/s40263-016-0347-2.
97. Weiner WJ, Minagar A, Shulman LM. Pramipexole in progressive supranuclear palsy. Neurology. 1999;52(4):873–4.
98. Scelzo E, Lozano AM, Hamani C, Poon YY, Aldakheel A, Zadikoff C, Lang AE, Moro E. Peduncolopontine nucleus stimulation in progressive supranuclear palsy: a randomised trial. J Neurol Neurosurg Psychiatry. 2017;88(7):613–6. https://doi.org/10.1136/jnnp-2016-315192.
99. Lamb R, Rohrer JD, Lees AJ, Morris HR. Progressive supranuclear palsy and corticobasal degeneration: pathophysiology and treatment options. Curr Treat Options Neurol. 2016;18(9):42. https://doi.org/10.1007/s11940-016-0422-5.
100. Clerici I, Ferrazzoli D, Maestri R, Bossio F, Zivi I, Canesi M, Pezzoli G, Frazzitta G. Rehabilitation in progressive supranuclear palsy: effectiveness of two multidisciplinary treatments. PLoS One. 2017;12(2):e0170927. https://doi.org/10.1371/journal.pone.0170927.
101. Slade SC, Finkelstein DI, McGinley JL, Morris ME. Exercise and physical activity for people with progressive supranuclear palsy: a systematic review. Clin Rehabil. 2020;34(1):23–33. https://doi.org/10.1177/0269215519877235.
102. Sadowski B. An optical device for patients with downgaze problems shown in a patient suffering from Steele-Richardson-Olszewski syndrome. Neuro-Ophthalmology. 2000;24(1):311–4. https://doi.org/10.1076/0165-8107(200008)2411-vft311.
103. Bates GP, Dorsey R, Gusella JF, Hayden MR, Kay C, Leavitt BR, Nance M, Ross CA, Scahill RI, Wetzel R, Wild EJ, Tabrizi SJ. Huntington disease. Nat Rev Dis Primers. 2015;1:15005. https://doi.org/10.1038/nrdp.2015.5.
104. The Huntington's Disease Collaborative Research Group. A novel gene containing a trinucleotide repeat that is expanded and unstable on Huntington's disease chromosomes. Cell. 1993;72(6):971–83. https://doi.org/10.1016/0092-8674(93)90585-e.
105. Hogarth P, Kayson E, Kieburtz K, Marder K, Oakes D, Rosas D, Shoulson I, Wexler NS, Young AB, Zhao H. Interrater agreement in the assessment of motor manifestations of Huntington's disease. Mov Disord. 2005;20(3):293–7. https://doi.org/10.1002/mds.20332.
106. Huntington Study Group. Unified Huntington's disease rating scale: reliability and consistency. Mov Disord. 1996;11(2):136–42. https://doi.org/10.1002/mds.870110204.
107. Quarrell OW, Nance MA, Nopoulos P, Paulsen JS, Smith JA, Squitieri F. Managing juvenile Huntington's disease. Neurodegener Dis Manag. 2013;3(3) https://doi.org/10.2217/nmt.13.18.
108. Ross CA, Aylward EH, Wild EJ, Langbehn DR, Long JD, Warner JH, Scahill RI, Leavitt BR, Stout JC, Paulsen JS, Reilmann R, Unschuld PG, Wexler A, Margolis RL, Tabrizi SJ. Huntington disease: natural history, biomarkers and prospects for therapeutics. Nat Rev Neurol. 2014;10(4):204–16. https://doi.org/10.1038/nrneurol.2014.24.
109. Cummings DM, Milnerwood AJ, Dallérac GM, Waights V, Brown JY, Vatsavayai SC, Hirst MC, Murphy KP. Aberrant cortical synaptic plasticity and dopaminergic dysfunction in a mouse model of Huntington's disease. Hum Mol Genet. 2006;15(19):2856–68. https://doi.org/10.1093/hmg/ddl224.
110. Rosenblatt A, Kumar BV, Mo A, Welsh CS, Margolis RL, Ross CA. Age, CAG repeat length, and clinical progression in Huntington's disease. Mov Disord. 2012;27(2):272–6. https://doi.org/10.1002/mds.24024.
111. André VM, Cepeda C, Levine MS. Dopamine and glutamate in Huntington's disease: a balancing act. Version 2. CNS Neurosci Ther. 2010;16(3):163–78. https://doi.org/10.1111/j.1755-5949.2010.00134.x.

112. Blumenstock S, Dudanova I. Cortical and striatal circuits in Huntington's disease. Front Neurosci. 2020;14:82. https://doi.org/10.3389/fnins.2020.00082.
113. Huntington Study Group. Tetrabenazine as antichorea therapy in Huntington disease: a randomized controlled trial. Neurology. 2006;66(3):366–72. https://doi.org/10.1212/01.wnl.0000198586.85250.13.
114. McGarry A, McDermott MP, Kieburtz K, Fung WLA, McCusker E, Peng J, de Blieck EA, Cudkowicz M, Huntington Study Group 2CARE Investigators and Coordinators. Risk factors for suicidality in Huntington disease: an analysis of the 2CARE clinical trial. Neurology. 2019;92(14):e1643–51. https://doi.org/10.1212/WNL.0000000000007244.
115. Schultz JL, Killoran A, Nopoulos PC, Chabal CC, Moser DJ, Kamholz JA. Evaluating depression and suicidality in tetrabenazine users with Huntington disease. Neurology. 2018;91(3):e202–7. https://doi.org/10.1212/WNL.0000000000005817.
116. Claassen DO, Carroll B, De Boer LM, Wu E, Ayyagari R, Gandhi S, Stamler D. Indirect tolerability comparison of Deutetrabenazine and Tetrabenazine for Huntington disease. J Clin Mov Disord. 2017;4:3. https://doi.org/10.1186/s40734-017-0051-5.
117. Huntington Study Group, Frank S, Testa CM, Stamler D, Kayson E, Davis C, Edmondson MC, Kinel S, Leavitt B, Oakes D, O'Neill C, Vaughan C, Goldstein J, Herzog M, Snively V, Whaley J, Wong C, Suter G, Jankovic J, Jimenez-Shahed J, Hunter C, Claassen DO, Roman OC, Sung V, Smith J, Janicki S, Clouse R, Saint- Hilaire M, Hohler A, Turpin D, James RC, Rodriguez R, Rizer K, Anderson KE, Heller H, Carlson A, Criswell S, Racette BA, Revilla FJ, Nucifora F Jr, Margolis RL, Ong M, Mendis T, Mendis N, Singer C, Quesada M, Paulsen JS, Brashers-Krug T, Miller A, Kerr J, Dubinsky RM, Gray C, Factor SA, Sperin E, Molho E, Eglow M, Evans S, Kumar R, Reeves C, Samii A, Chouinard S, Beland M, Scott BL, Hickey PT, Esmail S, Fung WL, Gibbons C, Qi L, Colcher A, Hackmyer C, McGarry A, Klos K, Gudesblatt M, Fafard L, Graffitti L, Schneider DP, Dhall R, Wojcieszek JM, LaFaver K, Duker A, Neefus E, Wilson-Perez H, Shprecher D, Wall P, Blindauer KA, Wheeler L, Boyd JT, Houston E, Farbman ES, Agarwal P, Eberly SW, Watts A, Tariot PN, Feigin A, Evans S, Beck C, Orme C, Edicola J, Christopher E. Effect of Deutetrabenazine on Chorea Among Patients With Huntington Disease: A Randomized Clinical Trial. JAMA. 2016;316(1):40–50. https://doi.org/10.1001/jama.2016.8655.
118. Claassen DO, Philbin M, Carroll B. Deutetrabenazine for tardive dyskinesia and chorea associated with Huntington's disease: a review of clinical trial data. Expert Opin Pharmacother. 2019;20(18):2209–21. https://doi.org/10.1080/14656566.2019.1674281.
119. Coppen EM, Roos RA. Current pharmacological approaches to reduce chorea in Huntington's disease. Drugs. 2017;77(1):29–46. https://doi.org/10.1007/s40265-016-0670-4.
120. Mestre TA, Ferreira JJ. An evidence-based approach in the treatment of Huntington's disease. Parkinsonism Relat Disord. 2012;18(4):316–20. https://doi.org/10.1016/j.parkreldis.2011.10.021.
121. Reilmann R. Pharmacological treatment of chorea in Huntington's disease-good clinical practice versus evidence-based guideline. Mov Disord. 2013;28(8):1030–3. https://doi.org/10.1002/mds.25500.
122. Testa CM, Jankovic J. Huntington disease: a quarter century of progress since the gene discovery. J Neurol Sci. 2019;396:52–68. https://doi.org/10.1016/j.jns.2018.09.022.
123. Brusa L, Versace V, Koch G, Bernardi G, Iani C, Stanzione P, Centonze D. Improvement of choreic movements by 1 Hz repetitive transcranial magnetic stimulation in Huntington's disease patients. Ann Neurol. 2005;58(4):655–6. https://doi.org/10.1002/ana.20613.
124. Groiss SJ, Netz J, Lange HW, Buetefisch CM. Frequency dependent effects of rTMS on motor and cognitive functions in Huntington's disease. Basal Ganglia. 2012;2(1):41–8. https://doi.org/10.1016/j.baga.2011.12.001.
125. Hartmann CJ, Groiss SJ, Vesper J, Schnitzler A, Wojtecki L. Brain stimulation in Huntington's disease. Neurodegener Dis Manag. 2016;6(3):223–36. https://doi.org/10.2217/nmt-2016-0007.
126. Quinn L, Kegelmeyer D, Kloos A, Rao AK, Busse M, Fritz NE. Clinical recommendations to guide physical therapy practice for Huntington disease. Neurology. 2020;94(5):217–28. https://doi.org/10.1212/WNL.0000000000008887.

127. Gilman S, Wenning GK, Low PA, Brooks DJ, Mathias CJ, Trojanowski JQ, Wood NW, Colosimo C, Dürr A, Fowler CJ, Kaufmann H, Klockgether T, Lees A, Poewe W, Quinn N, Revesz T, Robertson D, Sandroni P, Seppi K, Vidailhet M. Second consensus statement on the diagnosis of multiple system atrophy. Neurology. 2008;71(9):670–6. https://doi.org/10.1212/01.wnl.0000324625.00404.15.
128. Jellinger KA. Multiple system atrophy: an oligodendroglioneural synucleinopathy1. J Alzheimers Dis. 2018;62(3):1141–79. https://doi.org/10.3233/JAD-170397.
129. Koga S, Parks A, Uitti RJ, van Gerpen JA, Cheshire WP, Wszolek ZK, Dickson DW. Profile of cognitive impairment and underlying pathology in multiple system atrophy. Mov Disord. 2017;32(3):405–13. https://doi.org/10.1002/mds.26874.
130. Stankovic I, Krismer F, Jesic A, Antonini A, Benke T, Brown RG, Burn DJ, Holton JL, Kaufmann H, Kostic VS, Ling H, Meissner WG, Poewe W, Semnic M, Seppi K, Takeda A, Weintraub D, Wenning GK, Movement Disorders Society MSA (MODIMSA) Study Group. Cognitive impairment in multiple system atrophy: a position statement by the neuropsychology task force of the MDS multiple system atrophy (MODIMSA) study group. Mov Disord. 2014;29(7):857–67. https://doi.org/10.1002/mds.25880.
131. Hughes AJ, Colosimo C, Kleedorfer B, Daniel SE, Lees AJ. The dopaminergic response in multiple system atrophy. J Neurol Neurosurg Psychiatry. 1992;55(11):1009–13.
132. Low PA, Reich SG, Jankovic J, Shults CW, Stern MB, Novak P, Tanner CM, Gilman S, Marshall FJ, Wooten F, Racette B, Chelimsky T, Singer W, Sletten DM, Sandroni P, Mandrekar J. Natural history of multiple system atrophy in the USA: a prospective cohort study. Lancet Neurol. 2015;14(7):710–9. https://doi.org/10.1016/S1474-4422(15)00058-7.
133. Wenning GK, Ben Shlomo Y, Magalhães M, Daniel SE, Quinn NP. Clinical features and natural history of multiple system atrophy. An analysis of 100 cases. Brain. 1994;117(Pt 4):835–45.
134. Wenning GK, Tison F, Ben Shlomo Y, Daniel SE, Quinn NP. Multiple system atrophy: a review of 203 pathologically proven cases. Mov Disord. 1997;12(2):133–47.
135. Wenning GK, Geser F, Krismer F, Seppi K, Duerr S, Boesch S, Köllensperger M, Goebel G, Pfeiffer KP, Barone P, Pellecchia MT, Quinn NP, Koukouni V, Fowler CJ, Schrag A, Mathias CJ, Giladi N, Gurevich T, Dupont E, Ostergaard K, Nilsson CF, Widner H, Oertel W, Eggert KM, Albanese A, del Sorbo F, Tolosa E, Cardozo A, Deuschl G, Hellriegel H, Klockgether T, Dodel R, Sampaio C, Coelho M, Djaldetti R, Melamed E, Gasser T, Kamm C, Meco G, Colosimo C, Rascol O, Meissner WG, Tison F, Poewe W, European Multiple System Atrophy Study Group. The natural history of multiple system atrophy: a prospective European cohort study. Lancet Neurol. 2013;12(3):264–74. https://doi.org/10.1016/S1474-4422(12)70327-7.
136. Wenning GK, Ben-Shlomo Y, Hughes A, Daniel SE, Lees A, Quinn NP. What clinical features are most useful to distinguish definite multiple system atrophy from Parkinson's disease? J Neurol Neurosurg Psychiatry. 2000;68(4):434–40.
137. Köllensperger M, Geser F, Ndayisaba JP, Boesch S, Seppi K, Ostergaard K, Dupont E, Cardozo A, Tolosa E, Abele M, Klockgether T, Yekhlef F, Tison F, Daniels C, Deuschl G, Coelho M, Sampaio C, Bozi M, Quinn N, Schrag A, Mathias CJ, Fowler C, Nilsson CF, Widner H, Schimke N, Oertel W, Del Sorbo F, Albanese A, Pellecchia MT, Barone P, Djaldetti R, Colosimo C, Meco G, Gonzalez-Mandly A, Berciano J, Gurevich T, Giladi N, Galitzky M, Rascol O, Kamm C, Gasser T, Siebert U, Poewe W, Wenning GK, EMSA-SG. Presentation, diagnosis, and management of multiple system atrophy in Europe: final analysis of the European multiple system atrophy registry. Mov Disord. 2010;25(15):2604–12. https://doi.org/10.1002/mds.23192.
138. Klos KJ, Bower JH, Josephs KA, Matsumoto JY, Ahlskog JE. Pathological hypersexuality predominantly linked to adjuvant dopamine agonist therapy in Parkinson's disease and multiple system atrophy. Parkinsonism Relat Disord. 2005;11(6):381–6.
139. Perez-Lloret S, Rascol O. Dopamine receptor agonists for the treatment of early or advanced Parkinson's disease. CNS Drugs. 2010;24(11):941–68. https://doi.org/10.2165/11537810-000000000-00000.

140. Wenning GK, Working Group on Atypical Parkinsonism of the Austrian Parkinson's Society. Placebo-controlled trial of amantadine in multiple-system atrophy. Clin Neuropharmacol. 2005;28(5):225–7.
141. Poewe W, Seppi K, Fitzer-Attas CJ, Wenning GK, Gilman S, Low PA, Giladi N, Barone P, Sampaio C, Eyal E, Rascol O, Rasagiline-for-MSA investigators. Efficacy of rasagiline in patients with the parkinsonian variant of multiple system atrophy: a randomised, placebo-controlled trial. Lancet Neurol. 2015;14(2):145–52. https://doi.org/10.1016/S1474-4422(14)70288-1.
142. Rey MV, Perez-Lloret S, Pavy-Le Traon A, Meissner WG, Tison F, Rascol O. A cross-sectional study on drug use in multiple system atrophy. CNS Drugs. 2014;28(5):483–90. https://doi.org/10.1007/s40263-014-0159-1.
143. Perez-Lloret S, Flabeau O, Fernagut PO, Pavy-Le Traon A, Rey MV, Foubert-Samier A, Tison F, Rascol O, Meissner WG. Current concepts in the treatment of multiple system atrophy. Mov Disord Clin Pract. 2015;2(1):6–16. https://doi.org/10.1002/mdc3.12145.
144. Santens P, Vonck K, De Letter M, Van Driessche K, Sieben A, De Reuck J, Van Roost D, Boon P. Deep brain stimulation of the internal pallidum in multiple system atrophy. Parkinsonism Relat Disord. 2006;12(3):181–3.
145. Tarsy D, Apetauerova D, Ryan P, Norregaard T. Adverse effects of subthalamic nucleus DBS in a patient with multiple system atrophy. Neurology. 2003;61(2):247–9.
146. Landers M, Adams M, Acosta K, Fox A. Challenge-oriented gait and balance training in sporadic olivopontocerebellar atrophy: a case study. J Neurol Phys Ther. 2009;33(3):160–8. https://doi.org/10.1097/NPT.0b013e3181b511f4.
147. Wedge F. The impact of resistance training on balance and functional ability of a patient with multiple system atrophy. J Geriatr Phys Ther. 2008;31(2):79–83.

11 Management of Sleep Disorders in Patients with Dementia

Geert Mayer and Helmut Frohnhofen

Abbreviations

AD	Alzheimer's disease
AHI	Apnoea–hypopnea index
APOE	*Apolipoprotein* E
Aß	Beta amyloid
CI	Confidence interval
CPAP	Continuous positive airway pressure
CSF	Cerebrospinal Fluid
EDS	Excessive daytime sleepiness
EEG	Electroencephalography
EOG	Electrooculography
EMG	Electromyography
FTD	Frontotemporal dementia
LBD	Lewy body disease
MCI	Mild cognitive impairment
MMSE	Mini-Mental State Examination
OR	Odds ratio
OSA	Obstructive sleep apnoea

G. Mayer (✉)
Hephata Klinik, Schwalmstadt, Germany

Department of Neurology, Philipps-Universität Marburg, Marburg, Germany

H. Frohnhofen
Fakultät für Gesundheit, Department Humanmedizin, Universität Witten-Herdecke, Witten, Germany

Klinik für Neurologie, Universitätsklinikum Essen, Essen, Germany

K. S. Frederiksen, G. Waldemar (eds.), *Management of Patients with Dementia*,
https://doi.org/10.1007/978-3-030-77904-7_11

PET	Positron emission tomography
PSG	Polysomnography
RAVLT	Rey Auditory Verbal Learning Test
RBD	Rapid eye movement sleep behaviour disorder
RLS	Restless leg syndrome
RSBSQ	REM Sleep Behavior Disorder Screening Questionnaire
SA	Sleep apnoea
TST	Total sleep time

Introduction

Refreshing and sufficient sleep are a prerequisite for well-being, daytime functioning and cognitive performance at any age. Furthermore, disturbed sleep can lead to a reduction in quality of life, depressed mood and cognitive impairment. Sleep disturbances are common in people who are elderly, suggesting that sleep is affected by ageing itself. Additionally, neurodegeneration causes a breakdown in the neuronal networks that control sleep function. Therefore, disturbed sleep may also be a sequela of dementia. However, epidemiological evidence suggests that the relationship appears to be mutual. Sleep research has shown that sleep disorders may (1) increase the risk of dementia, (2) deteriorate the course of dementia, (3) have symptoms similar to dementia, (4) be an early marker of dementia. It is therefore essential to search for and recognise sleep disorders in patients with dementia, to establish differential diagnoses and initiate treatment for these and other comorbid conditions to positively influence the course of dementia.

These issues are of pivotal importance since sleep disorders are potentially modifiable [1].

Sleep disorders encompass a variety of disorders like insomnia, sleep disordered breathing, restless leg syndrome (RLS), hypersomnia, circadian rhythm disorders and rapid eye movement (REM) sleep behavior disorder (RBD) (Table 11.1). Since treatment differs according to the type of sleep disorder a careful evaluation of sleep is mandatory before any treatment is initiated [2].

The aim of treating sleep disorders is (1) the prevention of cognitive decline and development of dementia in older subjects without dementia and (2) to mitigate sleep-related symptoms and suffering in patients with dementia and their caregivers.

Regulation of Sleep and Wakefulness

Sleep and wakefulness result from an interaction between several nuclei and neuronal networks located in the brain stem, the basal ganglia and the forebrain. Furthermore, various neurotransmitters, molecular and genetic factors, and input from the organism and the environment have an impact on sleep regulation. This complex interaction generates circadian rhythmicity and electrical brain activity that define different stages, like wakefulness, REM sleep and three non-REM sleep

Table 11.1 Classification according to the International Classification of Sleep Disorders and core symptoms of relevant sleep disorders

Classification	Sleep disorder	Core symptoms
Insomnia	Insomnia – Acute – Chronic	Difficulties initiating or maintaining sleep more than 2–3 times per week – Acute <3 months – Chronic >3 months
Sleep-related breathing disorders	Obstructive/central sleep apnoea	Apnoeas and hypopneas caused by partial or complete collapse of the upper airways; in central apnoea there is a lack of respiratory airflow despite open upper airways
Hypersomnias of central origin	Narcolepsy	Excessive daytime sleepiness (>3 months), cataplexy, hypnagogic/hypnopompic hallucinations, sleep paralysis, fragmented night sleep
	Idiopathic hypersomnia	Nocturnal sleep >10 h, excessive daytime sleepiness
	Kleine–Levin syndrome	Episodes of hypersomnia with changes in personality, eating and sometimes sexual behaviour
Circadian sleep-wake rhythm disorders (all >3 months)	Sleep-phase advance syndrome	Advanced sleep times, normal sleep structure
	Sleep-phase delay syndrome	Delayed sleep time, normal sleep structure
	Non-24-h syndrome	Misalignment with the 24-h dark-light cycle
Parasomnias	Non-rapid eye movement parasomnia, sleepwalking, night terror	Emerging from slow-wave sleep, dissociated behaviour, screaming with partial or complete amnesia, inappropriate responsiveness
	Rapid eye movement parasomnias Rapid eye movement sleep behaviour disorder	Complex motor behaviours during rapid eye movement sleep, dream enactment
	Nightmare disorder	Awakening from dysphoric dreams
	Isolated sleep paralysis	Inability to move the complete body upon awakening
Sleep-related movement disorders	Restless leg syndrome	Sensory misperception of the limbs with the urge to move the limbs occurring predominantly at nighttime
Sleep disorders in neurological diseases	Fatal familial insomnia Sleep-related epilepsy Sleep-related headaches	Prion disease, insomnia and complete breakdown of sleep-wake structure Epilepsy at sleep onset, offset or during sleep Headaches at sleep onset, offset or during sleep

stages N1, N2 (light sleep) and N3 (deep slow-wave sleep). More specifically, circadian and homeostatic processes generate the sleep-wake cycle. The nucleus suprachiasmaticus is the central generator of the circadian rhythms that regulate the interactions of the "clock genes" (e.g. PER1/2/3, CRY1/2, BMAL1, CLOCK).

Altered circadian rhythmicity, which depends on behaviour, light exposure, age and genetic disposition, can induce circadian rhythm sleep disorders. The circadian rhythm is best measured by plasma melatonin, cortisol levels and core body temperature over time.

The hypothalamic sleep-wake switch is a widely accepted model that relies on the evidence that sleep-promoting neurons of the ventral lateral preoptic nucleus and wake-promoting neurons in the monoaminergic cell groups inhibit each other. The lateral hypothalamus contains the neuropeptide orexin (synonymous with hypocretin), which projects to almost the entire brain and stabilises this switch. The firing of orexin neurons stimulates awakening and the classic arousal neurons of the brain (histamine, serotonin and noradrenaline neurons).

The pathophysiology of frequently occurring RBD (e.g. in Lewy body disease (LBD)) is not yet fully understood. Intermittent release of glutamate activates non-N-methyl-D-aspartate receptors and excites motoneurons, causing muscle twitches in normal REM sleep. Glutamatergic neurons, especially in the subcoeruleus nucleus, are active during REM sleep and project to the ventromedial medulla and to the spinal cord, whereas gamma aminobutyric acid and glycine neurons inhibit motoneurons leading to REM sleep with atonia. Animal models have shown that lesions in the brainstem nuclei, specifically the subcoeruleus nucleus, cause a REM sleep behavioural phenotype with increased muscle tone and abnormal excessive motor activities, resembling the dream-like behaviours of RBD.

The sleep stages show a regular sequence that starts with light sleep (N1 and N2), followed by deep sleep (N3) and that terminates with REM sleep. This type of sequence is called a sleep cycle, which lasts 60–90 min. The number of sleep cycles is age-dependent and comprises three to five cycles. As the night proceeds, the amount of deep sleep diminishes and the amount of REM sleep increases.

Figure 11.1 contains a hypnogram showing a sequence of nocturnal electrical brain activity or macrostructure of sleep.

Deep sleep (N3) is presumed to be responsible for consolidation of declarative memory, REM sleep for procedural and emotional memory. Animal experiments indicate that information accumulated throughout the day is replayed during the night. Slow-wave oscillation generated in cortical areas coordinates the replay in the hippocampus (sharp wave/ripple activity) and plasticity-promoting spindle activity in the thalamus [3, 4]. The reduction of NREM sleep, especially reduced slow-wave

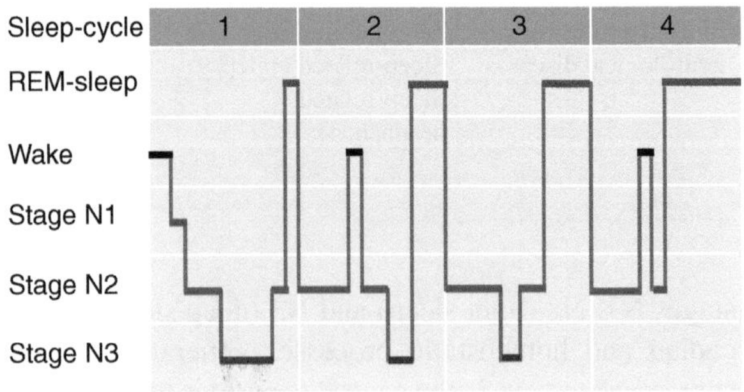

Fig. 11.1 Hypnogram of a healthy adult. (see Appendix Fig. 1). 1–4: quartiles of the time spent in sleep. REM: rapid eye movement; stage N1 and stage N2: light sleep; stage N3: deep sleep

sleep, may cause a decrease in memory consolidation and generate a feedback loop. Memory consolidation occurs normally after 3 h of sleep, but after a complete night of sleep, consolidation is much better. Daytime sleep lasting a few minutes consolidates memories, though 60–90-min naps lead to the best consolidation [4]. Sleep deprivation generally worsens encoding. The shorter the interval between learning and going to sleep, the better the recall.

Sleep Changes and Sleep Disorders in the Elderly

There are two main reasons for altered sleep in the elderly: (1) changes in sleep physiology with age and (2) comorbid conditions.

Changes in Sleep Physiology

In the elderly, the need for sleep in terms of hours needed does not change significantly, whereas the ability to get enough sleep changes. Sleep macrostructure, as presented in a hypnogram, shows a reduction in slow-wave sleep and REM sleep. Latency to slow-wave sleep (N3) and REM sleep is increased, and total sleep time (TST) is reduced. On the other hand, light sleep (N2) and wake after sleep onset are increased [5]. These changes occur mainly between the sixth and seventh decade of life in healthy humans [6]. Meta-analyses examining sleep changes in middle-aged people in their sixties found only small differences between this and younger age groups, i.e. the differences were rather small, insignificant and mainly concerned the circadian distribution [6]. Gender differences are reported, but the findings are conflicting [7].

Common Sleep Disorders in the Elderly

One of the most frequent comorbid sleep disorders is sleep apnoea (SA), mainly of the obstructive type. Obstructive SA (OSA) is characterised by apnoeas and hypopnoeas during sleep. Apnoeas and hypopnoeas lead to intermittent hypoxemia and sleep fragmentation. The apnoea–hypopnoea index (AHI), which indicates the number of apnoea–hypopnoea periods (> 10 s, desaturation >4%) per hour, is used as a measure of the severity of OSA. An AHI < 5/h is considered normal. An AHI of 5–15 events per hour is considered mild SA, an AHI of 15–0 events per hour is considered moderate SA, while severe SA shows 30 or more events per hour. The Sleep Health Heart Study reported clinically relevant AHI of >15 events per hour in 19% of people 60–69 years of age, 21% aged 70–79 and 20% aged 80–89 [8]. Various medications may further aggravated SA, e.g. sedatives and antidepressants. Immobility may destabilise the circadian rhythm and further lead to an increase in body mass index, which worsens SA. Continuous and intermittent hypoxemia and the reduction of slow-wave sleep due to apnoea-related arousals may enhance the process of developing cognitive deficits leading to dementia. Patients with dementia have a high frequency of intermittent nocturnal hypoxemia [9] and a fivefold higher risk for OSA [10].

Patients with RLS have the urge to move their legs during periods of rest, especially in the evening and at night, to relieve uncomfortable or painful sensations in the calves, causing impaired sleep onset. Periodic leg movements during sleep in the majority of patients contribute to sleep disruption and a reduced quality of life. Secondary forms of RLS may be caused by iron deficiency, pregnancy and end-stage renal disease and associated morbidity, such as increased cardiovascular risk. RLS is the most frequent neurological sleep disorder that increases with age (up to 10% of the elderly in North America and Europe). Since patients with dementia are often not able to report symptoms, observable behaviours such as rubbing of legs or feet together, kicking, flexing against surfaces or as if pushing a gas pedal, stretching, crossing and uncrossing the legs or feet, and fidgeting may also be indicative of RLS [11].

A typical disorder of older age, RBD is most commonly seen in α-synucleinopathies like Parkinson disease, multiple system atrophy and LBD [12]. Its conversion rate into neurodegenerative diseases is 6.3% per year [13], but it has no major impact on sleep quality. RBD is characterised by the loss of physiological muscle atonia during REM sleep (REM sleep without atonia). Patients with RBD act out vivid dreams during REM sleep. RBD may be misdiagnosed on clinical interview alone in patients with LBD due to the high rate of nocturnal activity in these patients [2]. With a known prevalence of 76%, RBD should always be suspected in LBD patients. The REM Sleep Behavior Disorder Screening Questionnaire (RSBSQ) provides more evidence for the diagnosis [14], which requires video-polysomnography [15]. Since RBD is an important issue with a high potential for injury of patients and bed partners, and video-polysomnography is not broadly available, treatment for RBD should pragmatically be initiated based on RSBSQ results. RBD usually responds well to clonazepam, but clonazepam belongs to the benzodiazepines, which may worsen cognition and SA [16]. Melatonin is an alternative treatment for RBD without major adverse reactions [17].

People who are elderly frequently suffer from insomnia, which is very frequent in patients with all types of dementia [2]. Depression is a precursor for insomnia and vice versa. Insomnia with sleep maintenance problems in people >75 years without primary cognitive impairment increases the risk of cognitive decline [18].

Pathophysiology of Sleep Disturbances

It has been suggested that several mechanisms in sleep disturbances promote neurodegeneration. These mechanisms constitute increased generation and deposition of beta amyloid (Aβ) and reduced glymphatic clearance of Aβ. In addition, circadian dysfunction, sleep fragmentation, neuro-inflammation and the generation of oxidative stress via reactive oxygen species contribute to synaptic damage and neurodegeneration.

Neuronal damage may cause different sleep disorders, irrespective of the type of damage. This may explain why several types of sleep disorders may occur in the same individual and why the appearance and severity of sleep disorders change as neurodegeneration progresses.

The individual risk of developing dementia is related to several genetic factors, but emerging evidence has shown that lifestyle factors, such as sleep disturbance may also increase an individual's risk [19]. However, despite this appealing hypothesis, many unanswered questions remain. Most of the evidence about the relationship between sleep disturbances, cognitive decline, dementia and neurodegeneration derives from animal experiments, and observational, cross-sectional studies in humans. Importantly, these studies have provided insight into pathophysiological mechanisms linking sleep disorders, neuronal damage and cognitive decline with Aβ accumulation, glymphatic clearance and inflammation being the most recognised mechanisms [20–22].

Neurodegenerative dementia disorders are progressive diseases which may start with subjective cognitive impairment before developing into mild cognitive impairment (MCI) and finally dementia [23]. A study [24] examining the relationship between sleep, cerebrospinal fluid (CSF) tau and Aß, and neuropsychological results of patients with subjective cognitive impairment, MCI, mild Alzheimer's disease (AD) (Mini-Mental State Examination (MMSE) > 21) and severe AD (MMSE < 21) to those of healthy controls using polysomnography in the sleep analysis showed that TST, sleep efficiency, slow-wave sleep (N3) and REM sleep were significantly reduced in mild and severe AD. Mean TST for mild AD was 318.82 ± 44.16 min, in severe AD 252.93 ± 47.77 min and in controls 367.22 ± 60.93 min MMSE and the Rey Auditory Verbal Learning Test (RAVLT) results were significantly lower than in the other groups. A component analysis (Bartlett's test of sphericity), including sleep architecture (REM, N1, N3 and TST), CSF $A\beta_{42}$ levels, MMSE and RAVLT, was highly significant ($p < 0.001$), confirming that sleep fragmentation with reduced REM and N3 sleep is associated with Aβ pathology and with tau neurodegeneration. The changes of sleep structure in patients with subjective cognitive impairment show that these changes may be early markers of dementia [25]. However, sleep may not only be one factor in the neurodegenerative cascade culminating in cognitive decline and dementia, but neurodegeneration and the ensuing dementia itself change sleep, indicating a bidirectional relationship. Furthermore, these studies give proof to the relationship between sleep and cognitive impairment that has been described in recent years [25].

Tau protein and Aß42 in CSF show a circadian rhythm with high levels during daytime and low levels during the night [26]. Sleep fragmentation and the reduction of slow-wave sleep (N3) may cause an accumulation of these proteins via diminished glymphatic clearance during nighttime [21]. With the worsening of sleep structure and accumulation of amyloids, a vicious cycle is initiated that needs to be recognised early to interrupt its progression (Fig. 11.2).

Aggregation of Aβ begins about 20 years prior to onset of AD. Factors that promote progression of amyloid deposition are age, genetic predisposition (apolipoprotein E epsilon 4 (APOE4) and lifestyle (e.g. physical inactivity, diet and sleep).

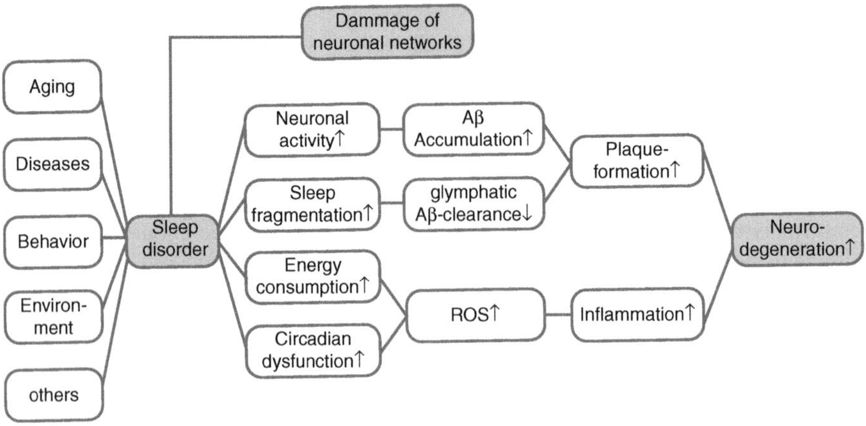

Fig. 11.2 Interaction of sleep and brain protein clearance

Deposition of Aβ starts in the entorhinal cortex and spreads to the hippocampus and the temporal lobe [3]. These structures are important for cognitive and motor functions.

Another major cause for the changes in sleep pattern in the elderly is the dampening of the circadian rhythm. This rhythm is associated with the circadian melatonin expression, which among other external factors (also called zeitgebers) is dependent on exposure to light, specifically the blue light spectrum. The low light exposure that many elderly and people with dementia live under is the result of reduced outdoor activities and low light intensity levels in homes or senior homes. This effect may be further deteriorated by the loss of melanopsin retinal ganglion cells due to amyloid deposition, also in the retina and the optic nerve in AD [27].

Comorbid diseases such as sleep-related breathing disorders and depression may contribute to the development of dementia. Patients with OSA have similar changes in sleep pattern as patients with dementia, e.g. slowing of slow-wave sleep and REM sleep, sleep fragmentation and a reduction in sleep spindles [28]. Furthermore, epidemiological studies in humans identified untreated OSA as an independent risk factor for dementia [29]. Animal studies have shown that intermittent hypoxia—which is a frequent sequela of sleep apnoea—causes an increase of Aß [30]. In a study investigating Aß1–40 and Aß1–42 in patients with severe OSA (AHI => 30/h), moderate OSA (AHI 5–30/h) and controls (AHI < 5/h) Aß1–40 was significantly higher in the severe OSA group (age, sex, obesity, diabetes, hypertension and chronic heart failure were ruled out) and correlated with nocturnal hypoxemia [31]. No group differences were found for Aß1–42. Other studies found increases in Aß1–40 and Aß1–42 [32]. A longitudinal study of 2.52 ± 0.51 years using amyloid positron emission tomography (PET) imaging compared elderly patients with normal cognition, patients with MCI and AD with OSA and without OSA. In cognitively normal people and MCI groups, patients with OSA experienced a faster annual increase in florbetapir (a PET tracer with affinity to amyloid plaques) uptake and decrease in CSF Aβ-42 levels, as well as increases in CSF T-tau and P-tau compared with participants without OSA, indicating faster accumulation of AD pathology. In the AD group no significant changes in biomarkers were observed [33]. OSA-induced pressure changes in the upper airway and the brain may cause a reduced glymphatic clearance [34] of these proteins.

Insomnia and sleep fragmentation are also considered to be associated with an increased risk for AD. This association is bidirectional as AD leads to sleep fragmentation and insomnia. To explore this relationship in detail 615 (36.5%) middle-aged, cognitively unimpaired individuals from the Alzheimer Family Study with insomnia were compared to those with no insomnia [35]. Patients underwent neuropsychological testing, MRI, diffusion weighted imaging, voxel-based morphometry, APOE genotype and the World Health Organisation's World Mental Health Survey Initiative version of the Composite International Diagnostic Interview for the assessment of insomnia. APOE-e4 carriers with insomnia displayed lower grey matter volumes in regions that also affect patients with AD. This finding underpins the importance of insomnia in the development of AD. Diffusion tensor imaging revealed that some white matter tracts were affected.

Furthermore, patients with long-standing insomnia aged 50–65 years had a higher risk of dementia (OR, 5.22; 95% confidence interval (CI), 2.62–10.41) than over 65-year-old patients without insomnia (HR, 2.33; 95% CI, 1.90–2.88). In addition, the use of high dose hypnotics with a long half-life increases risk of dementia [36].

In a population-based Italian study, 86 out of 750 people over 65 years of age were classified as having dementia according to Diagnostic and Statistical Manual IV. Of them, 84.7% reported insomnia, 26.2% snoring and apnoeas, 25.7% nocturnal leg movements and 30.6% excessive daytime sleepiness (EDS). EDS was the only predictive factor for cognitive deterioration [37].

Another sleep questionnaire study with almost 500 patients with early stages of LBD, AD and Parkinson's dementia found insomnias in 29.9%, nocturnal cramps in 24.1%, EDS in 22.6%, RLS in 20.7% and RBD in 18.5% of all patients. Patients with Alzheimer's dementia had less sleep problems than the other forms [38].

In patients >55 years of age with MCI of a mean duration of 5.4 years, 29% developed AD dementia. In people with comorbid affective disorders the risk of developing AD dementia was reduced significantly (odds ratio (OR) 0.35, $p < 0.001$). Symptoms of depression and anxiety showed the same tendency [39].

The cited studies show the relevance of various sleep disorders as comorbid disorders as well as possible predictors for neurodegenerative diseases and dementias in particular.

Figure 11.3 presents putative mechanisms involved in the complex interplay of sleep disorders and neurodegeneration.

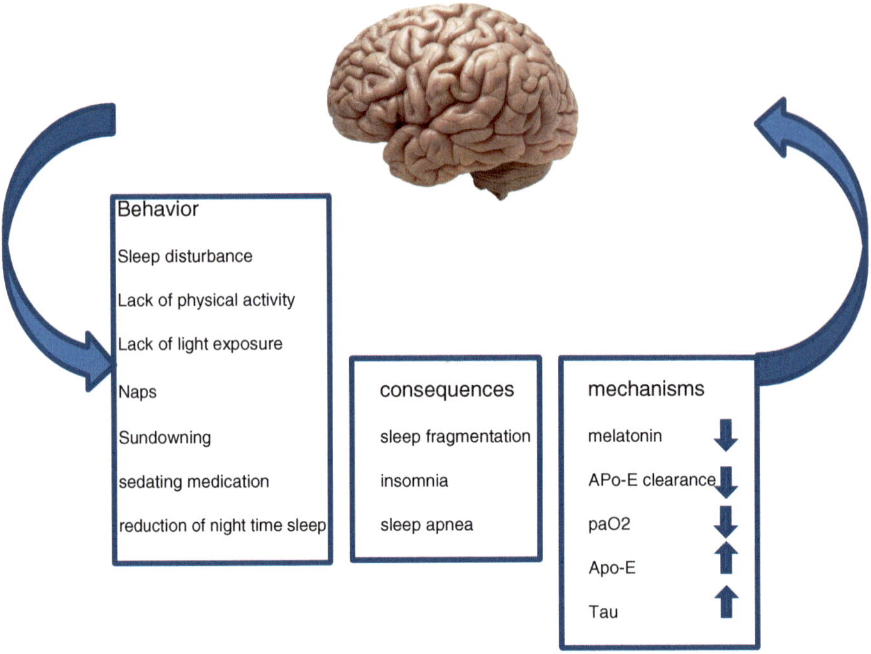

Fig. 11.3 Simplified presentation of putative mechanisms linking sleep disorders and neurodegeneration. *ROS* reactive oxygen species; *Aβ* beta amyloid; ↑: increase; ↓: decrease

Sleep in Patients with Dementia

Sleep and the circadian rhythm are disturbed in most patients with dementia regardless of the subtype of dementia [2]. Furthermore, these disturbances worsen as the disease progresses. Rest activity rhythms may be stable in the early stages of dementia but deteriorate when the disease progresses. Patients with dementia often display fragmentation in their sleep-wake patterns, such that they frequently wake up during the night and frequently fall asleep during the day. In end-stage dementia there is a complete breakdown of sleep wakefulness regulation in which sleep occurs only sporadically across the 24-h day. The cause of this breakdown is a progressive neuropathological change in brain centres involved in sleep regulation [40]. In advanced dementia patients often show little evidence of any rhythmicity.

However, in the early stages of dementia, the prevalence and type of sleep disturbances differ somewhat between subtypes of dementia. Importantly, most patients with dementia usually suffer from a mixture of sleep disorders at the same time.

Sleep Disturbance and Comorbidities in Different Types of Dementia

Alzheimer's Disease (AD)

Sleep disturbances in patients with AD are qualitatively similar to those seen in older persons. However, the severity of the changes is usually greater, and REM sleep has specific alterations. The prevalence of any sleep disorder is estimated to range from 30 to 60% [2]. Sleep is usually more disrupted, with an increasing amount of wakefulness during the night, resulting in shorter TST, reduced sleep efficacy and a lower percentage of slow-wave sleep. Furthermore, characteristics of sleep stage N2, such as k-complexes and spindles become poorly formed with lower amplitude and lower frequencies. These alterations in sleep quality deteriorate as the dementia progresses.

The main change in sleep in AD is the intrusion of wakefulness into sleep time. Furthermore, REM sleep diminishes very early in patients with amyloid deposition and might be a very early biomarker for impending dementia [25]. Other sleep disorders in mild AD patients are sleep disordered breathing (54%), EDS (45%), insomnia (48%), REM sleep behaviour disorder (21%) and RLS (6%) [2]. Since Aβ plaques are also present in the retina and the optic nerve, circadian rhythm may be affected additionally in these patients.

A further important issue in sleep disturbance in patients with AD and other types of dementia is sundowning, which occurs in 2.4–66% of patients with AD [41]. Not all patients with dementia sundown, but nearly all patients with sundowning have dementia [42]. Sundowning is diagnosed clinically. Signs and symptoms of sundowning cover a wide variety of cognitive, affective and behavioural patterns. Furthermore, the abnormalities are usually temporal, with worsening of symptoms in the late evening or in the night. The time course of sundowning allows differentiation from delirium. Although the exact cause of sundowning is unknown so far, both delirium and sundowning seem to share some common risk factors [43]. Unfortunately, there is very little research on sundowning in terms of genesis, prognosis and treatment [44, 45]. Therefore, treatments focused on prevalent clinical signs and symptoms are discussed in more detail elsewhere.

Sleep in Patients with Vascular Dementia

About 80% of patients with mild vascular dementia show any sleep disorder [2]. The most frequent disorder is OSA, with a frequency of more than 70%. OSA causes daytime sleepiness, insomnia, agitation and cognitive and functional impairment. The comorbidities of patients with vascular dementia are insomnia disorder (67%), EDS (58%), REM sleep behaviour disorders (25%) and RLS (5%) [2].

Sleep in Patients with Frontotemporal Dementia

Sleep disorders are present in about 70% of patients with early frontotemporal dementia (FTD). These patients more often show an advancement of the circadian rhythm. Furthermore, sleep disordered breathing (68%), EDS (64%), insomnia (48%) and RLS (8%) are frequent findings [2]. A study with 14 FTD patients confirmed significantly increased sleep duration measured by actigraphy at night and more EDS than the caregivers who served as controls [46]. In addition, a small study compared sleep patterns of patients with FTD, AD and healthy controls with polysomnography [47]. In this study cognitive impairment of patients with AD and FTD was comparable. Also, sleep complaints did not differ between patient groups, but sleep parameters and sleep macrostructure were better preserved in patients with AD.

Sleep in Patients with Lewy Body Dementia

The prevalence of any sleep disorder reaches nearly 90% in patients with LBD. Patients show sleep disordered breathing (76%), EDS (71%), insomnia (67%), REM sleep behaviour disorder (48%) and RLS (0%). According to the revised criteria for the clinical diagnosis of probable and possible LBD [48] sleep disturbance is a core clinical feature in REM sleep behaviour disorder and a supportive feature with hypersomnia.

Assessment of Sleep Disorders in Patients with Dementia

Subjective Measures of Sleep and Wakefulness

Based on current guidelines the management of sleep disorders in patients with and without dementia does not differ in principle [49]. However, cognitive and behavioural symptoms in patients with advanced dementia often require individualised diagnostic and treatment procedures.

The basic diagnostic measure in any patient with presumed sleep disorders is to take a complete history on sleep habits and daytime functioning. Table 11.2 provides a list of relevant questions to ask [49]. Contributing factors should also be assessed, including depression and anxiety, pain, comorbidities that cause awakenings, prescribed medication with an impact on sleep, living and sleep arrangements, degree and frequency of physical activity, including outdoor activity, daytime structure and exposure to light during the day and the night. Of note, in patients with moderate to advanced dementia, a proxy should also always be inquired too, because some patients with dementia may lack insight or may not be able to remember details about their sleeping patterns.

Table 11.3 shows results from pharmacological treatment trials of sleep disorders in patients with dementia.

Table 11.2 Relevant questions when taking a complete history on sleep habits and daytime functioning

Question	Presumed sleep disorder
What time do you normally go to bed at night?	Poor sleep hygiene, circadian rhythm disturbance REM sleep behaviour disorder
What time do you normally wake up in the morning?	Circadian rhythm disturbance, depression
Do you often have trouble falling asleep at night?	Insomnia with difficulties in terms of sleep initiation, depression
About how many times do you wake up in the night?	Insomnia with difficulties in terms of sleep maintenance, nocturia, somatic disorder
If you do wake up during the night, do you usually have trouble falling back asleep?	Insomnia with difficulties in terms of sleep maintenance, depression
Does your bed partner say that you frequently snore, gasp for air or stop breathing?	Sleep disordered breathing, sleep apnoea
Does your bed partner say that you kick or thrash about while asleep?	Parasomnia, restless leg syndrome, REM sleep behaviour disorder
Are you sleepy or tired during much of the day?	Clinical sequelae of a relevant sleep disorder, excessive daytime sleepiness
Do usually take one or more naps during the day?	Clinical sequelae of a relevant sleep disorder, excessive daytime sleepiness
Do you usually doze off without planning to during the day?	Clinical sequelae of a relevant sleep disorder, excessive daytime sleepiness
How much sleep do you need to feel alert and function well?	Subjective sleep need
Are you currently taking any medication or other preparations to help you sleep?	Insomnia, use of hypnotics

Table 11.3 Results from pharmacological treatment trials of sleep disorders in patients with dementia

Drug name	Doses applied in trials	Trial results for disturbed sleep in dementia and comorbid disorders	References
Melatonin	10 mg 2.5 mg slow release	Efficacy for disturbed night sleep and comorbid RBD	[50, 51]
Trazodone	50 mg	Efficacy for disturbed night sleep	[52]
Mirtazapine	15 mg	Not indicated due to lack of effect	[53]
Modafinil	200 mg	Not indicated due to lack of effect and side effects (EDS, apathy, severe side effects)	[54]
Benzodiazepines	Multiple doses	Not indicated due to lack of effect	[55]
Suvorexant	Multiple doses	Not indicated due to lack of effect	[56]

The next step is to document the above-mentioned sleep habits in a sleep diary for about 2 weeks by a proxy. This type of a diary provides pivotal basic information, and it is needed to evaluate changes over time due to therapeutic interventions.

Furthermore, there are many validated retrospective questionnaires available to assess subjective sleep. However, despite the current lack of questionnaire validated in patients with dementia, it appears possible to apply retrospective questionnaires in patients with MCI or with mild dementia. In moderate and severe dementia, the application of observational tools is meaningful.

Scales and questionnaires typically applied to evaluate sleep are the Pittsburgh Sleep Quality Index [57] for the measurement of sleep quality and the Epworth Sleepiness Scale [58] to assess daytime sleepiness. However, despite a lack of validation of these scales in patients with dementia, using them if the dementia is mild appears reasonable [59].

In patients with more advanced dementia, behavioural symptoms often preclude the application of a questionnaire. Of note, a validated and meaningful observational tool to assess daytime sleepiness in older subjects with dementia of any stage is the Epworth Sleepiness Scale [60].

Proxies may report additional sleep disturbances with an obvious impact on daytime function and wakefulness in the night, reflecting also caregiver burden. However, there is no consensus on the best way to measure sleep disturbances in people with dementia.

Objective Measures of Sleep and Wakefulness as Assessed by Polysomnography

Sleep and wake states are usually measured by electroencephalography (EEG), electrooculography and electromyography. The last two measurements allow detection of rapid eye movements and muscle atonia that represent REM sleep. Electrical brain activity is the gold standard of the objective measurement of sleep [61].

Polysomnography (PSG) measures EEG, eye movements, muscle activity, breathing, blood oxygenation, snoring, body position and leg movement. PSG performed in a sleep laboratory is used to confirm the diagnosis of sleep disorders, e.g. sleep-related breathing disorders, parasomnias, sleep-related epileptic seizures and periodic limb movement disorders. In subjects with insomnia and RLS, PSG is not the first-line diagnostic procedure and used only in unclear and complex clinical situations in need of further clarification.

PSG provides a great amount of useful information about sleep, but it is expensive and difficult to obtain. Importantly, it is uncomfortable for the patient and therefore only useful in mildly demented patients [62]. PSG requires analysis and interpretation based on special expertise in sleep medicine.

Actigraphy, a method designed to profile sleep-wake behaviour over days and weeks, is cost effective and much more convenient than full PSG. Actigraphy results correlate highly with PSG data. Actigraphy records movement using a watch-like device worn on the non-dominant hand over a given threshold [62]. An event marker is used to score bedtime, awakenings during the night, getting up time in the morning, daytime sleep and also napping. These data can be used to estimate sleep-wake patterns in all subjects with dementia irrespective of disease severity.

The steering committee of the American Academy of Sleep Medicine recommends the routine use of actigraphy and sleep diaries to assess irregular sleep-wake rhythms in dementia and RLS [63].

Treatment

Non-pharmacological Treatment (Table 11.4)

The treatment of sleep disorders in people with dementia is similar to that in individuals without dementia. However, primary and secondary sleep disorders must be identified before any treatment is initiated.

Non-pharmacological interventions are the first choice of treatment for sleep disorders, also in patients with dementia. However, evidence for this approach is scare since there is a lack of large studies of good quality [64]. But the advantage of a non-pharmacological approach to sleep disorders is that interventions are free of any adverse reactions, which is why they should be applied despite the lack of evidence.

The first step is to search for and to remove personal or environmental factors with a negative impact on sleep. Optimal sleep hygiene (going to bed at regular sleep times, avoiding heavy meals and strong physical activity prior to bedtime, using the bedroom exclusively for sleep) constitutes the basic procedure before any other treatment is initiated. Additionally, regular daily routines, physical activity, bright light exposure and social interactions improve daytime alertness and night-time sleep [65]. For example, a combination of walking and light exposition >4 days/week over 6 months in AD dementia patients improved sleep time measured by actigraphy [66]. A recent meta-analysis considering non-pharmacological interventions in patients with dementia and sleep disorders concluded that multifactorial approaches are most likely to be successful. However, high quality intervention trials and strong evidence for any non-pharmacological intervention are not available. Further studies are warranted. An on-going study called the DISCO trial aims to show if remote online cognitive behavioural therapy for insomnia intervention can improve cognition [67].

Light exposure interventions, which have a definite biological action, are looked upon as a non-invasive, low-cost therapy [50]. However, study results are inconsistent due to the high heterogeneity of the studies [64]. Furthermore, light exposure is applied over a prolonged period of time (typically 30 min or more daily), causing a considerable treatment burden of time, effort and organisation to control adherence. Adherence (to any therapy) has a major impact on health, well-being and quality of life and should not be ignored [68].

Behavioural treatments like cognitive behavioural therapy for insomnia or sleep restriction require sufficient compliance by the patient and therefore may only be applied successfully in people with mild dementia.

Table 11.4 Non-pharmacological treatment for sleep disorders

Sleep hygiene
Daytime activity
Social interaction
Bright light exposure
Cognitive behavioural therapy
Complementary alternative procedures

Treatment of patients with various types of dementia with OSA with continuous positive airway pressure (CPAP) breathing is feasible if dementia is mild, and if patients can tolerate and adhere to the therapy. Effective PAP treatment with different modifications (CPAP, bi-level PAP, automatic PAP) may remove daytime sleepiness and improve physical and cognitive function [59].

Alternative medicine procedures like acupuncture and acupressure, a child-like robot for older women or taking a bath before bedtime were investigated in small studies with small to moderate effectiveness [69]. Double-blind, randomised trials are difficult to perform in patients with dementia and are therefore not available. Nevertheless, non-pharmacological interventions should always be used irrespective of evidence, since individual effectiveness is possible and adverse reactions are nearly absent [70].

Pharmacological Treatment

Pharmacological treatment for sleep disorders must be applied with caution in patients with dementia, who frequently have many co-medications and can tolerate only lower doses due to their age and a general tendency to be more sensitive in terms of drugs affecting the brain. Hypnotics such as benzodiazepines and benzodiazepine receptor inhibitors are contraindicated because they can cause nocturnal falls and delirium. Many antidepressants with sleep-inducing properties have anticholinergic properties and can cause delirium. Only very few evidence-based studies targeting sleep have been performed. Given the importance of sleep in people with dementia the need for such studies is high.

Treatment with melatonin, up to 10 and 2.5 mg slow release has no effect on sleep disorders in AD dementia [52]. In an additional study, melatonin [50] improved sleep onset latency and TST, cognitive and emotional performance and daily sleep-wake cycles. Side effects can be a depressed mood and withdrawal behaviour. In combination with bright light, 2500 Lux reduced the side effects of melatonin.

A meta-analysis on the efficacy of melatonin showed a significant prolongation of TST but sleep efficiency did not improve (McCleery). Of note, the cut-off value to constitute normal sleep efficiency was 85% and may be inappropriate for patients with dementia.

Trazodone 50 mg improves TST and sleep efficiency but does not have an effect on sleep fragmentation and wake after sleep onset [52]. Patients who did not use trazodone had a 2.6-fold faster decline on the MMSE in this 4-year retrospective study. Long-term use of trazodone therefore seems to be promising [71].

A placebo-controlled study using 15 mg mirtazapine at 9 pm for 2 weeks in patients with AD with sleep disturbance as assessed by actigraphy showed no beneficial effects on sleep. Instead patients on mirtazapine were sleepier during daytime than those on placebo. Due to the very low number of patients (mirtazapine (n = 8), placebo (n = 16)) the study's findings should be interpreted with caution [53].

Unfortunately, there is no literature on the impact of cholinesterase inhibitors, which are frequently used for treatment of cognitive decline, on sleep in patients with dementia, but they may cause lucid, disturbing dreams [72]. Dosing in the morning may improve such side effects.

Medications for EDS in patients with dementia have not explicitly been studied. In two studies reporting on apathy in patients with AD, one study had 23 patients with mild to moderate dementia who received 200 mg of modafinil in addition to cholinesterase inhibitors. Modafinil did not improve the activities of daily life or apathy compared to the patients on placebo [54]. In the other study, a 6-week double-blind, placebo-controlled multi-centre randomised trial with 60 patients, 29 received 20 mg methylphenidate and 31 placebo. Apathy scores improved in two out of three efficacy outcomes and showed significant improvement [73].

Modafinil may cause agitation and hallucinations in patients with DLB [74]. In a meta-analysis on the use of benzodiazepines in patients with dementia (i.e. meeting the authors criteria for dementia) 18 out of 657 articles were included. Benzodiazepines were used in 8.5–20% of all patients. Lorazepam was the most frequently used medication (35%). Benzodiazepines were found to cause deterioration in cognition. There was no effect at all on sleep problems [55]. Another issue regarding benzodiazepines is risk of daytime sleepiness, increased risk of falls and a paradoxical reaction in some elderly, leading to agitation, depression and anxiety.

A review by Schroeck et al. [56] on safety and the efficacy of sleep medicines in older adults highlighted suvorexant as a possible therapy with few adverse events and only mild sedation during daytime. However, the results have not been confirmed in patients with dementia.

There are no studies investigating the effect of drugs for the treatment of RBD in patients with dementia. Since melatonin is among the first-line medications for RBD and has little or no side effects, it may be tried [51].

Conclusion

Growing evidence derived from large epidemiological studies suggests that any sleep disturbance in humans is associated with an increased risk for the development of cognitive decline or dementia. The ORs range from 1.3 to 2.5 and vary between the distinct types of sleep disorders.

Further, animal studies yield compelling evidence that deposition of βA, neuroinflammation and reactive oxygen species cause synaptic dysfunction and neurodegeneration. It is tempting to hypothesise that the treatment for sleep disorders in middle-aged people without cognitive impairment may prevent the development of cognitive decline or dementia. However, to prove this hypothesis large prospective randomised controlled trials are needed. However, this type of trial would involve leaving the sleep disorders of many patients untreated. Since effective treatments for sleep disorders are available, such a trial appears to be unethical. Nevertheless, the available evidence warrants vigilance on the part of the clinician to be attentive to possible symptoms and signs of sleep disorders and to treat them with the intention to prevent cognitive decline.

Only few studies have rigorously investigated the occurrence of specific sleep disorders in patients with dementia. However, these studies have shown that sleep disorders are very common in people with dementia and that one or more comorbid sleep disorders in the same patient is more the rule than the exception. Sleep disorders can have detrimental effects on patients with dementia and should be treated.

A careful evaluation should be performed before treatment of sleep disorders is started. Several validated questionnaires for the assessment of sleep disorders are available and should be applied in patients with MCI or mild dementia. In patients with advanced dementia an interview of proxies is required. The use of diagnostic tools like polysomnography, polygraphy and actigraphy should be used in patients with dementia who can cooperate. In most cases, this means that the investigations are limited to patients in the early stages of dementia and in MCI.

The multifactorial aetiology and co-existence of various sleep disorders in people with dementia imply that the use of complex multimodal treatment strategies is required. Non-pharmacological treatments for sleep disorders show no adverse effects in patients with dementia and are first-line treatments (modification of the environment, sleep hygiene, bright light therapy, reduction of time in bed, activation during daytime and education of the caregiver) despite the lack of convincing evidence available. Furthermore, the evidence for pharmacological treatment of sleep disorders in patients with dementia is also very poor since large randomised controlled trials with sufficient duration are scarce. Furthermore, the side effects of this type of pharmacological treatment are common and may be serious, warranting caution.

References

1. Spira AP, Gamaldo AA, An Y, Wu MN, Simonsick EM, Bilgel M, et al. Self-reported sleep and β-amyloid deposition in community-dwelling older adults. JAMA Neurol. 2013;70(12):1537–43. https://doi.org/10.1001/jamaneurol.2013.4258.
2. Guarnieri B, Adorni F, Musicco M, Appollonio I, Bonanni E, Caffarra P, et al. Prevalence of sleep disturbances in mild cognitive impairment and dementing disorders: a multicenter Italian clinical cross-sectional study on 431 patients. Dement Geriatr Cogn Disord. 2012;33(1):50–8. https://doi.org/10.1159/000335363.
3. Braak H, Del Tredici K. Spreading of tau pathology in sporadic Alzheimer's disease along cortico-cortical top-down connections. Cereb Cortex. 2018;28(9):3372–84. https://doi.org/10.1093/cercor/bhy152.
4. Feld GB, Diekelmann S. Sleep smart-optimizing sleep for declarative learning and memory. Front Psychol. 2015;6:622. https://doi.org/10.3389/fpsyg.2015.00622.
5. Neikrug AB, Ancoli-Israel S. Sleep disorders in the older adult—a mini-review. Gerontology. 2010;56(2):181–9. https://doi.org/10.1159/000236900.
6. Ohayon MM. Interactions between sleep normative data and sociocultural characteristics in the elderly. J Psychosom Res. 2004;56(5):479–86. https://doi.org/10.1016/j.psychores.2004.04.365.
7. Ohayon MM. Sleep and the elderly. J Psychosom Res. 2004;56(5):463–4. https://doi.org/10.1016/j.jpsychores.2004.03.001.

8. Young T, Shahar E, Nieto FJ, Redline S, Newman AB, Gottlieb DJ, et al. Predictors of sleep-disordered breathing in community-dwelling adults: the Sleep Heart Health Study. Arch Intern Med. 2002;162(8):893–900. https://doi.org/10.1001/archinte.162.8.893.
9. Frohnhofen H, Roffe C. Intermittent nocturnal hypoxemia in individuals with dementia: prevalence and relationship with functional status. J Am Geriatr Soc. 2012;60(10):1997–9. https://doi.org/10.1111/j.1532-5415.2012.04183.x.
10. Emamian F, Khazaie H, Tahmasian M, Leschziner GD, Morrell MJ, Hsiung G-YR, et al. The association between obstructive sleep apnea and Alzheimer's disease: a meta-analysis perspective. Front Aging Neurosci. 2016;8:78. https://doi.org/10.3389/fnagi.2016.00078.
11. Richards KC, Bost JE, Rogers VE, Hutchison LC, Beck CK, Bliwise DL, et al. Diagnostic accuracy of behavioral, activity, ferritin, and clinical indicators of restless legs syndrome. Sleep. 2015;38(3):371–80. https://doi.org/10.5665/sleep.4492.
12. Boeve BF. REM sleep behavior disorder: updated review of the core features, the REM sleep behavior disorder-neurodegenerative disease association, evolving concepts, controversies, and future directions. Ann N Y Acad Sci. 2010;1184:15–54. https://doi.org/10.1111/j.1749-6632.2009.05115.x.
13. Postuma RB, Iranzo A, Hu M, Högl B, Boeve BF, Manni R, et al. Risk and predictors of dementia and Parkinsonism in idiopathic REM sleep behaviour disorder: a multicentre study. Brain. 2019;142(3):744–59. https://doi.org/10.1093/brain/awz030.
14. Stiasny-Kolster K, Mayer G, Schäfer S, Möller JC, Heinzel-Gutenbrunner M, Oertel WH. The REM sleep behavior disorder screening questionnaire—a new diagnostic instrument. Mov Disord. 2007;22(16):2386–93. https://doi.org/10.1002/mds.21740.
15. Zhang Y, Ren R, Yang L, Sanford LD, Tang X. Polysomnographically measured sleep changes in idiopathic REM sleep behavior disorder: a systematic review and meta-analysis. Sleep Med Rev. 2020;54:101362. https://doi.org/10.1016/j.smrv.2020.101362.
16. McCarter SJ, St Louis EK, Boswell CL, Dueffert LG, Slocumb N, Boeve BF, et al. Factors associated with injury in REM sleep behavior disorder. Sleep Med. 2014;15(11):1332–8. https://doi.org/10.1016/j.sleep.2014.06.002.
17. McGrane IR, Leung JG, St Louis EK, Boeve BF. Melatonin therapy for REM sleep behavior disorder: a critical review of evidence. Sleep Med. 2015;16(1):19–26. https://doi.org/10.1016/j.sleep.2014.09.011.
18. Johar H, Kawan R, Emeny RT, Ladwig K-H. Impaired sleep predicts cognitive decline in old people: findings from the prospective KORA age study. Sleep. 2016;39(1):217–26. https://doi.org/10.5665/sleep.5352.
19. Livingston G, Sommerlad A, Orgeta V, Costafreda SG, Huntley J, Ames D, et al. Dementia prevention, intervention, and care. Lancet. 2017;390(10113):2673–734. https://doi.org/10.1016/S0140-6736(17)31363-6.
20. Mander BA, Winer JR, Jagust WJ, Walker MP. Sleep: a novel mechanistic pathway, biomarker, and treatment target in the pathology of Alzheimer's disease? Trends Neurosci. 2016;39(8):552–66. https://doi.org/10.1016/j.tins.2016.05.002.
21. Xie L, Kang H, Xu Q, Chen MJ, Liao Y, Thiyagarajan M, et al. Sleep drives metabolite clearance from the adult brain. Science. 2013;342(6156):373–7. https://doi.org/10.1126/science.1241224.
22. Yang Q, Wang Y, Feng J, Cao J, Chen B. Intermittent hypoxia from obstructive sleep apnea may cause neuronal impairment and dysfunction in central nervous system: the potential roles played by microglia. Neuropsychiatr Dis Treat. 2013;9:1077–86. https://doi.org/10.2147/NDT.S49868.
23. Molinuevo JL, Rabin LA, Amariglio R, Buckley R, Dubois B, Ellis KA, et al. Implementation of subjective cognitive decline criteria in research studies. Alzheimers Dement. 2017;13(3):296–311. https://doi.org/10.1016/j.jalz.2016.09.012.
24. Liguori C, Placidi F, Izzi F, Spanetta M, Mercuri NB, Di Pucchio A. Sleep dysregulation, memory impairment, and CSF biomarkers during different levels of neurocognitive functioning in Alzheimer's disease course. Alzheimers Res Ther. 2020;12(1):5. https://doi.org/10.1186/s13195-019-0571-3.

25. Mander BA, Winer JR, Walker MP. Sleep and Human Aging. Neuron. 2017;94(1):19–36. https://doi.org/10.1016/j.neuron.2017.02.004.
26. Lucey BP, Fagan AM, Holtzman DM, Morris JC, Bateman RJ. Diurnal oscillation of CSF Aβ and other AD biomarkers. Mol Neurodegener. 2017;12(1):36. https://doi.org/10.1186/s13024-017-0161-4.
27. Feng R, Li L, Yu H, Liu M, Zhao W. Melanopsin retinal ganglion cell loss and circadian dysfunction in Alzheimer's disease (review). Mol Med Rep. 2016;13(4):3397–400. https://doi.org/10.3892/mmr.2016.4966.
28. Polsek D, Gildeh N, Cash D, Winsky-Sommerer R, Williams SCR, Turkheimer F, et al. Obstructive sleep apnoea and Alzheimer's disease: in search of shared pathomechanisms. Neurosci Biobehav Rev. 2018;86:142–9. https://doi.org/10.1016/j.neubiorev.2017.12.004.
29. Liguori C, Maestri M, Spanetta M, Placidi F, Bonanni E, Mercuri NB, Guarnieri B. Sleep-disordered breathing and the risk of Alzheimer's disease. Sleep Med Rev. 2020;55:101375. https://doi.org/10.1016/j.smrv.2020.101375.
30. Sun X, He G, Qing H, Zhou W, Dobie F, Cai F, et al. Hypoxia facilitates Alzheimer's disease pathogenesis by up-regulating BACE1 gene expression. Proc Natl Acad Sci U S A. 2006;103(49):18727–32. https://doi.org/10.1073/pnas.0606298103.
31. Przybylska-Kuć S, Zakrzewski M, Dybała A, Kiciński P, Dzida G, Myśliński W, et al. Obstructive sleep apnea may increase the risk of Alzheimer's disease. PLoS One. 2019;14(9):e0221255. https://doi.org/10.1371/journal.pone.0221255.
32. Sharma RA, Varga AW, Bubu OM, Pirraglia E, Kam K, Parekh A, et al. Obstructive sleep apnea severity affects amyloid burden in cognitively normal elderly. A longitudinal study. Am J Respir Crit Care Med. 2018;197(7):933–43. https://doi.org/10.1164/rccm.201704-0704OC.
33. Bubu OM, Pirraglia E, Andrade AG, Sharma RA, Gimenez-Badia S, Umasabor-Bubu OQ, et al. Obstructive sleep apnea and longitudinal Alzheimer's disease biomarker changes. Sleep. 2019; https://doi.org/10.1093/sleep/zsz048.
34. Ju Y-ES, Finn MB, Sutphen CL, Herries EM, Jerome GM, Ladenson JH, et al. Obstructive sleep apnea decreases central nervous system-derived proteins in the cerebrospinal fluid. Ann Neurol. 2016;80(1):154–9. https://doi.org/10.1002/ana.24672.
35. Grau-Rivera O, Operto G, Falcón C, Sánchez-Benavides G, Cacciaglia R, Brugulat-Serrat A, et al. Association between insomnia and cognitive performance, gray matter volume, and white matter microstructure in cognitively unimpaired adults. Alzheimers Res Ther. 2020;12(1):4. https://doi.org/10.1186/s13195-019-0547-3.
36. Chen P-L, Lee W-J, Sun W-Z, Oyang Y-J, Fuh J-L. Risk of dementia in patients with insomnia and long-term use of hypnotics: a population-based retrospective cohort study. PLoS One. 2012;7(11):e49113. https://doi.org/10.1371/journal.pone.0049113.
37. Merlino G, Piani A, Gigli GL, Cancelli I, Rinaldi A, Baroselli A, et al. Daytime sleepiness is associated with dementia and cognitive decline in older Italian adults: a population-based study. Sleep Med. 2010;11(4):372–7. https://doi.org/10.1016/j.sleep.2009.07.018.
38. Rongve A, Boeve BF, Aarsland D. Frequency and correlates of caregiver-reported sleep disturbances in a sample of persons with early dementia. J Am Geriatr Soc. 2010;58(3):480–6. https://doi.org/10.1111/j.1532-5415.2010.02733.x.
39. Ramakers IH, Visser PJ, Aalten P, Kester A, Joes J, Verhey FR. Affective symptoms as predictors of Alzheimer's disease in subjects with mild cognitive impairment: a 10-year follow-up study. Psychol Med. 2010;40(7):1193–201.
40. van Erum J, van Dam D, de Deyn PP. Sleep and Alzheimer's disease: a pivotal role for the suprachiasmatic nucleus. Sleep Med Rev. 2018;40:17–27. https://doi.org/10.1016/j.smrv.2017.07.005.
41. Devanand DP, Brockington CD, Moody BJ, Brown RP, Mayeux R, Endicott J, Sackeim HA. Behavioral syndromes in Alzheimer's disease. Int Psychogeriatr. 1992;4(Suppl 2):161–84.
42. Duckett S. Managing the sundowning patient. J Rehabil. 1993;1:24–8.
43. Lipowski ZJ. Transient cognitive disorders (delirium, acute confusional states) in the elderly. Am J Psychiatry. 1983;140(11):1426–36. https://doi.org/10.1176/ajp.140.11.1426.

44. Grabowski J. Sun-downing and integration for the advancement of science and therapeutics: the National Institute on substance use disorders (NISUD). Addiction. 2010;105(12):2044–9. https://doi.org/10.1111/j.1360-0443.2010.03071.x.
45. Scarmeas N, Brandt J, Blacker D, Albert M, Hadjigeorgiou G, Dubois B, et al. Disruptive behavior as a predictor in Alzheimer disease. Arch Neurol. 2007;64(12):1755–61. https://doi.org/10.1001/archneur.64.12.1755.
46. Merrilees J, Hubbard E, Mastick J, Miller BL, Dowling GA. Sleep in persons with frontotemporal dementia and their family caregivers. Nurs Res. 2014;63(2):129–36. https://doi.org/10.1097/NNR.0000000000000024.
47. Bonakis A, Economou N-T, Paparrigopoulos T, Bonanni E, Maestri M, Carnicelli L, et al. Sleep in frontotemporal dementia is equally or possibly more disrupted, and at an earlier stage, when compared to sleep in Alzheimer's disease. J Alzheimers Dis. 2014;38(1):85–91. https://doi.org/10.3233/JAD-122014.
48. McKeith IG, Boeve BF, Dickson DW, Halliday G, Taylor J-P, Weintraub D, et al. Diagnosis and management of dementia with Lewy bodies: fourth consensus report of the DLB Consortium. Neurology. 2017;89(1):88–100. https://doi.org/10.1212/WNL.0000000000004058.
49. Bloom HG, Ahmed I, Alessi CA, Ancoli-Israel S, Buysse DJ, Kryger MH, et al. Evidence-based recommendations for the assessment and management of sleep disorders in older persons. J Am Geriatr Soc. 2009;57(5):761–89. https://doi.org/10.1111/j.1532-5415.2009.02220.x.
50. Dowling GA, Burr RL, van Someren EJW, Hubbard EM, Luxenberg JS, Mastick J, Cooper BA. Melatonin and bright-light treatment for rest-activity disruption in institutionalized patients with Alzheimer's disease. J Am Geriatr Soc. 2008;56(2):239–46. https://doi.org/10.1111/j.1532-5415.2007.01543.x.
51. Högl B, Stefani A. REM sleep behavior disorder: update on diagnosis and treatment. Somnologie. 2017;21:1–8.
52. McCleery J, Cohen DA, Sharpley AL. Pharmacotherapies for sleep disturbances in dementia. Cochrane Database Syst Rev. 2016;11:CD009178. https://doi.org/10.1002/14651858.CD009178.pub3.
53. Scoralick FM, Louzada LL, Quintas JL, Naves JOS, Camargos EF, Nóbrega OT. Mirtazapine does not improve sleep disorders in Alzheimer's disease: results from a double-blind, placebo-controlled pilot study. Psychogeriatrics. 2017;17(2):89–96. https://doi.org/10.1111/psyg.12191.
54. Frakey LL, Salloway S, Buelow M, Malloy P. A randomized, double-blind, placebo-controlled trial of modafinil for the treatment of apathy in individuals with mild-to-moderate Alzheimer's disease. J Clin Psychiatry. 2012;73(6):796–801. https://doi.org/10.4088/JCP.10m06708.
55. Defrancesco M, Marksteiner J, Fleischhacker WW, Blasko I. Use of benzodiazepines in Alzheimer's disease: a systematic review of literature. Int J Neuropsychopharmacol. 2015;18(10):pyv055. https://doi.org/10.1093/ijnp/pyv055.
56. Schroeck JL, Ford J, Conway EL, Kurtzhalts KE, Gee ME, Vollmer KA, Mergenhagen KA. Review of safety and efficacy of sleep medicines in older adults. Clin Ther. 2016;38(11):2340–72. https://doi.org/10.1016/j.clinthera.2016.09.010.
57. Buysse DJ, Reynolds CF, Monk TH, Berman SR, Kupfer DJ. The Pittsburgh Sleep Quality Index: a new instrument for psychiatric practice and research. Psychiatry Res. 1989;28(2):193–213. https://doi.org/10.1016/0165-1781(89)90047-4.
58. Johns MW. Daytime sleepiness, snoring, and obstructive sleep apnea. The Epworth Sleepiness Scale. Chest. 1993;103(1):30–6. https://doi.org/10.1378/chest.103.1.30.
59. Chong MS, Ayalon L, Marler M, Loredo JS, Corey-Bloom J, Palmer BW, et al. Continuous positive airway pressure reduces subjective daytime sleepiness in patients with mild to moderate Alzheimer's disease with sleep disordered breathing. J Am Geriatr Soc. 2006;54(5):777–81. https://doi.org/10.1111/j.1532-5415.2006.00694.x.
60. Frohnhofen H, Fulda S, Frohnhofen K, Popp R. Validation of the essener questionnaire of age and sleepiness in the elderly using pupillometry. Adv Exp Med Biol. 2013;755:125–32. https://doi.org/10.1007/978-94-007-4546-9_17.

61. Kushida CA, Chang A, Gadkary C, Guilleminault C, Carrillo O, Dement WC. Comparison of actigraphic, polysomnographic, and subjective assessment of sleep parameters in sleep-disordered patients. Sleep Med. 2001;2(5):389–96. https://doi.org/10.1016/s1389-9457(00)00098-8.
62. Ancoli-Israel S, Cole R, Alessi C, Chambers M, Moorcroft W, Pollak CP. The role of actigraphy in the study of sleep and circadian rhythms. Sleep. 2003;26(3):342–92. https://doi.org/10.1093/sleep/26.3.342.
63. Morgenthaler T, Alessi C, Friedman L, Owens J, Kapur V, Boehlecke B, et al. Practice parameters for the use of actigraphy in the assessment of sleep and sleep disorders: an update for 2007. Sleep. 2007;30(4):519–29. https://doi.org/10.1093/sleep/30.4.519.
64. O'Caoimh R, Mannion H, Sezgin D, O'Donovan MR, Liew A, Molloy DW. Non-pharmacological treatments for sleep disturbance in mild cognitive impairment and dementia: a systematic review and meta-analysis. Maturitas. 2019;127:82–94. https://doi.org/10.1016/j.maturitas.2019.06.007.
65. McCurry SM, Gibbons LE, Logsdon RG, Vitiello MV, Teri L. Nighttime insomnia treatment and education for Alzheimer's disease: a randomized, controlled trial. J Am Geriatr Soc. 2005;53(5):793–802. https://doi.org/10.1111/j.1532-5415.2005.53252.x.
66. McCurry SM, Pike KC, Vitiello MV, Logsdon RG, Larson EB, Teri L. Increasing walking and bright light exposure to improve sleep in community-dwelling persons with Alzheimer's disease: results of a randomized, controlled trial. J Am Geriatr Soc. 2011;59(8):1393–402. https://doi.org/10.1111/j.1532-5415.2011.03519.x.
67. Kyle SD, Hurry M.E., Emsley A, Luik X, Omline K, Spiegelhalder K, et al. Effects of digital cognitive behavioral therapy for insomnia on cognitive function: study protocol for a randomized controlled trial. Trials 2017:18 281.
68. Faulkner SM, Dijk D-J, Drake RJ, Bee PE. Adherence and acceptability of light therapies to improve sleep in intrinsic circadian rhythm sleep disorders and neuropsychiatric illness: a systematic review. Sleep Health. 2020; https://doi.org/10.1016/j.sleh.2020.01.014.
69. Deguchi A, Nakamura S, Yoneyama S, Hamaguchi H, Kawamura Y, Horio S, et al. Improving symptoms of senile dementia by a night-time spa bathing. Arch Gerontol Geriatr. 1999;29(3):267–73. https://doi.org/10.1016/s0167-4943(99)00039-4.
70. Ooms S, Ju Y-E. Treatment of sleep disorders in dementia. Curr Treat Options Neurol. 2016;18(9):40. https://doi.org/10.1007/s11940-016-0424-3.
71. La AL, Walsh CM, Neylan TC, Vossel KA, Yaffe K, Krystal AD, et al. Long-term trazodone use and cognition: a potential therapeutic role for slow-wave sleep enhancers. J Alzheimers Dis. 2019;67(3):911–21. https://doi.org/10.3233/JAD-181145.
72. LaBerge S, LaMarca K, Baird B. Pre-sleep treatment with galantamine stimulates lucid dreaming: a double-blind, placebo-controlled, crossover study. PLoS One. 2018;13(8):e0201246. https://doi.org/10.1371/journal.pone.0201246.
73. Rosenberg PB, Lanctôt KL, Drye LT, Herrmann N, Scherer RW, Bachman DL, et al. Safety and efficacy of methylphenidate for apathy in Alzheimer's disease: a randomized, placebo-controlled trial. J Clin Psychiatry. 2013;74(8):810–6. https://doi.org/10.4088/JCP.12m08099.
74. Prado E, Paholpak P, Ngo M, Porter V, Apostolova LG, Marrocos R, Ringman JM. Agitation and psychosis associated with dementia with Lewy bodies exacerbated by modafinil use. Am J Alzheimers Dis Other Dement. 2012;27(7):468–73. https://doi.org/10.1177/1533317512456450.

Seizures and Epilepsy in Dementia: Diagnosis and Management

12

Laura Mantoan Ritter and Christer Nilsson

List of Abbreviations

AD	Alzheimer's Disease
ADL	Activities of daily life
AED	Antiepileptic drugs
APP	Amyloid-beta precursor protein
CBZ	Carbamazepine
CJD	Creutzfeld-Jakob Disease
CR	Controlled-release
CSF	Cerebrospinal fluid
CT	Computed tomography
DLB	Dementia with Lewy bodies
DMN	Default mode network
EEG	Electroencephalogram
FTD	Frontotemporal dementia
HD	Huntington's Disease
IED	Interictal epileptiform discharges

L. Mantoan Ritter (✉)
Clinical Neurosciences Department, Epilepsy Centre, King's College NHS Foundation Trust, London, UK

Maurice Wohl Clinical Neuroscience Institute, Institute of Psychiatry, Psychology and Neuroscience, King's College London, London, UK
e-mail: laura.mantoan@kcl.ac.uk

C. Nilsson
Department of Neurology, Rehabilitation, Memory Disorders and Geriatrics, Skåne University Hospital, Malmö, Sweden

Department of Clinical Sciences, Clinical Memory Research Unit, Lund University, Lund, Sweden
e-mail: christer.f.nilsson@skane.se

K. S. Frederiksen, G. Waldemar (eds.), *Management of Patients with Dementia*,
https://doi.org/10.1007/978-3-030-77904-7_12

IL	Interleukin
LEV	Levetiracetam
LTG	Lamotrigine
MCI	Mild cognitive impairment
MMSE	Mini-mental state examination
MRI	Magnetic resonance imaging
NCSE	Non-convulsive status epilepticus
PB	Phenobarbital
PDD	Parkinson's disease dementia
PS1	Presenilin 1
PSP	Progressive supranuclear palsy
SE	Status epilepticus

Pathophysiology of Epilepsy in Dementia

A wide range of pathologies can cause dementia, these include vascular, infectious, traumatic, metabolic, and inflammatory causes. For the purposes of this chapter, we will focus on the most common neurodegenerative aetiologies, which is where much of the epidemiological and experimental evidence originates.

A large body of epidemiological studies suggests that late-onset epilepsy is common [1, 2]: ~25% of new onset epilepsy occurs in individuals older than 65 years [3]. After cerebrovascular disease (~50–70% of late-onset epilepsy; [4, 5]) and trauma (~20% [6, 7], dementia and neurodegenerative disorders are the third most common causes of late-onset epilepsy, with 10–20% of cases attributed to these aetiologies [8]. Furthermore, individuals with a recent diagnosis of epilepsy (under 10 years), have an increased relative risk of developing dementia (RR 2.5) and being diagnosed 1 year after epilepsy diagnosis: this risk not thought to be due to cumulative effect of seizures [9, 10]. Conversely, patients with dementia are known to have an increased risk of epilepsy [11]. Patients with Alzheimer's Disease (AD) and those aged >65 years have a tenfold higher risk of epilepsy and seizures [12, 13]. This is also the case in patients with a diagnosis of vascular dementia [14].

Seizures and Dementia Share Common Risk Factors and Pathological Features

An important observation that may explain the common co-occurrence of epilepsy and dementia is that both share common risk factors [15]: these include hypertension, diabetes mellitus, obesity, smoking, and low physical activity levels [16, 17]. Whilst patients with early [18] and late-onset epilepsy have higher burden of cerebrovascular disease [19], it remains unclear if modification of vascular risk factors would reduce seizures (beyond prevention of strokes) and/or mitigate cognitive decline. Interestingly, a recent study in religious groups that refrain from alcohol and tobacco showed reduced incidence of AD but not epilepsy [20]. A further important observation is that epilepsy and AD-type dementia share pathological markers: temporal lobectomy tissue from temporal lobe epilepsy patients harbours increased levels of amyloid-beta precursor protein (APP) [21]. Of note, seizures are particularly prominent in patients with AD due to APP duplication. Temporal lobe epilepsy specimen also showed age accelerated presence of senile amyloid plaques [22], and abnormal hippocampal tau immunohistochemistry [23]. Increased tau was also found in surgical specimens with focal cortical dysplasia lesions [24]. Conversely, hippocampal sclerosis, which is sometimes reported in patients with AD (but also frontotemporal dementia, primary age-related tauopathy, and limbic-predominant age-related TDP-43 encephalopathy) differs regarding pathology and subfield localization in the hippocampus, relative to hippocampal sclerosis seen in temporal lobe epilepsy [25, 26].

It remains to be elucidated, how this variety of risk factors interact, although some pathologies appear to be worse than others for cognition and seizures (e.g. vascular risk factors) [15].

A Bidirectional Relationship: Dementia Increases Risk of Seizures and Seizures Worsen Cognitive Function

More recent evidence suggests that rather than just sharing the same risk factors, the pathophysiology underlying dementia itself increases the risk of seizures, and that frequent seizures worsen cognitive performance, as has been widely studied in patients undergoing epilepsy surgery [27]. Seizures can therefore be interpreted as one manifestation of the pathophysiological process underlying dementia. For example, seizures are common in the prodromal phase of neurodegenerative disease [28]. Cognitive decline may begin several years earlier in individuals with AD who suffer from seizures compared to those who do not [29, 30]. In patients with familial AD, seizures occur in >45% cases [31], suggesting that younger people (50–59 years) with AD are at highest risk of developing seizures, and that therefore disease duration in itself is not crucial for epileptogenesis. In late onset AD, epilepsy may be associated with faster cognitive decline [32], but overall, lack of population based studies and common definitions of dementia used in studies make estimates difficult [33]. Whether epilepsy, especially late-onset epilepsy may lower brain reserve and facilitate manifestation of dementia [15] or if epilepsy in itself produces dementia (e.g. by frequent seizures and subsequent network disruption) remains unclear.

Animal Models of Network Disruption and Epilepsy in Alzheimer's Disease

Much of the preclinical evidence of epileptogenesis and dementia comes from animal models of AD. These are characterized by overexpression of amyloid precursor protein (APP), presenilin 1 (PS1) or both, and therefore mimic familial forms of AD

[34, 35]. Within the same individual, the relative contribution of amyloid beta, APP and its metabolites, and tau, however, remain unclear [35]. Box 12.1 summarizes currently available evidence from experimental data (Box 12.1).

Epileptogenesis in mouse models of AD is different from other experimental models of epilepsy [35]. Firstly, fibrillary amyloid beta appears to act as a trigger for epileptiform activity, disrupting neuronal membranes [36, 37] and the balance of excitation and inhibition across brain networks [38]. Secondly, both endogenous and experimentally mutated tau (in order to increase tau production/reduce clearance) modulates seizure susceptibility and network excitability in a dose-dependent manner [35]. Interestingly, knocking out tau improves deficits in spatial memory and protects mice against excitotoxicity in a human APP (hAPP) mouse model, without effect on amyloid deposition [39].

Recent evidence suggests that amyloid beta initiates neuronal hyperactivation by suppressing glutamate reuptake [40]: Active neurons at baseline are particularly susceptible to excessively increased activity. Further evidence indicates that neuronal hyperactivity increases amyloid beta and tau secretion, thereby establishing a vicious cycle of disease protein secretion and aberrant aggregation [41, 42].

Finally, it is interesting to note that antiepileptic drugs (AED) interfere in the disease process: Levetiracetam and Topiramate reduced amyloid plaques in a double transgenic mouse model of AD (APP23xPS45: overexpressing APP and mutant PS1) and improved spatial memory in the water maze [43]. In the hAPP model, Levetiracetam but no other AEDs reduced abnormal spike activity on electroencephalogram (EEG) and improved memory performance in vivo, whereas, in acute slices, levetiracetam reversed deficits in synaptic transmission restoring long-term potentiation [44].

Box 12.1 Proposed Mechanisms of Epileptogenesis in Alzheimer's Disease

1. Extrasynaptic glutamate spillover due to impaired glial or neuronal glutamate transporters [45, 46]
2. Tau-induced enhancement of presynaptic glutamate release [47].
3. Reduced axonal and dendritic transport of cargoes (e.g. mitochondria) that regulate neuronal excitability [48–50]
4. Altered trafficking and surface expression of postsynaptic α-amino-3-hydroxy-5-methyl-4-isoxazolepropionic acid receptor and *N*-methyl-D aspartate receptors [51, 52]
5. Altered amounts of voltage-gated ion channels in the brain [52–54]
6. Fyn-mediated alterations in *N*-methyl-D aspartate activity [39, 51, 55, 56]
7. Selective impairment of GABAergic interneurons in the hippocampus and parietal cortex [46, 53, 57–60]
8. Shortened dendrites, lowering threshold for action potential generation [61]
9. Impaired cortical input to the reticular thalamic nucleus and subsequent disinhibition of thalamic relay nuclei and their cortical and limbic targets [62]

10. Increases in cholinergic tone before the degeneration of cholinergic pathways [63]
11. Induction of intracellular neuronal expression of ApoE4 in GABA-ergic interneurons and subsequent ApoE4-mediated toxicity through a tau-dependent mechanism, which leads to their dysfunction and eventual death, with resulting network hyperexcitability [64]

Reproduced with amendments and permission from Elsevier [35]

The Role of Interictal Epileptiform Discharges

Whilst it is widely appreciated that recurrent seizures and status epilepticus impact upon cognition regardless of their aetiology [65], more recent findings in animal models and humans suggest that even interictal epileptiform discharges (IED) can affect cognitive function [66, 67]. During the presurgical evaluation of 67 patients, IEDs worsened recall on a memory task even if originating outside the ictal onset zone [68]. These findings suggest that both seizures and IEDs can affect cognition by long-range network disruption. Whether cognitive function is affected if network disruption involves critical areas, has been the subject of recent investigations and the default mode network (DMN) has emerged as a critical ensemble [69]. The default mode network comprises the posterior cingulate cortex, precuneus, lateral parietal, and medial frontal regions with strong links to the hippocampus [70]. Blood oxygen level-dependent signals detected on functional magnetic resonance imaging (MRI) demonstrate that the DMN is active at rest and deactivates during goal-directed behaviour [71]. Greater DMN deactivation and stronger functional connectivity within DMN regions correlate positively with better cognitive performance [15, 72, 73]. Intriguingly, simultaneous functional MRI-EEG studies of temporal lobe epilepsy patients, detected hippocampal hyperactivity during IEDs, as well as decreased resting functional connectivity of the DMN [74–76]. A similar pattern has also emerged in individuals with mild cognitive impairment (MCI) and therefore at risk of developing AD [77, 78]. Furthermore, greater hippocampal hyperactivity and reduced DMN deactivation correlates with greater amyloid deposition even in healthy individuals [79, 80].

In two patients with established AD but no clinical seizures, EEG recordings employing foramen ovale electrodes revealed not only the presence of IEDs but also of silent hippocampal seizure activity [81]. Recording patients with standard EEG overnight increases the yield in detecting IEDs: Vossel et al. demonstrated that ~42% of patients with established AD and no history of seizures had detectable IEDs on overnight Video-EEG [82]. Patients with IEDs did not differ clinically from those without, nor was there any significant differences in brain atrophy, suggesting that the severity of AD is not useful in distinguishing between the two [82].

An important question arising from these investigations is whether excessive hippocampal activity is pathological or represents an early compensatory mechanism. Bakker et al. addressed the hypothesis that suppressing excessive neuronal activity leads to improved cognitive performance: 2 weeks of low dose levetiracetam (LEV 62.5 or 125 mg BD but not 250 mg BD) suppressed aberrant hippocampal dentate gyrus/cornu ammonis 3 blood oxygen level-dependent signal and significantly improved memory performance in early MCI [78]. These results suggest that hippocampal hyperactivity more likely represents abnormal activity, in keeping with similar findings in animal models of AD [83].

Epilepsy in Other Forms of Dementia

The incidence of epilepsy in other forms of neurodegeneration and dementia is higher than in the general population [84]: Epidemiological studies reveal tenfold increased seizure incidence rates in AD and dementia with Lewy bodies (DLB), and sixfold in frontotemporal dementia (FTD) [85]. Myoclonus is also more common in these disorders with an increase in relative myoclonus rates with earlier age at onset of dementia in AD, DLB, and FTD [85]. Seizures may be an important feature in patients with frontotemporal dementia (FTD) with hippocampal sclerosis and FTD and parkinsonism linked to chromosome 17 with a P301S MAPT gene mutation [86]. Patients with progressive supranuclear palsy (PSP) may also be at higher risk of developing seizures [84, 87].

Whilst the pathogenesis of epilepsy in these forms of neurodegeneration is less extensively studied, a transgenic mouse model of FTD with parkinsonism linked to chromosome 17 recapitulates some of the clinical features, including a propensity for spontaneous seizures on EEG [88]. In this model of human mutant tau overexpression, reactive microglia and astrocytes in the hippocampus precede the appearance of neurofibrillary tangles, and epilepsy develops in the absence of Aβ pathology.

Seizures can be a presenting feature of sporadic Creutzfeld-Jakob Disease (CJD), with focal onset seizures, generalized convulsive and non-convulsive status epilepticus (NCSE) all reported, in addition to myoclonic jerks which are a very common feature in CJD. Animal models of CJD demonstrate that loss of the prion protein (nPrP knockout mice) leads to neocortical and hippocampal hyperexcitability and synchronized activity [89], possibly through facilitated *N*-methyl-D aspartate receptor-mediated excitation in the hippocampus. A more recent study in a mouse model expressing a mutated and misfolding prion protein (Tg(CJD) mice) has shown that abnormal hippocampal *N*-methyl-D aspartate-dependent synaptic plasticity and susceptibility to seizures results from a combination of both gain and loss of function of the prion protein [90]. In addition, astrocytic interleukin (IL)-1beta plays an important role in modulating susceptibility to seizures, as treatment with the IL1 antagonist anakinra, reduces seizure susceptibility and normalizes hippocampal neurotransmission, thereby establishing an important link between neurodegeneration and inflammation [90].

Epilepsy may also be feature of Huntington's Disease (HD) [91], with a 30–40% incidence in juvenile HD [92]. Higher number of CAG repeats are correlated with younger age of onset and increased seizure risk [91], although the exact mechanism by which seizures are caused remains unknown. In adult onset HD, incidence of epilepsy is only 1–2% [92], with an adult onset HD phenotype with epilepsy more commonly caused by dentato-rubro-pallido-luysian atrophy.

Opportunities for Translational Research

Past research on the pathophysiology of epilepsy in dementia highlights a number of important areas for future research with immediate translational potential. These include the investigation of whether more aggressive management of vascular risk factors is protective for both development of dementia and epilepsy, and whether antiepileptic drug therapy in AD patients without seizures has beneficial effect on cognitive function. Ongoing trials may yield important information in due course (NCT02002819, NCT01044758). Finally, some of the difficulties in developing good epilepsy and dementia guidelines arise from the heterogeneous data available from clinical trials, e.g. using a multitude of cognitive scales to define cognitive impairment. Large-scale patient registers, harmonized cognitive assessments and multi-centre collaborations [93] will be instrumental in achieving better quality and meaningful data.

Clinical Seizure Semiology and Differential Diagnosis

Seizure Semiology

As new-onset epilepsy in dementia can be considered a structural form of epilepsy, the clinical features of seizures will depend on the anatomical location of seizure onset and whether there is secondary spreading to adjacent regions or both hemispheres. In both AD and FTD, the underlying neurodegenerative pathology can be present in large parts of the brain at an early stage, providing a basis for seizure generation outside the brain regions involved at onset of cognitive symptoms [94]. In AD, seizures usually originate in the medial temporal or frontal lobes [30, 95–97], with corresponding seizure semiology as described below [35]. There is less data on seizure semiology in frontotemporal dementia (FTD), although the distribution of the underlying pathology would suggest that seizures will usually start in the frontal or temporal lobes [85, 98]. In vascular dementia, cortical infarcts commonly cause post-stroke seizures and can be located in different cortical regions. The diagnosis of specific types of dementia does not rest on the presence or type of seizure. In a large retrospective study of almost 2000 patients with AD, DLB, and FTD, seizures lacked distinguishing clinical features, providing no evidence for specific seizure semiology in different types of neurodegenerative dementia [85]. In clinical practice, many patients will present either after generalized tonic-clonic seizures or non-motor seizures with decreased consciousness, which will not allow the clinician to determine in which brain region the seizures started. On the other hand, it is important to be aware of the common types of seizures in dementia, especially in

AD [35]: based mostly on studies in AD, the most common clinical presentation of epilepsy are focal impaired awareness seizures (previously termed complex partial seizures) with or without secondary generalization [35]. Focal onset aware seizures (i.e. without impairment of consciousness, previously called simple partial seizures) are less common [35].

In AD, focal impaired awareness seizures (complex partial seizures) with non-motor onset and can manifest as recurrent, stereotyped attacks of decreased awareness, speech arrest, more pronounced amnesia, déjà vu, unexplained expressions of emotion, or sensory symptoms [35]. Seizures can induce tachycardia, bradycardia, or even asystole requiring pacemaker implantation, possibly due to involvement of insular cortical regions [30]. These attacks reflect epileptic activity in the hippocampus and medial temporal lobes and have similar features as in common temporal lobe epilepsy in patients without dementia. The recognition of these symptoms as possible epileptic seizures will depend on the degree of cognitive impairment, especially amnesia, changes in emotion and, to some degree, decreased verbal fluency are common cognitive features in AD.

While transient changes in consciousness and behaviour will often be a manifestation of epilepsy in persons with normal cognition and recognized as such by both bystanders and clinical professionals, similar symptoms in persons with dementia might go unnoticed or be misinterpreted by carers and clinicians. In addition, cardiac or other causes for transient loss of awareness or alertness are common, especially in certain types of dementia as described below.

Generalized seizures may be more common in DLB [85], but data on this disease is scarce. In a study on Huntington's disease with juvenile onset, generalized tonic-clonic seizures were the most common types of seizures, followed by tonic seizures and seizures with spells of staring [91].

Myoclonus is a common feature in early-onset (<65 years) and atypical forms of AD, as well as in DLB [85]. Whilst myoclonus can be expression of either cortical or subcortical hyperexcitability, in patients with dementia and stereotyped cognitive or behavioural changes, it should prompt an evaluation for possible seizures. Although most seizures will be self-limiting, non-convulsive status epilepticus (NCSE) is not uncommon and can be particularly difficult to both diagnose and treat [4].

Obtaining a Good Seizure History in Dementia Patients: Common Challenges

Reliance on information and observations from caregivers play a central role for reliable information on seizure activity. While generalized seizures will always be noted, partial or nocturnal seizures might go unnoticed. It is important to ask specifically for signs of fluctuating cognition or consciousness, speech arrest, staring, motor automatisms, and if these episodes are followed by unusual tiredness. However, all these signs could have other causes than epilepsy as is further detailed below and in Table 12.1.

Table 12.1 Differential diagnoses of seizures in dementia

Diagnosis	Clinical features	Useful investigations
Epilepsy (seizures)	*Duration*: Short (seconds-minutes; longer in Todd's paresis[a]) *Characteristics*: Acute onset, recurring, stereotypical, unprovoked *Symptoms*: Episodes of confusion or behavioural change, loss or impairment of consciousness, involuntary movements or sensory disturbances in a body part, visual disturbances, agitation, anxiety, recurrent episodes of sleep disturbances (motor, vocal), frequent falls which the patient does not remember afterwards	EEG
Epilepsy (NCSE)[b]	*Duration*: Medium-long (hours-weeks) *Characteristics*: Acute or gradual onset, fluctuating symptoms *Symptoms*: Change in cognition and behaviour, varying degrees of impaired consciousness	EEG
Transient global amnesia (TGA)	*Duration*: Medium (hours, <24 h) *Characteristics*: Acute onset, isolated amnesia, often provoked by mental or physical stress *Symptoms*: Isolated anterograde and varying degrees of retrograde amnesia	
Cardiac arrhythmia	*Duration*: Brief to short (seconds-minutes) *Characteristics*: Acute onset, recurring, provoked, or unprovoked *Symptoms*: Syncope, dizziness, feeling faint, shortness of breath	ECG Holter-ECG
Postural hypotension	*Duration*: Short to medium (depending on severity) *Characteristics*: Positional, always in a standing position (in very severe cases also while sitting) *Symptoms*: Syncope, dizziness, feeling faint, confusion, cognitive worsening, leg weakness	Orthostatic BP or tilt testing
Transient ischemic attacks (TIA)	*Duration*: Short to medium (minutes-hours, <24 h) *Characteristics*: Acute onset, single to multiple episodes, varying severity and symptoms *Symptoms*: Mostly preserved consciousness, manifestations vary (motor, sensory, speech etc.)	CT/MRI
Stroke	*Duration*: Long (days-months) *Characteristics*: Acute onset, duration >24 h *Symptoms*: Manifestations vary (motor, sensory, speech, visual, brain stem etc.)	CT/MRI
Migraine aura	*Duration*: Medium (hours up to 1–2 days) *Characteristics*: Gradual onset (minutes), first attack onset <50 years *Symptoms*: Visual, motor, sensory (headache phase can become less prominent with ageing)	
Delirium	*Duration*: Long (days-weeks) *Characteristics*: Gradual onset, often provoked by infection, metabolic or environmental factors *Symptoms*: Cognitive or behavioural change, impaired attention, perception, and consciousness, Hallucinations	Blood tests EEG Lumbar puncture

(continued)

Table 12.1 (continued)

Diagnosis	Clinical features	Useful investigations
Psychosis	*Duration*: Long (weeks-months) *Characteristics*: Gradual onset, often permanent part of pre-existing condition (psychiatric illness or dementia), varying degrees of severity *Symptoms*: hallucinations, delusions, agitation, anxiety	
Fluctuations in dementia	*Duration*: Short to medium (minutes-hours) *Characteristics*: Acute or gradual onset, fluctuating condition *Symptoms*: worsening of cognitive problems, impaired attention and speech, normal muscle tone	EEG
Metabolic disturbance[c]	*Duration*: Short to long depending on condition *Characteristics*: Sudden or gradual onset depending on condition *Symptoms*: Feeling faint or dizzy, syncope (in hypoglycaemia), worsening of cognitive problems	Blood tests
Paroxysmal movement disorders[d]	*Duration*: Short to medium depending on condition *Characteristics*: Focal, stereotypical, varying in severity, duration, and distribution *Symptoms*: Brief (myoclonus) or fluctuating motor symptoms (tremor, dyskinesia, dystonia)	
Intoxication[e]	*Duration*: Medium to long (days-weeks) *Characteristics*: Attacks occur, but mostly fluctuating change in general condition *Symptoms*: Variable, attacks occur, but usually fluctuating change in cognition, behaviour, attention, consciousness	Blood and urine tests
Sleep disorder[f]	*Duration*: Brief (seconds) to short (minutes) *Characteristics*: Recurring, nocturnal *Symptoms*: Complex movements and speech in sleep (REM-sleep behaviour disorder; RBD) or twitching focal leg movements (Periodic leg movements in sleep; PLS)	Polysomnography Video-EEG

[a]Todd's paresis is a transient paresis during the post-ictal phase after an epileptic seizure, not caused by ischaemia
[b]Non-convulsive status epilepticus
[c]Hypoglycaemia, hyperglycaemia, electrolyte disturbance
[d]Tremor, myoclonus, dyskinesia, dystonia
[e]Drugs or toxins
[f]REM-sleep behaviour disorder (RBD), Paroxysmal leg-movements in sleep (PLS)

Persons with dementia might have varying degrees of language impairment or lack of insight. In these cases, it might be even more difficult for the patient and carers to recognize changes in awareness, speech and behaviour, and consultation due to possible seizure activity will not be sought unless in cases of partial motor seizures, loss of consciousness, and generalized tonic-clonic seizures. In progressive supranuclear palsy (PSP), verbal fluency can be severely impaired, with periods of speech arrest that can be misunderstood as partial seizures. In the presence of other clinical features of PSP such as postural problems with falls, vertical gaze palsy, and general psychomotor slowing, episodes of speech arrest should be seen as a cognitive symptom and not a manifestation of epilepsy.

Persons with dementia with Lewy bodies (DLB), Parkinson's disease dementia (PDD), and vascular dementia, often have pronounced subcortical dysfunction which often leads to fluctuations in cognition, awareness, and even consciousness that can last from a few minutes to almost an hour. Muscle tone is often preserved, and the patient can remain in a sitting position but is unable to respond to the environment. These manifestations of decreased cortical activation are difficult to distinguish from epileptic seizures and a common reason for misdiagnosis of epilepsy in these types of dementia. The key to diagnosis is the presence of a subcortical type of dementia, concomitant fluctuations in cognition often lasting several hours and the absence of other suspected epileptic features, such as motor manifestations.

Differential Diagnosis

Diagnosing epilepsy in dementia can be challenging due to many factors. Patients are often elderly, have single or multiple comorbidities, including cardiovascular disease, polypharmacy, and the inherent cognitive impairment, which makes it more difficult to distinguish changes in cognition and behaviour. Possible differential diagnoses are summarized in Table 12.1. In general, and irrespective of age or underlying conditions, epileptic seizures tend to be brief in duration (minutes), stereotypical, recurring, and not dependent on situation or body position. The most important differential diagnoses to identify or exclude are cardiac arrhythmias, postural hypotension, stroke or transient ischemic attacks, and delirium. After a generalized seizure, patients with dementia can have a prolonged post-ictal phase lasting from a few days up to 2 weeks [99, 100]. On the other hand, NCSE can present as delirium which can be misinterpreted as worsening of cognitive decline inherent to a progressive dementia disorder. Stroke can present with focal symptoms from an area of cerebral ischaemia, which at the same time can provoke an epileptic seizure (acute symptomatic seizure [101]). An epileptic seizure can result in a Todd's paresis, which in dementia may be prolonged and can mimic a stroke. The coexistence of neurodegenerative and ischemic pathology in mixed AD and vascular dementia increases the risk of epilepsy and further complicates the differential diagnosis and treatment of the different conditions.

Status Epilepticus in Patients with Dementia

Although most seizures in patients with dementia are self-limiting, some seizures may continue unabated, and are then considered a separate entity, status epilepticus (SE). SE is a condition "resulting either from the failure of the mechanisms responsible for seizure termination or from the initiation of mechanisms which lead to abnormally prolonged seizures. It is a condition that can have long-term consequences, including neuronal death, neuronal injury, and alteration of neuronal networks, depending on the type and duration of seizures" [102]. While convulsive SE is clinically apparent and a medical emergency which requires immediate and rapidly escalating therapeutic interventions, non-convulsive status epilepticus (NCSE) can be challenging to diagnose, as it might manifest only as delirium or a slightly decreased level of awareness or consciousness [103], and its diagnosis relies on EEG criteria [104, 105]. The incidence of non-convulsive status epilepticus increases with age [103]. Up to 16% of persons older than 60 years that present in the emergency department with confusion or an altered mental state were found to have NCSE [106] and it is of great importance to perform an EEG early in the diagnostic process, to determine whether NCSE is present. Treatment can be very difficult for both convulsive and non-convulsive status, as patients often are old and frail, and may not tolerate higher doses of AEDs, sedatives, or anaesthesia. EEG is also helpful to identify if SE has been successfully treated. Admission to an intensive or an intermediate care unit (preferably with the possibility of continuous or repeated EEG monitoring) may become necessary if SE is not controlled with first- or second-line agents. In younger persons, NCSE frequently results as an exacerbation from the patient's pre-existing underlying epilepsy and has a better prognosis [107]. In contrast, in older people with NCSE prognosis is much worse, with significant morbidity and a mortality of up to 50% [103, 106].

Making a Diagnosis

As discussed in section "Clinical Seizure Semiology and Differential Diagnosis", the diagnosis of epilepsy in patients with dementia can be challenging and may be delayed, particularly in the elderly population: in a subgroup analysis of the Veterans Affairs Cooperative Study of seizures in people >60 years old, the time to correct diagnosis was significantly delayed, with a mean of 2.3 years [108]. Whilst there is no evidence base to guide which investigations to adopt in patients with dementia and possible seizures, the following pragmatic approach appears sensible, by extrapolating from research in younger people and elderly patients without dementia [109]: We recommend routinely enquiring about seizure markers at each clinic appointment and to teach carers to detect and document possible ictal features. After careful history taking in the presence of a caregiver, preferably a person who has regular contact with the patient and who observed the suspected seizure (section "Clinical Seizure Semiology and Differential Diagnosis"), a thorough clinical examination should establish if there is residual focal neurological involvement, evidence of cardiac disease (e.g. a heart murmur, an arrhythmia) or additional clues as to the underlying diagnosis (e.g. a rash, liver stigmata) and potential risk of seizure recurrence (e.g. signs of meningism or raised intracranial pressure). Further, routine baseline observations, such as heart rate, blood pressure, and temperature should be part of the clinical assessment. History and clinical examinations are aimed at establishing an aetiological diagnosis but also, importantly, at excluding causes for acute symptomatic seizures (acute brain and metabolic precipitants). With this in mind, whilst there is no evidence supporting extensive laboratory tests in patients who have fully recovered, a basic set of investigations is recommended [109–111] to rule out easily treatable precipitants. These include serum glucose, electrolytes (Na, K, Ca), and urea, as well as a routine screen including baseline markers of renal and liver function and a septic screen including a full blood count and C-reactive protein. A 12-lead electrocardiogram should always be performed to rule out cardiac arrhythmias or any abnormalities precluding the use of certain anticonvulsants.

Recommended Investigations

Acute Setting

Residual focal neurology should prompt urgent brain imaging: Computed tomography (CT) is the preferred imaging modality, as it is easily available, rapid, detects bony abnormalities (e.g. fractures), and identifies blood earlier than MRI. A lumbar puncture should be considered in the acute setting, if the differential diagnosis includes infection, subarachnoid haemorrhage, or malignancy [112].

Outpatient Setting

A patient with dementia who has fully recovered from a seizure, and where acute precipitants have been excluded, should be referred to an appropriate outpatient setting with expertise in epilepsy within an acceptable time frame (2–4 weeks depending on national guidelines [110, 113]).

Whilst the diagnosis of epilepsy is predominantly clinical, the following investigations may help ruling out non-epileptic and dangerous causes of transient loss of consciousness, if suggested by the clinical history: carotid and basilar artery ultrasonography, orthostatic blood pressure measurement, and Holter monitoring of the electrocardiogram. A useful aid for the clinician may also be a video capture of the event, e.g. on a mobile phone, and family and carers should be encouraged to video the suspected seizure, providing the patient's safety is maintained. However, despite extensive investigations, often the diagnosis will be uncertain, unless a typical event is recorded with simultaneous EEG and electrocardiogram monitoring.

Imaging

MRI of the brain is the imaging modality of choice in epilepsy, as it demonstrates higher sensitivity than CT [114] and is particularly important in patients with refractory focal onset seizures. Despite the lack of prospective data on the diagnostic yield of imaging in the population with dementia and seizures, it should be recommended in any new-onset epilepsy patient regardless of age, to rule out hippocampal sclerosis, tumours, or dual pathology [115].

Despite these recommendations, a few points relevant to clinical practice are worth discussing: Firstly, many patients with dementia may already have undergone a recent MRI in the work-up for dementia. Secondly, a typical epilepsy protocol

MRI takes 15–20 min to acquire: the requirement to lie immobile for such an extended length of time in a noisy environment may be unattainable for some patients, especially in more advanced stages of disease. Finally, MRI may not be ubiquitously available and may be expensive. In such cases, we feel CT imaging may be a viable option to exclude new or acute causes of seizures, keeping MRI (possibly with general anaesthesia or sedation) as an option only if there is a pressing clinical need.

Electroencephalography

To correctly determine the value of electroencephalography in evaluating a patient with dementia and suspected seizures, the following important points need to be highlighted: Firstly, interictal routine scalp EEG (i.e. 20–30 min) recordings greatly underestimate subclinical hyperexcitability in AD: in patients with episodic confusion, a fluctuating course or a seizure-like event, a normal EEG does not exclude epilepsy or subclinical seizures [81]. Secondly, subclinical seizures and spikes are activated in sleep [81]. In a study of 33 patients with AD and no seizures, subclinical epileptiform activity was detected in 42.4% of AD patients on overnight video telemetry [82]: AD patients with epileptiform activity did not differ clinically from those without such activity but showed faster rates of cognitive decline. Whilst subclinical seizures and spikes can cause significant cognitive impairments [67, 116], it is currently unknown whether treatment of interictal epileptiform discharges improves cognitive function in patients with dementia or mild cognitive impairment and is the subject of ongoing clinical trials (see Sect. "The Role of Interictal Epileptiform Discharges").

Finally, misdiagnosis of "benign" EEG patterns (e.g. wicket spikes, *hypnagogic* hypersynchronicity, hyperventilation induced slowing) is common when EEGs are interpreted by physicians without specialized training [117, 118]. In addition, non-specific patterns are commonly seen in the elderly, making a distinction between "normal" and "abnormal" even more challenging [119].

In conclusion, the "gold-standard" investigation in problematic cases is to capture a typical event on video-EEG. Whilst this may not be ubiquitously feasible, available or indicated, the EEG evaluation in the population with dementia should at minimum include sleep [35] and be reported by a certified electroencephalographer, especially in difficult cases.

Diagnosing Non-convulsive Status Epilepticus

As discussed in section "Clinical Seizure Semiology and Differential Diagnosis", a diagnosis of non-vascular dementia is an independent risk factor for status epilepticus [120]. Diagnosing non-convulsive status epilepticus (NCSE) can be particularly challenging in the elderly population, and even more so in patients with dementia. Diagnosing non-convulsive status is difficult, but whilst there are now consensus electrographic criteria [121], there are no defining clinical parameters. Elderly patients may simply present with confusion of unknown origin or delirium [122–124], although acute onset (i.e. within 24 h) and lack of clinical response to simple commands were reported to be associated with NCSE rather than an alternative diagnosis [122]. Prion Disease Dementia has been reported to be associated with NCSE [125–127] and generalized status epilepticus [128, 129].

In conclusion, whilst NCSE should be considered in all elderly patients when sudden and transient cognitive fluctuations appear [130], diagnosing NCSE in dementia patients, who frequently have cognitive fluctuations at baseline, remains challenging. A low index of suspicion remains key: quick progression of cognitive deterioration or subtle ictal features (minor twitching of the face or limbs, nystagmoid eye movements) should be screened for and Video-EEG monitoring instituted as the best and probably only modality helping to make a diagnosis.

Management Approaches

General Principles of Epilepsy Management in Dementia

The general principles for management of epilepsy in persons with dementia are not different from other patient groups. However, there are many factors to take into consideration in new-onset epilepsy in the elderly population, which are especially important in persons with cognitive impairment and dementia. The ageing brain, in combination with coexisting focal lesions or regional neurodegeneration found in dementia, is especially sensitive to both the effects of seizures and the pharmaceutical treatments given to prevent further seizures. In addition, elderly patients, commonly suffer from comorbidities affecting their general physical condition, including balance, gait, and muscle strength, which will further increase the risk of falls and fractures in connection with seizures. Falls may also be related to adverse events from antiepileptic drugs (AED). Medication taken to treat medical comorbidities, also increases the risk for interactions with AEDs. Other considerations to take into account include the consequences of the cognitive problems (e.g. strategies to remember to take medication) and different psychosocial factors (e.g. education of carers, safety of accommodation) involved in dementia.

When a diagnosis of epilepsy is made in a person with dementia there are several issues that have to be addressed. Due to the patient's cognitive impairment, information about the diagnosis and its consequences should be given both orally and in writing, not only to the patient, but also to family and other caregivers. It is important to educate caregivers on signs that can indicate seizures, in which circumstances emergency medication should be given (if relevant) and when it is important to seek medical advice or call an ambulance. Contact information to a specialist service should be available, especially if the patient is living at home. Rapid follow-up should be arranged, either at a clinic or by phone, to ensure that the information given has been understood, to check whether there are repeated seizures and, if treatment with AEDs has been started, ensure that there is no worsening of cognitive function or the general condition due to adverse effects, see further below.

As with all cases of newly diagnosed epilepsy, treatment with an AED should be started if there are frequent generalized tonic-clonic seizures (especially nocturnal, as this increases the risk of sudden unexpected death in epilepsy [131]). Further, treatment should be commenced if there is a risk for recurrent seizures that might increase the risk for falls or other traumatic events, accentuate the cognitive impairment, or lead to behavioral disturbances that could be negative to the patient or caregivers. However, these risks have to be balanced against the risk of side effects from the treatment, which is especially common in cognitively impaired patients and might lead to poor compliance to treatment. While the primary goal of treating epilepsy in a cognitively healthy and independent person will always be to achieve seizure freedom, this goal has to be modified in persons with dementia and one should always take into consideration the risk of decreasing the quality of life when treating with an AED. In a person with moderate-to-severe dementia with occasional focal seizures that do not lead to falls, severe behavioural changes, or other potentially dangerous situations, active treatment can be postponed. On the other hand, it is important to inform patients and caregivers that if treatment with an AED is initiated, seizure freedom on low or moderate doses of AEDs can often be achieved. In the elderly, seizure freedom of 60–90% with treatment has been reported [132]. There is also some evidence that treatment with an AED can improve cognitive function in some patients [35, 133]. This could be due to a decrease in interictal seizure activity or a direct positive effect on hippocampal function as demonstrated with low doses of levetiracetam in one study in patients with mild cognitive impairment [134]. Drug treatment, including choice of AED, is discussed in more detail below.

Due to their cognitive problems, patients with dementia often find it difficult to self-report seizures, recognize and express the nature of adverse events, and remember to take their medication. Arrangements should be made both for supervision of the patient's general condition, signs of new seizures and to ensure that prescribed medications are taken. The latter can be facilitated by using drug dispensers or supervision of drug intake. A driving ban due to epilepsy is seldom an issue in patients with an established dementia diagnosis but might need to be addressed in patients with mild cognitive impairment and seizures. Both patients and caregivers should be given practical and psychological support to handle other psychosocial aspects of newly diagnosed epilepsy in dementia: Issues include anxiety both for the patient and for the caregiver, due to fear of new seizures and possible side effects of AEDs, social isolation, stigma and uncertainty concerning the diagnosis and its practical aspects for daily life. Some of these issues might have a greater impact on the caregiver's situation and general well-being than on the person with dementia and epilepsy. Clear written information and contact details to a specialist service will decrease worry and increase confidence in those affected.

General Aspects of Drug Treatment

After deciding to treat a person with epilepsy in dementia with an AED, there are a number of factors to consider. While drug absorption, protein binding, and hepatic clearance are not substantially affected by normal ageing [4], this is often the case

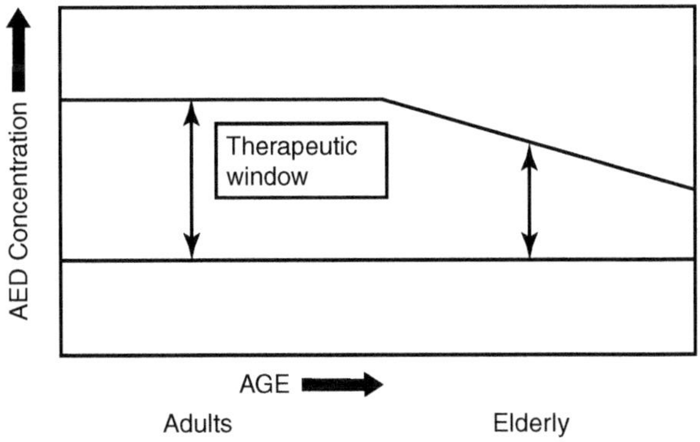

Fig. 12.1 Effect of age on therapeutic ranges: The elderly have a narrower therapeutic window (the range between the lowest effective concentration and the maximal tolerated concentration (Source: Bergey [135]; reproduced with permission from Wolters Kluver Health)

in patients with dementia that are frail, possibly malnourished, and often have comorbidities that might affect these aspects of the patient's condition. Renal clearance decreases with age and dosage need to be adjusted for AEDs that are primarily metabolized by renal excretion, such as levetiracetam and gabapentin. Pharmacodynamic aspects are also very important. Due to a decline in homeostatic mechanisms in the ageing brain, older people are very sensitive to adverse effects of psychoactive drugs [4]: the therapeutic window is typically narrower in the elderly (Fig. 12.1, reproduced from [135]). This is even more important in dementia, where the cerebral changes of ageing are compounded by neurodegenerative or other lesions.

Polypharmacy is common in persons with dementia, due to multiple concomitant medical conditions. For example, secondary prophylactic treatment is given after transient ischaemic attack/stroke, while the cognitive, affective and behavioural symptoms in dementia might require symptomatic treatment with antidepressants, anxiolytics, antipsychotics, and antidementia medications (choline esterase inhibitors, memantine). In addition, persons with dementia are often older and are prone to general medical comorbidities such as cardiovascular disease, diabetes, gastrointestinal conditions, and pain. Consequently, a careful review of the patient's list of medications is needed before initiating treatment with an AED. Especially the risk for interactions and additive adverse effects on cognition and wakefulness need to be taken into account.Additionally, patients with epilepsy who receive long-term monotherapy with enzyme inducing AEDs (carbamazepine, phenytoin, or valproate) exhibit altered circulatory markers of vascular risk (increased total cholesterol and homocysteine, reduced folate, increased common carotid artery intima media thickness), which is significantly associated with the duration of AED monotherapy and may contribute to acceleration of the atherosclerotic process [136]. Recent large population-based cohort studies have also demonstrated that persons with AD treated with AEDs are at increased relative risk of death (mainly due to dementia and more so on older AEDs) [137] and of stroke (regardless of AED used) [138], highlighting the need to use AEDs judiciously in this vulnerable population. Box 12.2 summarizes desirable features of AEDs for dementia patients (reproduced from [135]).

Box 12.2 Summary of Desirable Features of an AED for Use in the Elderly and Persons with Dementia

No interaction with other medications
No interaction with other AEDs
Can be introduced at therapeutic doses
No metabolism
No protein binding
Once or twice daily dosing
Laboratory monitoring not necessary
Excellent safety record
Good side-effect profile
High therapeutic index
Little effect on cognitive function
Psychoactive benefits

Source: Bergey [135]; reproduced with permission from Wolters Kluver Health

AEDs with minimal interactions should be chosen (see further below) and decreased dosage of other psychoactive drugs should be attempted when starting treatment with an AED. Newer AEDs have lower cognitive and sedative effects than older AEDs and should be drugs of first choice [133, 139–142]. Finally, oral intake might be compromised by dysphagia, decreased appetite, or behavioural issues in the patient with dementia. In these cases, AEDs where tablets can be divided in smaller pieces or crushed, or are available as granules or liquid formulations, might be preferred.

The following steps should be followed when starting treatment with an AED in dementia:

1. *Assess cognitive function before starting treatment.* In order to evaluate whether introduction of an AED affects the patients' cognition and general condition, baseline assessment of cognitive and activities of daily living (ADL) functions should be performed before starting treatment. Depending on whether the patient has a mild, moderate, or severe dementia, different methods of assessment can be utilized. As a minimum, this should include a cognitive screening test such as Mini-mental state evaluation (MMSE) and a structured interview with family members and other caregivers.
2. *Treatment is started with a low dose and titrated slowly to a minimum effective dose.* When treating epilepsy in dementia a lower dose of AED can be used than which is usually required in younger or otherwise healthy older patients with epilepsy. For example, a daily dose of 100 mg lamotrigine or 500 mg levetiracetam is often sufficient [133]. Careful evaluation of efficacy and adverse effects should be made before further increases in dosage.

3. *Rapid follow-up of the patient after starting treatment.* The importance of rapid follow-up cannot be overemphasized and should be performed within 2–3 weeks, much faster than is often the case in follow up of epilepsy treatment in cognitively intact patients who can self-report any adverse events. The initial follow-up can be done by phone and should include an interview with a caregiver, focusing on cognitive and general ADL function, as well as sedative and other adverse effects. The same principle should be applied when starting treatment with other psychoactive drugs such as antidepressants or antipsychotics. Adherence issues should also be addressed. Check if the patient is taking the medication and if supervision or a drug dispenser is needed.
4. *Long-term follow-up.* Follow-up in person should be scheduled within 1–3 months and include assessment of further seizures, cognition (with renewed cognitive screening test for objective comparison), ADL function, changes in behaviour (e.g. sedation, apathy, depression, irritability, disinhibition), balance and general well-being. Always interview a caregiver who knows the patient well, in person or by phone, as an accompanying person at a clinic visit might not be closely acquainted with the patient. Provide caregivers with contact details and encourage them to contact the clinic if there are changes in the patient's condition.
5. *Length of treatment.* Seizure control is often good when treating epilepsy in patients with dementia and older people in general, with 60–90% of patients becoming seizure free or have a greater than 95% reduction in seizure frequency and less than 3 seizures per year (up to 79% in a retrospective study of 39 patients with various dementia syndromes [95]). However, seizure recurrence is possible and should be carefully monitored for [95, 132]. In addition, the underlying dementia disorder remains and progresses, and treatment should most often be continued long-term providing there are no adverse effects or other factors that might require stopping or reducing the dose of the AED.

Antiepileptic Drugs Used in Patients with Dementia

The evidence base to guide the choice of antiepileptic treatment in patients with seizures and dementia is limited due to paucity of randomized clinical trials [143], and relies mainly on other studies in the elderly with or without dementia.

Taken together with limited data from randomized controlled studies in older people [139, 142, 144, 145] the newer anticonvulsants (including levetiracetam and lamotrigine) should be considered as a first line in the treatment of epilepsy in patients with dementia due to their lower potential for drug interactions, lower incidence of adverse effects and linear pharmacokinetics [93].

The following section and Table 12.2 summarize commonly used AEDs in patients with dementia, their metabolism, interactions, efficacy and tolerability, and adverse effects [35, 146].

Table 12.2 Commonly prescribed antiepileptic drugs in older patients with cognitive impairment

	Dose (mg per day)	Tolerability	Efficacy	Metabolism/ Excretion/ Elimination half-life (hours)[a]	Cognitive side-effects?	Adverse reactions (including those of concern in cognitive impairment)	Other uses
Levetiracetam	250–500	Excellent	Excellent	Enzymatic hydrolysis of acetamide group/ renal unchanged/6–8	No	Aggression, asthenia, dizziness, fatigue, headache, irritability, and nausea	Treatment of myoclonus
Lamotrigine	25–500	Excellent	Excellent	Liver (mostly UGT1A4-mediated)/ urine (70%), faeces (2%)/2–5	No	Asthenia, ataxia, blurred vision, diarrhea, diplopia, dizziness, hypersensitivity reaction, incoordination, insomnia, nausea, rash, somnolence, Stevens-Johnson syndrome, and tremor	Mood stabilization
Gabapentin	300–1500	Good	Good	Not significantly metabolized/ renal/5–9	Possible	Ataxia, dizziness, fatigue, nystagmus, nausea, peripheral oedema, somnolence, and weight gain	Treatment of insomnia, peripheral neuropathy, postherpetic neuralgia, and migraine prophylaxis
Carbamazepine	600	Fair	Good	Hepatic (CYP3A4)/ urine (72%), faeces (28%)/5–26 (autoinduction and reduced half-life on repeat dosing)	Yes	Agranulocytosis, asthenia, ataxia, blurred vision, cardiac dysrhythmia, constipation, decreased bone density, dizziness, hepatotoxicity, hypersensitivity reaction, hyponatraemia, nausea, rash, somnolence, and xerostomia	Mood stabilization, and treatment of trigeminal neuralgia

	Dose (mg per day)	Tolerability	Efficacy	Metabolism/ Excretion/ Elimination half-life (hours)[a]	Cognitive side-effects?	Adverse reactions (including those of concern in cognitive impairment)	Other uses
Valproic acid	250–1000	Fair	Good	Hepatic-glucuronidation (50%), beta-oxidation (40%), hydroxylation (10%)/renal/13–16	Yes	Alopecia, asthenia, ataxia, constipation, diarrhoea, diplopia, dizziness, gait disturbance, headache, hepatotoxicity, indigestion, nausea, nervousness, nystagmus, peripheral oedema, rash, somnolence, tinnitus, tremor, weakness, and weight gain	Mood stabilization, migraine prophylaxis, and treatment of myoclonus
Phenytoin	200–300	Poor	Good	Hepatic/mainly bil, <5% unmetabolized in urine/7–80 (mean 20 at 10–20 mg/L)	Yes	Ataxia, constipation, decreased bone density, dizziness, dysarthria, gingival hyperplasia, hepatotoxicity, hypersensitivity reaction, incoordination, lethargy, muscle hypotonia, nausea, nervousness, nystagmus, and sedation or drowsiness	None
Phenobarbital	50–100	Poor	Excellent	Liver (CYP2C19)/ renal (25%)and Feacal/70–130	Yes	Asthenia, barbiturate withdrawal, decreased bone density, hypersensitivity reaction, somnolence, and syncope	Long-term sedation

Reproduced with permission from Elsevier with amendments [35]

[a]Elimination half-life in healthy adults (from Shorvon et al. [146])

Newer Antiepileptic Drugs

Levetiracetam

Levetiracetam (LEV) is a broad-spectrum AED thought to exert its function by binding synaptic vesicle protein 2A [147], thereby reducing neurotransmitter release during repetitive stimulation on rapidly firing neurons [148]. Its main advantages are the broad-spectrum activity, the availability of oral and parenteral formulations, and the lack of clinically significant drug interactions.

The use of LEV in the treatment of seizures in patients with AD is supported by strong evidence [133, 149]: In an open-label observational study of LEV, Belcastro and colleagues [149] administered LEV daily (1000–1500 mg) to 25 patients with advanced AD and new-onset epilepsy: 72% were seizure free for at least 1 year, 16% discontinued due to side effects, 8% were unresponsive, 4% were lost to follow-up. Cumbo et al. [133] performed a prospective, randomized, three-arm parallel-group, case-control study of 95 patients with AD and seizures: Three treatment groups (LEV $n = 38$, phenobarbital $n = 28$, lamotrigine $n = 29$) were compared to a control group ($n = 68$) to evaluate cognitive effects of AEDs. The study revealed that LEV (500–2000 mg/day) is effective in treating focal onset seizures in patients with AD: at 12 months, 71% were responders (seizure reduction of at least 50%) and 29% had become seizure free. Importantly, efficacy was observed at low doses (mean 1343.7 mg/day), justifying the use of lower doses in elderly patients with dementia. There was no difference in the efficacy of all three anticonvulsants but LEV was associated with fewer adverse events. Additionally, LEV improved cognitive performance (especially attention level and oral fluency) measurable clinically by MMSE and Alzheimer's disease Assessment Scale-cognitive scoring. Patients treated with LEV experienced less depression than patients treated with phenobarbital, but more so than those treated with lamotrigine.

LEV is available as modified release formulation, useful in patients who have compliance issues. Serum level monitoring and blood monitoring are usually not required, although it would be advisable to determine serum creatinine and creatinine clearance prior to starting in the elderly to establish correct dosing [150].

Lamotrigine

Lamotrigine (LTG) is another broad-spectrum anticonvulsant with efficacy against multiple seizure types and with good tolerability [151]. It exerts its action predominantly by blocking voltage-dependent sodium and calcium channels, preventing action potential propagation [152, 153] and the release of neurotransmitters, mainly excessive glutamate [154, 155] from excitatory neurons, which may be a relevant mechanism in the pathophysiology of AD.

With LEV, LTG is supported by the strongest available evidence for the treatment of focal onset seizures in AD: as mentioned in the section above, Cumbo et al. [133] demonstrated that LTG (25–200 mg/day) is equivalent to LEV and phenobarbital (PB) at achieving seizure reduction at 1 year (LTG response rate 59%). Like LEV, LTG has fewer adverse effects and a better cognitive outcome compared to PB. Additionally, LTG improved mood. In a small crossover trial of LTG, Tekin et al. [156] demonstrated that 300 mg/day of LTG improved word recognition, naming, and depressed mood in AD patients without epilepsy on Alzheimer's disease Assessment Scale behavioural subscale after 8 weeks of treatment. In the Veterans Administration Cooperative Study, Rowan and colleagues [140] showed that LTG (150 mg/day) and gabapentin (1500 mg/day; see section below) were better tolerated than carbamazepine (CBZ) (600 mg/day) in a 12-month efficacy and tolerability study of 593 adults (mean age 72 years) with new-onset epilepsy. Efficacy and seizure freedom rates of around 50% were comparable in all three groups.

LTG is non-sedating and does not cause significant cognitive dysfunction [157, 158]. LTG is not highly protein bound, nor an hepatic enzyme inducer, resulting in minimal drug interactions except for when it is given with enzyme-inducing drugs (lowering LTG levels) or valproate (resulting in two to threefold higher LTG levels) [151]. The main disadvantage of lLTG is the need for slow dose escalation, due to the risk of hypersensitivity reactions if the dose is escalated too rapidly [159].

Gabapentin

Gabapentin (GBP) is a well-tolerated anticonvulsant with modest efficacy, which has good tolerability, including in the elderly and lacks major drug interactions [160]. The predominant effect of GBP is as a selective inhibitor of voltage-gated calcium channels containing the $\alpha2$-$\delta1$ subunit [161]. Additionally, GBP reduces the release of a number of neurotransmitters, including, among others, glutamate, noradrenaline, and acetylcholine, but their effect on seizures remains to be elucidated [162]. The Veterans Administration Cooperative Study [140], a randomized, double-blind, double dummy, parallel study of 593 elderly subjects with newly diagnosed seizures, demonstrated that GBP (up to 1500 mg/day) was better tolerated than carbamazepine (CBZ) and was as efficacious as both LTG and CBZ at seizure control, with more than 50% of participants seizure free at 12 months.

GBP is renally excreted without being metabolized in the liver, and does not induce hepatic enzymes. The only reported drug interactions are antacids containing aluminium or magnesium hydroxide, as they reduce absorption of the drug by about 20%. Their administration should be separated by at least 2 h [163].

Oxcarbazepine and Eslicarbazepine

Oxcarbazepine (OXC) is a 10-keto analogue of CBZ [164], whilst eslicarbazepine (ESL) is a prodrug of (*S*)-(+)-licarbazepine [165, 166]. Both act mainly via inhibition of voltage-gated sodium channels. Both are licensed for adjunctive and monotherapy of focal-onset and secondarily generalized seizures [166]. OXC can be more rapidly uptitrated than CBZ, and is also available as extended-release formulation that can be administered once daily. Eslicarbazepine only requires once daily dosing, too. No evidence is available on the safety and efficacy of these two drugs in patients with dementia, although both are being used successfully in the treatment of elderly patients. Efficacy of OXC appears to be similar to CBZ when used in older patients, whilst ESL showed improved efficacy (62% in >65 years vs. 48.8% in 65 years, ESL was found to cause low rates of hyponatraemia [168], possibly due to the lower mean doses used in this subgroup (850 mg/day in >65 years vs. 1032.6 mg/day in <65 years), hence serum sodium monitoring is always recommended when using OXC and ESL in the elderly population. Discontinuation rates due to adverse effects among elderly patients were similar to those of younger individuals for OXC [169], but higher for ESL [168]. The most common adverse effects for both drugs included dizziness and nausea [164, 168]. The tolerability profile improved in patients who switched from CBZ or OXC to ESL due to adverse effects [168].

Enzyme-inducing antiepileptic drugs reduce levels of the active metabolite monohydroxycarbazepine and of ESL [164], whilst both may increase serum levels of phenytoin.

Lacosamide

Lacosamide (LCS) is a later generation antiepileptic drug, which enhances the slow inactivation of voltage-gated Na channels with comparable efficacy to other antiepileptic drugs licenced in the last decade [170]. There is no available evidence of its use in patients with dementia. Most of the evidence of its use in the elderly comes from retrospective case series [171–173], a subgroup analysis of a non-inferiority trial vs. controlled-release (CR) carbamazepine [174] and from its use in neuropathic pain trials, which enrolled higher numbers of elderly patients [175]: Overall LCS is well tolerated and no dose reduction is recommended in older patients (unless there are known renal problems). LCS has similar efficacy to CBZ-CR (6-and 12-month seizure freedom) and is better tolerated than CBZ-CR. There is, however, a higher incidence of cardiac disorder adverse effects with higher discontinuation rates because of any adverse effect in the 400–600 mg/day groups. LCS can induce a dose-dependent prolongation of the PR interval, with occasional reports of atrioventricular block and alterations in cardiac rhythm reported when the drug was used at high doses in patients with pre-existing cardiac disease risk factors, in which caution is mandated in using this drug. Psychiatric side effects including psychosis, agitation, and suicidality have rarely been reported in post-marketing studies [176]. LCS has several properties that make it an attractive choice in patients with dementia and their comorbidities: LCS is available as tablet, syrup, and iv preparation with bioequivalence between the formulations making direct conversions possible [177]. Further, LCS has linear pharmacokinetics, is not affected by food and has a low potential for clinically relevant pharmacokinetic drug–drug interactions with AEDs and other common medications [167].

Topiramate, Perampanel, and Brivaracetam (BRV)

Of the newer anticonvulsants, Topiramate (TPM) and Perampanel (INN) are less suitable for treatment of seizures in dementia due to their cognitive and psychiatric side effects.

TPM alleviates behavioural deficits in mouse models of AD [43] and is effective in older adults as monotherapy or add-on for the treatment of one or more focal seizures [178]. However, cognitive side effects are a significant disadvantage: they appear to impact particularly on working memory, short-term verbal memory, language skills, verbal IQ, attention/concentration, processing speed, complex visuomotor ability, and perception [179]. Cognitive side effects can be minimized by slow uptitration but there is a proportion of patients very sensitive to cognitive side effects of TPM regardless of how cautiously it is introduced. Furthermore, cognitive side effects, albeit reversible on drug withdrawal, may appear at low doses and persist throughout treatment. TPM can also have negative side effects on mood and cause psychosis [180].

INN is a selective non-competitive antagonist at the α-amino-3-hydroxy-5--methyl-4-isoxazolepropionic acid receptor (AMPA) receptor, an ionotropic glutamate receptor. Its mechanism of action is unique among anticonvulsants and it requires only once daily dosing. No data is available to support its use in older patients with epilepsy, as there were not sufficient numbers of subjects aged 65 years and over enrolled in the trials. A significant drawback is the occurrence of common psychiatric side effects [181] including aggression, but also thoughts of harming others, physical assault, threatening behaviour, and suicidal ideation, which prompted the FDA to issue a black box warning against INN. Careful consideration of these important side effects and particular care should be taken when considering INN for patients with dementia.

BRV is one of the latest anticonvulsants licenced, where no or very little data exists on its use in the elderly population: BRV is the 4R-propyl analogue of LEV. Like LEV it binds to synaptic vesicle protein 2A but with 15- to 30-fold higher binding affinity than LEV, possibly at a different binding site and interacting with different conformational states of the synaptic vesicle protein 2A protein [182]. Its efficacy in older adults is comparable to that in younger subjects and no dosage adjustment is required [183]. One of the major advantages of BRV is that no initial dose titration is needed and efficacy is seen on day 1 of oral use in a significant percentage of patients [182]. Parenteral and oral formulations are available and side effect profile is similar to that of LEV, with irritability, agitation, anxiety, insomnia, aggression, and depression the commonest dose-dependent side effects, which are typically mild to moderate. Whilst post-marketing data is being collected, to date, the psychiatric side effects of BRV have been reported as being perhaps less frequent and less severe compared to LEV [182].

Older Antiepileptic Drugs

Carbamazepine

Carbamazepine (CBZ) is a blocker of voltage-sensitive sodium channels and a widely prescribed anticonvulsant [184]. In respect to the elderly and patients with dementia, it has a less than favourable pharmacokinetic profile: as a hepatic enzyme inducer it may have numerous drug–drug interactions, and hyponatraemia has been more frequently reported in elderly patients taking CBZ [185]. In the Veterans Administration Cooperative Study [140], Rowan and colleagues demonstrated that cCBZ (600 mg/day) was less well tolerated than lLTG or gGBP for the treatment of new-onset seizures in older patients, although the efficacy rates were comparable among the three groups.

Phenytoin

Data on the use of phenytoin (PHT), a potent blocker of voltage-gated sodium channels, in AD derives from observational studies, which have demonstrated high rates of adverse effects (up to 40% [186]) including worsening of cognitive symptoms, ataxia, delirium and sedation [30, 95, 187] and variable efficacy on seizure control. Individuals with Down Syndrome and epilepsy, for example, respond well to PHT when treated early in life but develop cognitive side-effects when treated for late-onset seizures [187]. The adverse effects of PHT on cognition and seizures may be due to blockage of NaV1.1 channels predominantly in parvalbumin-positive inhibitory interneurons, thereby causing network hyperexcitability, findings replicated in the APP–J20 mouse model [53].

Phenobarbital

The use of phenobarbital (PB) in patients with AD was evaluated in a randomized three-group parallel case control study [133] of LEV, LTG, and PB (described in the previous section): There were no differences in responder rates among the 95 patients treated with either of the three AEDs. There was, however, higher incidence of adverse events on PB (43%), most commonly somnolence and asthenia, and high withdrawal rates (17%). More than half of patients on PB experienced side effects (61%). The authors concluded that despite its efficacy, due to its side effects of ataxia, somnolence, and central nervous system depression causing further cognitive impairment, PB is not a good choice in elderly patients [133].

Valproic Acid

Valproic acid (VPA) was evaluated in a multicentre, randomized, double-blind, placebo-controlled trial of 313 patients with moderate AD without epilepsy, to determine whether treatment with VPA 10–12 mg/kg/day could delay/prevent the onset of agitation or psychosis [188]. This study revealed not only that VPA did not delay onset of agitation and psychosis but showed that the valproate group had higher rates of toxic effects including somnolence, gait disturbance, tremor, diarrhoea, and weakness. It also showed that there was greater hippocampal volume loss in the valproate group when imaged at 12 months [189]. These results should caution on the use of VPA at these doses in patients with AD with or without epilepsy. A further concern is a development of valproate-induced parkinsonism and of valproate encephalopathy, an idiosyncratic drug reaction, characterized by impaired cognition, drowsiness, and apathy, which typically resolves on stopping the drug [112, 190, 191]; see section "Valproate Encephalopathy").

Benzodiazepines: Chronic Use

Chronic benzodiazepine use in older patients remains high in developed countries (7–43% [192]), although international guidelines [193] discourage its use due to the inherent risks of withdrawal symptoms, making dose reduction difficult, and the risk of withdrawal seizures on forgetting medication even in healthy individuals. A recent study has additionally shown a 50% higher risk of developing dementia upon lifetime use of >90 doses of benzodiazepines, equivalent to two doses a week for

1 year [192]. The use of chronic benzodiazepines is therefore discouraged in the management of epilepsy in dementia, whilst acute benzodiazepine use maintains its role in treating prolonged seizures in the acute phase (see section "Acute Seizure Treatment with Benzodiazepines").

Aspects Requiring Special Consideration

Bone Health

Several AEDs have negative effects on bone metabolism and might increase osteoporosis in the already susceptible population of older people, especially in dementia where physical activity often is limited. A recent meta-analysis found that first-generation AEDs, including valproate, phenobarbital, phenytoin, and carbamazepine, as well as the second-generation AED lamotrigine, could decrease bone density, while levetiracetam did not [4, 194]. This may be especially important in patients with manifest osteoporosis. Due consideration for follow-up of bone density and risk for fractures is needed during long-term treatment with an AED, and prophylaxis with calcium and vitamin D started as needed. On the other hand, in patients with progressive dementia and shorter expected survival, this issue might not be of major importance.

Acute Seizure Treatment with Benzodiazepines

Elderly patients are very sensitive to the sedative effects of benzodiazepines, especially long-acting ones. If given in the acute setting to curtail an ongoing seizure, in a hospital, or by an ambulance service, iv formulations are often used. This may lead to depression of respiration and might result in intubation and need of intensive care. Benzodiazepines should therefore be used with caution and ideally reserved for cases of convulsive status epilepticus. In prolonged seizures or seizure clusters, short-acting bensodiazepines such as alprazolam and iv treatment with, e.g. LEV, VPA, or LCS should be considered as first-line treatment. Diazepam easily accumulates in the elderly with risk for long-term sedation, while LEV, VPA, and LCS have less risk for acute falls in blood pressure compared to phenytoin or fos-phenytoin, which is another commonly used iv treatment for prolonged seizures and status epilepticus. In a person with dementia with frequent generalized seizures, it can be advisable to have acute medication available that can be given in cases of prolonged seizures. Traditionally, rectal diazepam has been given, but entails some problems with administration. Liquid midazolam is available in syringes and can more easily be administered orally between the teeth and the inside of the cheek. Although respiratory depression is less of an issue with rectal or oral administration, post-ictal sedation and delirium remain problematic.

Valproate Encephalopathy

A number of case reports and smaller case series have described cognitive decline and extrapyramidal motor symptoms during long-term treatment with valproic acid [195–199]. Although rare, valproate encephalopathy can affect both younger and older patients. The clinical symptoms of valproate encephalopathy are usually related to introducing the drug but onset can occur several years after starting treatment. As VPA concentrations most often are within the therapeutic range, the reaction appears to be idiosyncratic, although the exact mechanism remains to be determined. Valproate encephalopathy is unrelated to derangement in liver function tests, but is typically associated with raised levels of ammonia, which can be screened for. Valproate encephalopathy is a reversible condition and often accompanied by pseudoatrophy, with normalization of brain volumes and cognitive function after valproate is discontinued [199]. In summary, a diagnosis of valproate encephalopathy should be considered in patients with more rapid cognitive decline and ammonia levels screened for. Treatment with VPA should be avoided in the elderly, especially in patients with dementia.

Case Scenarios and Summary Teaching Points

The final section of this chapter presents three real-life case scenarios to illustrate and summarize the major teaching points arising from the sections above.

Case 1

An 85-year-old man with mixed AD and vascular dementia had a self-limiting generalized seizure of 1–2 min duration and a post-ictal state lasting several hours. He was admitted to hospital and started on treatment with levetiracetam 500 mg daily. After discharge, he was followed up by a general practitioner at the care facility where he lived. There were no further seizure episodes during the following year.

> **Teaching Points**
> Epilepsy in dementia is common and risk of seizure recurrence is fairly high. The institution of treatment with an AED should therefore be considered already after a first seizure. Low doses of a newer AED are often sufficient and leads to seizure freedom in a majority of cases.

Case 2

An 82-year-old single woman was referred to the Neurology Outpatient Clinic after two episodes of generalized seizures. She was started on carbamazepine but developed severe lethargy and stopped the medication. After having a few focal onset impaired awareness seizures (complex partial seizures), she was started on lamotrigine 100 mg daily but again developed sedative adverse effects, as well as dizziness. Treatment was changed to gabapentin 300 mg three times daily, which was well tolerated. There remained occasional short-lasting focal onset impaired awareness seizures but no further generalized seizures during 2 years of follow-up.

Teaching Points

Elderly people, with or without dementia, can be very sensitive to adverse effects of AEDs, even at low doses. A risk-benefit assessment should always be made when starting, changing, or terminating treatment. Complete seizure freedom cannot always be attained.

Case 3

A 68-year-old male was admitted to hospital for new-onset delirium and urinary voiding. He was married, university educated, a non-smoker with moderate alcohol consumption. He had localized prostate cancer and a 4-year history of progressive problems with gait, general psychomotor slowing and problems with executive function. He had been operated on for a lumbar spinal stenosis 1 year previously with improvement of pain but not gait.

On admission, EEG showed focal epileptiform activity in both frontal lobes but no signs of NCSE. He was diagnosed with epilepsy and treatment with valproate was initiated. This led to cognitive worsening and lethargy and his AED treatment was changed to carbamazepine. His condition improved and he was discharged to his home with assistance and alternate-weekly stays in a care facility. He was referred to a Memory Clinic pending follow-up of his epilepsy at the Neurology Outpatient Clinic. During the hospital stay an MRI was performed that showed mild atrophy of the frontal lobes and mesencephalon, while cerebrospinal fluid (CSF) analysis showed no signs of inflammation but a mildly raised level of Neurofilament light protein of 3740 ng/L (<1850 ng/L) and an increased Albumin CSF/serum ratio, while biomarkers for AD were normal.

On examination at the Memory Clinic, 3 months after he was started on carbamazepine but before follow-up at the Neurology Outpatient Clinic, he showed severe psychomotor slowing and could not participate in conversation or cognitive testing. He had a horizontal and vertical gaze palsy, bilateral but asymmetric rigidity and bradykinesia. He could only stand and walk with the aid of two persons. A diagnosis of a neurodegenerative disorder caused by probable progressive supranuclear palsy (PSP) was made. The patient was also suspected to have an encephalopathy caused by carbamazepine (700 mg per day), in spite of carbamazepine levels of 30 μmol/L (therapeutic range 20–40), with worsening of pre-existing gait and cognitive symptoms. An EEG was repeated and showed a slight increase in the focal bifrontal epileptiform activity seen previously but no electrographic seizures. The patient's AED treatment was changed to levetiracetam 1000 mg daily.

At follow-up 1 month after the switch to levetiracetam, the patient was much better, and he talked and joked spontaneously. He did not want to spend time in a respite home any longer and home assistance had been stopped. He walked independently but with a broad-based gait and had decreased postural reflexes, but showed no bradykinesia, rigidity, or gaze palsy. A cognitive screening test showed MMSE 23/30, but he was unable to draw a three-dimensional cube or a clock. He had no further seizures but progressed in his cognitive and motor symptoms. After 6 years, he had progressed to the same clinical state as he had originally presented with and he died of pneumonia 7 years after onset of epilepsy and first presentation to our Memory Clinic. No autopsy was performed but the clinical diagnosis of PSP was maintained.

Teaching Points

When starting treatment with an AED in patients with an underlying neurodegenerative disorder, rapid clinical follow-up is essential to exclude adverse effects, especially worsening of cognitive function. Severe cognitive side effects are common and can occur in spite of AED levels within the therapeutic range. The risk of negative effects on cognition is more common with older AEDs.

References

1. Annegers JF, Dubinsky S, Coan SP, Newmark ME, Roht L. The incidence of epilepsy and unprovoked seizures in multiethnic, urban health maintenance organizations. Epilepsia. 1999;40:502–6.
2. Hussain SA, Haut SR, Lipton RB, Derby C, Markowitz SY, Shinnar S. Incidence of epilepsy in a racially diverse, community-dwelling, elderly cohort: results from the Einstein aging study. Epilepsy Res. 2006;71:195–205.
3. Joint Epilepsy Council. Epilepsy prevalence, incidence and other statistics. London: Joint Epilepsy Council; 2011.
4. Brodie MJ, Elder AT, Kwan P. Epilepsy in later life. Lancet Neurol. 2009;8:1019–30.
5. Choi H, Pack A, Elkind MSV, Longstreth WT, Ton TGN, Onchiri F. Predictors of incident epilepsy in older adults: the Cardiovascular Health Study. Neurology. 2017;88:870–7.
6. Annegers JF, Hauser WA, Coan SP, Rocca WA. A population-based study of seizures after traumatic brain injuries. N Engl J Med. 1998;338:20–4.
7. Bruns J, Hauser WA. The epidemiology of traumatic brain injury: a review. Epilepsia. 2003;44:2–10.
8. Stefan H. Epilepsy in the elderly: facts and challenges. Acta Neurol Scand. 2011;124: 223–37.
9. Breteler MM, van Duijn CM, Chandra V, Fratiglioni L, Graves AB, Heyman A, Jorm AF, Kokmen E, Kondo K, Mortimer JA. Medical history and the risk of Alzheimer's disease: a collaborative re-analysis of case-control studies. EURODEM Risk Factors Research Group. Int J Epidemiol. 1991;20(Suppl 2):S36–42.
10. Breteler MM, de Groot RR, van Romunde LK, Hofman A. Risk of dementia in patients with Parkinson's disease, epilepsy, and severe head trauma: a register-based follow-up study. Am J Epidemiol. 1995;142:1300–5.
11. Zelano J, Brigo F, Garcia-Patek S. Increased risk of epilepsy in patients registered in the Swedish Dementia Registry. Eur J Neurol. 2020;27:129–35.

12. Hommet C, Mondon K, Camus V, De Toffol B, Constans T. Epilepsy and dementia in the elderly. Dement Geriatr Cogn Disord. 2008;25:293–300.
13. Pandis D, Scarmeas N. Seizures in Alzheimer disease: clinical and epidemiological data. Epilepsy Curr. 2012;12:184–7.
14. Imfeld P, Bodmer M, Schuerch M, Jick SS, Meier CR. Risk of incident stroke in patients with Alzheimer disease or vascular dementia. Neurology. 2013;81:910–9.
15. Sen A, Capelli V, Husain M. Cognition and dementia in older patients with epilepsy. Brain. 2018;141:1592–608.
16. Hamed SA. Atherosclerosis in epilepsy: its causes and implications. Epilepsy Behav. 2014;41:290–6.
17. Keezer MR, Sisodiya SM, Sander JW. Comorbidities of epilepsy: current concepts and future perspectives. Lancet Neurol. 2016;15:106–15.
18. Sillanpää M, Anttinen A, Rinne JO, Joutsa J, Sonninen P, Erkinjuntti M, Hermann B, Karrasch M, Saarinen M, Tiitta P, Shinnar S. Childhood-onset epilepsy five decades later. A prospective population-based cohort study. Epilepsia. 2015;56:1774–83.
19. Maxwell H, Hanby M, Parkes LM, Gibson LM, Coutinho C, Emsley HCA. Prevalence and subtypes of radiological cerebrovascular disease in late-onset isolated seizures and epilepsy. Clin Neurol Neurosurg. 2013;115:591–6.
20. Thygesen LC, Gimsing LN, Johansen C. Chronic neurodegenerative illnesses and epilepsy in Danish adventists and baptists: a nationwide cohort study. J Alzheimers Dis. 2017;56:1429–35.
21. Sheng JG, Boop FA, Mrak RE, Griffin WS. Increased neuronal beta-amyloid precursor protein expression in human temporal lobe epilepsy: association with interleukin-1 alpha immunoreactivity. J Neurochem. 1994;63:1872–9.
22. Mackenzie IR, Miller LA. Senile plaques in temporal lobe epilepsy. Acta Neuropathol. 1994;87:504–10.
23. Tai XY, Koepp M, Duncan JS, Fox N, Thompson P, Baxendale S, Liu JYW, Reeves C, Michalak Z, Thom M. Hyperphosphorylated tau in patients with refractory epilepsy correlates with cognitive decline: a study of temporal lobe resections. Brain. 2016;139:2441–55.
24. Sen A, Thom M, Martinian L, Harding B, Cross JH, Nikolic M, Sisodiya SM. Pathological tau tangles localize to focal cortical dysplasia in older patients. Epilepsia. 2007;48:1447–54.
25. Hatanpaa KJ, et al. Hippocampal sclerosis in dementia, epilepsy, and ischemic injury: differential vulnerability of hippocampal subfields. J Neuropathol Exp Neurol. 2014;73:136–42.
26. Nelson PT, et al. New old pathologies: AD, PART, and cerebral age-related TDP-43 with sclerosis (CARTS). J Neuropathol Exp Neurol. 2016;75(6):482–98.
27. Helmstaedter C, Witt J-A. Epilepsy and cognition—a bidirectional relationship? Seizure. 2017;49:83–9.
28. Cretin B, Philippi N, Dibitonto L, Blanc F. Epilepsy at the prodromal stages of neurodegenerative diseases. Geriatr Psychol Neuropsychiatr Vieil. 2017;15:75–82.
29. Irizarry MC, Jin S, He F, Emond JA, Raman R, Thomas RG, Sano M, Quinn JF, Tariot PN, Galasko DR, Ishihara LS, Weil JG, Aisen PS. Incidence of new-onset seizures in mild to moderate Alzheimer disease. Arch Neurol. 2012;69:368–72.
30. Vossel KA, Beagle AJ, Rabinovici GD, Shu H, Lee SE, Naasan G, Hegde M, Cornes SB, Henry ML, Nelson AB, Seeley WW, Geschwind MD, Gorno-Tempini ML, Shih T, Kirsch HE, Garcia PA, Miller BL, Mucke L. Seizures and epileptiform activity in the early stages of Alzheimer disease. JAMA Neurol. 2013;70:1158–66.
31. Zarea A, Charbonnier C, Rovelet-Lecrux A, Nicolas G, Rousseau S, Borden A, Pariente J, Le Ber I, Pasquier F, Formaglio M, Martinaud O, Rollin-Sillaire A, Sarazin M, Croisile B, Boutoleau-Bretonnière C, Ceccaldi M, Gabelle A, Chamard L, Blanc F, Sellal F, Paquet C, Campion D, Hannequin D, Wallon D, et al. Seizures in dominantly inherited Alzheimer disease. Neurology. 2016;87:912–9.
32. Amatniek JC, Hauser WA, DelCastillo-Castaneda C, Jacobs DM, Marder K, Bell K, Albert M, Brandt J, Stern Y. Incidence and predictors of seizures in patients with Alzheimer's disease. Epilepsia. 2006;47:867–72.

33. Subota A, Pham T, Jetté N, Sauro K, Lorenzetti D, Holroyd-Leduc J. The association between dementia and epilepsy: a systematic review and meta-analysis. Epilepsia. 2017;58:962–72.
34. Scharfman HE. Alzheimer's disease and epilepsy: insight from animal models. Future Neurol. 2012;7:177–92.
35. Vossel KA, Tartaglia MC, Nygaard HB, Zeman AZ, Miller BL. Epileptic activity in Alzheimer's disease: causes and clinical relevance. Lancet Neurol. 2017;16:311–22. https://doi.org/10.1016/S1474-4422(17)30044-3.
36. Westmark CJ, Westmark PR, Beard AM, Hildebrandt SM, Malter JS. Seizure susceptibility and mortality in mice that over-express amyloid precursor protein. Int J Clin Exp Pathol. 2008;1:157–68.
37. Minkeviciene R, Rheims S, Dobszay MB, Zilberter M, Hartikainen J, Fülöp L, Penke B, Zilberter Y, Harkany T, Pitkänen A, Tanila H. Amyloid beta-induced neuronal hyperexcitability triggers progressive epilepsy. J Neurosci. 2009;29:3453–62.
38. Busche MA, Eichhoff G, Adelsberger H, Abramowski D, Wiederhold K-H, Haass C, Staufenbiel M, Konnerth A, Garaschuk O. Clusters of hyperactive neurons near amyloid plaques in a mouse model of Alzheimer's disease. Science (New York, NY). 2008;321:1686–9.
39. Roberson ED, Halabisky B, Yoo JW, Yao J, Chin J, Yan F, Wu T, Hamto P, Devidze N, Yu G-Q, Palop JJ, Noebels JL, Mucke L. Amyloid-β/Fyn-induced synaptic, network, and cognitive impairments depend on tau levels in multiple mouse models of Alzheimer's disease. J Neurosci. 2011;31:700–11.
40. Zott B, Simon MM, Hong W, Unger F, Chen-Engerer H-J, Frosch MP, Sakmann B, Walsh DM, Konnerth A. A vicious cycle of β amyloid-dependent neuronal hyperactivation. Science (New York, N.Y.). 2019;365:559–65.
41. Yamamoto K, Tanei Z-I, Hashimoto T, Wakabayashi T, Okuno H, Naka Y, Yizhar O, Fenno LE, Fukayama M, Bito H, Cirrito JR, Holtzman DM, Deisseroth K, Iwatsubo T. Chronic optogenetic activation augments aβ pathology in a mouse model of Alzheimer disease. Cell Rep. 2015;11:859–65.
42. Wu JW, Hussaini SA, Bastille IM, Rodriguez GA, Mrejeru A, Rilett K, Sanders DW, Cook C, Fu H, Boonen RACM, Herman M, Nahmani E, Emrani S, Figueroa YH, Diamond MI, Clelland CL, Wray S, Duff KE. Neuronal activity enhances tau propagation and tau pathology in vivo. Nat Neurosci. 2016;19:1085–92.
43. Shi J-Q, Wang B-R, Tian Y-Y, Xu J, Gao L, Zhao S-L, Jiang T, Xie H-G, Zhang Y-D. Antiepileptics topiramate and levetiracetam alleviate behavioral deficits and reduce neuropathology in APPswe/PS1dE9 transgenic mice. CNS Neurosci Ther. 2013;19:871–81.
44. Sanchez PE, Zhu L, Verret L, Vossel KA, Orr AG, Cirrito JR, Devidze N, Ho K, Yu G-Q, Palop JJ, Mucke L. Levetiracetam suppresses neuronal network dysfunction and reverses synaptic and cognitive deficits in an Alzheimer's disease model. Proc Natl Acad Sci U S A. 2012;109:E2895–903.
45. Li S, Hong S, Shepardson NE, Walsh DM, Shankar GM, Selkoe D. Soluble oligomers of amyloid Beta protein facilitate hippocampal long-term depression by disrupting neuronal glutamate uptake. Neuron. 2009;62:788–801.
46. Lei M, Xu H, Li Z, Wang Z, O'Malley TT, Zhang D, Walsh DM, Xu P, Selkoe DJ, Li S. Soluble Aβ oligomers impair hippocampal LTP by disrupting glutamatergic/GABAergic balance. Neurobiol Dis. 2016;85:111–21.
47. Decker JM, KrÃŒger L, Sydow A, Dennissen FJ, Siskova Z, Mandelkow E, Mandelkow E-M. The Tau/A152T mutation, a risk factor for frontotemporal-spectrum disorders, leads to NR2B receptor-mediated excitotoxicity. EMBO Rep. 2016;17:552–69.
48. Vossel KA, Zhang K, Brodbeck J, Daub AC, Sharma P, Finkbeiner S, Cui B, Mucke L. Tau reduction prevents Abeta-induced defects in axonal transport. Science (New York, N.Y.). 2010;330:198.
49. Vossel KA, Xu JC, Fomenko V, Miyamoto T, Suberbielle E, Knox JA, Ho K, Kim DH, Yu G-Q, Mucke L. Tau reduction prevents Aβ-induced axonal transport deficits by blocking activation of GSK3β. J Cell Biol. 2015;209:419–33.

50. Zempel H, Luedtke J, Kumar Y, Biernat J, Dawson H, Mandelkow E, Mandelkow E-M. Amyloid-β oligomers induce synaptic damage via Tau-dependent microtubule severing by TTLL6 and spastin. EMBO J. 2013;32:2920–37.
51. Um JW, Nygaard HB, Heiss JK, Kostylev MA, Stagi M, Vortmeyer A, Wisniewski T, Gunther EC, Strittmatter SM. Alzheimer amyloid-β oligomer bound to postsynaptic prion protein activates Fyn to impair neurons. Nat Neurosci. 2012;15:1227–35.
52. Corbett BF, Leiser SC, Ling H-P, Nagy R, Breysse N, Zhang X, Hazra A, Brown JT, Randall AD, Wood A, Pangalos MN, Reinhart PH, Chin J. Sodium channel cleavage is associated with aberrant neuronal activity and cognitive deficits in a mouse model of Alzheimer's disease. J Neurosci. 2013;33:7020–6.
53. Verret L, Mann EO, Hang GB, Barth AMI, Cobos I, Ho K, Devidze N, Masliah E, Kreitzer AC, Mody I, Mucke L, Palop JJ. Inhibitory interneuron deficit links altered network activity and cognitive dysfunction in Alzheimer model. Cell. 2012;149:708–21.
54. Hall AM, Throesch BT, Buckingham SC, Markwardt SJ, Peng Y, Wang Q, Hoffman DA, Roberson ED. Tau-dependent Kv4.2 depletion and dendritic hyperexcitability in a mouse model of Alzheimer's disease. J Neurosci. 2015;35:6221–30.
55. Ittner LM, Ke YD, Delerue F, Bi M, Gladbach A, van Eersel J, Wölfing H, Chieng BC, Christie MDJ, Napier IA, Eckert A, Staufenbiel M, Hardeman E, Götz J. Dendritic function of tau mediates amyloid-beta toxicity in Alzheimer's disease mouse models. Cell. 2010;142:387–97.
56. Kaufman AC, Salazar SV, Haas LT, Yang J, Kostylev MA, Jeng AT, Robinson SA, Gunther EC, van Dyck CH, Nygaard HB, Strittmatter SM. Fyn inhibition rescues established memory and synapse loss in Alzheimer mice. Ann Neurol. 2015;77:953–71.
57. Andrews-Zwilling Y, Bien-Ly N, Xu Q, Li G, Bernardo A, Yoon SY, Zwilling D, Yan TX, Chen L, Huang Y. Apolipoprotein E4 causes age- and Tau-dependent impairment of GABAergic interneurons, leading to learning and memory deficits in mice. J Neurosci. 2010;30:13707–17.
58. Krantic S, Isorce N, Mechawar N, Davoli MA, Vignault E, Albuquerque M, Chabot J-G, Moyse E, Chauvin J-P, Aubert I, McLaurin J, Quirion R. Hippocampal GABAergic neurons are susceptible to amyloid-β toxicity in vitro and are decreased in number in the Alzheimer's disease TgCRND8 mouse model. J Alzheimers Dis. 2012;29:293–308.
59. Baglietto-Vargas D, Moreno-Gonzalez I, Sanchez-Varo R, Jimenez S, Trujillo-Estrada L, Sanchez-Mejias E, Torres M, Romero-Acebal M, Ruano D, Vizuete M, et al. Calretinin interneurons are early targets of extracellular amyloid-β pathology in PS1/AβPP Alzheimer mice hippocampus. J Alzheimers Dis. 2010;21(1):119–32.
60. Hazra A, Gu F, Aulakh A, Berridge C, Eriksen JL, Žiburkus J. Inhibitory neuron and hippocampal circuit dysfunction in an aged mouse model of Alzheimer's disease. PLoS One. 2013;8(5):e64318.
61. Šišková Z, Justus D, Kaneko H, Friedrichs D, Henneberg N, Beutel T, Pitsch J, Schoch S, Becker A, von der Kammer H, Remy S. Dendritic structural degeneration is functionally linked to cellular hyperexcitability in a mouse model of Alzheimer's disease. Neuron. 2014;84:1023–33.
62. Hazra A, Corbett BF, You JC, Aschmies S, Zhao L, Li K, Lepore AC, Marsh ED, Chin J. Corticothalamic network dysfunction and behavioral deficits in a mouse model of Alzheimer's disease. Neurobiol Aging. 2016;44:96–107.
63. Kam K, Duffy ÁM, Moretto J, LaFrancois JJ, Scharfman HE. Interictal spikes during sleep are an early defect in the Tg2576 mouse model of β -amyloid neuropathology. Sci Rep. 2016;6:20119.
64. Najm R, Jones EA, Huang Y. Apolipoprotein E4, inhibitory network dysfunction, and Alzheimer's disease. Mol Neurodegener. 2019;14:24.
65. Holmes GL. Cognitive impairment in epilepsy: the role of network abnormalities. Epileptic Disord. 2015;17:101–16.
66. Kleen JK, Scott RC, Holmes GL, Lenck-Santini PP. Hippocampal interictal spikes disrupt cognition in rats. Ann Neurol. 2010;67(2):250–7.

67. Kleen JK, Scott RC, Holmes GL, Roberts DW, Rundle MM, Testorf M, Lenck-Santini P-P, Jobst BC. Hippocampal interictal epileptiform activity disrupts cognition in humans. Neurology. 2013;81(1):18–24.
68. Ung H, Cazares C, Nanivadekar A, Kini L, Wagenaar J, Becker D, Krieger A, Lucas T, Litt B, Davis KA. Interictal epileptiform activity outside the seizure onset zone impacts cognition. Brain. 2017;140(8):2157–68.
69. Raichle ME. The brain's default mode network. Annu Rev Neurosci. 2015;38:433–47.
70. Vincent JL, Snyder AZ, Fox MD, Shannon BJ, Andrews JR, Raichle ME, Buckner RL. Coherent spontaneous activity identifies a hippocampal-parietal memory network. J Neurophysiol. 2006;96:3517–31.
71. Fahoum F, Zelmann R, Tyvaert L, Dubeau F, Gotman J. Epileptic discharges affect the default mode network—FMRI and intracerebral EEG evidence. PLoS One. 2013;8(6):e68038.
72. Sambataro F, Murty VP, Callicott JH, Tan H-Y, Das S, Weinberger DR, Mattay VS. Age-related alterations in default mode network: impact on working memory performance. Neurobiol Aging. 2010;31:839–52.
73. Dang LC, O'Neil JP, Jagust WJ. Genetic effects on behavior are mediated by neurotransmitters and large-scale neural networks. NeuroImage. 2013;66:203–14.
74. Laufs H, Hamandi K, Salek-Haddadi A, Kleinschmidt AK, Duncan JS, Lemieux L. Temporal lobe interictal epileptic discharges affect cerebral activity in "default mode" brain regions. Hum Brain Mapp. 2007;28:1023–32.
75. Zhang Z, Lu G, Zhong Y, Tan Q, Chen H, Liao W, Tian L, Li Z, Shi J, Liu Y. fMRI study of mesial temporal lobe epilepsy using amplitude of low-frequency fluctuation analysis. Hum Brain Mapp. 2010;31:1851–61.
76. Liao W, Zhang Z, Pan Z, Mantini D, Ding J, Duan X, Luo C, Wang Z, Tan Q, Lu G, Chen H. Default mode network abnormalities in mesial temporal lobe epilepsy: a study combining fMRI and DTI. Hum Brain Mapp. 2011;32:883–95.
77. Dickerson BC, Salat DH, Greve DN, Chua EF, Rand-Giovannetti E, Rentz DM, Bertram L, Mullin K, Tanzi RE, Blacker D, Albert MS, Sperling RA. Increased hippocampal activation in mild cognitive impairment compared to normal aging and AD. Neurology. 2005;65:404–11.
78. Bakker A, Krauss GL, Albert MS, Speck CL, Jones LR, Stark CE, Yassa MA, Bassett SS, Shelton AL, Gallagher M. Reduction of hippocampal hyperactivity improves cognition in amnestic mild cognitive impairment. Neuron. 2012;74:467–74.
79. Sperling RA, Laviolette PS, O'Keefe K, O'Brien J, Rentz DM, Pihlajamaki M, Marshall G, Hyman BT, Selkoe DJ, Hedden T, Buckner RL, Becker JA, Johnson KA. Amyloid deposition is associated with impaired default network function in older persons without dementia. Neuron. 2009;63:178–88.
80. Mormino EC, Brandel MG, Madison CM, Marks S, Baker SL, Jagust WJ. Aβ deposition in aging is associated with increases in brain activation during successful memory encoding. Cereb Cortex. 2012;22:1813–23.
81. Lam AD, Deck G, Goldman A, Eskandar EN, Noebels J, Cole AJ. Silent hippocampal seizures and spikes identified by foramen ovale electrodes in Alzheimer's disease. Nat Med. 2017;23:678–80.
82. Vossel KA, Ranasinghe KG, Beagle AJ, Mizuiri D, Honma SM, Dowling AF, Darwish SM, Berlo V, Victoria B, Deborah E, Mantle M, Karydas AM, Coppola G, Roberson ED, Miller BL, Garcia PA, Kirsch HE, Mucke L, Nagarajan SS. Incidence and impact of subclinical epileptiform activity in Alzheimer's disease. Ann Neurol. 2016;80:858–70.
83. Palop JJ, Mucke L. Network abnormalities and interneuron dysfunction in Alzheimer disease. Nat Rev Neurosci. 2016;17:777–92.
84. Sánchez MP, García-Cabrero AM, Sánchez-Elexpuru G, Burgos DF, Serratosa JM. Tau-induced pathology in epilepsy and dementia: notions from patients and animal models. Int J Mol Sci. 2018;19:1092.
85. Beagle AJ, Darwish SM, Ranasinghe KG, La AL, Karageorgiou E, Vossel KA. Relative incidence of seizures and myoclonus in Alzheimer's disease, dementia with lewy bodies, and frontotemporal dementia. J Alzheimers Dis. 2017;60:211–23.

86. Bugiani O, Murrell JR, Giaccone G, Hasegawa M, Ghigo G, Tabaton M, Morbin M, Primavera A, Carella F, Solaro C, Grisoli M, Savoiardo M, Spillantini MG, Tagliavini F, Goedert M, Ghetti B. Frontotemporal dementia and corticobasal degeneration in a family with a P301S mutation in tau. J Neuropathol Exp Neurol. 1999;58:667–77.
87. Nygaard TG, Duvoisin RC, Manocha M, Chokroverty S. Seizures in progressive supranuclear palsy. Neurology. 1989;39:138–40.
88. García-Cabrero AM, Guerrero-López R, Giráldez BG, Llorens-Martín M, Avila J, Serratosa JM, Sánchez MP. Hyperexcitability and epileptic seizures in a model of frontotemporal dementia. Neurobiol Dis. 2013;58:200–8.
89. Walz R, Amaral OB, Rockenbach IC, Roesler R, Izquierdo I, Cavalheiro EA, Martins VR, Brentani RR. Increased sensitivity to seizures in mice lacking cellular prion protein. Epilepsia. 1999;40:1679–82.
90. Bertani I, Iori V, Trusel M, Maroso M, Foray C, Mantovani S, Tonini R, Vezzani A, Chiesa R. Inhibition of IL-1β signaling normalizes NMDA-dependent neurotransmission and reduces seizure susceptibility in a mouse model of Creutzfeldt-Jakob disease. J Neurosci. 2017;37:10278–89.
91. Cloud LJ, Rosenblatt A, Margolis RL, Ross CA, Pillai JA, Corey-Bloom J, Tully HM, Bird T, Panegyres PK, Nichter CA, Higgins DS, Helmers SL, Factor SA, Jones R, Testa CM. Seizures in juvenile Huntington's disease: frequency and characterization in a multicenter cohort. Mov Dis. 2012;27:1797–800.
92. Barker RA, Squiteri F. The clinical phenotype of juvenile Huntington's disease. In: OWJ Q, Brewer HM, Squitieri F, Barker RA, Nance MA, Landwehrmeyer BG, editors. juvenile Huntington's disease and other trinucleotide repeat disorders. New York: Oxford University Press; 2009.
93. Frederiksen KS, Cooper C, Frisoni GB, Lutz F, Jean G. A European Academy of Neurology guideline on medical management issues in dementia. Eur J Neurol. 2020; https://doi.org/10.1111/ene.14412.
94. Jack CR, Holtzman DM. Biomarker modeling of Alzheimer's disease. Neuron. 2013;80:1347–58.
95. Rao SC, Dove G, Cascino GD, Petersen RC. Recurrent seizures in patients with dementia: frequency, seizure types, and treatment outcome. Epilepsy Behav. 2009;14:118–20.
96. Cretin B, Sellal F, Philippi N, Bousiges O, Di Bitonto L, Martin-Hunyadi C, Blanc F. Epileptic prodromal Alzheimer's disease, a retrospective study of 13 new cases: expanding the spectrum of Alzheimer's disease to an epileptic variant? J Alzheimers Dis. 2016;52:1125–33.
97. Sarkis RA, Dickerson BC, Cole AJ, Chemali ZN. Clinical and neurophysiologic characteristics of unprovoked seizures in patients diagnosed with dementia. J Neuropsychiatry Clin Neurosci. 2016;28:56–61.
98. Arnaldi D, Donniaquio A, Mattioli P, Massa F, Grazzini M, Meli R, Filippi L, Grisanti S, FamÃ F, Terzaghi M, Girtler N, Brugnolo A, Doglione E, Pardini M, Villani F, Nobili F. Epilepsy in neurodegenerative dementias: a clinical, epidemiological, and EEG study. J Alzheimers Dis. 2020;74:865–74.
99. Ramsay RE, Rowan AJ, Pryor FM. Special considerations in treating the elderly patient with epilepsy. Neurology. 2004;62:S24–9.
100. Cloyd J, Hauser W, Towne A, Ramsay R, Mattson R, Gilliam F, Walczak T. Epidemiological and medical aspects of epilepsy in the elderly. Epilepsy Res. 2006;68(Suppl 1):S39–48.
101. Beghi E, Carpio A, Forsgren L, Hesdorffer DC, Malmgren K, Sander JW, Tomson T, Hauser WA. Recommendation for a definition of acute symptomatic seizure. Epilepsia. 2010;51:671–5.
102. Trinka E, Cock H, Hesdorffer D, Rossetti AO, Scheffer IE, Shinnar S, Shorvon S, Lowenstein DH. A definition and classification of status epilepticus—report of the ILAE Task Force on Classification of Status Epilepticus. Epilepsia. 2015;56:1515–23.
103. Manfredonia F, Saturno E, Lawley A, Gasverde S, Cavanna AE. Prevalence and clinical correlates of non-convulsive status epilepticus in elderly patients with acute confusional state: a systematic literature review. J Neurol Sci. 2020;410:116674.

104. Beniczky S, Hirsch LJ, Kaplan PW, Pressler R, Bauer G, Aurlien H, Brøgger JC, Trinka E. Unified EEG terminology and criteria for nonconvulsive status epilepticus. Epilepsia. 2013;54(Suppl 6):28–9.
105. Leitinger M, Trinka E, Giovannini G, Zimmermann G, Florea C, Rohracher A, Kalss G, Neuray C, Kreidenhuber R, Höfler J, Kuchukhidze G, Granbichler C, Dobesberger J, Novak HF, Pilz G, Meletti S, Siebert U. Epidemiology of status epilepticus in adults: a population-based study on incidence, causes, and outcomes. Epilepsia. 2019;60:53–62.
106. Leppik IE. Status epilepticus in the elderly. Epilepsia. 2018;59(Suppl 2):140–3.
107. Holtkamp M, Meierkord H. Nonconvulsive status epilepticus: a diagnostic and therapeutic challenge in the intensive care setting. Ther Adv Neurol Disord. 2011;4:169–81.
108. Spitz M, Banbridge J, Winzenburg K, et al. Observations on the delay in diagnosis of seizures in the elderly: update 3. Epilepsia. 2003;44(suppl 9):18.
109. Mantoan L, Kullmann DM. Evaluating first seizures in adults in primary care. Practitioner. 2011;255:25–8, 2–3.
110. NICE. Epilepsies: diagnosis and management. Clinical guideline [CG137]. 2012. Last updated Feb 2020.
111. SIGN. Diagnosis and management of epilepsy in adults. 2015.
112. Mahmoud F, Tampi RR. Valproic acid-induced parkinsonism in the elderly: a comprehensive review of the literature. Am J Geriatr Pharmacother. 2011;9:405–12.
113. Swedish National guidelines on epilepsy. National Board on Health and Welfare, Sweden. 2019.
114. Duncan JS. Brain imaging in epilepsy. Pract Neurol. 2019;19:438–43.
115. Haider HA, Hirsch LJ. Management of epilepsy in the elderly. 2016.
116. Binnie CD. Cognitive impairment during epileptiform discharges: is it ever justifiable to treat the EEG? Lancet Neurol. 2003;2:725–30.
117. Benbadis SR, Tatum WO. Overintepretation of EEGs and misdiagnosis of epilepsy. J Clin Neurophysiol. 2003;20:42–4.
118. Krauss GL, Abdallah A, Lesser R, Thompson RE, Niedermeyer E. Clinical and EEG features of patients with EEG wicket rhythms misdiagnosed with epilepsy. Neurology. 2005;64:1879–83.
119. Smith J. Clinical neurophysiology in the elderly. In: Tallis R, editor. 1989.
120. Canouï-Poitrine F, Bastuji-Garin S, Alonso E, Darcel G, Verstichel P, Caillet P, Paillaud E. Risk and prognostic factors of status epilepticus in the elderly: a case-control study. Epilepsia. 2011;52:1849–56.
121. Leitinger M, Beniczky S, Rohracher A, Gardella E, Kalss G, Qerama E, Höfler J, Hess Lindberg-Larsen A, Kuchukhidze G, Dobesberger J, Langthaler PB, Trinka E. Salzburg Consensus Criteria for Non-Convulsive Status Epilepticus—approach to clinical application. Epilepsy Behav. 2015;49:158–63.
122. Veran O, Kahane P, Thomas P, Hamelin S, Sabourdy C, Vercueil L. De novo epileptic confusion in the elderly: a 1-year prospective study. Epilepsia. 2010;51:1030–5.
123. Naeije G, Depondt C, Meeus C, Korpak K, Pepersack T, Legros B. EEG patterns compatible with nonconvulsive status epilepticus are common in elderly patients with delirium: a prospective study with continuous EEG monitoring. Epilepsy Behav. 2014;36:18–21.
124. Chen L-A, Jou S-B. Status epilepticus in the elderly. Int J Gerontol. 2016;10(1):2–5.
125. Rees JH, Smith SJ, Kullmann DM, Hirsch NP, Howard RS. Creutzfeldt-Jakob disease presenting as complex partial status epilepticus: a report of two cases. J Neurol Neurosurg Psychiatry. 1999;66:406–7.
126. Cohen D, Kutluay E, Edwards J, Peltier A, Beydoun A. Sporadic Creutzfeldt-Jakob disease presenting with nonconvulsive status epilepticus. Epilepsy Behav. 2004;5:792–6.
127. Fernández-Torre JL, Solar DM, Astudillo A, Cereceda R, Acebes A, Calatayud MT. Creutzfeldt-Jakob disease and non-convulsive status epilepticus: a clinical and electroencephalographic follow-up study. Clin Neurophysiol. 2004;115:316–9.
128. Neufeld MY, Talianski-Aronov A, Soffer D, Korczyn AD. Generalized convulsive status epilepticus in Creutzfeldt-Jakob disease. Seizure. 2003;12:403–5.

129. Karatas H, Dericioglu N, Kursun O, Saygi S. Creutzfeldt-Jakob disease presenting as hyperparathyroidism and generalized tonic status epilepticus. Clin EEG Neurosci. 2007;38:203–6.
130. Chiara C, Giovanni A, Giovanni P, Antonella B, Federica A, Francesca U, Fabrizio V, Mario T. Nonconvulsive seizures and dementia: a case report. Int J Alzheimer's Dis. 2011;2011:690305.
131. Sveinsson O, Andersson T, Mattsson P, Carlsson S, Tomson T. Clinical risk factors in SUDEP: a nationwide population-based case-control study. Neurology. 2020;94:e419–29.
132. Vu LC, Piccenna L, Kwan P, O'Brien TJ. New-onset epilepsy in the elderly. Br J Clin Pharmacol. 2018;84:2208–17.
133. Cumbo E, Ligori LD. Levetiracetam, lamotrigine, and phenobarbital in patients with epileptic seizures and Alzheimer's disease. Epilepsy Behav. 2010;17:461–6.
134. Bakker A, Albert MS, Krauss G, Speck CL, Gallagher M. Response of the medial temporal lobe network in amnestic mild cognitive impairment to therapeutic intervention assessed by fMRI and memory task performance. NeuroImage Clin. 2015;7:688–98.
135. Bergey GK. Initial treatment of epilepsy: special issues in treating the elderly. Neurology. 2004;63:S40–8.
136. Chuang YC, Chuang HY, Chan SH. Effects of long-term antiepileptic drug monotherapy on vascular risk factors and atherosclerosis. Epilepsia. 2012;53(1):120–8.
137. Sarycheva T, Lavikainen P, Tolppanen AM. Antiepileptic drug use and mortality among community-dwelling persons with Alzheimer disease. Neurology. 2020;94:e2099–108.
138. Sarycheva T, Lavikainen P, Tolppanen AM. Antiepileptic drug use and the risk of stroke among community-dwelling people with Alzheimer disease: a matched cohort study. J Am Heart Assoc. 2018;7(18):e009742.
139. Brodie MJ, Overstall PW, Giorgi L. Multicentre, double-blind, randomised comparison between lamotrigine and carbamazepine in elderly patients with newly diagnosed epilepsy. The UK Lamotrigine Elderly Study Group. Epilepsy Res. 1999;37:81–7.
140. Rowan AJ, Ramsay RE, Collins JF, Pryor F, Boardman KD, Uthman BM, Spitz M, Frederick T, Towne A, Carter GS, Marks W, Felicetta J, Tomyanovich ML, V.A. Cooperative Study 428 Group. New onset geriatric epilepsy: a randomized study of gabapentin, lamotrigine, and carbamazepine. Neurology. 2005;64:1868–73.
141. Saetre E, Perucca E, Isojärvi J, Gjerstad L, L.A.M. 40089 Study Group. An international multicenter randomized double-blind controlled trial of lamotrigine and sustained-release carbamazepine in the treatment of newly diagnosed epilepsy in the elderly. Epilepsia. 2007;48:1292–302.
142. Werhahn KJ, Trinka E, Dobesberger J, Unterberger I, Baum P, Deckert-Schmitz M, Kniess T, Schmitz B, Bernedo V, Ruckes C, Ehrlich A, Krämer G. A randomized, double-blind comparison of antiepileptic drug treatment in the elderly with new-onset focal epilepsy. Epilepsia. 2015;56:450–9.
143. Liu J, Wang L-N, Wu L-Y, Wang Y-P. Treatment of epilepsy for people with Alzheimer's disease. Cochrane Database Syst Rev. 2018;12:CD011922.
144. Ferrendelli JA, French J, Leppik I, Morrell MJ, Herbeuval A, Han J, Magnus L. Use of levetiracetam in a population of patients aged 65 years and older: a subset analysis of the KEEPER trial. Epilepsy Behav. 2003;4:702–9.
145. Kutlu G, Gomceli YB, Unal Y, Inan LE. Levetiracetam monotherapy for late poststroke seizures in the elderly. Epilepsy Behav. 2008;13:542–4.
146. Shorvon S, Perucca E, Engel J Jr. The treatment of epilepsy. London: Wiley Blackwell; 2016.
147. Lynch BA, Lambeng N, Nocka K, Kensel-Hammes P, Bajjalieh SM, Matagne A, Fuks B. The synaptic vesicle protein SV2A is the binding site for the antiepileptic drug levetiracetam. Proc Natl Acad Sci U S A. 2004;101:9861–6.
148. Meehan AL, Yang X, McAdams BD, Yuan L, Rothman SM. A new mechanism for antiepileptic drug action: vesicular entry may mediate the effects of levetiracetam. J Neurophysiol. 2011;106:1227–39.

149. Belcastro V, Costa C, Galletti F, Pisani F, Calabresi P, Parnetti L. Levetiracetam monotherapy in Alzheimer patients with late-onset seizures: a prospective observational study. Eur J Neurol. 2007;14:1176–8.
150. Chong DJ, French JA. Levetiracetam. London: Wiley Blackwell; 2016.
151. Riaz A, Matsuo F. Lamotrigine. London: Wiley Blackwell; 2016.
152. Cheung H, Kamp D, Harris E. An in vitro investigation of the action of lamotrigine on neuronal voltage-activated sodium channels. Epilepsy Res. 1992;13:107–12.
153. Lang DG, Wang CM, Cooper BR. Lamotrigine, phenytoin and carbamazepine interactions on the sodium current present in N4TG1 mouse neuroblastoma cells. J Pharmacol Exp Ther. 1993;266:829–35.
154. Meldrum BS, Leach M. The mechanism of action of lamotrigine. Rev Contemp Pharmacother. 1994;5:107–14.
155. Cunningham MO, Jones RS. The anticonvulsant, lamotrigine decreases spontaneous glutamate release but increases spontaneous GABA release in the rat entorhinal cortex in vitro. Neuropharmacology. 2000;39:2139–46.
156. Tekin S, Aykut-Bingöl C, Tanridağ T, Aktan S. Antiglutamatergic therapy in Alzheimer's disease—effects of lamotrigine. Short communication. J Neural Transm (Vienna). 1996;105(1998):295–303.
157. Blum D, Meador K, Biton V, Fakhoury T, Shneker B, Chung S, Mills K, Hammer A, Isojärvi J. Cognitive effects of lamotrigine compared with topiramate in patients with epilepsy. Neurology. 2006;67:400–6.
158. Pressler RM, Binnie CD, Coleshill SG, Chorley GA, Robinson RO. Effect of lamotrigine on cognition in children with epilepsy. Neurology. 2006;66:1495–9.
159. Mockenhaupt M, Messenheimer J, Tennis P, Schlingmann J. Risk of Stevens-Johnson syndrome and toxic epidermal necrolysis in new users of antiepileptics. Neurology. 2005;64:1134–8.
160. Somerville ER, Michell AW, Sen A. Gabapentin. London: Wiley Blackwell; 2016.
161. Marais E, Klugbauer N, Hofmann F. Calcium channel alpha(2)delta subunits-structure and Gabapentin binding. Mol Pharmacol. 2001;59:1243–8.
162. Taylor CP, Angelotti T, Fauman E. Pharmacology and mechanism of action of pregabalin: the calcium channel alpha2-delta (alpha2-delta) subunit as a target for antiepileptic drug discovery. Epilepsy Res. 2007;73:137–50.
163. Johannessen SI, Battino D, Berry DJ, Bialer M, Krämer G, Tomson T, Patsalos PN. Therapeutic drug monitoring of the newer antiepileptic drugs. Ther Drug Monit. 2003;25:347–63.
164. Faught E, Kim H. Oxcarbazepine. London: Wiley Blackwell; 2016.
165. Tambucci R, Basti C, Maresca M, Coppola G, Verrotti A. Update on the role of eslicarbazepine acetate in the treatment of partial-onset epilepsy. Neuropsychiatr Dis Treat. 2016;12:1251–60.
166. Trinka E, Ben-Menachem E, Kowacs PA, Elger C, Keller B, Löffler K, Rocha JF, Soares-da-Silva P. Efficacy and safety of eslicarbazepine acetate versus controlled-release carbamazepine monotherapy in newly diagnosed epilepsy: a phase III double-blind, randomized, parallel-group, multicenter study. Epilepsia. 2018;59:479–91.
167. Sachdeo RC, Wasserstein A, Mesenbrink PJ, D'Souza J. Effects of oxcarbazepine on sodium concentration and water handling. Ann Neurol. 2002;51:613–20.
168. Gómez-Ibáñez A, Serratosa JM, Guillamón E, Garcés M, Giráldez BG, Toledo M, Salas-Puig J, López-González FJ, Rodríguez-Uranga J, Castillo A, Mauri JA, Camacho JL, López-Gomáriz E, Giner P, Torres N, Palau J, Molins A, Villanueva V. Efficacy and safety of eslicarbazepine-acetate in elderly patients with focal epilepsy: case series. Seizure. 2017;48:53–6.
169. Kutluay E, McCague K, D'Souza J, Beydoun A. Safety and tolerability of oxcarbazepine in elderly patients with epilepsy. Epilepsy Behav. 2003;4:175–80.
170. Bauer S, Willems LM, Paule E, Petschow C, Zöllner JP, Rosenow F, Strzelczyk A. The efficacy of lacosamide as monotherapy and adjunctive therapy in focal epilepsy and its use in status epilepticus: clinical trial evidence and experience. Ther Adv Neurol Disord. 2017;10:103–26.

171. Wong PA, Bainbridge J, Spitz M, Frey L, Dees C, et al. Retrospective study of lacosamide in the elderly (≥60 years of age). Clin Ther. 2015;37:e134.
172. Sarkis RA, Nicolas J, Lee JW. Tolerability of lacosamide or zonisamide in elderly patients with seizures. Seizure. 2017;49:1–4.
173. Rainesalo S, Mäkinen J, Raitanen J, Peltola J. Clinical management of elderly patients with epilepsy; the use of lacosamide in a single center setting. Epilepsy Behav. 2017;75:86–9.
174. Rosenow F, Toledo M, Baulac M, et al. Efficacy and tolerability of lacosamide monotherapy in elderly patients with newly diagnosed epilepsy: subgroup analysis of a non-inferiority trial versus controlled-release carbamazepine (P5.232). Neurology. 2017.
175. Bainbridge J, Backer D, Marc E, Klaus T, Frank B, Sabine S, David W, Konrad J, Shaibani A, Faught E. Safety and tolerability of lacosamide monotherapy in the elderly: a subgroup analysis from lacosamide trials in diabetic neuropathic pain. Epilepsia Open. 2017;2:415–23.
176. UCBPharma. Lacosamide summary of product characteristics. 2019.
177. Cawello W, Bonn R, Boekens H. Bioequivalence of intravenous and oral formulations of the antiepileptic drug lacosamide. Pharmacology. 2012;90:40–6.
178. Ramsay RE, Uthman B, Pryor FM, Rowan AJ, Bainbridge J, Spitz M, Sirven JI, Frederick TE. Topiramate in older patients with partial-onset seizures: a pilot double-blind, dose-comparison study. Epilepsia. 2008;49:1180–5.
179. Cross HJ, Riney CJ. Topiramate. London: Wiley Blackwell; 2016.
180. Mula M, Trimble MR, Lhatoo SD, Sander JWAS. Topiramate and psychiatric adverse events in patients with epilepsy. Epilepsia. 2003;44:659–63.
181. European Medicines Agency. Fycompa summary of product characteristics. 2016.
182. Stephen LJ, Brodie MJ. Brivaracetam: a novel antiepileptic drug for focal-onset seizures. Ther Adv Neurol Disord. 2018;11:1756285617742081.
183. Brodie MJ, Whitesides J, Schiemann J, D'Souza J, Johnson ME. Tolerability, safety, and efficacy of adjunctive brivaracetam for focal seizures in older patients: a pooled analysis from three phase III studies. Epilepsy Res. 2016;127:114–8.
184. Tomson T, Johannessen SI. Carbamazepine. London: Wiley Blackwell; 2016.
185. Van Amelsvoort T, Bakshi R, Devaux CB, Schwabe S. Hyponatremia associated with carbamazepine and oxcarbazepine therapy: a review. Epilepsia. 1994;35:181–8.
186. Sander JW. The use of antiepileptic drugs—principles and practice. Epilepsia. 2004;45(Suppl 6):28–34.
187. Tsiouris JA, Patti PJ, Tipu O, Raguthu S. Adverse effects of phenytoin given for late-onset seizures in adults with Down syndrome. Neurology. 2002;59:779–80.
188. Tariot PN, Schneider LS, Cummings J, Thomas RG, Raman R, Jakimovich LJ, Loy R, Bartocci B, Fleisher A, Ismail MS, Porsteinsson A, Weiner M, Jack CR, Thal L, Aisen PS, Alzheimer's Disease Cooperative Study Group. Chronic divalproex sodium to attenuate agitation and clinical progression of Alzheimer disease. Arch Gen Psychiatry. 2011;68:853–61.
189. Fleisher AS, Truran D, Mai JT, Langbaum JBS, Aisen PS, Cummings JL, Jack CR, Weiner MW, Thomas RG, Schneider LS, Tariot PN, Alzheimer's Disease Cooperative Study. Chronic divalproex sodium use and brain atrophy in Alzheimer disease. Neurology. 2011;77:1263–71.
190. Perucca E. Pharmacological and therapeutic properties of valproate: a summary after 35 years of clinical experience. CNS Drugs. 2002;16:695–714.
191. Verrotti A, Trotta D, Morgese G, Chiarelli F. Valproate-induced hyperammonemic encephalopathy. Metab Brain Dis. 2002;17:367–73.
192. Billioti de Gage S, Pariente A, Bégaud B. Is there really a link between benzodiazepine use and the risk of dementia? Expert Opin Drug Saf. 2015;14:733–47.
193. By the 2019 American Geriatrics Society Beers Criteria® Update Expert Panel. American Geriatrics Society 2019 Updated AGS Beers Criteria® for potentially inappropriate medication use in older adults. J Am Geriatr Soc. 67(2019):674–94.
194. Fu J, Peng L, Li J, Tao T, Chen Y. Effects of second-generation antiepileptic drugs compared to first-generation antiepileptic drugs on bone metabolism in patients with epilepsy: a meta-analysis. Horm Metab Res = Hormon- und Stoffwechselforschung = Hormones et metabolisme. 2019;51:511–21.

195. Guerrini R, Belmonte A, Canapicchi R, Casalini C, Perucca E. Reversible pseudoatrophy of the brain and mental deterioration associated with valproate treatment. Epilepsia. 1998;39:27–32.
196. Ziyeh S, Thiel T, Spreer J, Klisch J, Schumacher M. Valproate-induced encephalopathy: assessment with MR imaging and 1H MR spectroscopy. Epilepsia. 2002;43:1101–5.
197. Ristić AJ, Vojvodić N, Janković S, Sindelić A, Sokić D. The frequency of reversible parkinsonism and cognitive decline associated with valproate treatment: a study of 364 patients with different types of epilepsy. Epilepsia. 2006;47:2183–5.
198. Beyenburg S, Back C, Diederich N, Lewis M, Reuber M. Is valproate encephalopathy underrecognised in older people? A case series. Age Ageing. 2007;36(3):344–6.
199. Evans MD, Shinar R, Yaari R. Reversible dementia and gait disturbance after prolonged use of valproic acid. Seizure. 2011;20(6):509–11.

Physical and Cognitive Exercise for Patients with Dementia

13

Kristian Steen Frederiksen

List of Abbreviations

AD	Alzheimer's disease
ADL	Activities of daily living
BDNF	Brain-derived neurotrophic factor
CS	Cognitive stimulation
EEG	Electroencephalography
MCI	Mild cognitive impairment
QoL	Quality of life
RCT	Randomized controlled trial
rs-fMRI	Resting state functional MRI

Introduction

Physical and cognitive exercise (in this chapter, cognitive exercise refers to cognitive stimulation and cognitive training) for patients with dementia encompass a somewhat heterogeneous group of interventions which vary greatly with regard to design, implementation, targeted population, and efficacy. The term non-pharmacological treatments may at times be used to encompass these types of specific interventions. Although it is difficult to define what is meant by non-pharmacological treatment, it is implicit that such treatments do not include stand-alone pharmacological treatment, and usually also do not include invasive

K. S. Frederiksen (✉)
Danish Dementia Research Centre, Department of Neurology, Rigshospitalet, University of Copenhagen, Copenhagen, Denmark
e-mail: Kristian.steen.frederiksen@regionh.dk

K. S. Frederiksen, G. Waldemar (eds.), *Management of Patients with Dementia*,
https://doi.org/10.1007/978-3-030-77904-7_13

procedures such as surgery. They are rarely alternatives to pharmacological treatment but are often adjuvants to it, e.g. by interacting with pharmacological treatments, mitigating side-effects or improving compliance. This is also true for physical and cognitive exercise.

This chapter will give an overview of the evidence that exists regarding possible effects of physical and cognitive exercise in dementia.

Methodological Considerations

Physical and cognitive exercise may be considered complex interventions. Complex interventions have several interacting components (e.g., exercise may have an effect on the cardiorespiratory system, coordination/balance and may also have an effect by the social interaction) and may include behaviors by those who deliver and receive the intervention which have a high degree of difficulty. Indeed, some interventions may not be immediately implementable in clinical practice in a particular center or nursing home but may require staff training or training of caregivers or the need for adaptation of the usual clinical routine in order to accommodate the treatment [1, 2]. Moreover, some degree of flexibility may be necessary in order to ensure the ability of the treatment to be implemented in variable settings.

This also raises the issue of how such interventions can be evaluated for efficacy as the methodology used in randomized controlled trials (RCTs) of pharmacological treatments may be inappropriate or not transferable to the evaluation of exercise interventions. Physical and cognitive exercise interventions, together with other non-pharmacological treatments should ideally be evidence-based and thus despite obstacles to the evaluation, rigor in the assessment must be maintained and insisted upon. This is also important from a patient safety point of view, since although the interventions are generally considered safe and with relatively few adverse effects, such cannot be ruled out before evaluation. Moreover, implementing non-pharmacological treatments will often be associated with resource-consumption which will prohibit other activities, and it is obviously counter-productive to introduce treatments for which there is evidence of no effect.

For the aforementioned reasons, the UK Medical Research Counsel has developed a methodological framework for the evaluation of complex interventions, such as physical and cognitive exercise, from hypothesis generation to implementation, and also suggests various study designs and other methodologies (e.g., consideration of alternative endpoints or study designs) adjusted to the evaluation of complex interventions [3]. In this vein it should also be kept in mind for clinicians and others evaluating the literature on exercise and other non-pharmacological treatments in dementia that the usual gold standard for the evaluation of pharmacological treatments, i.e. a double-blinded RCT, will be unattainable for interventions such as physical exercise. Indeed, it may be an inappropriate methodology for evaluating a large proportion of non-pharmacological interventions.

Physical Exercise

For many years, exercise has received increasing attention as an important factor in maintaining health and wellbeing for humans of all ages. From an evolutionary point of view, being physically active has always been a stable of human existence as the vast majority of our time as a species have been spent as hunter-gatherers employing a strategy which involved traveling large distances by foot at a relatively high speed [4]. It is, therefore, not surprising that physical activity may impact on many organs and organ systems, and that physical inactivity may have detrimental impact on health. In other words, physical activity is a prerequisite for good health even in old age and in the presence of chronic diseases. In this vein, and specifically related to the brain it is interesting to note that the evolution of Homo Sapiens from apes coincided with a remodeling and growth of skeletal muscle and the brain in parallel further highlighting a linkage between muscle and brain [4]. This goes beyond the mere control of muscle which is subserved by a number of central and peripheral nervous system parts. However, this evolutionary perspective is more indicative of the role of physical exercise in the prevention of the occurrence of disease, and less so to the treatment of an acquired diseases such as dementia. Nevertheless, an interest in this aspect with regard to dementia and mild cognitive impairment (MCI) has become an increasing focal point in research within recent years as evidence has accumulated of an effect of physical exercise on the brain and symptoms of dementia. Physical activity has been defined according to the World Health Organization stating that "physical activity as any bodily movement produced by skeletal muscles that requires energy expenditure. Physical activity refers to all movement including during leisure time, for transport to get to and from places, or as part of a person's work" [5], whereas physical exercise is physical activity that is planned, structured, and repetitive for the purpose of conditioning any part of the body. Thus, some persons may have a very physically active life but enjoy little physical exercise, whereas for others, the physical activity in their lives consists of exercise. For patients with dementia, having a physically active life may be difficult due to impairments prohibiting engagement in normal activities such as gardening and housekeeping or walking, and physical exercise may not be accessible to patients with dementia. For example, for persons with dementia exercise may need to be specifically tailored, or they may reside in assisted living facilities where physical exercise may not be made available.

Exercise and the Brain: Effects and Underlying Mechanisms

A large number of studies using different methods of investigation such as electroencephalography (EEG), brain scans, cognitive testing, biochemical analysis, and genetic and epigenetic analysis have studied the effects of exercise on the brain and possible underlying mechanisms (Fig. 13.1).

It has become evident from a number of studies using structural MR scans of the brain that being physically active affects the structural properties of the brain.

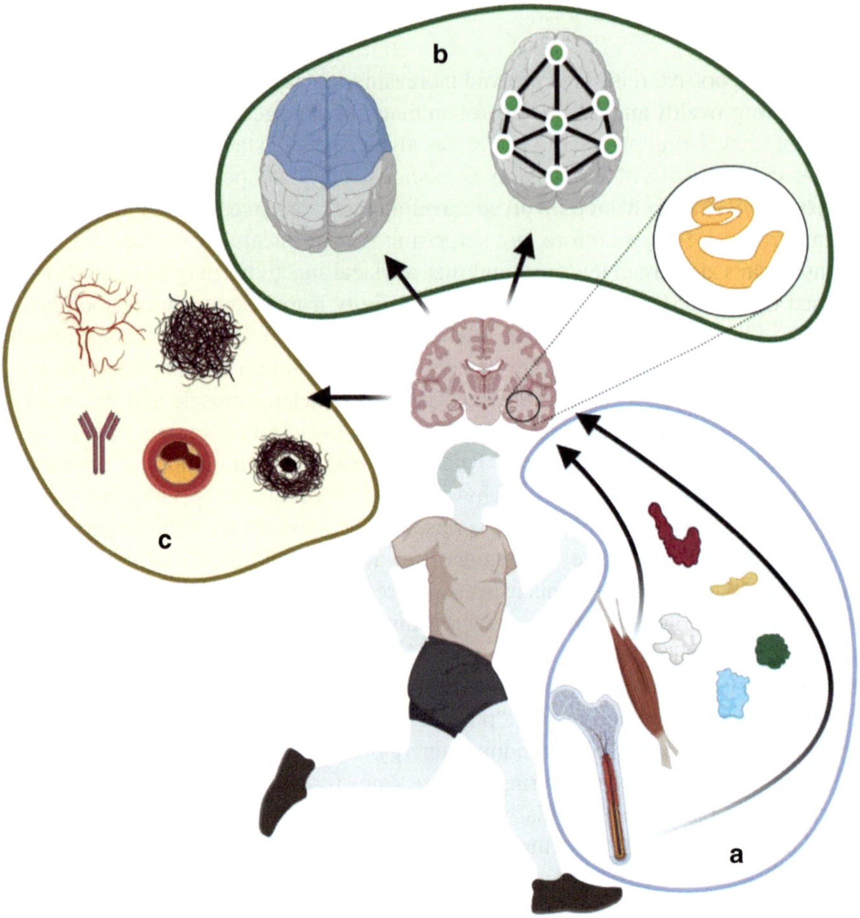

Fig. 13.1 Role of exerkines in the effects of exercise on the brain. A number of exerkines (**a**) such as brain-derived neurotrophic factor (BDNF), irisin, cathepsin B, interleukine-6, and other molecules from muscle and osteocalcin from bone may be released into the blood stream and enter the brain (brain–muscle cross-talk). Evidence from animal and human studies suggest a possible effect of exercise on a number of brain regions (**b**) such as the hippocampus, frontal cortical areas, and brain networks. Other effects may be mediated through an effect on beta-amyloid, vascular pathology, angiogenesis, neurogenesis, and anti-inflammatory effects

Evidence comes from observational studies offering indirect evidence, but data from interventional studies also support this. A relatively large focus has been on the hippocampus with earlier studies finding the hippocampus to be especially responsive to exercise in terms of volume change [6–8]. Subsequent studies in humans have however, been less convincing, and a relatively recent meta-analysis pooling 14 studies failed to find convincing evidence for an effect [9]. Intriguingly, the hippocampus is one of the few areas in the brain where adult neurogenesis has been shown to occur in humans [10], and it has been speculated that an effect may be mediated through stimulation of neurogenesis [11]. Animal studies support the notion that exercise preserves adult neurogenesis in the dentate gyrus in Alzheimer's disease (AD) mice, and thus may also hint at a role in patients with AD regarding exercise [12]. Studies examining hippocampal subfields have not been able to find that exercise specifically stimulates volume changes in the dentate gyrus [13, 14], where adult neurogenesis takes place [10]. Maass et al. investigated whether vascular plasticity in the hippocampus was affected by a 3-month aerobic exercise program in sedentary older adults (60–77 years) and found that perfusion increased in the oldest participants and that change was correlated with improvements in hippocampus-dependent cognitive tasks [15]. This thus indicates that an effect of exercise on the hippocampus may be mediated by other mechanisms than volumetric changes. Long-term potentiation, which is believed to be the cellular basis of memory formation, and alterations in neurocircuitry may be other changes induced in the hippocampus by exercise which may not lead to volume changes [16], but may nevertheless improve hippocampal function such as memory.

Other areas of the brain are also possibly affected by exercise including frontal areas and the white matter. Regarding the white matter, fractional anisotropy, a measure of microstructural integrity derived from diffusion-weighted MRI, in the corpus callosum was cross-sectionally correlated with peak oxygen uptake in one study [17], but findings in the corpus callosum are not consistent across studies [18]. In a large observational study, measures of cardiorespiratory fitness and whole brain white matter integrity 5 years after assessment were found to be associated [19], and in another large study, self-reported physical activity was associated with preserved integrity of frontal lobe tracts including the genu of corpus callosum, uncinate fasciculus, external capsule, and anterior limb of the internal capsule [20]. Lastly, and in a smaller study, amount of physical activity was associated with higher integrity of white matter of the left fornix [21]. Moving to intervention studies, whole brain white matter atrophy in older women was attenuated following a 2 year resistance exercise program [22], and in another study, 1 year of weekly aerobic exercise also improved white matter microstructure in frontal areas [23]. As interventions of shorter duration did not lead to changes in the white matter [24, 25], it may be speculated that longer interventions may be needed to affect white matter. Since the primary function of white matter tracts is as structural connections between different cortical and subcortical areas, assessing the effects of exercise on neural networks may be an indirect way to assess white matter function. Two commonly applied methods to assess networks are resting state functional MRI (rs-fMRI) and resting state EEG. Gramkow et al. reviewed the literature regarding the effects of acute exercise interventions on resting state EEG and found that in general, studies were small, with varying methodologies and low methodological quality [26]. It was not possible to arrive at any conclusion regarding effects on networks, and an effect of exercise on the delta band was the most consistent finding [26]. Regarding rs-fMRI, Dorsman et al. longitudinally investigated 212 healthy elderly persons and found that inter-network inter-subject synchronicity in subcortical and frontal-subcortical networks increased with amount of self-reported physical activity over time. There was no association between other networks and physical activity, including the default-mode network [27]. A small number of intervention studies have also investigated the effects of exercise on network connectivity and other metrics, and effects have been reported for the sensori-motor network [28], default-mode network [29, 30], and fronto-parietal network [29].

A comprehensive review of the literature regarding exercise and cognition in older adults is not possible in this chapter, but the evidence has recently been reviewed in a systematic review [31] and a meta-analysis [32]. Especially executive functions are improved by exercise, but also attention and processing speed [33] are affected. These cognitive functions are primarily reliant on frontal brain areas as well as more distributed brain networks, and thus in line with findings from MRI studies. This further highlights the notion that these parts of the brain are amenable to exercise. Also yoga [34] and Tai-Chi [35] seem to improve attention and processing speed. Indeed both aerobic, stretching and Tai-Chi are effective [32]. Chen et al. in their meta-analysis [32] found a possible dose-response effect for both frequency, intensity, duration and session duration. Whether memory is affected by exercise is less certain [36], but cannot be ruled out [37].

Despite the evidence suggesting a positive effect of exercise on brain structure and function, it remains largely unknown exactly what underlying mechanisms couple exercise and the brain. One intriguing possibility is that signaling molecules from peripheral tissues outside the brain such as muscle and bone are released into the blood stream and induce the changes. Skeletal muscle is metabolically very active during exercise, but also bone is activated by exercise, and both release molecules with autocrine, paracrine, and endocrine functions [38]. For muscle, these substances have been termed myokines, or, to reflect their relationship with exercise, exerkines [39] (Fig. 13.1). These include brain-derived neurotrophic factor (BDNF), irisin, cathepsin B, interleukine-6, and other molecules. BDNF has been most extensively investigated regarding an effect on the brain [39–43]. For bone and brain interaction, osteocalcin has been investigated [38, 44] and other candidates have been reviewed previously [38, 45]. Animal and cellular studies have shown that BDNF is associated with hippocampal function and is actively secreted [46]. In humans, a polymorphism in the gene coding for BDNF which leads to either a valine or methionine amino acid in BDNF has been shown to confer an increased risk of AD [47], and to modulate the protective effects of exercise on incident dementia [48] and interacts with the relationship between physical activity and hippocampal and temporal lobe volume [49]. Interestingly, in one study using a transgenic mouse model transfected with the methionine polymorphism, activation-induced secretion was reduced indicating that levels of BDNF protein have an important role [46]. A number of animal studies have further demonstrated that production and secretion of BDNF is induced by exercise. In humans, an acute bout of exercise in patients with depression increased serum BDNF [50], but a meta-analysis of chronic interventions in the same patient group did not find a similar increase [51]. This indicates that there may be a transient and immediate increase of BDNF following exercise but that the more tonic secretion is not affected by exercise. This may hint at two fundamentally different effects of exercise on the brain, i.e. an acute effect possibly mediated through exerkines/myokines and a chronic effect partly mediated by other mechanisms (e.g., vascular, anti-inflammatory), but this remains speculative. BDNF has been coupled to a number of effects in the brain most principally neurogenesis [52], but also beta-amyloid production [53] and hippocampal dendritic spine density [54], and the exact linkage between exercise, BDNF, and the brain remains elusive. The evidence for a link between other myokines/exerkines and the brain remains less well examined.

Effects of Exercise in MCI and Dementia

The interest in exercise as a possible adjunctive therapy in dementia and especially AD is to some degree motivated by two lines of evidence. Firstly, animal studies have shown that exercise may remove pathological aggregates of protein and may ameliorate other pathological changes in the brain, and thus that being physically active reduces the risk of dementia and AD through these mechanisms [55]. Secondly, in observational studies physical activity has been shown to reduce the risk of cognitive decline [56].

In animal models of AD, exercise seems to effectively reduce the pathological deposition of beta-amyloid, a protein which is believed to be a central player in AD pathophysiology. This may happen through increased clearance, promotion of the non-amyloidogenic pathway, and reduced production of beta-amyloid [57–60]. Moreover, exercise also modulates tau protein and hippocampal volume, two other pathological hallmarks of AD [61, 62]. However, evidence remains scarce regarding this effect in humans. In a study of 16 weeks of aerobic exercise compared to usual care in patients with AD, cortical beta-amyloid was not reduced [63]. This to date remains the only study in which the hypothesis has been tested, and the negative finding may be due to the short intervention warranting further studies. Data on this issue from observational studies is inconclusive and neither support nor negate that physical activity is associated with reduced beta-amyloid (reviewed in [64]). Two studies examined the effects of exercise on hippocampus in AD patients [65, 66] and were not able to show an effect. Similarly, observational studies have not been able to establish a connection between physical activity and hippocampal volume in AD patients [67, 68].

Several studies have found that exercise mitigates symptoms of dementia and AD dementia. Exercise has been found to both reduce behavioral and psychological symptoms of dementia, improve activities of daily living (ADL) and improve cognition, and not only in patients with AD (e.g., [69–72]). This clearly demonstrates the potential of exercise as a component in the treatment of dementia. As in elderly persons without cognitive impairment, exercise seems to affect executive functions more than memory, but also general cognition [73]. Moderate to high intensity exercise is feasible in AD patients [74] and there may be a dose-dependent effect [70], although relatively low-intensity exercise has also been reported to improve cognition [75]. The effect on ADL may be mediated through an effect on physical function, but may also be mediated through an effect on executive function [76]. Moreover, this may be due to a differential effect on more difficult ADL, so-called instrumental ADL, which may be more reliant on cognitive functions, and thus be less affected by exercise [77].

Planning and Adapting Exercise to Patients with Cognitive Impairment and Dementia

One of the advantages of physical exercise as an intervention in patients with dementia is that it may be modified and adapted to fit different needs such as preferences and abilities of patients, and available equipment and physical surroundings. It may also be combined with other interventions. Both aerobic, strength exercise, flexibility and balance training may be beneficial for patients with dementia. Moreover, exercise may be carried out inside or outside, in groups or individually, at home, in care facilities or in gyms. Some patients may prefer fitness training, whereas others prefer soccer, badminton, swimming, or other sports.

Some patients in the MCI or mild dementia stage will be able to participate in exercise and sports on equal terms with patients without cognitive impairment. However, a large share of patients will be dependent on a degree of adaptation of the activities to accommodate impairments in cognition and physical disability in order to exercise.

A myriad of different forms of exercise are feasible and acceptable to patients with dementia, such as moderate-to-high intensity aerobic exercise [36, 78], Tai-Chi [79], telemedicine based exercise interventions [80], strength exercise [81], and walking programs [82], but it is important to be aware of possible barriers to participation. In a systematic review, the following groupings of barriers were found for patients with dementia in care homes: physical health and mental wellbeing related reasons (e.g., acute illness, anxiety, fear of injury and frailty, low levels of previous activity level), relationship dynamics (e.g., disagreement within the group, family miscommunication), and socioeconomic reasons (e.g., low staffing levels). Similarly, a number of facilitators were identified: bio-medical benefits and benefits related to physical ability (e.g., physiological benefits, wellbeing), feelings and emotions and confidence improvements (e.g., mastery of engagement, empowerment, self-worth, regaining control), therapist, staff, and group relationship dynamics (e.g., anticipating challenges, availability of staff, motivating nursing assistants), activity related (e.g., allowing space for gaming approach, flexible approach, tailoring its approach and its safeness) [83]. A piloting phase may be advisable also outside research settings [74] as this will help adjust the exercise program to the specific needs of individual patients and patient group.

Another relevant consideration is whether exercise should be group-based or individual. Group-based exercise has a social component, which may give additional benefit. Many patients will need some guidance and assistance, and group-based exercise will enable a single instructor to oversee more patients at once than is possible with individual training, which may thus be more cost effective.

Unsupervised exercise may be feasible in some patients [84] but may also be associated with lower adherence [85]. Group-based exercise will usually be conducted outside the home for community dwelling patients. This may function as a "break" for family caregivers living with the patient, but also necessitates transport to the place where the activity will be organized. Prevention of injuries will include proper warm-up, adequate training, supervision by trained personnel, adequate equipment and clothing, and adaptation of the exercises to participants' cognitive impairment [74]. In this regard it is also important to be mindful of the risk of weight-loss which is often unwanted in patients with dementia as the disease itself means that patients are at risk of unwanted weight-loss (e.g., due to loss of appetite and forgetfulness regarding meals) (Table 13.1).

It is not possible from the literature to establish a lower limit to the exercise intensity or frequency of exercise which may elicit a benefit for patients with dementia. In this regard it is important to emphasize that apart from an effect on specific symptoms of dementia such as cognitive impairment, patients with

Table 13.1 Consideration regarding delivery of exercise programs to patients with dementia

Before an exercise program
Intended target population
• Degree of cognitive impairment and specific cognitive impairment (e.g., language comprehension problems, visuospatial) • Other symptoms of dementia (e.g., aggression, agitation) • Comorbidities and medication (e.g., musculoskeletal problems, beta-blockers (limits pulse increase)) • Community dwelling or assisted living • Motivations and previous experience with exercise
Setting and organization
• Individualized or group-based, at home or in a gym or other facility • Supervision and qualifications of those supervising • Need for transportation
Type of exercise
• Aerobic, strength, stretching, balance • On exercise machines, team sports, outside, indoors
Identify facilitatory and barriers
• Economic, resources, lack of previous experience, lack of a caregiver • Motivational factors (e.g., social element, providing music for exercise, small competitive elements, defining individual goals)
Consider safety
• Provide information about proper shoes and clothing • Information about warming up • Designing a ramp-up period in the intervention
During an exercise program
Make room for adaptation on the individual basis Consider barriers and facilitatory factors that may become evident during the program Be mindful of injuries Be mindful of caregiver burden associated with the patient's participation
After an exercise program
Give advice on maintenance of exercise habits

dementia will of course also benefit in other areas typically associated with engagement in exercise such as improved physical function and decreased risk of cardiovascular disease. In one study, patients with mild dementia improved cardiorespiratory fitness following a moderate-to-high intensity aerobic exercise intervention of 1-h session 3 times weekly for 16 weeks [86]. In a subset of patients participating in more than 66.7% of the offered sessions, improvements in walking speed and timed-up-and-go (a mobility measure) were observed [86]. Interestingly, in the same study, only those participants engaging in most of the offered exercise sessions improved on the cognitive outcome measure [86]. Two messages may be gleaned from these observations: (1) as for persons without dementia, there is a dose-response regarding improvements of physical fitness such as cardiorespiratory, and that ideally, one should engage in exercise a minimum of 2 times weekly, (2) that improvements in cognition may only be evident in patients who exercise at a relatively high intensity and frequency. However, this assumes that a possible effect on cognition is mediated either through improvement in cardiorespiratory fitness or a process which improves parallel with cardiorespiratory fitness. This remains speculative and needs to be examined in further studies examining the underlying mechanisms linking exercise and the brain.

Conclusion

Physical exercise is undoubtedly a prerequisite for health and longevity in humans. In patients with dementia, there may be an additional effect, as studies have found an effect of exercise on cognitive function and other symptoms. Processing speed, mental speed, and executive function may be especially sensitive to an effect of exercise, but memory may also be improved. Underlying mechanisms remain undetermined, but effects on frontal brain regions are plausible, whereas data for an effect on the hippocampus is less convincing. The role of myokines remains to be investigated. Exercise is a very flexible intervention which is applicable to any stage of the disease including in the severe stages of a dementia disorder, but appropriate measures to facilitate and to limit barriers for persons with dementia to exercise must be taken.

Cognitive Stimulation and Training

Cognitive stimulation (CS), cognitive training, and cognitive rehabilitation (latter covered in Chap. 14) are sometimes used interchangeable in research literature and in writings on their practical implementation. This has led to some confusion, and at present there are no definitions which are uniformly accepted. Indeed, elements of the three practices also overlap. However, a number of distinct characteristics unique for each of the approaches may be stated which has some validity and function, in that they relate to different underlying theoretical, conceptual assumptions, core elements and target populations, and therefore may have utility. All three

Table 13.2 Cognitive stimulation, cognitive training, cognitive rehabilitation

	Intervention—description	Target population	Setting	Possible mechanism of action	Goal
Cognitive stimulation	General activities believed to stimulate cognition	MCI, mild, dementia, moderate dementia	Usually in groups	General stimulation of cognition	Prevent decline ("use it or loose it")
Cognitive training	Tasks designed to train cognitive functions	MCI, mild dementia (moderate dementia)	Group or individ-ualized	Targets impairment in cognitive functions	Restoration of specific cognitive functions and subsequent improvement in functions
Cognitive rehabil-itation	Training in real-word situations	MCI, mild dementia	Individ-ualized	Development and training of compensatory/adaptive mechanisms	Performance and functioning

approaches share the characteristic that they are focused on improving cognitive functions or to abate deficits in functioning caused by cognitive impairment [87].

CS usually refers to activities in which participants take part in a variety of activities that are often group based and viewed as being able to stimulate cognitive engagement (e.g., discussions, lectures, games), whereas cognitive training involves exercises or tasks which are designed to target specific cognitive functions. Through incremental increases in difficulty, cognitive training aims to improve the individual's level of ability within the domain being targeted. Cognitive rehabilitation is the development of strategies which are aimed at helping the participant to achieve specific goals (e.g., being able to keep appointments, participating in specific activities) usually set out by the participant. Therefore, cognitive rehabilitation is directed at improving performance in everyday life in contrast to cognitive training where the focus is on specific cognitive functions which may in turn improve performance [88] (Table 13.2).

Cognitive Stimulation

CS has a long history within therapies aimed at patients with dementia [89]. The basic tenet behind CS is to view the brain as a muscle in the sense that you "use it or loose it" [90]. Initially, CS was devised as a group-based activity, but in recent years, efforts to develop individualized CS have been underway [91]. CS is designed to stimulate general cognition, i.e. not specific cognitive domains in isolation (e.g., memory), the argument for this approach being that cognitive functions are not used in isolation, and therefore stimulation needs to target several brain functions at once [89].

Different types of activities and content have been used in CS. The initial RCT on CS in dementia, for example, used images and tasks related to the images to stimulate discussion. In one example from the study participants were presented with the dotted outline of an umbrella, with participants being asked to connect the dots. Subsequently, they were asked to draw an umbrella from a different perspective as well as a closed umbrella. This was followed by discussions with the umbrella as a starting point (e.g., about rain/the weather, parts of France where it rained a lot, etc.). An improvement in general cognition and memory function (measured by the Mini Mental State Examination and AD Assessment Scale—Cognitive Subscale) was found following this 5-week intervention study [89]. Building on this promising finding as well as further including techniques from reality orientation, reminiscence therapy, and multisensory therapy, Spector et al. developed a 7-week, twice weekly 45 min session program (15 sessions in total) which was piloted [92]. This type of CS is specifically referred to as CS therapy, and may only be practiced by trained therapists (see also International Cognitive Stimulation Therapy Centre website). The program could be implemented in care homes, and had sessions on "Current affairs," "Number games," "Food," "Being creative," "Faces/scenes," "Word game," and others [93]. The program was tested in an RCT with 201 persons with dementia (mild to moderate range), and was found to improve general cognition and QoL [94]. There were no between-group effects on measures of depression, anxiety, communication, behavior, or global functioning. A number of subsequent studies have been carried out on the effects of CS, but the aforementioned studies remain one of the largest with other studies ranging from a few participants to around 70–100 participants [95].

Two fairly recent meta-analyses [95, 96] have examined the effects of CS on AD and dementia in general, and have arrived at somewhat different conclusions. Oltra-Cucarella et al. [96] were able to include 14 studies in their analysis, all relatively small studies ranging from 4 to 20 participants. They did not find a significant effect of CS on general cognitive function, memory, or ADL when pooling data from the included studies. An important caveat in the interpretation of this finding is that as well as small sample sizes, the authors of the meta-analysis reported that in general risk of bias was high for a number of the studies included. Thus, caution in ruling out an effect in AD based on these findings is warranted. Huntley et al. in their meta-analysis [95] were able to include a total of 33 studies including the relatively large study by Spector et al. [94] and other larger studies [97–99] given the fact that they looked at dementia and not subtypes. Significant effects of CS on the Mini Mental State Examination and AD Assessment Scale—Cognitive Subscale was found. It seems reasonable to assume that the different conclusions in the two meta-analyses are due to the number of studies and sizes of included studies rather than a differential effect in general dementia versus in AD. This is also supported by findings in a third meta-analysis looking at CS in combination with acetylcholinesterase inhibitor treatment versus acetylcholinesterase inhibitor treatment alone in patients with AD, in which the former showed superiority regarding both cognitive function and behavior [100].

Huntley et al. [95] also examined a number of other factors by meta-regression analysis. The analyses revealed that format (inpatient vs outpatient; group vs individual), dose (length, intensity of intervention in hours per week), or participant characteristics (dementia severity) were not associated with differences in effects [95]. Moreover, results did on differ depending on whether active or passive control situations were used [95].

A small number of studies have also investigated the effect of CS in MCI patients. Gomez-Soria et al. [101] tested a 10-week CS program in 155 patients characterized as MCI patients. The group-based intervention included reality orientation (questions about date, time and place, using calendars, etc.), practical exercises targeted at specific cognitive domains paired with an explanation of the cognitive aspect that was going to be focused on in each session, and finally group-based corrections of the exercises. There were no significant between-group differences in cognition, ADL, anxiety, or depression. In a much smaller study in patients with MCI due to Parkinson's disease (n=20), 7 weeks of individual CS improved cognition and some items related to ADL. However, patients were younger (age under 40 was an inclusion criteria), and replication in a larger study is needed. Two other studies examined whether CS in combination with exercise was beneficial [102, 103] in MCI patients. In the largest of the two, 555 patients were randomized to either cognitive stimulation, physical exercise, a combination, or social group (control). The interventions were based on 33 activities from Chinese culture (the study was conducted in Hong Kong) which were divided into cognitively activating, physically strenuous, or primarily social. The intervention could be completed in an activity center or at home and lasted for 12 months. All three interventions were found to improve measures of verbal fluency, delayed recall, and general cognition measured on the ADAS-cog. Subgroup analysis revealed that combined CS and exercise was superior to the others in improving verbal fluency. There were no effects on ADL, depression, or general function.

A number of modified approaches of the initial program of CS (i.e., CS therapy) have also been suggested, and in some instances tested. One modification has been the development of the maintenance CS therapy program. Initial studies of CS therapy had indicated that 3 months following the intervention effect of the intervention were minimal or not present [104], and were not detectable after 10 months [105]. Therefore, a program was developed [106] where the 7-week program [92] was followed by a maintenance program with once weekly sessions over 16 weeks. New sessions were added such as "Art discussions" and "Household treasures." A subsequent pragmatic RCT which included 236 care-home residents with dementia was conducted. At the 6-month follow-up significant improvements in self-rated Quality of Life-AD compared with the control group (7 week CS, but no maintenance). At the 3-month follow-up the proxy-rated QoL by carers, and daily activities showed improvements. There were no significant effects on cognitive scores or behavioral symptoms [107]. Maintenance CS therapy did likewise not improve the health of family caregivers of patients with dementia undergoing the intervention [108].

Another modified approach is individual CS therapy. An individualized approach has a number of advantages over group-based ones. Patients may have preferences that are not compatible with group-based activities, may have difficulty in interacting with groups, an individualized approach may be more easily implemented at home and may be more implementable in areas where resources are scarce [109]. Orrell et al. [91] found that individual CS therapy improved the quality of the caregiving relationship and caregivers' QoL, but found no effect on cognitive function or patient QoL. The intervention consisted of a manual, and sessions were done at home with a caregiver. Each session had a theme, beginning with warm-up sessions (orientation using aids, current events) and moving on to the main session which could use artifacts from the home and were based on a specific theme which changed from session to session. The intervention was generally well accepted by participants and their caregivers, but was found to be best suited for those with less need for intensive support with barriers to participation being life commitments [110]. A high degree of acceptability is in line with previous findings including across different cultural settings [102, 111]. Lastly, it is worth mentioning that CS may also be delivered via computer [112] or telemedicine [113, 114] in an effective manner.

In conclusion, CS seems effective in improving general cognitive function and improving QoL in patients with dementia in mild to moderate stage and may have beneficial effects on family caregiver health. The most solid evidence exists for CS therapy. For this reason, the therapy has been recommended in the World Alzheimer's Report 2014 for patients with dementia as well as by the National Institute for Health & Clinical Excellence guidelines (2006) in the UK for treating cognitive symptoms of dementia. CS may also be effective in MCI, but the evidence base is smaller. In general, CS is well accepted by patients and is flexible in that it may be carried out in groups or individual, in care homes or in residential homes. Guidelines for adaptation of CS in different cultural settings have been developed [115] as has guidance on staff training [116], although the impact of such training is uncertain [117]. Cost effectiveness analyses indicate that CS therapy is most cost effective for those living alone and with higher cognitive function [118].

Cognitive Training

Cognitive training, sometimes referred to as "brain training," "retraining," or "remediation," is a process which uses a program or series of tasks, usually of incremental difficulty, that are designed to train cognitive functions. Cognitive functions usually refer to relatively specific cognitive domains such as memory, problem-solving, attention, or planning. The training targets one domain or domains which from a theoretical point of view are often used together. Cognitive training may be performed as a group activity or individually and may be performed as pen-and-paper exercises or computerized. As the intervention targets cognitive abilities, it has been suggested that the method may work better when combined with pharmacological treatment which improves cognitive function such as acetylcholine esterase inhibitors, but findings have not been convincing [119, 120].

A number of theoretical assumptions lie behind cognitive training. As previously mentioned, cognitive training is aimed at improving or maintaining underlying cognitive functions. In this connection "underlying" refers to those cognitive processes which are a prerequisite for the performance of ADL and therefore by extension, that cognitive training results in improved functioning. This requires that cognitive functions are indeed trainable in the sense that they will either not worsen (i.e., remain stable) or even improve following training. The mechanism of neural plasticity is often referred to as a possible underlying biological mechanism, but evidence to support that cognitive training (or CS) is able to induce or promote neural plasticity, is scarce. Another assumption is that the effects of training will generalize, i.e. that the individual undergoing training not only improves on the specific task being trained (e.g., a memory task), but that this generalizes to other situations in which the individual engages memory. However, this last assumption has been difficult to prove [121]. Factors such as age and baseline cognitive performance have been shown to predict the effectiveness of the technique [122] and thus may explain why the effect is more pronounced in cognitively unimpaired individuals compared to cognitively impaired. Generalizability may be divided into near transfer (i.e., to positively affect cognitive functions closely related to or resembling that being trained) or far transfer (i.e., to positively affect cognitive functions no related to or resembling that being trained). The distinction between cognitive training and cognitive rehabilitation may at times be difficult, especially since cognitive training may be designed to draw on elements from a real-world setting (e.g., shopping).

It has been suggested to subdivide cognitive training into those programs which focus on training specific cognitive domains, and those which aim to train cognition optimizing strategies. One example of the latter is mental imagery. Mental imagery draws on the fact that images are more effectively encoded into memory than words (the picture superiority effect), and that spontaneous mental imagery may be elicited by words. Encoding of imagery versus words has been suggested to be subserved by different brain regions. Specifically, word encoding activates frontal and temporoparietal regions, whereas mental imagery activates visual areas [123], and thus may be less reliant on areas affected in, e.g. AD. However, while this strategy is effective in improving memory in elderly persons [124], this does not seem to apply to patients with AD [125]. Other cognitive training methods which have been tested in patients with AD include Trial and error, where the individual tries to guess the target which is to be recalled, and will receive fee-back on wrong guesses; Errorless learning, which involves reduction of the element of guessing by providing clues prior to performing the target task and Modeling with spaced retrieval, where the individual is asked to remember a sequence of steps in a task and after a delay reproduce the sequence. This may include both physical tasks and no-physical tasks. In a direct comparison of all three methods in mild to moderate AD, all three were found to be equally effective with regard to improving the ability to perform an instrumental ADL [126]. However, due to a lack of a control situation, and since generalizability was not tested, it is difficult to evaluate the effectiveness of the methods. A number of methods concerned with non-memory cognitive domains, including attention, written and spoken language, reasoning, concentration, praxis, and gnosis have also been tested in dementia populations [127–129].

In a recent Cochran review, Bahar-Fuchs et al. reviewed and meta-analyzed intervention studies of cognitive training in dementia [130]. An operational definition of cognitive training in the review was that the training had to target one or more cognitive processes rather than a skill, and that the intervention was specifically designed to deliver the training. Further, the intervention could combine other components than strictly cognitive training. A total of 33 studies were included, with number of participants per study ranging from 12 to 653. The included studies varied greatly with regard to dosing such as length (from 2 weeks to 104 weeks), number of sessions (from, e.g., weekly sessions to more than one session per day), and duration of sessions (e.g., from 30 min to 1.5 h). Most studies included patients with mild to moderate dementia, with the intervention being delivered by either trained staff or caregivers. Pooled results showed an effect on global cognitive function when compared to control, and the effect seemed to last at least 3–12 months. However, there was no effect when cognitive training was compared to an active control (in contrast to a passive control situation). Data also showed an effect on specific cognitive domains including attention, language, and executive function. However, apart from effects on delayed memory and verbal fluency, the quality of evidence was low to very low. With regard to verbal fluency, subgroup analysis revealed that the effect was only present if the intervention was delivered more than three times a week and for interventions which targeted multiple domains. For ADL, caregiver burden and depression, the intervention was not effective. A single study reported data on caregiver wellbeing and mood for which there was an effect [131].

To conclude, cognitive training has yet to be shown to be effective but may carry some benefit for patients with mild dementia in regard to improving cognitive functions. Cognitive training may consist of different types of tasks, but data suggests a threshold of more than 3 sessions per week to be effective and should target more than one cognitive domain. Effects may be seen immediately following treatment and may be effective for up to 12 months. Cognitive training may be combined with, e.g., acetylcholine esterase inhibitors, but there does not seem to be an additional effect of this.

Conclusion

Treatment and management of dementia symptoms includes the appropriate use of non-pharmacological interventions such as those presented in this chapter. The interventions are safe and flexible meaning that they may be applied in diverse settings and taking the individual persons' preferences and abilities into consideration. Some interventions require staff training and adaptation to the specific setting. When implementing physical and cognitive exercise, knowledge of efficacy as well as barriers and facilitatory factors is necessary. Despite the obstacle to a rigorous evaluation of the efficacy and safety of physical and cognitive exercise, a growing evidence base exists to inform the physician about its effectiveness.

References

1. Lam LCW, Lee JSW, Chung JCC, Lau A, Woo J, Kwok TCY. A randomized controlled trial to examine the effectiveness of case management model for community dwelling older persons with mild dementia in Hong Kong. Int J Geriatr Psychiatry. 2010;25(4):395–402. Available from: http://doi.wiley.com/10.1002/gps.2352
2. Khan F, Curtice M. Non-pharmacological management of behavioural symptoms of dementia. Br J Community. 2011;16(9):441–9. Available from: http://www.magonlinelibrary.com/doi/10.12968/bjcn.2011.16.9.441
3. Council M. Developing and evaluating complex interventions: new guidance. Med Res Counc. 2009 [cited 2011 Nov 19]. Available from: http://scholar.google.com/scholar?hl=en&btnG=Search&q=intitle:Developing+and+evaluating+complex+interventions+:+new+guidance#1
4. Bramble DM, Lieberman DE. Endurance running and the evolution of Homo. Nature. 2004;432(7015):345–52. Available from: http://www.nature.com/articles/nature03052
5. https://www.who.int/news-room/fact-sheets/detail/physical-activity. Accessed 26 Nov 2020.
6. Erickson KI, Voss MW, Prakash RS, Basak C, Szabo A, Chaddock L, et al. Exercise training increases size of hippocampus and improves memory. Proc Natl Acad Sci U S A. 2011 [cited 2011 Jul 11];108(7):3017–22. Available from: http://www.pubmedcentral.nih.gov/articlerender.fcgi?artid=3041121&tool=pmcentrez&rendertype=abstract
7. Colcombe SJ, Erickson KI, Raz N, Webb AG, Cohen NJ, McAuley E, et al. Aerobic fitness reduces brain tissue loss in aging humans. J Gerontol A Biol Sci Med Sci. 2003;58(2):176–80. Available from: http://www.ncbi.nlm.nih.gov/pubmed/12586857
8. Colcombe SJ, Erickson KI, Scalf PE, Kim JS, Prakash R, McAuley E, et al. Aerobic exercise training increases brain volume in aging humans. J Gerontol A Biol Sci Med Sci. 2006 [cited 2011 Nov 1];61A(11):1166–70. Available from: http://biomedgerontology.oxfordjournals.org/content/61/11/1166.short
9. Firth J, Stubbs B, Vancampfort D, Schuch F, Lagopoulos J, Rosenbaum S, et al. Effect of aerobic exercise on hippocampal volume in humans: a systematic review and meta-analysis. Neuroimage. 2018;166(April 2017):230–8. Available from: https://doi.org/10.1016/j.neuroimage.2017.11.007
10. Eriksson PS, Perfilieva E, Björk-Eriksson T, Alborn AM, Nordborg C, Peterson DA, et al. Neurogenesis in the adult human hippocampus. Nat Med. 1998;4(11):1313–7. Available from: http://www.ncbi.nlm.nih.gov/pubmed/9809557
11. van Praag H. Neurogenesis and exercise: past and future directions. NeuroMolecular Med. 2008;10(2):128–40.
12. Mirochnic S, Wolf S, Staufenbiel M, Kempermann G. Age effects on the regulation of adult hippocampal neurogenesis by physical activity and environmental enrichment in the APP23 mouse model of Alzheimer disease. Hippocampus. 2009;19(10):1008–18.
13. Varma VR, Tang X, Carlson MC. Hippocampal sub-regional shape and physical activity in older adults. Hippocampus. 2016;26(8):1051–60.
14. Wagner G, Herbsleb M, La Cruz FD, Schumann A, Brünner F, Schachtzabel C, et al. Hippocampal structure, metabolism, and inflammatory response after a 6-week intense aerobic exercise in healthy young adults: a controlled trial. J Cereb Blood Flow Metab. 2015;35(10):1570–8. Available from: http://www.nature.com/doifinder/10.1038/jcbfm.2015.125
15. Maass A, Duzel S, Goerke M, Becke A, Sobieray U, Neumann K, et al. Vascular hippocampal plasticity after aerobic exercise in older adults. Mol Psychiatry. 2015;20(5):585–93. Available from: http://www.nature.com/mp/journal/v20/n5/pdf/mp2014114a.pdf
16. Moore D, Loprinzi PD. Exercise influences episodic memory via changes in hippocampal neurocircuitry and long-term potentiation. Eur J Neurosci. 2020;(March):1–12. https://doi.org/10.1111/ejn.14728

17. Johnson NF, Kim C, Clasey JL, Bailey A, Gold BT. Cardiorespiratory fitness is positively correlated with cerebral white matter integrity in healthy seniors. Neuroimage. 2012;59(2):1514–23.
18. Loprinzi PD, Harper J, Ikuta T. The effects of aerobic exercise on corpus callosum integrity: systematic review. Phys Sportsmed. 2020;48:1–7. Available from: https://www.tandfonline.com/doi/full/10.1080/00913847.2020.1758545
19. Zhu N, Jacobs DRJ, Schreiner PJ, Launer LJ, Whitmer RA, Sidney S, et al. Cardiorespiratory fitness and brain volume and white matter integrity: the CARDIA Study. Neurology. 2015;84(23):2347–53.
20. Strömmer JM, Davis SW, Henson RN, Tyler LK, Campbell KL. Physical activity predicts population-level age-related differences in frontal white matter. Journals Gerontol Ser A Biol Sci Med Sci. 2020;75(2):236–43.
21. Smith JC, Lancaster MA, Nielson KA, Woodard JL, Seidenberg M, Durgerian S, et al. Interactive effects of physical activity and APOE-ε4 on white matter tract diffusivity in healthy elders. Neuroimage. 2016;131(12):102–12. Available from: https://linkinghub.elsevier.com/retrieve/pii/S1053811916312148
22. Best JR, Chiu BK, Liang Hsu C, Nagamatsu LS, Liu-Ambrose T. Long-term effects of resistance exercise training on cognition and brain volume in older women: results from a randomized controlled trial. J Int Neuropsychol Soc. 2015;21(10):745–56. Available from: http://www.journals.cambridge.org/abstract_S1355617715000673
23. Tabei KI, Satoh M, Ogawa JI, Tokita T, Nakaguchi N, Nakao K, et al. Physical exercise with music reduces gray and white matter loss in the frontal cortex of elderly people: the mihama-kiho scan project. Front Aging Neurosci. 2017;9(Jun):1–12.
24. Clark CM, Guadagni V, Mazerolle EL, Hill M, Hogan DB, Pike GB, et al. Effect of aerobic exercise on white matter microstructure in the aging brain. Behav Brain Res. 2019;373(July):112042. Available from: https://doi.org/10.1016/j.bbr.2019.112042
25. Fissler P, Müller HP, Küster OC, Laptinskaya D, Thurm F, Woll A, et al. No evidence that short-term cognitive or physical training programs or lifestyles are related to changes in white matter integrity in older adults at risk of dementia. Front Hum Neurosci. 2017;11(March):1–13.
26. Gramkow MH, Hasselbalch SG, Waldemar G, Frederiksen KS. Resting state EEG in exercise intervention studies: a systematic review of effects and methods. Front Hum Neurosci. 2020;14:155.
27. Dorsman KA, Weiner-Light S, Staffaroni AM, Brown JA, Wolf A, Cobigo Y, et al. Get moving! Increases in physical activity are associated with increasing functional connectivity trajectories in typically aging adults. Front Aging Neurosci. 2020;12(April):1–10.
28. Rajab AS, Crane DE, Middleton LE, Robertson AD, Hampson M, Macintosh BJ. A single session of exercise increases connectivity in sensorimotor-related brain networks : a resting-state fMRI study in young healthy adults. Front Hum Neurosci. 2014;8(August):1–9.
29. Voss MW, Prakash RS, Erickson KI, Basak C, Chaddock L, Kim JS, et al. Plasticity of brain networks in a randomized intervention trial of exercise training in older adults. Front Aging Neurosci. 2010;2(Aug):1–17.
30. Li MY, Huang MM, Li SZ, Tao J, Zheng GH, Chen LD. The effects of aerobic exercise on the structure and function of DMN-related brain regions: a systematic review. Int J Neurosci. 2017;127(7):634–49.
31. Quigley A, MacKay-Lyons M, Eskes G. Effects of exercise on cognitive performance in older adults: a narrative review of the evidence, possible biological mechanisms, and recommendations for exercise prescription. J Aging Res. 2020;2020:1407896.
32. Chen FT, Etnier JL, Chan KH, Chiu PK, Hung TM, Chang YK. Effects of exercise training interventions on executive function in older adults: a systematic review and meta-analysis. Sport Med. 2020;50(8):1451–67.
33. Smith PJ, Blumenthal JA, Hoffman BM, Cooper H, Strauman TA, Welsh-Bohmer K, et al. Aerobic exercise and neurocognitive performance: a meta-analytic review of randomized controlled trials. Psychosom Med. 2010;72(3):239–52.

34. Gothe NP, McAuley E. Yoga and cognition: a meta-analysis of chronic and acute effects. Psychosom Med. 2015;77(7):784–97.
35. Kelly ME, Loughrey D, Lawlor BA, Robertson IH, Walsh C, Brennan S. The impact of exercise on the cognitive functioning of healthy older adults: a systematic review and meta-analysis. Ageing Res Rev. 2014;16(1):12–31. Available from: https://doi.org/10.1016/j.arr.2014.05.002
36. Frederiksen K, Verdelho A, Madureira S, Bäzner H, O'Brien JT, Fazekas F, et al. Physical activity in the elderly is associated with improved executive function and processing speed: the LADIS Study. Int J Geriatr Psychiatry. 2014 [cited 2014 Nov 11]; Available from: http://www.ncbi.nlm.nih.gov/pubmed/25363336
37. Groot C, Hooghiemstra AM, Raijmakers PGHM, van Berckel BNM, Scheltens P, Scherder EJA, et al. The effect of physical activity on cognitive function in patients with dementia: a meta-analysis of randomized control trials. Ageing Res Rev. 2016;25(2016):13–23. Available from: https://linkinghub.elsevier.com/retrieve/pii/S1568163715300349
38. Nakamura M, Imaoka M, Takeda M. Interaction of bone and brain: osteocalcin and cognition. Int J Neurosci. 2020:1–17. Available from: https://doi.org/10.1080/00207454.2020.1770247.
39. Tsai CL, Ukropec J, Ukropcová B, Pai MC. An acute bout of aerobic or strength exercise specifically modifies circulating exerkine levels and neurocognitive functions in elderly individuals with mild cognitive impairment. NeuroImage Clin. 2018;17(1):272–84. Available from: https://doi.org/10.1016/j.nicl.2017.10.028
40. Eaton M, Granata C, Barry J, Safdar A, Bishop D, Little JP. Impact of a single bout of high-intensity interval exercise and short-term interval training on interleukin-6, FNDC5, and METRNL mRNA expression in human skeletal muscle. J Sport Heal Sci. 2018;7(2):191–6.
41. Kabak B, Belviranli M, Okudan N. Irisin and myostatin responses to acute high-intensity interval exercise in humans. Horm Mol Biol Clin Investig. 2018;35(3):1–7.
42. Briken S, Rosenkranz SC, Keminer O, Patra S, Ketels G, Heesen C, et al. Effects of exercise on Irisin, BDNF and IL-6 serum levels in patients with progressive multiple sclerosis. J Neuroimmunol. 2016;299(2016):53–8. Available from: https://doi.org/10.1016/j.jneuroim.2016.08.007
43. Young MF, Valaris S, Wrann CD. A role for FNDC5/Irisin in the beneficial effects of exercise on the brain and in neurodegenerative diseases. Prog Cardiovasc Dis. 2019;62(2):172–8. Available from: https://doi.org/10.1016/j.pcad.2019.02.007
44. Bradburn S, Mcphee JS, Bagley L, Sipila S, Stenroth L, Narici MV, et al. Association between osteocalcin and cognitive performance in healthy older adults. Age Ageing. 2016;45(6):844–9.
45. Obri A, Khrimian L, Karsenty G, Oury F. Osteocalcin in the brain: from embryonic development to age-related decline in cognition. Nat Rev Endocrinol. 2018;14(3):174–82. Available from: http://www.nature.com/articles/nrendo.2017.181
46. Egan MF, Kojima M, Callicott JH, Goldberg TE, Kolachana BS, Bertolino A, et al. The BDNF val66met polymorphism affects activity-dependent secretion of BDNF and human memory and hippocampal function. Cell. 2003;112(2):257–69. Available from: http://www.ncbi.nlm.nih.gov/pubmed/12553913
47. Riemenschneider M, Schwarz S, Wagenpfeil S, Diehl J, Müller U, Förstl H, et al. A polymorphism of the brain-derived neurotrophic factor (BDNF) is associated with Alzheimer's disease in patients lacking the Apolipoprotein E epsilon4 allele. Mol Psychiatry. 2002 [cited 2011 Aug 25];7(7):782–5. Available from: http://www.ncbi.nlm.nih.gov/pubmed/12192623
48. Kim J-M, Stewart R, Bae K-Y, Kim S-W, Yang S-J, Park K-H, et al. Role of BDNF val66met polymorphism on the association between physical activity and incident dementia. Neurobiol Aging. 2011 [cited 2011 Aug 1];32(3):551.e5–12. Available from: http://www.ncbi.nlm.nih.gov/pubmed/20172629
49. Brown BM, Bourgeat P, Peiffer JJ, Burnham S, Laws SM, Rainey-Smith SR, et al. Influence of BDNF Val66Met on the relationship between physical activity and brain volume. Neurology. 2014;83(15):1345–52.

50. Kallies G, Rapp MA, Fydrich T, Fehm L, Tschorn M, Terán C, et al. Serum brain-derived neurotrophic factor (BDNF) at rest and after acute aerobic exercise in major depressive disorder. Psychoneuroendocrinology. 2019;102(November 2018):212–5. Available from: https://www.sciencedirect.com/science/article/pii/S0306453018307911?dgcid=rss_sd_all
51. Dinoff A, Herrmann N, Swardfager W, Gallagher D, Lanctôt KL. The effect of exercise on resting concentrations of peripheral brain-derived neurotrophic factor (BDNF) in major depressive disorder: a meta-analysis. J Psychiatr Res. 2018;105(August 2018):123–31.
52. Pedersen BK. Physical activity and muscle–brain crosstalk. Nat Rev Endocrinol. 2019;15(7):383–92. Available from: https://doi.org/10.1038/s41574-019-0174-x
53. Nigam SM, Xu S, Kritikou JS, Marosi K, Brodin L, Mattson MP. Exercise and BDNF reduce Aβ production by enhancing α-secretase processing of APP. J Neurochem. 2017;142(2):286–96.
54. Stranahan AM, Lee K, Martin B, Maudsley S, Golden E, Cutler RG, et al. Voluntary exercise and caloric restriction enhance hippocampal dendritic spine density and BDNF levels in diabetic mice. Hippocampus. 2009 [cited 2012 Aug 14];19(10):951–61. Available from: http://www.pubmedcentral.nih.gov/articlerender.fcgi?artid=2755651&tool=pmcentrez&rendertype=abstract
55. Adlard P, Perreau VM, Pop V, Cotman CW. Voluntary exercise decreases amyloid load in a transgenic model of Alzheimer's disease. J Neurosci. 2005;25(17):4217–21.
56. Sofi F, Valecchi D, Bacci D, Abbate R, Gensini GF, Casini A, et al. Physical activity and risk of cognitive decline: a meta-analysis of prospective studies. J Intern Med. 2011 [cited 2011 Jul 12];269(1):107–17. Available from: http://www.ncbi.nlm.nih.gov/pubmed/20831630
57. Alkadhi KA, Dao AT. Exercise decreases BACE and APP levels in the hippocampus of a rat model of Alzheimer's disease. Mol Cell Neurosci. 2018;86(February 2017):25–9. Available from: https://doi.org/10.1016/j.mcn.2017.11.008
58. Moore K, Girens R, Larson S, Jones M, Restivo J, Holtzman D, et al. A spectrum of exercise training reduces soluble Abeta in a dose-dependent manner in a mouse model of Alzheimer's disease. Neurobiol Dis. 2015;85:218–24.
59. Moore KM, Girens RE, Larson SK, Jones MR, Restivo JL, Holtzman DM, et al. A spectrum of exercise training reduces soluble Aβ in a dose-dependent manner in a mouse model of Alzheimer's disease. Neurobiol Dis. 2016;85(2016):218–24. Available from: https://doi.org/10.1016/j.nbd.2015.11.004
60. Koo JH, Kang EB, Oh YS, Yang DS, Cho JY. Treadmill exercise decreases amyloid-β burden possibly via activation of SIRT-1 signaling in a mouse model of Alzheimer's disease. Exp Neurol. 2017;288:142–52. Available from: https://doi.org/10.1016/j.expneurol.2016.11.014
61. Belarbi K, Burnouf S, Fernandez-gomez F, Laurent C, Lestavel S, Figeac M, et al. Neurobiology of Disease Beneficial effects of exercise in a transgenic mouse model of Alzheimer' s disease-like Tau pathology. Neurobiol Dis. 2011;43(2):486–94. Available from: https://doi.org/10.1016/j.nbd.2011.04.022
62. Lin T, Shih Y, Chen S, Lien C, Chang C, Huang T, et al. Running exercise delays neurodegeneration in amygdala and hippocampus of Alzheimer's disease (APP/PS1) transgenic mice. Neurobiol Learn Mem. 2015;118:198–7.
63. Frederiksen K, Madsen K, Andersen BB, Beyer N, Garde E, Høgh P, et al. Moderate- to high-intensity exercise does not modify cortical β-amyloid in Alzheimer's disease. Alzheimer's Dement Transl Res Clin Interv. 2019;5:208–15.
64. Frederiksen K, Gjerum L, Waldemar G, Hasselbalch SG. Physical activity as a moderator of Alzheimer pathology: a systematic review of observational studies. Curr Alzheimer Res. 2019; Available from: http://www.ncbi.nlm.nih.gov/pubmed/30873924
65. Morris JK, Vidoni ED, Johnson DK, Van Sciver A, Mahnken JD, Honea RA, et al. Aerobic exercise for Alzheimer's disease: a randomized controlled pilot trial. PLoS One. 2017;12(2):1–14. Available from: https://doi.org/10.1371/journal.pone.0170547
66. Frederiksen K, Larsen CT, Hasselbalch SG, Christensen AN, Høgh P, Wermuth L, et al. A 16-week aerobic exercise intervention does not affect hippocampal volume and cortical thickness in mild to moderate Alzheimer's disease. Front Aging Neurosci.

2018;10(September):1–10. Available from: https://www.frontiersin.org/article/10.3389/fnagi.2018.00293/full
67. Honea RA, Thomas GP, Harsha A, Anderson HS, Donnelly JE, Brooks WM, et al. Cardiorespiratory fitness and preserved medial temporal lobe volume in Alzheimer disease. Alzheimer Dis Assoc Disord. 2009;23(3):188–97. Available from: http://www.pubmedcentral.nih.gov/articlerender.fcgi?artid=2760037&tool=pmcentrez&rendertype=abstract
68. Vidoni ED, Honea R, Billinger S, Swerdlow RH, Burns JM. Cardiorespiratory fitness is associated with atrophy in Alzheimer's and aging over 2 years. Neurobiol Aging. 2012 [cited 2012 Oct 29];33(8):1624–32. Available from: http://www.ncbi.nlm.nih.gov/pubmed/21531480
69. Forbes D, Forbes SC, Blake CM, Thiessen EJ, Forbes S. Exercise programs for people with dementia. Cochrane Database Syst Rev. 2015;4:CD006489.
70. Hoffmann K, Frederiksen KS, Sobol NA, Beyer N, Vogel A, Simonsen AH, et al. Preserving cognition, quality of life, physical health and functional ability in Alzheimer's disease: the effect of physical exercise (ADEX Trial): rationale and design. Neuroepidemiology. 2013 [cited 2014 Jan 8];41(3–4):198–207. Available from: http://www.ncbi.nlm.nih.gov/pubmed/24135720
71. Rolland Y, Pillard F, Klapouszczak A, Reynish E, Thomas D, Andrieu S, et al. Exercise program for nursing home residents with Alzheimer's disease: a 1-year randomized, controlled trial. J Am Geriatr Soc. 2007 [cited 2011 Jul 24];55(2):158–65. Available from: http://doi.wiley.com/10.1111/j.1532-5415.2007.01035.x
72. Eggermont LHP, Swaab DF, Hol EM, Scherder EJ. Walking the line: a randomised trial on the effects of a short term walking programme on cognition in dementia. JNNP. 2009;80(7):802–4.
73. Venegas-Sanabria LC, Martínez-Vizcaino V, Cavero-Redondo I, Chavarro-Carvajal DA, Cano-Gutierrez CA, Álvarez-Bueno C. Effect of physical activity on cognitive domains in dementia and mild cognitive impairment: overview of systematic reviews and meta-analyses. Aging Ment Heal. 2020. https://doi.org/10.1080/13607863.2020.1839862
74. Frederiksen KS, Sobol N, Beyer N, Hasselbalch S, Waldemar G. Moderate-to-high intensity aerobic exercise in patients with mild to moderate Alzheimer's disease: a pilot study. Int J Geriatr Psychiatry. 2014 [cited 2014 May 7];29(12):1242–8. Available from: http://www.ncbi.nlm.nih.gov/pubmed/24733599
75. Vidoni ED, Johnson DK, Morris JK, Van Sciver A, Greer CS, Billinger SA, et al. Dose-response of aerobic exercise on cognition: a community-based, pilot randomized controlled trial. Fukumoto Y, editor. PLoS One. 2015;10(7):e0131647. Available from: https://dx.plos.org/10.1371/journal.pone.0131647
76. Yu F, Chen Y, Mathiason MA, Wan Q, Lin FV. Cognitive and physical factors affecting daily function in Alzheimer's disease: a cross-sectional analysis. Nurs Health Sci. 2018;(April 2017):1–7. Available from: http://doi.wiley.com/10.1111/nhs.12426
77. Clemmensen FK, Hoffmann K, Siersma V, Sobol N, Beyer N, Andersen BB, et al. The role of physical and cognitive function in performance of activities of daily living in patients with mild-to-moderate Alzheimer's disease—a cross-sectional study. BMC Geriatr. 2020;20(1):1–9.
78. Hoffmann K, Sobol NA, Frederiksen KS, Beyer N, Vogel A, Vestergaard K, et al. Moderate-to-high intensity physical exercise in patients with Alzheimer's disease: a randomized controlled trial. J Alzheimers Dis. 2016;50(2):443–53.
79. Barrado-Martín Y, Heward M, Polman R, Nyman SR. Acceptability of a dyadic tai chi intervention for older people living with dementia and their informal carers. J Aging Phys Act. 2019;27(2):166–83. Available from: https://journals.humankinetics.com/doi/10.1123/japa.2017-0267
80. Dal Bello-Haas VPM, O'Connell ME, Morgan DG, Crossley M. Lessons learned: feasibility and acceptability of a telehealth-delivered exercise intervention for rural-dwelling individuals with dementia and their caregivers. Rural Remote Health. 2014;14(3):2715. Available from: http://www.ncbi.nlm.nih.gov/pubmed/25081991
81. Judge KS, Yarry SJ, Orsulic-Jeras S. Acceptability and feasibility results of a strength-based skills training program for dementia caregiving dyads. Gerontologist. 2010 [cited 2011 Nov

19];50(3):408–17. Available from: http://www.pubmedcentral.nih.gov/articlerender.fcgi?artid=2867494&tool=pmcentrez&rendertype=abstract
82. Cott CA, Dawson P, Sidani S, Wells D. The effects of a walking/talking program on communication, ambulation, and functional status in residents with Alzheimer disease. Alzheimer Dis Assoc Disord. 2002;16(2):81–7. Available from: http://onlinelibrary.wiley.com/o/cochrane/clcentral/articles/340/CN-00389340/frame.html
83. Vseteckova J, Deepak-gopinath M, Borgstrom E, Holland C, Draper J, Pappas Y, et al. Barriers and facilitators to adherence to group exercise in institutionalized older people living with dementia : a systematic review. Eur Rev Aging Phys Act. 2018;3:1–11.
84. Steinberg M, Leoutsakos J-MS, Podewils LJ, Lyketsos CG. Evaluation of a home-based exercise program in the treatment of Alzheimer's disease: the maximizing Independence in dementia (MIND) study. Int J Geriatr Psychiatry. 2009;24(7):680–5.
85. Di Lorito C, Bosco A, Booth V, Goldberg S, Harwood RH, Van der Wardt V. Adherence to exercise interventions in older people with mild cognitive impairment and dementia: a systematic review and meta-analysis. Prev Med Rep. 2020;19(May):101139. Available from: https://doi.org/10.1016/j.pmedr.2020.101139
86. Sobol NA, Hoffmann K, Frederiksen KS, Vogel A, Vestergaard K, Braendgaard H, et al. Effect of aerobic exercise on physical performance in patients with Alzheimer's disease. Alzheimer's Dement. 2016;12(12):1207–15. Available from: http://www.ncbi.nlm.nih.gov/pubmed/27344641
87. Bahar-Fuchs A, Clare L, Woods B. Cognitive training and cognitive rehabilitation for persons with mild to moderate dementia of the Alzheimer's or vascular type: a review. Alzheimer's Res Ther. 2013;5(4):35.
88. Clare L, Woods B. Cognitive rehabilitation and cognitive training for early-stage Alzheimer's disease and vascular dementia. In: Clare L, editor. Chichester: Wiley. 2003, p. 6. Available from: http://doi.wiley.com/10.1002/14651858.CD003260
89. Breuil V, De Rotrou J, Forette F, Tortrat D, Ganansia-Ganem A, Frambourt A, et al. Cognitive stimulation of patients with dementia: preliminary results. Int J Geriatr Psychiatry. 1994;9(3):211–7.
90. Salthouse TA. Mental exercise and mental aging: evaluating the validity of the "use it or lose it" hypothesis. Perspect Psychol Sci. 2006;1(1):68–87. Available from: http://www.ncbi.nlm.nih.gov/pubmed/26151186
91. Orrell M, Yates L, Leung P, Kang S, Hoare Z, Whitaker C, et al. The impact of individual Cognitive Stimulation Therapy (iCST) on cognition, quality of life, caregiver health, and family relationships in dementia: a randomised controlled trial. PLoS Med. 2017;14(3):1–22.
92. Spector A, Orrell M, Davies S, Woods B. Can reality orientation be rehabilitated? Development and piloting of an evidence-based programme of cognition-based therapies for people with dementia. Neuropsychol Rehabil. 2001;11(3–4):377–97. Available from: https://www.tandfonline.com/doi/full/10.1080/09602010143000068
93. Rai H, Yates L, Orrell M. Cognitive stimulation therapy for dementia. Clin Geriatr Med. 2018;34(4):653–65. Available from: https://doi.org/10.1016/j.cger.2018.06.010
94. Spector A, Thorgrimsen L, Woods B, Royan L, Davies S, Butterworth M, et al. Efficacy of an evidence-based cognitive stimulation therapy programme for people with dementia: randomised controlled trial. Br J Psychiatry. 2003;183(Sept.):248–54.
95. Huntley JD, Gould RL, Liu K, Smith M, Howard RJ. Do cognitive interventions improve general cognition in dementia ? A meta-analysis and meta-regression. 2015;(table 1):1–12.
96. Oltra-Cucarella J, Ferrer-Cascales R, Clare L, Morris SB, Espert R, Tirapu J, et al. Differential effects of cognition-focused interventions for people with Alzheimer's disease: a meta-analysis. Neuropsychology. 2018;32(6):664–79.
97. Baldelli MV, Boiardi R, Fabbo A, Pradelli JM, Neri M. The role of reality orientation therapy in restorative care of elderly patients with dementia plus stroke in the subacute nursing home setting. Arch Gerontol. 2002;35:15–22. Available from: https://linkinghub.elsevier.com/retrieve/pii/S0167494302000985

98. Onder G, Zanetti O, Giacobini E, Frisoni GB, Bartorelli L, Carbone G, et al. Reality orientation therapy combined with cholinesterase inhibitors in Alzheimer's disease: randomised controlled trial. Br J Psychiatry. 2005;187(5):450–5. Available from: https://www.cambridge.org/core/product/identifier/S0007125000168394/type/journal_article
99. Wang J-J. Group reminiscence therapy for cognitive and affective function of demented elderly in Taiwan. Int J Geriatr Psychiatry. 2007;22(12):1235–40. Available from: http://doi.wiley.com/10.1002/gps.1821
100. Chen J, Duan Y, Li H, Lu L, Liu J, Tang C. Different durations of cognitive stimulation therapy for Alzheimer's disease: a systematic review and meta-analysis. Clin Interv Aging. 2019;14:1243–54.
101. Gomez-Soria I, Peralta-Marrupe P, Plo F. Cognitive stimulation program in mild cognitive impairment a randomized controlled trial. Dement Neuropsychol. 2020;14(2):110–7.
102. Lam LCW, Chan WC, Leung T, Fung AWT, Leung EMF. Would older adults with mild cognitive impairment adhere to and benefit from a structured lifestyle activity intervention to enhance cognition? A cluster randomized controlled trial. PLoS One. 2015;10(3):1–17.
103. Binns E, Kerse N, Peri K, Cheung G, Taylor D. Combining cognitive stimulation therapy and fall prevention exercise (CogEx) in older adults with mild to moderate dementia: a feasibility randomised controlled trial. Pilot Feasibility Stud. 2020;6(1):1–16.
104. Woods B, Aguirre E, Ae S, Orrell M. Cognitive stimulation to improve cognitive functioning in people with dementia (Review). Cochrane Database Syst Rev. 2012; https://doi.org/10.1002/14651858.CD005562.pub2.
105. Chapman SB, Weiner MF, Rackley A, Hynan LS, Zientz J. Effects of cognitive-communication stimulation for Alzheimer's disease patients treated with donepezil. J Speech Lang Hear Res. 2004;47(5):1149–63. Available from: http://pubs.asha.org/doi/10.1044/1092-4388%282004/085%29
106. Aguirre E. Development of an evidence-based extended programme of maintenance cognitive stimulation therapy (cst) for people with dementia. Non-pharm Ther Dement. 2011;1(3):197–216.
107. Orrell M, Aguirre E, Spector A, Hoare Z, Woods RT, Streater A, et al. Maintenance cognitive stimulation therapy for dementia: single-blind, multicentre, pragmatic randomised controlled trial. Br J Psychiatry. 2014;204(6):454–61.
108. Aguirre E, Hoare Z, Spector A, Woods RT, Orrell M. The effects of a Cognitive Stimulation Therapy [CST] programme for people with dementia on family caregivers' health. BMC Geriatr. 2014;14(1):1–6.
109. Yates LA, Leung P, Orgeta V, Spector A, Orrell M. The development of individual cognitive stimulation therapy (iCST) for dementia. Clin Interv Aging. 2014;10:95–104.
110. Yates LA, Orgeta V, Leung P, Spector A, Orrell M. Field-testing phase of the development of individual cognitive stimulation therapy (iCST) for dementia. BMC Health Serv Res. 2016;16(1):1–11. Available from: https://doi.org/10.1186/s12913-016-1499-y
111. Toh HM, Ghazali SE, Subramaniam P. The acceptability and usefulness of cognitive stimulation therapy for older adults with dementia: a narrative review. Int J Alzheimers Dis. 2016;2016:5131570.
112. García-casal JA, Loizeau A, Csipke E, Franco M, Perea-Bartolomé MV, Orrell M, et al. Computer-based cognitive interventions for people living with dementia: a systematic literature review and meta-analysis. 2017;7863. Available from: https://doi.org/10.1080/13607863.2015.1132677.
113. Gately ME, Trudeau SA, Moo LR. In-home video telehealth for dementia management: implications for rehabilitation. Curr Geriatr Rep. 2019;8(3):239–49. Available from: http://link.springer.com/10.1007/s13670-019-00297-3
114. Jelcic N, Agostini M, Meneghello F, Bussè C, Parise S, Galano A, et al. Feasibility and efficacy of cognitive telerehabilitation in early Alzheimer's disease: a pilot study. Clin Interv Aging. 2014;9:1605–11.
115. Aguirre E, Spector A, Orrell M. Guidelines for adapting cognitive stimulation therapy to other cultures. Clin Interv Aging. 2014;9:1003–7.

116. Streater A, Spector A, Hoare Z, Aguirre E, Russell I, Orrell M. Staff training and outreach support for Cognitive Stimulation Therapy and its implementation in practice: a cluster randomised trial. Int J Geriatr Psychiatry. 2017;32(12):e64–71.
117. Cove J, Jacobi N, Donovan H, Orrell M, Stott J, Spector A. Effectiveness of weekly cognitive stimulation therapy for people with dementia and the additional impact of enhancing cognitive stimulation therapy with a carer training program. Clin Interv Aging. 2014;9:2143–50.
118. Brown H, D'Amico F, Knapp M, Orrell M, Rehill A, Vale L, et al. A cost effectiveness analysis of maintenance cognitive stimulation therapy (MCST) for people with dementia: examining the influence of cognitive ability and living arrangements. Aging Ment Heal. 2019;23(5):602–7. Available from: https://doi.org/10.1080/13607863.2018.1442410
119. Cahn-Weiner DA, Malloy PF, Rebok GW, Ott BR. Results of a randomized placebo-controlled study of memory training for mildly impaired Alzheimer's disease patients. Appl Neuropsychol. 2003;10(4):215–23. Available from: http://www.ncbi.nlm.nih.gov/pubmed/14690802
120. Loewenstein DA, Acevedo A, Czaja SJ, Duara R. Cognitive rehabilitation of mildly impaired Alzheimer disease patients on cholinesterase inhibitors. Am J Geriatr Psychiatry. 2004;12(4):395–402.
121. Owen AM, Hampshire A, Grahn JA, Stenton R, Dajani S, Burns AS, et al. Putting brain training to the test. Nature. 2010;465(7299):775–8. Available from: http://www.ncbi.nlm.nih.gov/pubmed/20407435
122. Zinke K, Zeintl M, Rose NS, Putzmann J, Pydde A, Kliegel M. Working memory training and transfer in older adults: effects of age, baseline performance, and training gains. Dev Psychol. 2014;50(1):304–15. Available from: http://www.ncbi.nlm.nih.gov/pubmed/23688173
123. Foley MA, Foy J. Pictorial encoding effects and memory confusions in the Deese-Roediger-McDermott paradigm: evidence for the activation of spontaneous imagery. Memory. 2008;16(7):712–27. Available from: http://www.ncbi.nlm.nih.gov/pubmed/18720219
124. Verhaeghen P, Marcoen A, Goossens L. Facts and fiction about memory aging: a quantitative integration of research findings. J Gerontol. 1993;48(4):P157–71. Available from: http://www.ncbi.nlm.nih.gov/pubmed/8315232
125. Hussey EP, Smolinsky JG, Piryatinsky I, Budson AE, Ally BA. Using mental imagery to improve memory in patients with Alzheimer disease: trouble generating or remembering the mind's eye? Alzheimer Dis Assoc Disord. 2012;26(2):124–34.
126. Bourgeois J, Laye M, Lemaire J, Leone E, Deudon A, Darmon N, et al. Relearning of activities of daily living: a comparison of the effectiveness of three learning methods in patients with dementia of the Alzheimer type. J Nutr Heal Aging. 2016;20(1):48–55.
127. Galante E, Venturini G, Fiaccadori C. Computer-based cognitive intervention for dementia: preliminary results of a randomized clinical trial. G Ital Med Lav Ergon. 29(3 Suppl B):B26–32. Available from: http://www.ncbi.nlm.nih.gov/pubmed/18575355
128. Bergamaschi S, Arcara G, Calza A, Villani D, Orgeta V, Mondini S. One-year repeated cycles of cognitive training (CT) for Alzheimer's disease. Aging Clin Exp Res. 2013;25(4):421–6. Available from: http://www.ncbi.nlm.nih.gov/pubmed/23784727
129. Fernández-Calvo B, Rodríguez-Pérez R, Contador I, Rubio-Santorum A, Ramos F. [Efficacy of cognitive training programs based on new software technologies in patients with Alzheimer-type dementia]. Psicothema. 2011;23(1):44–50. Available from: http://www.ncbi.nlm.nih.gov/pubmed/21266141
130. Bahar-Fuchs A, Clare L, Woods B. Cognitive training and cognitive rehabilitation for mild to moderate Alzheimer's disease and vascular dementia. Cochrane Database Syst Rev. 2013;2013(6):CD003260.
131. Quayhagen MP, Quayhagen M, Corbeil RR, Hendrix RC, Jackson JE, Snyder L, et al. Coping with dementia: evaluation of four nonpharmacologic interventions. Int psychogeriatrics. 2000;12(2):249–65. Available from: http://www.ncbi.nlm.nih.gov/pubmed/10937544

Promoting Functional Independence in Dementia

14

Andrew Sommerlad and Penny Rapaport

Abbreviations

AD	Alzheimer's disease
BADLs	Basic activities of daily living
bvFTD	Behavioural-variant frontotemporal dementia
CST	Cognitive stimulation therapy
DLB	Dementia with Lewy bodies
IADLs	Instrumental activities of daily living
RCT	Randomised controlled trial

Introduction

The presence of dementia inevitably indicates that there has been a loss of functional independence. The World Health Organisation's criteria for even mild dementia indicates that cognitive decline 'interferes with everyday activities' and once dementia reaches its moderate stages, there is expected to be 'serious handicap to independent living' [1]. However, it should be a goal of clinical management in dementia to minimise the loss of independence caused by dementia through environmental adaptations, psychological therapies and social support, involving both the patient with dementia and their wider milieu. These treatments have the

A. Sommerlad (✉)
Division of Psychiatry, University College London, London, UK

Camden and Islington NHS Foundation Trust, London, UK
e-mail: a.sommerlad@ucl.ac.uk

P. Rapaport
Division of Psychiatry, University College London, London, UK
e-mail: p.rapaport@ucl.ac.uk

K. S. Frederiksen, G. Waldemar (eds.), *Management of Patients with Dementia*,
https://doi.org/10.1007/978-3-030-77904-7_14

potential to improve the quality of life for the patient with dementia and their family members and to markedly reduce the high societal costs required to provide care.

A major focus of dementia care during the past 10–20 years has been making early diagnoses of people developing symptoms [2, 3] including, in some countries, incentivisation and targets [4] and case-finding in high-risk populations, such as older people admitted to hospital [5], for improving diagnostic rates. This approach has aimed to ensure that the condition is recognised, that treatment can be initiated, and that risky behaviour arising from cognitive impairment can be mitigated. However, there has been criticism that this rising rate of diagnosis has not yet been matched with development of post-diagnostic care [6] to support patients with dementia and their families to maintain functional independence and live well. Provision of high-quality psychosocial care has therefore been identified as a current global priority area [7].

Functional independence can be conceptualised and defined in several ways, as described in more detail below. For the purposes of this chapter, maintaining functional independence will refer to preservation of the ability of a person to complete one or more of a range of activities. As considered in previous research, [8] maintenance of functional independence can include the provision of support from family, friends or professional carers, which means that the patient with dementia is not acting entirely alone in their functional activities, but that there is a degree of interdependence between patients with dementia and their support networks, which enables patients with dementia to live relatively independently.

Dementia is linked to difficulties in maintaining function for several reasons. Cognitive decline impairs the ability to manage self-care, and other common neuropsychiatric symptoms such as agitation and apathy [9] further inhibit independence. Dementia is also associated with complex multimorbidity whereby around three-quarters of people diagnosed with dementia have at least two other chronic conditions [10, 11] and cognitive impairment in dementia influences the effect of physical illness on independence [12]. The interplay of cognitive decline, behavioural and psychological symptoms and physical ill-health combine to create challenges for a patient with dementia, as well as carers and practitioners aiming to support independence.

Functional independence is important for patients with dementia. Dependence on others, and the impact on personal relationships is one of the consequences of dementia most feared by people without dementia [13]. Impairment in activity of daily living functions is associated with poor quality of life, particularly in patients with more severe dementia [14, 15]. Impairment in social function correlates with poor quality of life in patients with dementia of all severity [16], and maintaining social relationships, a key component of social function, is an important predictor of better well-being [17]. Functional independence also matters to family members of patients with dementia, with difficulties in completing instrumental activities of daily living being strongly linked to higher rates of carer burden [18] and distress [19].

This chapter aims to describe the loss of functional independence in dementia, how this progresses over the disease course and what disease-related, social and psychological factors affect this. It will outline approaches to assessing functional independence and then consider evidence-based interventions addressing different domains of functional independence, including activities of daily living, social function and physical function. Finally, it will consider the application of interventions in different settings and mechanisms for delivery, such as remote delivery through internet-based approaches or other technology.

Functional Independence in Patients with Dementia

The range of functions impaired in dementia are commonly conceptualised as comprising basic activities of daily living (BADLs), which are simple self-maintenance activities such as bathing, toileting, dressing or eating; instrumental activities of daily living (IADLs) [20], which are more complex activities such as handling finances, navigating, shopping or preparing a meal; and social functions such as maintaining social contact with friends and relatives and participating in social hobbies and leisure activities [21]. This chapter will focus on clinical approaches to maximising independence in activities of daily living and social functions. We will also consider how maintaining physical functions, facilitating communication and supporting family members can facilitate independence.

Another conceptual approach is to consider independence as maintenance of current living circumstances, usually meaning the individual continuing to live in their own home for longer [22]. This is a potentially relevant marker of independence, as impairment in function is associated with patients with dementia having shorter time between diagnosis and moving from independent living into care settings [23, 24]. Another model suggests that rather than considering the level of independence as a domain of dementia, alongside cognition and behaviour, independence itself should be the unifying construct in defining dementia disease severity [25].

Loss of Independence Over the Disease Course

Loss of functional independence in dementia varies according to the activity or function being studied. This progressive loss, and factors which affect it, is summarised in Fig. 14.1. Dependence has been reported to occur for some complex activities very early in the course of dementia, such as in a study of Japanese elderly patients with very mild Alzheimer's disease (AD) where around half of people were noted to have difficulty in managing medication and preparing meals and 60% had lost independence in managing finances [26]. Other complex functional tasks such as maintaining social activity [27] and IADLs [28] may even be impaired during the prodromal stages of dementia, over 5 years before diagnosis.

In patients with established dementia, studies of patients with dementia in the UK [14] and Europe [29] examining six BADLs (bathing, dressing, toileting, transferring, continence and feeding) in over 1000 people with dementia suggested that bathing, continence and dressing were the activities most susceptible to loss of

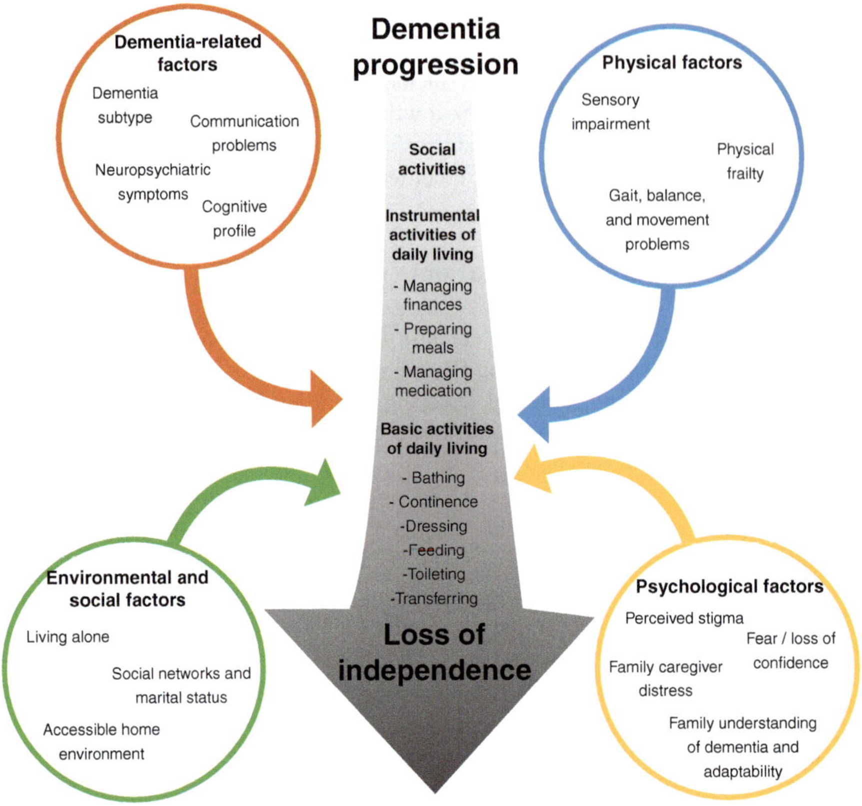

Fig. 14.1 Loss of functional independence during the course of dementia progression and disease-related, physical and environmental and social factors affecting independence

independence in early dementia, and that feeding, toileting and transferring were relatively preserved until the later stages of dementia. Bathing and continence were impaired in over half of patients with mild dementia, dressing became additionally impaired in the majority of patients with moderate dementia, and toileting and feeding were also impaired in over 50% of patients with severe dementia [14], findings which are supported by other research [30].

Studies which have examined the length of time until the person moves from living independently into a care home setting have reported varying results. For example, a German prospective cohort study of older people living in private homes found that median time from dementia onset to residing in a nursing home was 2.75 years [31] and mean time for patients with dementia onset after 65 years in the Netherlands was 4 years [32].In addition, half of patients in a US sample were institutionalised over 2.5 years [24], and Australian studies have reported institutionalisation in 25% of people 3 years after diagnosis [23] and 76% of people 5 years after diagnosis [33]. This variation across different study populations and settings likely reflects differences in baseline patient characteristics—some may have been diagnosed with dementia at a later stage. The diverse findings are also explained by societal differences such as different approaches to state provision of care and cultural differences [34], whereby it is customary in some settings for older people to live within wider family units where support can be given informally by the family, and in others to live alone in older age, where there is less support at hand to maintain current living circumstances.

Several factors appear to make institutionalisation more likely, and therefore should be of interest to clinicians aiming to prolong living at home, including being widowed or divorced compared to being married [24, 31], neuropsychiatric symptoms [23, 32, 35], rapid dementia progression and family caregiver psychological morbidity [33, 34].

Some aspects of social function appear to decline during the course of dementia. A cross-sectional study of ratings by family carers of 299 patients with dementia of varying disease severities [16] found that mean score in social functioning domains related to 'spending time with other people' and 'communicating with other people' declined significantly with increasing dementia severity. This suggests that patients with more severe dementia may be less motivated to maintain social activity, possibly related to apathy, have difficulty in arranging social engagements, maintaining communication [36], or be concerned about the potential challenges of these situations and so avoid these. Perceived stigma for a patient with dementia who anticipates that will struggle with functional and social activities [37] and anxiety of family members who have limited knowledge of dementia and difficulties adapting to their relative's condition are additional barriers to functional independence [8].

Other Factors Affecting Loss of Independence in Dementia

There is variation between patients with dementia in maintaining independence. Several factors which can be classified as relating to the dementia process, including dementia subtype, profile of cognitive deficit and neuropsychiatric symptoms; physical health including level of sensory impairment and physical frailty; and wider environmental and social factors affect the progressive loss of independence. These contributory factors are summarised in Fig. 14.1.

Variations in functioning have been reported according to dementia subtype. Patients with mild AD were rated by family carers as performing better on a range of IADLs than a comparator group with mild vascular dementia [38]. Those with AD also are more independent than patients with dementia with Lewy bodies (DLB) on BADLs and IADLs [39]. Comparison of patients with AD and behavioural-variant frontotemporal dementia (bvFTD) in financial calculations and errors found that patients with AD were more likely to make errors related to poor memory, but those with bvFTD advocated spending excessively with less concern for negative consequences [40]. Loss of independence in social functions related to impairments in social behaviour is also characteristic of bvFTD and has been shown to be worse in patients with bvFTD than in those with AD [41, 42].

These differences according to dementia type are likely to be related to several disease-related factors. Firstly, the profile of cognitive impairment such as the prominence of amnesia in AD compared to executive function and behavioural symptoms in bvFTD. Secondly, associated neuropsychiatric symptoms are clearly linked to worse ADL function [23, 32], so the higher rate of hallucinations in DLB [43] or apathy in bvFTD [44] are likely important drivers of functional decline in these conditions. Thirdly, associated somatic symptoms such as Parkinsonism in DLB or stroke-related impairments in vascular dementia increase frailty which impairs independence. Some studies have endeavoured to describe the detailed neural correlates of functional dependence [45] finding, for example, that impairment in IADLs in Alzheimer's disease is linked to lower medial frontal cortex volume [12], but the complexity of many functional tasks makes it difficult to conclude that these are localised in specific brain regions.

Physical frailty is a risk factor for losing functional independence in those with and without dementia [46, 47]. A Canadian longitudinal study of activity of daily living independence in patients with mild dementia at baseline found that 18% of the sample did not lose functional independence over 5 years follow-up. Those who maintained independence were likely to have no problems with gait, balance or movement, and have maintained sensory functions [48]. Other factors associated with independence were age, the presence of extrapyramidal symptoms and having less education.

Finally, environmental and social factors are key considerations in assessing propensity to lose independence of patients with dementia. As discussed previously, living alone and being unmarried are risk factors for institutionalisation as there is an absence of a carer to support previous levels of function. Wider social networks, including the availability of friends and relatives who are aware of, and can make reasonable adjustments to, the patient with dementia's impairments are particularly important in maintaining social functions [37]. The level of psychological distress and burden on family relatives is also important, making it a relevant area to assess when approaching clinical management, and having an accessible and adaptable home environment may also facilitate maintenance of independence. Box 14.1 describes two case vignettes with different factors affecting loss of independence in dementia.

Box 14.1 Case Vignettes: Factors Affecting Independence in Dementia

Mr. A is a 76-year-old widowed man who was diagnosed 3 months ago with mild Alzheimer's disease after complaining to his primary care doctor that he had become forgetful and was having difficulty navigating when driving his car. He lives alone in a second-floor apartment, and has family living 100 miles away who he speaks to regularly on the telephone although this is difficult due to hearing impairment. He is feeling lonely as he has stopped going regularly to his local social club.

Mrs. B is an 82 -year-old married woman who was diagnosed with dementia with Lewy bodies 4 years ago and has developed rigidity, bradykinesia and a stooped posture affecting her balance and gait. She has distressing visual hallucinations which are worse in the evenings and she cannot manage to wash or dress independently. Her husband, with whom she lives, is struggling with low mood and anxiety symptoms and no longer leaves her alone in the house.

Assessment of Functional Independence in Dementia

Approaches to maximise functional independence in dementia require the clinician to have an accurate appraisal of existing ability, especially considering that individuals vary in which domains are impaired and retained. There are several approaches to this assessment, including using proxy-report scales and observing performance on functional tasks [45], and there is potential for future approaches to further improve the assessment of function in dementia. Box 14.2 illustrates key approaches to assessing functional independence in the case vignettes.

Box 14.2 Case Vignettes: Assessment of Functional Independence

Mr. A was assessed by the occupational therapist who completed the UCSD performance-skills assessment. It was identified that Mr. A had difficulties in using the telephone related to hearing impairments, and that he struggled to manage navigation in unfamiliar settings. Safety assessment, including telephone conversation with his daughter, indicated that Mr. A's apartment did not have functioning smoke sensors, and that he may not be able to drive safely due to difficulties with navigation. He was willing to stop driving but identified his primary goal as wanting to continue to meet his friends at his local club. He explained that he had gradually stopped going because he was worried about getting there but also that he found it difficult to keep up with conversations once he arrived.

Mrs. B's husband completed the Bristol Activities of Daily Living Scale where it was noted that she had deficits in several basic ADLs, including dressing and hygiene, and instrumental ADLs such as preparing food and managing finances. Mrs. B had previously fallen in her home, where the lighting was poor, and she did not wear a safety alarm and she was observed in her home to have poor safety practices when attempting to prepare a cup of coffee using a gas cooker. Mrs. B's husband was seen by a psychologist who assessed his stress and burden; he explained that he worried a great deal about her safety and so found it easier to do things for her rather than getting her to try for herself. Mr. and Mrs. B identified several goals related to doing pleasurable activities out of the house together, and increasing social contact with others.

Proxy-Report Scales

There are a large range of scales which are used in clinical and research settings to assess levels of functional independence and ability. These usually rely on asking an informant—a relative or friend who knows the patient well, or a professional carer or other healthcare professional—about the patient's daily functioning, as it is usually thought that a patient with dementia would not be able to accurately gauge their own performance. A range of scales and their aims is presented in Table 14.1.

Table 14.1 Examples of assessment scales for measuring function in dementia

Domain of function	Scale	Aim
Basic or instrumental activities of daily living	Instrumental activities of daily living scale [49]	Assesses ability in eight daily living tasks, e.g. shopping, housekeeping, and takes 5 min for completion. Commonly used in dementia assessment services
	Bristol activities of daily living scale [50]	Questionnaire assessing 25 activities of daily living and completed by professional or family carer, taking around 15 min. Sensitive to change and can be used in clinical practice or research settings including clinical trials
	Disability Assessment for Dementia [51]	Interview-based questionnaire with a proxy respondent aiming to evaluate functional disability in community-dwelling patients with Alzheimer disease. Assesses 40 domains including leisure activities
	Functional independence measure [52]	Assesses overall disability, covering self-care, continence, mobility, communication, and psychosocial and cognitive function. Can be used in hospital settings, particularly inpatient rehabilitation
	Katz index of Independence in activities of daily living [53]	Assesses independence in six key areas of daily living activity including bathing, dressing. Rated by an informant and completed in less than 5 min. Designed for general population of older people but is frequently used in dementia clinical services
	Barthel Index [54]	Assesses functional ability for older people with a focus on physical functioning, and should be used only to assess impairments caused by physical function. Completed by an informant and has been widely translated and validated
Social function	Engagement and Independence in Dementia [55]	Self-report scale comprising 26 questions examining sense of independence and social engagement for a patient with dementia, with acceptable psychometric properties for research settings
	Social functioning in dementia scale [21]	Assesses 17 domains of social function in three key areas including spending time with others and communicating with others and has patient- and carer-rated versions. Primarily for use in research
Overall function	Informant Questionnaire on Cognitive Decline in the Elderly [56]	Administered to an informant to assess for presence of dementia by detecting changes in tasks, including recalling information and function, e.g. using new objects. Takes 10 min for completion

Scales assessing instrumental activities of daily living are considered useful in clinical settings, with a large pan-European study of memory clinics finding that the instrumental activities of daily living scale [49] were used in over one-third of these settings and the Katz scale [53] used in around one quarter. There is however limited evidence for the psychometric properties of many of these, and a systematic review found that only two were of overall moderate quality and that the rest were of lower quality [20]. The two scales favoured in this review were the Bristol Activities of Daily Living Scale, which aims to assesses change in ADLs in patients with early dementia as it lacks floor and ceiling effects and possible sensitivity to detect change, and the Disability Assessment for Dementia questionnaire, which assesses function in patients with dementia living in the general community which has established validity and reliability. Aspects of social function are often included within IADL scales, but few instruments specifically aim to assess social function.

Performance-Based Assessment

The other main approach to standardised assessment of functional independence is through directly assessing the performance of a patient with dementia in specific tasks [57]. This approach has potential to provide a more objective and valid evaluation than a scale completed by an informant and may be more qualitatively rich and informative. However, this process of assessment is more time-consuming and costly and may require the expertise of allied healthcare professionals including occupational therapists and physiotherapists. Assessments of this sort are often conducted in clinic or hospital settings although could be administered in the patient's own home.

Examples of scales which are validated in dementia include the Direct Assessment of Functional Status [58], which assesses a range of BADLs and IADLs, including dressing, feeding and shopping and takes around 45 min, the Performance ADL Test, which additionally assesses gross and fine motor control, the Erlangen Test of Activities of Daily Living [59] which assesses five activities such as eating and self-care, and the UCSD performance-based skills assessment [60] which assesses IADLs in around 30 min and is more sensitive in early disease. Other scales focus on specific functions, such as assessing in more detail ability to manage finances using the Financial Capacity Instrument [61].

Safety

A key consideration in assessing functional independence is the safety of the patient with dementia, meaning that risk should be evaluated and managed, ideally at home where unidentified areas of risk can be seen. Family members may have a different, often lower, threshold for tolerating risk than professionals or patients with dementia themselves as they may be the ones who are most affected, so assessment also needs to obtain different perspectives.

A common principle of risk management is to allow people to have acceptable level of risk to minimise restrictive strategies and permit patient autonomy, which usually requires assessing the mental capacity of the patient with dementia to make risky decisions related to poor judgement, apathy or forgetting and usually accompanied by lack of insight [62]. Key risks which should be evaluated are floods, fire or gas from leaving on cooking appliances, dehydration and malnutrition from forgetting or being unable to eat, forgetting to take medication, financial exploitation by others, unsafe driving and risk of getting lost or being harmed when out of the house, for example, due to poor road safety awareness [63].

Management of risk includes many of the measures and interventions discussed in the next section, as well as avoiding patients with dementia being left in dangerous situations, wearing personal pendant alarms, using medication aids, use of 'telecare' devices [64] and smoke, fire and gas sensors, and preventing people unable to drive safely from doing so. Risk changes throughout the course of dementia so need to be reassessed and managed regularly.

Other Approaches

There is significant potential for future technological approaches to improve the assessment of functional independence with greater ecological validity. Remote monitoring devices in the home including sensors to detect the interaction between a patient with dementia and their environment, such as their movement and use of appliances, have been tested in older people [65] and suggested for those with dementia [66] but are not used routinely in clinical settings. Mobile telephone technology could assess social functions such as time spent with or communicating with other people, and navigation [67]. Such technologies will require exploration of potential ethical issues related to privacy as well as evaluation of their accuracy and validity in this patient group.

Interventions for Promoting Functional Independence

The research evidence for the efficacy of interventions to promote functional independence is variable and there is no consistent evidence from high-quality research studies for any one particular approach. The studies which have shown efficacy in improving function for patients with dementia have all been delivered individually, rather than in group settings, allowing tailoring to the individual needs of patients with dementia [68]. This should therefore be the principle of clinical approaches to promoting independence and these may focus on supporting independent living, maintaining activities of daily living, promoting social function, maximising physical function and improving communication. Box 14.3 describes approaches to managing the case vignettes.

Supporting Independent Living

A recent systematic review found 11 randomised controlled trials (RCT) aiming to support patients with dementia to live at home for longer [22], two of which reported effective interventions. The Maximising Independence (MIND) at Home study focused on optimising the home environment and supporting family carers using a model based on the needs and goals of the patient with dementia. The MIND at Home study advocates that specific needs are identified and then mapped to a list of care strategies which can be carer-focused, self-management or involve other resources or services. This study used well-trained non-clinical staff as the coordinators of care, supported by clinicians such as nurses and physicians. This approach is potentially scalable to larger settings and findings of a RCT including 303 patients with dementia had 37% lower risk of moving from their homes during the 18 months following the intervention (median difference in time spent living at home between the intervention and control groups = 9.5 months), which may have been related to better safety management and advance care planning [69]. The intervention also improved quality of life relative to controls and led to less input being needed by family caregivers [70].

The other effective intervention was the New York University Spouse Caregiver Intervention which was primarily delivered to the family carer through two individual and four family sessions tailored to the caregiver's individual needs and with a focus on relationships and accommodating the dementia course to enable recovery, as well as providing telephone contact and support group participation. The intervention reduced nursing home placement risk in patients with dementia by 28% (median time to placement was 18.3 months longer for those receiving the intervention compared to controls) [71]and was most effective delivered for patients with mild or moderate dementia, rather than severe disease [72]. It has also been adapted to address the specific needs of adult-child caregivers of a parent with dementia, by changing the format of intervention delivery and incorporating additional sources of family support, and this adapted NYUCI showed maintained efficacy in a further RCT [73].

Other promising research which has shown encouraging pilot data is in process, such as the interdisciplinary home-based reablement program [74], a multicomponent intervention over 4 months including occupational therapist, nursing and other healthcare staff input, environmental adaptations to the home of the patient with dementia and carer support, and showed feasibility and potential for efficacy in a small pilot study [75]. The New interventions for Independence in dementia study [22] is also on-going and is an eight-session family carer-focused intervention aiming to support the patient with dementia to remain living independently at home. And the Promoting Independence in Dementia project [76] incorporates cognitive, physical and social activities delivered individually over three sessions and guided by a manual and can be delivered consistently and acceptably to patients with dementia [77].

Summary
Evidence from research interventions aiming to maintain a patient with dementia living in their own home therefore suggests that key components are that the clinician (1) identifies care needs and goals for the patient with dementia and their families; (2) prioritises these needs using therapy strategies aiming to minimise functional impairments and promoting self-management where possible; (3) offers support to family carers and gives them on-going support through a single point-of-contact; (4) forges links with other services and resources which are involved in patient care. These interventions are often relational, meaning that they are not simply about the patient with dementia continuing to do everything for themselves but involve building a supportive care environment which relies on interdependence for the patient with dementia and their informal and professional support networks.

Maintaining Activities of Daily Living

Several research studies have aimed specifically at improving a patient with dementia's ability to fulfil their activities of daily living. These tend to be occupational therapy-led interventions training patients with dementia to improve their performance at ADLs and, where function is impaired, developing compensatory strategies [68]. One US RCT found improvements in ADL function, which examined independence in ADLs as a secondary outcome in a study aiming primarily to reduce behavioural symptoms of dementia. The Tailored Activity Programme (TAP-VA) [78] involved eight sessions with occupational therapists in the homes of patients with dementia, tailored to the interests and abilities of the patients with dementia, aiming to customise activities and teach their family caregivers about dementia and how to maintain activities. In 160 dyads, the people receiving the intervention had fewer activities on which they were dependent on another person at 4 months follow-up, although this benefit did not extend to 8 months, possibly suggesting that gains from this intervention are lost and indicating the need to consider longer-term interventions or reassessment of needs at appropriate intervals.

Cognitive rehabilitation may be an effective approach to maximising ADL independence [79]; it aims to improve everyday function by helping patients with dementia to set individual goals and use strategies to achieve these. In a large RCT of 475 patients with mild dementia in the United Kingdom, the 'Goal-oriented cognitive rehabilitation for early-stage Alzheimer's and related dementias study', cognitive rehabilitation was given in ten therapy sessions over 3 months and then four maintenance sessions during the subsequent 6 months, delivered by occupational therapists or nurses to a patient with dementia and, during parts of the sessions, their caregiver. Sessions focused on three specified goals and aimed to model effective strategies and skills towards these goals, with encouragement for the patient and carer to continue these approaches between sessions. Improvements in participant-rated goal attainment, as rated by the patients and carers, were shown at 6 and 9 month follow-up, and this was considered to be cost-effective although there was no effect on secondary measures such as quality of life [80]. In another RCT, cognitive rehabilitation in patients with mild AD in 40 clinical sites in France resulted in better functional ability and delayed institutionalisation compared to usual care [81].

Other studies have examined before/after effects of interventions without comparator groups. For example, a small Spanish pilot study [82] of 21 patients with dementia found that an occupational therapist led 12 week programme of activities, cognitive stimulation, home modification and ADL training led to large increase in functional independence, and that top-up sessions 6 weeks later led to further improvements. However, the lack of control groups in studies such as these makes it impossible to know what aspect of this intervention may have been helpful.

Other studies have not reported significant improvement in ADL function. For example, an RCT which focused on ADL ability as primary outcome, using nine sessions of 'errorless learning', which guides people in activities to prevent them from making mistakes, and compared this to a simple trial-and-error approach to activities [83], did not find significant benefit of the therapeutic approach on task performance at 4–6 months in 161 patients with AD or mixed dementia. This type of intervention is sometimes referred to as cognitive training and is dealt with in Chap. 13. Another study which included occupational therapists working in patients' home settings over 5 weeks with patients and their caregivers to identify and encourage meaningful activities showed no difference in ADL performance for people who received the intervention compared to the control group [84].

Summary

The best approach to improving activity of daily living independence may be through cognitive rehabilitation. It appears likely that prolonged intervention over at least eight sessions is important and this may be best led by occupational therapists. As with interventions aiming to maintain independent living, it is likely that individualised approaches, involving family members, and setting appropriate patient-led goals are key to efficacy.

Promoting Social Function

Few studies have aimed primarily to promote social function in patients with dementia although improving social function is often a potential secondary outcome or mediator of other effective interventions. For example, group-based cognitive stimulation therapy (CST) [85] which involves group sessions led by a trained therapist consisting of social activities, cognitive exercise and reminiscence is recommended for all patients with mild dementia in the United Kingdom [86] due to the beneficial effects reported for cognitive outcomes. It may also confer benefits in social interactions, with moderate effect size [87], and therapeutic group-based interventions of this sort may be an appropriate first management step for patients with dementia whose social function is impaired. Individualised CST, delivered by a family caregiver with support and training, was not effective in improving cognition, but may improve the quality of family relationships [88]. CST is discussed further in Chap. 13. Other approaches such as support groups, which are popular with many patients and family carers, may also be beneficial in improving social function [89], and one RCT of support groups in the US reported improvements in quality of life which may have related to better social functioning [90].

Summary

There is no clear evidence for the best approaches to maximise social function in patients with dementia, but this may because few studies which have attempted to promote social activity alongside ADLs have considered social function as an outcome. Social function is a potential candidate for novel technological interventions as, for example, web-based communication has appeared promising in mild cognitive impairment [91], and social robots have been advocated for increasing the amount of social interaction for isolated people and those with advanced dementia [92].

Maximising Physical Function

Physical functioning is an important domain of function, which is closely linked to functional independence. Mobility, endurance, strength and balance all enable individuals to maintain daily functions, in particular basic activities of daily living, but these areas are also vulnerable for patients with dementia, who have high rates of other physical conditions, because of the bidirectional relationship between physical and cognitive health and shared risk factors for physical illnesses and dementia.

Several studies have shown efficacy in approaches to maximise physical function. Eight of nine RCTs of moderate or high quality which were included in a systematic review [93] found that intensive exercise improves physical functioning in patients with dementia. These studies tended to adopt more than one exercise modality, including strength and balance training or aerobic training, for example, using a stationary bicycle. Effective interventions had to be frequent (at least twice weekly), with progressive intensity, last at least 12 weeks, and be either individual or group-based.

There is variable evidence for the effect of these interventions on independence more broadly. Some have shown efficacy in improving BADL performance [94]. A Finnish RCT of a combination of either group-based exercise at day centres, or a goal-oriented tailored home exercise programme, each delivered once weekly for 1 h by specialist physiotherapists, focusing on endurance, strength, and balance and executive function tasks led to less functional decline those who received the intervention individually, but not in a group, compared to controls [93]. However, the Dementia And Physical Activity [95] trial of moderate to physiotherapist-delivered high intensity group-based exercise training in 494 patients with mild to moderate dementia found no improvements in ADL performance measured as a secondary outcome, and similar lack of efficacy was found in two other group-based interventions [96, 97]. See also Chap. 13 for further discussion on physical exercise and cognitive function.

Summary
There is strong evidence that intensive exercise interventions improve physical fitness and function in patients with dementia. Such interventions delivered in individual, but not group, settings may improve overall functional independence.

Supporting Sensory Function and Communication

As effective communication with others is an essential component of independence, supporting better sensory function including hearing and vision, and facilitating better communication is a potentially important facet of clinical care. As hearing is crucial to communicating with others, hearing loss should be identified and evaluated, and treated where appropriate with hearing aids, although the evidence for the efficacy of this as an intervention on function in patients with dementia is variable [98, 99].The increasing awareness that hearing impairment may confer negative effects on cognition, including elevating the risk of dementia [100], is likely to lead to more research in this area in future.

There is also limited research on the efficacy of correcting visual impairment, but this should be a priority of good quality clinical care, either by locating and cleaning existing spectacles, or assessment of visual acuity and provision of new glasses. Particular dementia types such as the posterior cortical atrophy variant of AD are associated with specific visual deficits [101] and these should also be assessed and environmental adaptations made to account for these to potentially improve function and reduce the risk of falls.

Several studies have aimed to improve communication between patients with dementia and their informal or professional carers. In a systematic review of these interventions in nursing home settings, approaches which were delivered to patients with dementia at set-times such as reminiscence, walking programmes including communication, or activity therapy, were ineffective, but those which aimed to incorporate improved communication into general daily care such as by training professional caregivers to provide better communication were effective in improving communication outcomes [102]. Particular problems with communication are encountered by those with rare dementia subtypes such as primary progressive aphasia and though there is currently a lack of clear research evidence and clinical pathways [103], approaches such as carrying picture books and cards may help in addition to structured therapeutic approaches [104].

Box 14.3 Case Vignettes: Management of Functional Independence
Mr. A attended a hearing assessment and was provided with hearing aids which improved his communication. He stopped driving and was provided with taxi transport to his local social club, which he was reminded to attend by a daily telephone call from his family. His hearing aid helped him to follow conversations better and he told one of his friends at the club about his dementia diagnosis which he had been worrying about. His family was signposted to local specialist dementia services. His apartment was fitted with functioning smoke sensors. Mr. A received regular review of his functional needs and goals.

Mrs. B's home underwent adaptations, with improved lighting to reduce falls risk, the gas cooker replaced by an electric alternative, and the installation of a telecare service including a 'pendant alarm' which Mrs. B wore to alert others to falls or injury. She received visits from a neighbour three times weekly to socialise and to enable Mr. B to leave the house alone to meet with a friend in a café. Mrs. B had pharmacological management of hallucinations optimised, and Mr. B continued to see the psychologist to receive structured therapy aiming to reduce his burden and stress and develop helpful strategies for supporting his wife.

Other Essential Considerations for Delivery of Interventions

In addition to considering the patient characteristics, needs and goals, clinicians should consider other important aspects related to the delivery of effective interventions including the setting, the mode of delivery and the role of different members of multidisciplinary teams.

Setting

In planning the delivery of interventions aiming to promote functional independence, clinicians should consider the setting in which these will be delivered. For example, maintaining functional independence in people living in independent homes is different to those who reside in settings with additional care support, such as residential homes or care homes. Although these settings by definition indicate that the patient with dementia has lost their independence to some extent, it remains an appropriate goal to maintain the current level of functional independence, which is likely to require collaborative working with care staff to devise, enact and maintain care strategies. Similarly, those who live in private homes alone compared to those who live with others will have different care needs and in these settings, having a supportive family member and/or high-quality professional care is important.

Rurality may also affect independence, as access to local amenities may be more impaired, in particular due to loss of driving ability [105]. Finally, there are international differences in current levels of post-diagnostic support for patients with dementia and models of care and funding for these, as well as significant disparities within countries for those from minority ethnic groups and deprived socio-economic backgrounds [6]. Promoting equity in healthcare should be a priority, meaning that those at greatest risk of losing functional independence should be most supported.

Mode of Delivery

As previously discussed, most evidence points towards individual, rather than group, treatments for patients with dementia, but there may be a role for group therapies where they are valued by patients and their family carers. Technological approaches to promoting functional independence include cognitive aids to remind people to take medication and prompt activities of daily living; robotic approaches to help with eating, washing and mobility; communication aids and technology to deliver music, images or video; and interventions to provide companionship [100]. These are in use already, primarily to maintain safety [64], and these are gaining increasing interest but there is a need for well-designed high-quality research evidence for these [106].

Assistive technology for supporting memory includes electronic pill dispensers or electronic diaries but in a recent Cochrane review, there were no high-quality studies meeting their predefined eligibility criteria examining functional independence, quality of life, or maintained independent living [107]. In a systematic review of qualitative studies, carers generally found use of assistive technology acceptable and viewed potential benefits in terms of promoting social interaction, maintaining autonomy and safety and therefore quality of life [108]; however, they reported potential barriers related to loss of personal aspects of caring and technical problems. A subsequent high-quality RCT comparing the effect on caregiver burden of provision of assistive technology and telecare following a structured needs assessment against simple safety measures such as smoke alarm and pendant alarm found no benefit for the technological approach [109]. However, the use of technology often does not reflect the recommendations of assessors [110] and a review found that lack of personalisation may adversely affect adoption of technological approaches for patients with dementia so this is an important future area for development [111].

Socially assistive robots, which have a social interface allowing interaction with a patient with dementia aiming to improve their well-being, take several forms, including human-like and animal robots. The most extensively research socially assistive robot is PARO, the seal-like companion robot which makes sounds and movements to interact with patients with dementia and there is provisional data suggesting that it is engaging for patients with dementia and reduces agitation [112]. Telepresence robots aim to promote social communication through interactive video calls between patients with dementia and their social contacts. Despite technical problems affecting their use in certain settings, they have generally been deemed acceptable by key stakeholders in small pilot studies [113, 114] though rigorous RCTs have not yet been conducted. Homecare assistive robots which provide supervision or monitoring to patients with dementia aiming to support BADLs and maintain safety have been described in the literature [115] and are viewed as feasible and acceptable [116] but there is scarce data on their efficacy.

The COVID-19 pandemic has accelerated the use of technology [117, 118] to provide remote care for people in settings where social and physical distancing has been necessary to reduce transmission of the disease. The evolution of care to address challenges is welcome, but may risk perpetuating isolation in patients with dementia so technological approaches should be evaluated and held to the high standards used for other non-pharmacological approaches, with consideration given to their acceptability to patients with dementia and potential adverse effects.

Role of Multidisciplinary Teams

There is a clear need for involvement of several members of the multidisciplinary team in managing promoting functional independence for patients with dementia. The role for physicians may be in clinical assessment of needs and risk and consideration of physical illness. Occupational therapists or physiotherapists may conduct performance-based assessment of function and lead or supervise interventions; specialist dementia nurses can offer additional support; neuropsychologists may evaluate cognitive profile in detail and clinical psychologists lead on delivery of psychological interventions for family carers and patients with dementia; speech and language therapists may assess communication and devise strategies to promote this. An aim of several research studies has been to develop scalable interventions [22, 70] which often mean that they are delivered directly by non-clinically trained staff, such as support workers, with supervision provided by more experienced staff, so there is role for other staff members with different levels of clinical experience. Collaborative working within and between teams is an essential component of clinical care.

Conclusions

Functional decline is one of the core features of dementia and so should be a focus of clinical care. Assessing areas of deficit allows clinicians to identify goals for improvement and develop strategies for promoting functional independence. The evidence base for interventions is growing, and the areas with strongest evidence for intervention, summarised in Fig. 14.2, appear to be multicomponent approaches which aim to tailor exercise programmes, cognitive rehabilitation approaches and home adaptations to dyads of patients with dementia and their family carers. There is a need to provide these treatments to people after the diagnosis of dementia and these have the potential to slow the loss of functional independence, save valuable resources and improve the quality of life of patients with dementia and their carers.

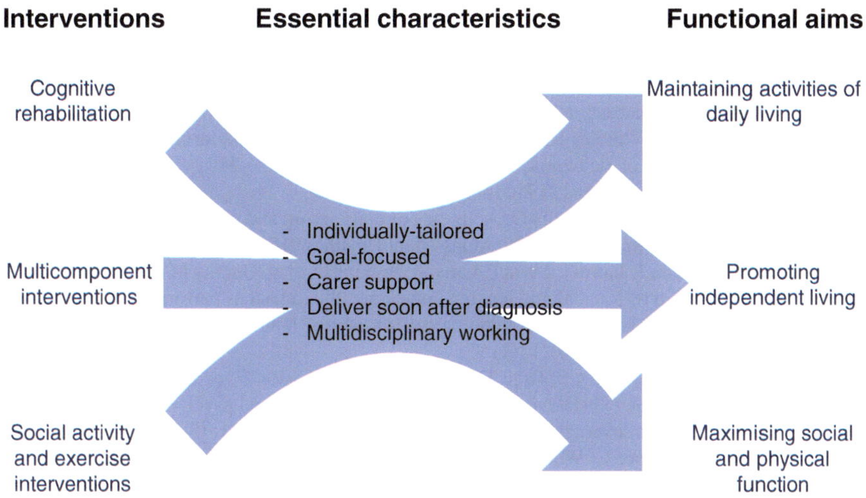

Fig. 14.2 Interventions to promote functional independence in dementia and essential characteristics of interventions

References

1. World Health Organization. International statistical classification of diseases and related health problems. Geneva: World Health Organization; 2004.
2. Laver K, Cumming R, Dyer S, Agar M, Beattie E, Brodaty H, et al. Clinical practice guidelines for dementia in Australia. Med J Aust. 2016;204(5):191–3. https://doi.org/10.5694/mja15.01.
3. Department of Health. Living well with dementia: a national dementia strategy. London: Department of Health; 2009.
4. Kmietowicz Z. Doctors condemn "unethical"£ 55 payment for every new dementia diagnosis. BMJ. 2014;349:g6424.
5. Shenkin SD, Russ TC, Ryan TM, MacLullich AM. Screening for dementia and other causes of cognitive impairment in general hospital in-patients. Oxford: Oxford University Press; 2014.
6. Giebel C. Current dementia care: what are the difficulties and how can we advance care globally? BMC Health Serv Res. 2020;20:414.
7. Shah H, Albanese E, Duggan C, Rudan I, Langa KM, Carrillo MC, et al. Research priorities to reduce the global burden of dementia by 2025. Lancet Neurol. 2016;15(12):1285–94.
8. Rapaport P, Burton A, Leverton M, Herat-Gunaratne R, Beresford-Dent J, Lord K, et al. "I just keep thinking that I don't want to rely on people." a qualitative study of how people living with dementia achieve and maintain independence at home: stakeholder perspectives. BMC Geriatr. 2020;20(1):5.
9. van der Linde RM, Dening T, Stephan BC, Prina AM, Evans E, Brayne C. Longitudinal course of behavioural and psychological symptoms of dementia: systematic review. Br J Psychiatry. 2016;209(5):366–77.
10. Browne J, Edwards DA, Rhodes KM, Brimicombe DJ, Payne RA. Association of comorbidity and health service usage among patients with dementia in the UK: a population-based study. BMJ Open. 2017;7(3):e012546.

11. Poblador-Plou B, Calderón-Larrañaga A, Marta-Moreno J, Hancco-Saavedra J, Sicras-Mainar A, Soljak M, et al. Comorbidity of dementia: a cross-sectional study of primary care older patients. BMC Psychiatry. 2014;14(1):84.
12. Vidoni ED, Honea RA, Burns JM. Neural correlates of impaired functional independence in early Alzheimer's disease. J Alzheimers Dis. 2010;19(2):517–27.
13. Olsen V, Taylor L, Whiteley K, Ellerton A, Kingston P, Bailey J. Exploring public perceptions and understanding of dementia: analysing narratives from the Mass Observation Project. Dementia. 2019;19:1471301219861468.
14. Giebel CM, Sutcliffe C, Challis D. Activities of daily living and quality of life across different stages of dementia: a UK study. Aging Ment Health. 2015;19(1):63–71.
15. Ballard C, O'brien J, James I, Mynt P, Lana M, Potkins D, et al. Quality of life for people with dementia living in residential and nursing home care: the impact of performance on activities of daily living, behavioral and psychological symptoms, language skills, and psychotropic drugs. Int Psychogeriatr. 2001;13(1):93.
16. Budgett J, Brown A, Daley S, Page TE, Banerjee S, Livingston G, et al. The social functioning in dementia scale (SF-DEM): exploratory factor analysis and psychometric properties in mild, moderate, and severe dementia. Alzheimers Dement. 2019;11:45–52.
17. Livingston G, Cooper C, Woods J, Milne A, Katona C. Successful ageing in adversity: the LASER–AD longitudinal study. J Neurol Neurosurg Psychiatry. 2008;79(6):641–5.
18. Kim H, Chang M, Rose K, Kim S. Predictors of caregiver burden in caregivers of individuals with dementia. J Adv Nurs. 2012;68(4):846–55.
19. Razani J, Kakos B, Orieta-Barbalace C, Wong JT, Casas R, Lu P, et al. Predicting caregiver burden from daily functional abilities of patients with mild dementia. J Am Geriatr Soc. 2007;55(9):1415–20.
20. Sikkes S, De Lange-de Klerk E, Pijnenburg Y, Scheltens P. A systematic review of Instrumental Activities of Daily Living scales in dementia: room for improvement. J Neurol Neurosurg Psychiatry. 2009;80(1):7–12.
21. Sommerlad A, Singleton D, Jones R, Banerjee S, Livingston G. Development of an instrument to assess social functioning in dementia: the Social Functioning in Dementia scale (SF-DEM). Alzheimers Dement. 2017;7:88–98.
22. Lord K, Beresford-Dent J, Rapaport P, Burton A, Leverton M, Walters K, et al. Developing the New Interventions for independence in Dementia Study (NIDUS) theoretical model for supporting people to live well with dementia at home for longer: a systematic review of theoretical models and Randomised Controlled Trial evidence. Soc Psychiatry Psychiatr Epidemiol. 2020;55(1):1–14.
23. Brodaty H, Connors MH, Xu J, Woodward M, Ames D, Group PS. Predictors of institutionalization in dementia: a three year longitudinal study. J Alzheimers Dis. 2014;40(1):221–6.
24. Severson MA, Smith GE, Tangalos EG, Petersen RC, Kokmen E, Ivnik RJ, et al. Patterns and predictors of institutionalization in community-based dementia patients. J Am Geriatr Soc. 1994;42(2):181–5.
25. McLaughlin T, Feldman H, Fillit H, Sano M, Schmitt F, Aisen P, et al. Dependence as a unifying construct in defining Alzheimer's disease severity. Alzheimers Dement. 2010;6(6):482–93.
26. Tabira T, Hotta M, Murata M, Yoshiura K, Han G, Ishikawa T, et al. Age-related changes in instrumental and basic activities of daily Living impairment in older adults with very mild Alzheimer's disease. Dement Geriatr Cogn Dis Extra. 2020;10(1):27–37.
27. Sommerlad A, Sabia S, Livingston G, Kivimäki M, Lewis G, Singh-Manoux A. Leisure activity participation and risk of dementia: 18 year follow-up of the Whitehall II Study. Neurology. 2020;95(20):e2803–15.
28. Amieva H, Le Goff M, Millet X, Orgogozo JM, Pérès K, Barberger-Gateau P, et al. Prodromal Alzheimer's disease: successive emergence of the clinical symptoms. Ann Neurol. 2008;64(5):492–8.
29. Giebel CM, Sutcliffe C, Stolt M, Karlsson S, Renom-Guiteras A, Soto M, et al. Deterioration of basic activities of daily living and their impact on quality of life across different cognitive stages of dementia: a European study. Int Psychogeriatr. 2014;26(8):1283.

30. Galasko D, Schmitt F, Thomas R, Jin S, Bennett D, Ferris S. Detailed assessment of activities of daily living in moderate to severe Alzheimer's disease. J Int Neuropsychol Soc. 2005;11(4):446–53.
31. Luck T, Luppa M, Weber S, Matschinger H, Glaesmer H, König H-H, et al. Time until institutionalization in incident dementia cases–results of the Leipzig Longitudinal Study of the Aged (LEILA 75+). Neuroepidemiology. 2008;31(2):100–8.
32. Bakker C, de Vugt ME, van Vliet D, Verhey FR, Pijnenburg YA, Vernooij-Dassen MJ, et al. Predictors of the time to institutionalization in young-versus late-onset dementia: results from the Needs in Young Onset Dementia (NeedYD) study. J Am Med Dir Assoc. 2013;14(4):248–53.
33. Brodaty H, McGilchrist C, Harris L, Peters KE. Time until institutionalization and death in patients with dementia: role of caregiver training and risk factors. Arch Neurol. 1993;50(6):643–50.
34. Mausbach BT, Coon DW, Depp C, Rabinowitz YG, Wilson-Arias E, Kraemer HC, et al. Ethnicity and time to institutionalization of dementia patients: a comparison of Latina and Caucasian female family caregivers. J Am Geriatr Soc. 2004;52(7):1077–84.
35. Dorenlot P, Harboun M, Bige V, Henrard JC, Ankri J. Major depression as a risk factor for early institutionalization of dementia patients living in the community. Int J Geriatr Psychiatry. 2005;20(5):471–8.
36. Williams CL, Newman D, Hammar LM. Preliminary psychometric properties of the verbal and nonverbal interaction scale: an observational measure for communication in persons with dementia. Issues Ment Health Nurs. 2017;38(5):381–90.
37. Singleton D, Mukadam N, Livingston G, Sommerlad A. How people with dementia and carers understand and react to social functioning changes in mild dementia: a UK-based qualitative study. BMJ Open. 2017;7(7):e016740.
38. Giebel CM, Burns A, Challis D. Taking a positive spin: preserved initiative and performance of everyday activities across mild Alzheimer's, vascular and mixed dementia. Int J Geriatr Psychiatry. 2017;32(9):959–67.
39. Ricci M, Guidoni SV, Sepe-Monti M, Bomboi G, Antonini G, Blundo C, et al. Clinical findings, functional abilities and caregiver distress in the early stage of dementia with Lewy bodies (DLB) and Alzheimer's disease (AD). Arch Gerontol Geriatr. 2009;49(2):e101–e4.
40. Chiong W, Hsu M, Wudka D, Miller BL, Rosen HJ. Financial errors in dementia: testing a neuroeconomic conceptual framework. Neurocase. 2014;20(4):389–96.
41. Gregory C, Lough S, Stone V, Erzinclioglu S, Martin L, Baron-Cohen S, et al. Theory of mind in patients with frontal variant frontotemporal dementia and Alzheimer's disease: theoretical and practical implications. Brain. 2002;125(4):752–64.
42. Kumfor F, Piguet O. Emotion recognition in the dementias: brain correlates and patient implications. Neurodegener Dis Manag. 2013;3(3):277–88.
43. Mueller C, Ballard C, Corbett A, Aarsland D. The prognosis of dementia with Lewy bodies. Lancet Neurol. 2017;16(5):390–8.
44. Kumfor F, Zhen A, Hodges JR, Piguet O, Irish M. Apathy in Alzheimer's disease and frontotemporal dementia: distinct clinical profiles and neural correlates. Cortex. 2018;103:350–9.
45. Marshall GA, Amariglio RE, Sperling RA, Rentz DM. Activities of daily living: where do they fit in the diagnosis of Alzheimer's disease? Neurodegener Dis Manag. 2012;2(5):483–91.
46. Abreu W, Tolson D, Jackson GA, Staines H, Costa N. The relationship between frailty, functional dependence, and healthcare needs among community-dwelling people with moderate to severe dementia. Health Soc Care Community. 2019;27(3):642–53.
47. Provencher V, Sirois MJ, Ouellet MC, Camden S, Neveu X, Allain-Boulé N, et al. Decline in activities of daily living after a visit to a Canadian emergency department for minor injuries in independent older adults: are frail older adults with cognitive impairment at greater risk? J Am Geriatr Soc. 2015;63(5):860–8.
48. Perrault A, Wolfson C, Egan M, Rockwood K, Hogan DB. Prognostic factors for functional independence in older adults with mild dementia: results from the Canadian study of health and aging. Alzheimer Dis Assoc Disord. 2002;16(4):239–47.

49. Lawton MP, Brody EM. Assessment of older people: self-maintaining and instrumental activities of daily living. Gerontologist. 1969;9(3_Part_1):179–86.
50. Bucks RS, Ashworth D, Wilcock G, Siegfried K. Assessment of activities of daily living in dementia: development of the Bristol Activities of Daily Living Scale. Age Ageing. 1996;25(2):113–20.
51. Gélinas I, Gauthier L, McIntyre M, Gauthier S. Development of a functional measure for persons with Alzheimer's disease: the disability assessment for dementia. Am J Occup Ther. 1999;53(5):471–81.
52. Keith R, Granger C, Hamilton B, Sherwin F. The functional independence measure: a new tool for rehabilitation. Adv Clin Rehabil. 1987;1:618.
53. Katz S, Ford AB, Moskowitz RW, Jackson BA, Jaffe MW. Studies of illness in the aged: the index of ADL: a standardized measure of biological and psychosocial function. JAMA. 1963;185(12):914–9.
54. Mahoney FI, Barthel DW. Functional evaluation: the Barthel Index: a simple index of independence useful in scoring improvement in the rehabilitation of the chronically ill. Maryland State Med J. 1965;14:61–5.
55. Stoner CR, Orrell M, Spector A. Psychometric properties and factor analysis of the engagement and independence in dementia questionnaire (EID-Q). Dement Geriatr Cogn Disord. 2018;46(3–4):119–27.
56. Jorm A, Jacomb P. The Informant Questionnaire on Cognitive Decline in the Elderly (IQCODE): socio-demographic correlates, reliability, validity and some norms. Psychol Med. 1989;19(4):1015–22.
57. Mlinac ME, Feng MC. Assessment of activities of daily living, self-care, and independence. Arch Clin Neuropsychol. 2016;31(6):506–16.
58. Loewenstein DA, Amigo E, Duara R, Guterman A, Hurwitz D, Berkowitz N, et al. A new scale for the assessment of functional status in Alzheimer's disease and related disorders. J Gerontol. 1989;44(4):P114–P21.
59. Graessel E, Viegas R, Stemmer R, Küchly B, Kornhuber J, Donath C. The Erlangen Test of Activities of Daily Living: first results on reliability and validity of a short performance test to measure fundamental activities of daily living in dementia patients. Int Psychogeriatr. 2009;21(1):103–12.
60. Gomar JJ, Harvey PD, Bobes-Bascaran MT, Davies P, Goldberg TE. Development and cross-validation of the UPSA short form for the performance-based functional assessment of patients with mild cognitive impairment and Alzheimer disease. Am J Geriatr Psychiatry. 2011;19(11):915–22.
61. Marson DC, Sawrie SM, Snyder S, McInturff B, Stalvey T, Boothe A, et al. Assessing financial capacity in patients with Alzheimer disease: a conceptual model and prototype instrument. Arch Neurol. 2000;57(6):877–84.
62. Starkstein SE, Jorge R, Mizrahi R, Adrian J, Robinson R. Insight and danger in Alzheimer's disease. Eur J Neurol. 2007;14(4):455–60.
63. Douglas A, Letts L, Richardson J. A systematic review of accidental injury from fire, wandering and medication self-administration errors for older adults with and without dementia. Arch Gerontol Geriatr. 2011;52(1):e1–e10.
64. Gibson G, Newton L, Pritchard G, Finch T, Brittain K, Robinson L. The provision of assistive technology products and services for people with dementia in the United Kingdom. Dementia. 2016;15(4):681–701.
65. Yang C-C, Hsu Y-L. Remote monitoring and assessment of daily activities in the home environment. J Clin Gerontol Geriatr. 2012;3(3):97–104.
66. Amiribesheli M, Bouchachia H. A tailored smart home for dementia care. J Ambient Intell Humaniz Comput. 2018;9(6):1755–82.
67. Kuntsche E, Labhart F. Using personal cell phones for ecological momentary assessment: an overview of current developments. Eur Psychol. 2013;18(1):3.
68. Scott I, Cooper C, Leverton M, Burton A, Beresford-Dent J, Rockwood K, et al. Effects of nonpharmacological interventions on functioning of people living with demen-

tia at home: a systematic review of randomised controlled trials. Int J Geriatr Psychiatry. 2019;34(10):1386–402.
69. Samus QM, Johnston D, Black BS, Hess E, Lyman C, Vavilikolanu A, et al. A multidimensional home-based care coordination intervention for elders with memory disorders: the maximizing independence at home (MIND) pilot randomized trial. Am J Geriatr Psychiatry. 2014;22(4):398–414.
70. Tanner JA, Black BS, Johnston D, Hess E, Leoutsakos J-M, Gitlin LN, et al. A randomized controlled trial of a community-based dementia care coordination intervention: effects of MIND at Home on caregiver outcomes. Am J Geriatr Psychiatry. 2015;23(4):391–402.
71. Mittelman MS, Haley WE, Clay OJ, Roth DL. Improving caregiver well-being delays nursing home placement of patients with Alzheimer disease. Neurology. 2006;67(9):1592–9.
72. Mittelman MS, Ferris SH, Shulman E, Steinberg G, Levin B. A family intervention to delay nursing home placement of patients with Alzheimer disease: a randomized controlled trial. JAMA. 1996;276(21):1725–31.
73. Gaugler JE, Reese M, Mittelman MS. Effects of the NYU caregiver intervention-adult child on residential care placement. The Gerontologist. 2013;53(6):985–97.
74. Jeon Y-H, Simpson JM, Low L-F, Woods R, Norman R, Mowszowski L, et al. A pragmatic randomised controlled trial (RCT) and realist evaluation of the interdisciplinary home-bAsed Reablement program (I-HARP) for improving functional independence of community dwelling older people with dementia: an effectiveness-implementation hybrid design. BMC Geriatr. 2019;19(1):199.
75. Jeon Y-H, Krein L, Simpson JM, Szanton SL, Clemson L, Naismith SL, et al. Feasibility and potential effects of interdisciplinary home-based reablement program (I-HARP) for people with cognitive and functional decline: a pilot trial. Aging Ment Health. 2019;24:1–10.
76. Yates L, Csipke E, Moniz-Cook E, Leung P, Walton H, Charlesworth G, et al. The development of the Promoting Independence in Dementia (PRIDE) intervention to enhance independence in dementia. Clin Interv Aging. 2019;14:1615.
77. Walton H, Spector A, Roberts A, Williamson M, Bhatt J, Tombor I, et al. Developing strategies to improve fidelity of delivery of, and engagement with, a complex intervention to improve independence in dementia: a mixed methods study. BMC Med Res Methodol. 2020;20(1):1–19.
78. Gitlin LN, Arthur P, Piersol C, Hessels V, Wu SS, Dai Y, et al. Targeting behavioral symptoms and functional decline in dementia: a randomized clinical trial. J Am Geriatr Soc. 2018;66(2):339–45.
79. Clare L, Woods RT. Cognitive training and cognitive rehabilitation for people with early-stage Alzheimer's disease: a review. Neuropsychol Rehabil. 2004;14(4):385–401.
80. Clare L, Kudlicka A, Oyebode JR, Jones RW, Bayer A, Leroi I, et al. Goal-oriented cognitive rehabilitation for early-stage Alzheimer's and related dementias: the GREAT RCT. Health Technol Assess. 2019;23(10):1–242.
81. Amieva H, Robert PH, Grandoulier A-S, Meillon C, De Rotrou J, Andrieu S, et al. Group and individual cognitive therapies in Alzheimer's disease: the ETNA3 randomized trial. Int Psychogeriatr. 2016;28(5):707–17.
82. Ávila A, De-Rosende-Celeiro I, Torres G, Vizcaíno M, Peralbo M, Durán M. Promoting functional independence in people with Alzheimer's disease: outcomes of a home-based occupational therapy intervention in Spain. Health Soc Care Community. 2018;26(5):734–43.
83. Voigt-Radloff S, de Werd MM, Leonhart R, Boelen DH, Rikkert MGO, Fliessbach K, et al. Structured relearning of activities of daily living in dementia: the randomized controlled REDALI-DEM trial on errorless learning. Alzheimers Res Ther. 2017;9(1):22.
84. Döpp CM, Graff MJ, Teerenstra S, Olde Rikkert MG, Nijhuis-van der Sanden MW, Vernooij-Dassen MJ. Effectiveness of a training package for implementing a community-based occupational therapy program in dementia: a cluster randomized controlled trial. Clin Rehabil. 2015;29(10):974–86.

85. Spector A, Thorgrimsen L, Woods B, Royan L, Davies S, Butterworth M, et al. Efficacy of an evidence-based cognitive stimulation therapy programme for people with dementia: randomised controlled trial. Br J Psychiatry. 2003;183(3):248–54.
86. Pink J, O'Brien J, Robinson L, Longson D. Dementia: assessment, management and support: summary of updated NICE guidance. BMJ. 2018;361:k2438.
87. Woods B, Aguirre E, Spector AE, Orrell M. Cognitive stimulation to improve cognitive functioning in people with dementia. Cochrane Database Syst Rev. 2012;(2):CD005562. https://doi.org/10.1002/14651858.CD005562.pub2.
88. Orrell M, Yates L, Leung P, Kang S, Hoare Z, Whitaker C, et al. The impact of individual Cognitive Stimulation Therapy (iCST) on cognition, quality of life, caregiver health, and family relationships in dementia: a randomised controlled trial. PLoS Med. 2017;14(3):e1002269.
89. Logsdon RG, McCurry SM, Teri L. Evidence-based interventions to improve quality of life for individuals with dementia. Alzheimers Care Today. 2007;8(4):309.
90. Logsdon RG, Pike KC, McCurry SM, Hunter P, Maher J, Snyder L, et al. Early-stage memory loss support groups: outcomes from a randomized controlled clinical trial. J Gerontol B Psychol Sci Soc Sci. 2010;65(6):691–7.
91. Dodge HH, Zhu J, Mattek NC, Bowman M, Ybarra O, Wild KV, et al. Web-enabled conversational interactions as a method to improve cognitive functions: results of a 6-week randomized controlled trial. Alzheimers Dement. 2015;1(1):1–12.
92. Valentí Soler M, Agüera-Ortiz L, Olazarán Rodríguez J, Mendoza Rebolledo C, Pérez Muñoz A, Rodríguez Pérez I, et al. Social robots in advanced dementia. Front Aging Neurosci. 2015;7:133.
93. Pitkälä K, Savikko N, Poysti M, Strandberg T, Laakkonen M-L. Efficacy of physical exercise intervention on mobility and physical functioning in older people with dementia: a systematic review. Exp Gerontol. 2013;48(1):85–93.
94. Blankevoort CG, Van Heuvelen MJ, Boersma F, Luning H, De Jong J, Scherder EJ. Review of effects of physical activity on strength, balance, mobility and ADL performance in elderly subjects with dementia. Dement Geriatr Cogn Disord. 2010;30(5):392–402.
95. Lamb SE, Sheehan B, Atherton N, Nichols V, Collins H, Mistry D, et al. Dementia And Physical Activity (DAPA) trial of moderate to high intensity exercise training for people with dementia: randomised controlled trial. BMJ. 2018;361:k1675.
96. Hoffmann K, Sobol NA, Frederiksen KS, Beyer N, Vogel A, Vestergaard K, et al. Moderate-to-high intensity physical exercise in patients with Alzheimer's disease: a randomized controlled trial. J Alzheimers Dis. 2016;50(2):443–53.
97. Padala KP, Padala PR, Lensing SY, Dennis RA, Bopp MM, Roberson PK, et al. Home-based exercise program improves balance and fear of falling in community-dwelling older adults with mild Alzheimer's disease: a pilot study. J Alzheimers Dis. 2017;59(2):565–74.
98. Adrait A, Perrot X, Nguyen M-F, Gueugnon M, Petitot C, Collet L, et al. Do hearing aids influence behavioral and psychological symptoms of dementia and quality of life in hearing impaired Alzheimer's disease patients and their caregivers? J Alzheimers Dis. 2017;58(1):109–21.
99. Allen NH, Burns A, Newton V, Hickson F, Ramsden R, Rogers J, et al. The effects of improving hearing in dementia. Age Ageing. 2003;32(2):189–93.
100. Livingston G, Sommerlad A, Orgeta V, Costafreda SG, Huntley J, Ames D, et al. Dementia prevention, intervention, and care. Lancet. 2017;390(10113):2673–734.
101. Yong KX, Shakespeare TJ, Cash D, Henley SM, Nicholas JM, Ridgway GR, et al. Prominent effects and neural correlates of visual crowding in a neurodegenerative disease population. Brain. 2014;137(12):3284–99.
102. Vasse E, Vernooij-Dassen M, Spijker A, Rikkert MO, Koopmans R. A systematic review of communication strategies for people with dementia in residential and nursing homes. Database of Abstracts of Reviews of Effects (DARE): Quality-assessed Reviews: Centre for Reviews and Dissemination (UK); 2010.

103. Volkmer A, Spector A, Warren JD, Beeke S. Speech and language therapy for primary progressive aphasia across the UK: a survey of current practice. Int J Lang Commun Dis. 2019;54(6):914–26.
104. Marshall CR, Hardy CJ, Volkmer A, Russell LL, Bond RL, Fletcher PD, et al. Primary progressive aphasia: a clinical approach. J Neurol. 2018;265(6):1474–90.
105. Marshall F, Basiri A, Riley M, Dening T, Gladman J, Griffiths A, et al. Scaling the Peaks Research Protocol: understanding the barriers and drivers to providing and using dementia-friendly community services in rural areas—a mixed methods study. BMJ Open. 2018;8(4):e020374.
106. Øksnebjerg L, Janbek J, Woods B, Waldemar G. Assistive technology designed to support self-management of people with dementia: user involvement, dissemination, and adoption. A scoping review. Int Psychogeriatr. 2020;32(8):937–53.
107. Van der Roest HG, Wenborn J, Pastink C, Dröes RM, Orrell M. Assistive technology for memory support in dementia. Cochrane Database Syst Rev. 2017;6(6):CD009627.
108. Sriram V, Jenkinson C, Peters M. Informal carers' experience of assistive technology use in dementia care at home: a systematic review. BMC Geriatr. 2019;19(1):160.
109. Davies A, Brini S, Hirani S, Gathercole R, Forsyth K, Henderson C, et al. The impact of assistive technology on burden and psychological well-being in informal caregivers of people with dementia (ATTILA Study). Alzheimers Dement. 2020;6(1):e12064.
110. Forsyth K, Henderson C, Davis L, Singh Roy A, Dunk B, Curnow E, et al. Assessment of need and practice for assistive technology and telecare for people with dementia—the ATTILA (Assistive Technology and Telecare to maintain Independent Living At home for people with dementia) trial. Alzheimers Dement. 2019;5(1):420–30.
111. Sanders D, Scott P. Literature review: technological interventions and their impact on quality of life for people living with dementia. BMJ Health Care Inform. 2020;27(1):e100064.
112. Moyle W, Jones CJ, Murfield JE, Thalib L, Beattie ERA, Shum DKH, et al. Use of a robotic seal as a therapeutic tool to improve dementia symptoms: a cluster-randomized controlled trial. J Am Med Dir Assoc. 2017;18(9):766–73.
113. Moyle W, Jones C, Cooke M, O'Dwyer S, Sung B, Drummond S. Connecting the person with dementia and family: a feasibility study of a telepresence robot. BMC Geriatr. 2014;14(1):7.
114. Moyle W, Jones C, Dwan T, Ownsworth T, Sung B. Using telepresence for social connection: views of older people with dementia, families, and health professionals from a mixed methods pilot study. Aging Ment Health. 2019;23(12):1643–50.
115. Martín F, Agüero CE, Cañas JM, Valenti M, Martínez-Martín P. Robotherapy with dementia patients. Int J Adv Robot Syst. 2013;10(1):10.
116. Law M, Sutherland C, Ahn HS, MacDonald BA, Peri K, Johanson DL, et al. Developing assistive robots for people with mild cognitive impairment and mild dementia: a qualitative study with older adults and experts in aged care. BMJ Open. 2019;9(9):e031937.
117. Wang H, Li T, Barbarino P, Gauthier S, Brodaty H, Molinuevo JL, et al. Dementia care during COVID-19. Lancet. 2020;395(10231):1190–1.
118. Goodman-Casanova JM, Dura-Perez E, Guzman-Parra J, Cuesta-Vargas A, Mayoral-Cleries F. Telehealth home support during COVID-19 confinement for community-dwelling older adults with mild cognitive impairment or mild dementia: survey study. J Med Internet Res. 2020;22(5):e19434.

Patients with Dementia in Hospital 15

Tomas J. Welsh and Roy W. Jones

Abbreviations

HR-QOL	Health Related-Quality of Life
NICE	The UK National Institute for Health and Clinical Excellence
NIHR	The UK National Institute of Health Research
TEAM	Trial of an Elderly Acute Care Medical and Mental Health Unit
CAM	Confusion Assessment Method

Introduction

Hospitals can be dangerous places [1, 2]. This is particularly true for people living with dementia where a change of environment and routine alone can be hugely disruptive and destabilising. Given that a hospital admission is likely to occur in the context of an intercurrent illness, then the well-documented risks of cognitive and physical decline are perhaps less surprising [3].

T. J. Welsh (✉)
The Research Institute for the Care of Older People, Bath, UK

Royal United Hospitals Bath NHS Foundation Trust, Bath, UK

University of Bristol, Bristol, UK
e-mail: tw695@bath.ac.uk

R. W. Jones
The Research Institute for the Care of Older People, Bath, UK

Royal United Hospitals Bath NHS Foundation Trust, Bath, UK

University of Bristol, Bristol, UK

University of Bath, Bath, UK
e-mail: r.w.jones@bath.ac.uk

K. S. Frederiksen, G. Waldemar (eds.), *Management of Patients with Dementia*,
https://doi.org/10.1007/978-3-030-77904-7_15

A view that hospital admission should be avoided, and hospital stay should be limited has become widespread. Certainly, people with dementia admitted to hospital will stay for longer than their cognitively intact peers with the same acute illness [3]. They will be more likely to become less mobile and be at higher risk of functional decline and institutionalisation [4]. The difficulty with this view is that it attenuates the responsibility of healthcare professionals to make hospital a better place for people with cognitive impairment and there is a risk that by prioritising early discharge longer term outcomes are adversely affected leading to recurrent admissions and functional decline [5, 6]. The hospital, its diagnostic facilities, and drug and non-drug therapies can be and should be as accessible to those with cognitive impairment as to those without. There are steps that can be taken to improve the care of people with dementia in hospital and the wider healthcare system but there needs to be the will to make those changes [7].

Up to 40% of people aged over 70 admitted to hospital may have a dementia (diagnosed or undiagnosed) [8], and this has been the case for many years, yet hospitals still struggle to meet the needs of people with dementia. Why is this? And what can be done to improve the situation?

This chapter sets out some of the principles that underpin good care for people with dementia. It will begin by discussing Person-Centred Care and Comprehensive Geriatric Assessment. It will discuss the importance of the hospital environment both social and physical. Next, it will discuss issues around care in some commonly occurring medical scenarios. Finally, we will discuss a specific case, which illustrates some of the challenges facing the physician managing the medical care of a patient with dementia in hospital.

Person-Centred Care

Even if they have cognitive impairment and communication difficulties, it seems self-evident that people with dementia are still individuals and should expect to be treated as such. Sadly, this has not always been the case and still, often unconsciously and with the best intentions, people with dementia can be 'disabled' by the behaviour of people around them. Tom Kitwood in 1997 identified and labelled ways in which people with dementia can be disabled referring to this as 'malignant social psychology' [9]. Such interactions commonly arise out of the stresses of a situation or unconsciously but may include actions such as: Labelling ('he always does that it's his dementia) or Withholding (ignoring someone calling out).

Person-Centred care 'founded on the ethic that all human beings are of absolute value and worthy of respect, no matter their disability, and on a conviction that people with dementia can lead fulfilling lives' provides an alternative approach [10]. It provides a framework for seeing people with dementia as equal partners in their care and putting people with dementia and their friends and family at the heart of decisions. The system should be moulded round the individual not the individual by the system.

Principles of Person-Centred care

1. Afford people dignity, respect and compassion
2. Offer coordinated care, support and treatment
3. Offer personalised care, support or treatment
4. Be enabling

Benefits

There is growing evidence around person-centred care approaches with improved outcomes for patient, carers and staff including: improved quality of life, better sleep patterns, less agitation and improved staff satisfaction [11].

How Can We Deliver Person-Centred Care for People in Hospital?

There are clear challenges in adopting a person-centred approach in hospitals [11]. Adapting the hospital routine to an individual's priorities may be particularly difficult but there is scope to do this in most cases. The first step is to have the relevant information to enable this and several approaches have been used. For example, one approach is the development of a 'This is me' document that travels with the patient and summarises key information to help understand who the person is and how best to tailor the approach to their care [12]. The document attempts to capture the life story of the person with dementia and can enable reminiscence and help provide a basis to personalise care and build rapport.

Handley and colleagues highlight additional potential interventions that could help promote patient-centred care for people with dementia including the use of dementia champions, staff training and education, dementia nurse specialists and liaison psychiatry teams [13].

Dementia Champions

Lack of training for healthcare professionals in the care of people with dementia is a major factor affecting the quality of inpatient care. Educational initiatives have sought to impart factual knowledge about the dementing process but the evidence that this results in sustained changes in behaviour and institutional culture is limited [14]. Programmes that stressed experiential learning, for instance meeting people with dementia outside of hospital, have received a more positive response [15]. A key part of this process is to cultivate empathy in healthcare staff and triggers a realisation of the challenges faced by someone with dementia in the hospital environment. A 'Dementia Champion' can help with this process and to focus on a sustained change in working patterns and culture. A dementia champion is a healthcare worker who, having completed the requisite training programme, provides peer support using 'change agent skills and knowledge to enhance and improve the care of people with dementia' [15].

Such a role can be complemented by a Dementia Coordinator who provides an in-reach service to hospital wards to improve the experience of patients and carers by engaging with and involving carers, helping plan for discharge and ensuring better support at home [16].

Volunteers

Healthcare workers increasingly report the feeling that they do not have adequate time to meet all of the complex needs of people with dementia in hospital. Historically volunteers provided much valued, additional support for people with dementia in hospital. Bateman and colleagues evaluated the impact of volunteers trained in the delivery of patient-centred care [17]. Staff and volunteers enjoyed the experience but no significant difference in length of stay, falls or mortality between intervention and control arms was reported. However, there is some evidence that volunteers do reduce the incidence of delirium, and may provide softer benefits such as a reduction in loneliness for patients and a feeling of increased safety amongst staff [18].

At the Royal United Hospital in Bath UK, the Friendly Faces project was launched in 2017 using volunteers to give support to people with dementia admitted to the hospital. The project was coordinated by the local Alzheimer's Society, which trained the volunteers who also worked closely with the hospital's team of three Dementia Coordinators. Fifty-nine volunteers by the end of 2018 were providing support regarded very positively by patients, their relatives and staff. It was thought to relieve pressure on the staff and the relationship between the volunteers and the patients was valued by the people themselves and their family carers and may well be therapeutic in the longer term [19].

Liaison Psychiatry/Mental Health Teams

Provision of specialist mental health liaison teams is common practice in many countries and one of the key competencies for such teams is the identification, assessment and diagnosis of dementia [20]. The teams are multidisciplinary in nature and are commonly composed of a mixture of mental health nurses and psychiatrists. In addition to providing specialist assessment they can provide training on dementia and other common mental health issues such as delirium and depression to ward staff. Such teams clearly have a wider remit than the provision of specific dementia related interventions and training but have been shown to be cost-effective through the reduction in length of stay [21]. They can provide additional specialist support for ward teams looking after people with dementia although there has been some concern that this may inadvertently de-skill ward teams [14].

Hospital Environment

Admission to hospital can be bewildering and frightening for anyone but for people with dementia this is especially likely. Hospitals are busy and often noisy places and the surroundings are unfamiliar. Most people with dementia are older and may already have visual and hearing difficulties [22, 23] which can then be compounded by the cognitive, perceptual and visuospatial problems associated with the particular dementia and its severity.

Constant movement and clinical activity round the clock can be disorientating. Signs and notices, sounds and lighting can be overwhelming in an unfamiliar environment.

In England the King's Fund Enhancing the Healing Environment programme worked with 26 NHS Trusts to develop more supportive design for people with dementia in hospital [24]. The evaluation found that relatively simple, cost-effective changes to the physical environment had positive effects in people with dementia and those using and working with the service. Too many patients still lose their independence in undertaking activities of daily living while they are in hospital making them unable to return home after completion of the acute episode of care.

When considering the hospital environment more generally, several aspects warrant consideration: the built environment; the internal design of the space including provision of support for carers; and the culture/working environment (see the earlier section on person-centred care).

Built Environment

The Centre for Excellence in Universal Design in Ireland promulgates: 'the design and composition of an environment so that it can be accessed, understood and used to the greatest extent possible by all people, regardless of age, size, ability or disability' [25]. A dementia-friendly design of the built environment can support people with dementia. This can be true for newly built or retrofitted hospitals. A dementia-friendly environment simultaneously acknowledges and accommodates the physical, psychological and cognitive difficulties of someone with dementia in the hospital [2].

One of the barriers preventing fuller integration of carers of people with dementia is that hospitals commonly lack support/facilities for them. The physical environment should be designed to afford space and support to carers where feasible to enable them to remain with the person with dementia. Physical space for meaningful activities should be provided either in the form of a communal space supported by an activity coordinator or at least an area where the patient and a carer can have a meaningful interaction in a more homely/familiar environment [26]; the design and decoration of such spaces are also of great importance [27].

Internal Design

A welcoming, comfortable and familiar environment can make all the difference to a person with dementia in hospital. A clear, hospital-wide, consistent colour scheme should be used and colours are carefully selected; certain colours appear to be more easily interpreted by people with dementia. In addition, due to age-related changes certain colours may appear 'washed out' due to natural thickening of the lens of the eye. Blues, greens and purples can be harder to differentiate as a result [28].

Signage should be clear and appropriately positioned. Visual clutter should be avoided. Any maps should be appropriately sized and accessible. Multiple modes of communication should be used, e.g. combining written and pictorial images, and using familiar styles and consistent simple language.

Within wards, the space should be decorated in a way that promotes orientation [29]. For instance, through the provision of large format clocks/calendars/video screens displaying the time, day, month, season and weather. Artwork should be carefully selected to help orientate but also to act as aids for conversation. Adequate sound insulation and sound absorbent material should be in place to reduce background noise and help promote sleep.

Medical Mental Health Units

Although the physical environment is important, of even greater importance is the experience and culture of the healthcare team involved in looking after people with dementia. Staff on general medical wards report that they lack specific training [30, 31] and carers not infrequently report poor communication with healthcare staff. One model which has been proposed to deal with some of these issues is a combined medical mental health unit. These units are designed to provide a specialist inpatient service for people with dementia and encompass enhanced components to care. An example of such a model was developed in the NIHR Trial of an Elderly Acute care Medical and mental health unit (TEAM) trial [32]. Enhanced care included: specialist mental health staff (nursing, occupational therapist, psychiatrist), additional physiotherapy, speech and language therapy, geriatrician time and activity coordinators; staff training in the recognition and management of delirium and dementia and the delivery of person-centred dementia care; a programme of organised therapeutic and diversionary activities; making the ward environment 'dementia-friendly'; and a proactive and inclusive approach to family carers. The NIHR TEAM trial compared the enhanced model against care on a standard geriatric medicine ward and demonstrated better patient experiences and greater carer satisfaction with care.

Comprehensive Geriatric Assessment

In addition to person-centred care and the hospital environment, it is also important to consider the framework within which medical care should be provided within the hospital to people with cognitive impairment and dementia. Comprehensive geriatric assessment is the most well-established and researched model for healthcare delivery to frail older patients. It has been shown to deliver measurable health improvements for frail older people [33]. These improvements hold true for people with dementia and comprehensive geriatric assessment should form the framework for their management in hospital.

What Is Comprehensive Geriatric Assessment?

Comprehensive geriatric assessment is often taken to be synonymous with 'geriatric medicine' but it is more than that. It is a process which is used to manage frail or vulnerable older people. It is interdisciplinary and multidimensional taking account not just of medical diagnoses but also functional impairments and the environmental and social issues which affect patient well-being. It produces problem lists and develops goal driven interventions to tackle these. Ultimately it provides and coordinates an integrated plan for treatment, rehabilitation, support and long-term care. A comprehensive assessment is not limited to disease states as a standard medical assessment would be, or to impairments, as a standard rehabilitation assessment might be, but instead consider a number of domains which include physical medical conditions, mental health conditions, function, social circumstances and environment. The full bio-psycho-social nature of a person's problems can thus be identified. Some clinicians formalise this process with standardised scales and tools but they can be time consuming and clinically constraining and may not always be helpful [34].

Comprehensive geriatric assessment has been shown to provide significant benefits in terms of increased independence, a reduction in mortality [35] and a higher chance of patients being alive and in their own home at 6 months post-discharge (number needed to treat 13 to avoid one death or admission to residential care) [36].

Accurate assessment is the first step to appropriate management and to avoiding over- and under-prescribing. Multimorbidity rises with age, resulting in complex clinical pictures which require a thorough response to avoid causing more harm. It is well recognised that frail older patients with dementia present a considerable clinical challenge as a consequence of polypharmacy, multimorbidity and presentations which have functional, psychological, social and environmental dimensions [37]. Comprehensive geriatric assessment provides a contrasting model of care to traditional approaches focussed on single problems by single clinicians, being multidimensional and multidisciplinary. Done well, it delivers effective health care to vulnerable groups that otherwise would have received an ineffective, inefficient and potentially unsafe response.

Sensory Impairment

Communication is extremely important and difficulties in vision and hearing are common in older people. Difficulties in language—both expressive and receptive—are also important especially in people with any of the dementias that particularly affect language.

The acute hospital ward or emergency department is not well suited to dealing with these issues as they tend to be noisy places. The rapid pace and technological focus of modern hospital care makes good clinical assessment and treatment more difficult for older people with dementia [38]. Wherever possible it is preferable to have a relatively quiet area set aside in the emergency department for assessing older people. As older people with dementia are often unable to communicate their needs, collateral information is essential from family and caregivers if possible. However, it is also vital not to assume someone cannot communicate adequately without checking that they can hear what is being said and that they can also see adequately [39], particularly in connection with any written information or any signs and notices in the hospital ward. Visual information can be aided by appropriate design of hospital wards, for example, by using a specific colour for toilet doors.

Since older adults with hearing loss have a greater risk of developing dementia [40], it is likely that people with dementia may also have hearing problems. Another reason is that age-related hearing loss is an increasingly important health problem affecting approximately one in three people between the ages of 65 and 74 and nearly half of those older than 75.

The primary clinical management interventions for people with hearing loss are hearing aids [41]; however, many people given a hearing aid either do not use them or do not wear them. McCormack and colleagues [41] considered studies from the UK, USA, Australia, Finland, Sweden and Switzerland. Several issues were identified including the hearing aid not being effective in noisy situations, and issues relating to the care and maintenance of the aid due to limitations in manual dexterity. Many people need help in changing the batteries or adjusting the volume control. Finally, it is worth checking whether there is condensation or wax in the hearing aid tubing or wax in the ear itself.

Using an assistive listening device such as a microphone and headset may overcome a hearing impediment as can writing questions down, though this is laborious. Reducing background noise, speaking clearly but not shouting and facing the patient (many of whom may use some element of lip reading, which may be a significant problem if the wearing of a face mask is essential) preferably at eye level are all important actions for people who are hard of hearing; rephrasing a question may also help.

Many people with dementia may appear to have or can be demonstrated to have problems with language expression and comprehension, and for some less common dementias language problems may be the dominant feature. Failure of language can, for example, make assessment of pain particularly difficult. Everyone working in a hospital needs to be aware of potential difficulties when speaking to, and communicating with, an older person who may have hearing or cognitive problems as well as anyone with dementia. It is important to remember the value of non-verbal communication including body language, facial expression and the use of gestures.

Issues that can arise in acute care communicating with people with dementia [42]:

Masking of language difficulties and loss of insight

- Except for patients with aphasia, patients with dementia can often express themselves quite fluently. They may be able to use social routines such as greetings and formulaic language (e.g. 'Oh right') even when their aphasia is severe. In a short interaction this can lead health staff to overestimate language ability and an overestimation of the level of comprehension is therefore common, for example, in assuming the patient has understood a specific question.
- Many people with moderate dementia may have reduced insight, which may also lead to misleading answers in response to questions. Loss of insight may also be an early and difficult feature in some people with a fronto-temporal dementia.

Unreliable 'yes/no' response

- Health staff may ask yes or no questions in a bid to be helpful but many patients do not have a reliable use of 'yes' and 'no'. People with dementia may tend towards always answering in the affirmative, or if they feel anxious and threatened, everything may be answered with 'no'.
- In some patients there may be binary (e.g. yes/no, Y/N) reversal which the patient may or may not self-correct. One way to check this is to ask a series of simple Y/N questions to which you know the answer (equally divided between Y/N). For example, 'is your name Mary?', 'are you a man?' and the patient may answer 10/10 questions with 'yes'.

Leading questions/intonation

- It is important to try and avoid asking leading questions with intonation that suggests the expected answer and then taking the response as factually correct. For example, 'and you're not in any pain?' or 'do you understand what I've been saying?'

Lack of knowledge of patient history

- In the community staff may know a patient's social history well but ward staff may know very little. Often when patients are confused or distressed there is an aspect of truth or an unmet need underlying what they are trying to communicate (for example, if the person is trying to find something, or is in pain, or needs to go to the toilet). This is easier to interpret if you know something of the personal circumstances/history and discussion with a family member or someone who knows them well can help.

Overall approach

– It is better to use short sentences and avoid jargon and double negatives. Speaking clearly and repeating a sentence if necessary is useful. The use of gestures, pictures or something written may also help.

Assessment by a speech therapist or a joint session with a speech therapist and the patient may help. For someone with a foreign first language, then a translator or family member may be necessary.

Eating and Drinking Including Oral Health

It is important to remember the vital link between good nutrition and hydration and general health and well-being and this is particularly likely to be overlooked in the acute general hospital situation. Several tools are available for the assessment of nutritional status and the most widely used of these is the Mini Nutritional Assessment (MNA) [43]. The patient must be given and, if necessary, helped to eat nutritious balanced meals, as well as having ready access to drinks. Providing help with this is time consuming and easily overlooked on a busy ward.

The Food for Life Partnership in the UK has produced a table of useful resources concerning nutrition in older people [44] and Healthcare Improvement Scotland Food, Fluid and Nutritional Care Standards for the care of older people in hospital [45]. Eating well is difficult without reasonable teeth and the quality of existing teeth should be checked as well as ensuring that a person with false teeth has them, that the teeth fit properly (e.g. it may be an issue after weight loss) and that they are using them.

Patients with Posterior Cortical Atrophy, which is usually due to underlying Alzheimer's disease pathology, are characterised by a progressive decline in visual processing skills. This may lead to difficulties in locating food on a plate or fluid in a cup or glass and grasping things such as cutlery; yet, superficially the person may seem relatively normal and, at least in the earlier stages of the disease, less obviously cognitively impaired.

Swallowing is a complex mechanism and dysphagia may occur for several reasons including stroke, ill-fitting or absent dentures, the presence of thrush (especially if they have previously received a course of antibiotics) and with specific dementing conditions such as Progressive Supranuclear Palsy. It may occur in all of the neurodegenerative dementia disorders in the very advanced stages. A person with significant dysphasia is also more likely to have dysphagia.

Formal assessment of swallowing by trained staff (e.g. a speech therapist) should be carried out whenever necessary and as soon as possible after admission to ensure good and safe nutrition is possible and the risk of aspiration pneumonia is reduced.

Subcutaneous infusion of fluids for hydration or nutrition may be useful as a bridge for frail older patients to recover from an intercurrent illness such as a delirium. The technique is simple and does not require venous access, the risk of complications especially infection is low, and the risk of fluid overload is minimised [46].

Undiagnosed or Unrecognised Dementia

Every person admitted to an acute hospital will have an admission assessment whether admitted from the emergency department or directly to a hospital ward. This assessment should cover past medical history including current medication, a systematic enquiry for symptoms and a physical examination to detect any abnormal pathology. Cognitive screening will potentially enable the identification of cognitive impairment at admission or may detect a previously undiagnosed person and prompt assessment for potential dementia. Cognitive impairment is one of the most significant risk factors for adverse events such as falls in older patients during hospitalisation and subjects at risk need to be identified on admission [47]. It is often recommended that screening for cognitive impairment be routinely carried out in all people over the age of 65. It certainly should be carried out in those over 70 where people with dementia represent some 42% of unplanned admissions to an acute hospital [48].

However, for an acutely unwell person, especially in the presence of pain and discomfort, such an assessment may be unreliable on admission. More importantly, the presence of delirium may make the situation more complicated [49] so a clinician should be cautious in making a precipitate diagnosis of dementia in such a case. Collateral history about the situation before admission including any previous concerns about the person's cognitive ability may help. The possibility of an underlying dementia may become clearer or can be reviewed later in the admission and include standard investigations such as a brain scan, which may be more accessible for a patient in hospital than subsequently as an outpatient. On the other hand, whilst in hospital it is often more relevant to identify and establish the presence of cognitive impairment and for any potential dementia diagnostic label to be established after discharge, for example, by referral to a memory clinic.

A reduced cognitive test score may be very helpful in a person with previously undiagnosed dementia if they do not have delirium or any other reason for such a reduction. This can be supported by a collateral history of cognitive or functional problems in the previous months or years. If a new diagnosis of dementia is made during an admission, there may be concerns about how and who should give details of the diagnosis to the patient (and their family where appropriate) and what support should then be offered, or information provided. Where available, older people's liaison mental health teams are ideally placed to provide this service [50] or it may sometimes be better for this to take place in the community after the person has been discharged.

Common Medical Issues in People with Dementia

The majority of people living with dementia will also have a number of physical health problems. Admission to secondary care facilities is common, outcomes are poorer, and readmission more likely in people with dementia [51]. Person-centred care and the framework of comprehensive geriatric assessment provide the general approach to the medical care of people with dementia in hospital. However, there are some specific and commonly occurring medical scenarios which warrant further discussion. These include multimorbidity and frailty, polypharmacy and anticholinergic burden, delirium, and osteoporosis and fractures. It is beyond the remit of this chapter to consider the specific medical treatments for these issues but only some of the specific issues that may arise in the context of a dementia.

Multimorbidity and Frailty

Multimorbidity, defined as the presence of two or more long-term health conditions, is typical of the majority of people living with dementia [52]. In the UK one observational study identified a mean of 4.6 comorbidities in addition to dementia [53]. Multimorbidity is important because it is associated with a poorer quality of life and increased risks of mortality, polypharmacy, adverse drug reactions, falls, and hospital admissions and readmissions [54]. It is more common in older people and in those living with socio-economic deprivation [55].

Dementia has a complex relationship with other long-term health conditions which can result in an accumulation of risks leading to an adverse health outcome. For instance, dementia is a risk factor not only for falls but also for osteoporosis resulting in a higher rate of fractures than might be expected from the falls rate alone. In addition dementia is associated with poorer recovery from fractures further compounding this issue [56]. Dementia changes the natural history of highly prevalent conditions such as hypertension. In contrast to the general population, systolic blood pressure has been observed to start falling up to 6 years before the development of clinically apparent dementia [57] and to continue to fall thereafter. The observed falls in blood pressure (of between 8 and 22 mmHg) would be sufficient to potentially move an individual below treatment thresholds. This has implications for the treatment and monitoring of blood pressure in people with dementia compared to the cognitively intact population [58].

The UK National Institute for Health and Clinical Excellence (NICE) multimorbidity guidance [55] acknowledges that the management of multimorbidity (already far from simple) is more complicated in the presence of dementia. It stresses a careful consideration of the benefits and harms of any interventions. However, clinicians are hampered by the exclusion of people with dementia from multiple trials—which extends even to trials of self-management of long-term health conditions [55]. Treatment goals of a person with dementia may change over time and the course of their cognitive diagnosis. Thus, when mildly impaired, preventative medications such as antihypertensives may be desired, but in later stages of the disease treatments which prioritise quality of life over quantity may be more valued. The potential benefits and risks of pharmacological and non-pharmacological interventions should be discussed and compared as part of routine care. Such conversations are not without difficulty—the capacity to make such a treatment decision, the treatment goal and perceived benefits and harms may change with time and this will continue to be an issue in supporting people with dementia.

Frailty

Defining frailty has proved difficult but is generally accepted as a vulnerability to deterioration in the face of a stressor [59]. Potential stressors include acute illness, iatrogenic factors (e.g. an operation or adverse drugs effect) and environmental changes, which could include admission to hospital.

There are two main models for evaluating frailty. The frailty phenotype [60] is based on assessment of five domains consisting of weak grip strength, slow walking speed, self-reported exhaustion, low energy expenditure and unintentional weight loss with three out of the five being required to meet the definition. The deficit accumulation model can use either a checklist of problems to produce a frailty index (operationalised with, for example, the Edmonton Frail Scale [61]) or the Clinical Frailty Scale which is a nine-point, ordinal, vignette-based scale based on the level of medical problems and disability (ranging from Very Fit, 1, to Terminally Ill, 9); the Clinical Frailty Scale is probably the most practical for use within the acute hospital setting.

The relationship between frailty and Health Related-Quality of Life (HR-QOL) in older individuals with Alzheimer's disease or mild cognitive impairment has been investigated [62]. Frailty and neuropsychiatric symptoms were the determinants of HR-QOL in the earlier stages of cognitive impairment, whereas functional limitation predicted HR-QOL in later stages. It was suggested that frailty may represent a novel modifiable target in early dementia to improve HR-QOL.

Frailty, and its severity, can predict other health outcomes including death, falls, hospitalisation and permanent institutionalisation [6]. Admission to an acute hospital for a frail older person, and especially for someone with dementia, represents a crisis that needs careful assessment to identify or exclude physical illness, to maintain or restore function and to make plans for the future, which may include a change of accommodation or end of life care.

Polypharmacy, Anticholinergic Burden and Deprescribing

With multimorbidity comes polypharmacy and polypharmacy has been a concern for longer than many might think [63]. Polypharmacy is associated with an increased risk of major morbidity and mortality in older people [64, 65]. Anticholinergic burden provides an a priori case for the risks of polypharmacy. Medications with anticholinergic properties are widely used for a variety of different indications. Some medications are used primarily for their anticholinergic effect whilst others exhibit this as a side effect. There has been growing concern about the adverse outcomes associated with cumulative exposure to medications with anticholinergic properties (anticholinergic burden). As reported in a review of reviews, a number of large scale database studies have shown a consistent association between increasing anticholinergic exposure and adverse outcomes such as falls, hospitalisation, delirium and death [66]. The risk is heightened in the case of someone with a pre-existing dementia [67] although the effect may be reversible when anticholinergic medications are discontinued [68].

Medication review with a view to deprescribing (i.e. stopping or reducing) potentially inappropriate medications is one of the key tools of geriatricians. Deprescribing is not a new concept. Guidance and tools for identifying and reducing potentially inappropriate medications have been available for several years, however their application in clinical practice is limited. Barriers to deprescribing include inertia; prescriber knowledge or skill deficits particularly when balancing the risks and benefits in older people with multimorbidity; patients' beliefs about their medication; and pressure to follow guidelines [69].

The most widely used deprescribing tools take the form of lists of recommendations for individual medicines in specific clinical scenarios and are based mainly on expert consensus [70, 71]. Whilst these tools are a useful starting point, they necessarily simplify the process as they cannot provide a definitive guide for all scenarios, nor do they provide a step-by-step process for deprescribing such as when, how or by whom it should be done. Patient-centred approaches have been proposed [72, 73], but these can be difficult to implement due to fragmented care and the time consuming process of documenting nuanced medication related decisions—another reason cited as increasing inertia to deprescribing [69, 74].

Evidence-based deprescribing guidelines are being developed [75, 76]. Guidance on deprescribing should be embedded in standard healthcare guidance to prompt discussions with patients when medication is initiated. Embedding the idea of deprescribing from the outset could help overcome many of the barriers already alluded to. A shared decision-making approach should involve a discussion of the rationale behind starting a treatment. This should include a discussion of the risks and benefits of starting treatment and it should also outline the circumstances under which the medication may need to be suspended or deprescribed and the potential for withdrawal symptoms when this is done. Clear, unambiguous discussion at the start of therapy may empower patients, carers and prescribers to question continuation of medication later; overcoming some of the barriers to deprescribing.

Delirium

Delirium is extremely common among inpatients with dementia and delirium itself may contribute or cause admission to hospital for older people with or without dementia. Delirium almost always causes deficits on standard cognitive tests and can therefore complicate the evaluation of older people with or without an underlying dementing condition.

It is characterised by disturbed consciousness and fluctuating changes in cognition, attention and perception. It is a serious condition and associated with poor outcomes. However, it can be prevented and treated if dealt with urgently [49]. It is important to be aware that delirium can be hypoactive as well as hyperactive and some people may show signs of both. With hypoactive delirium, the person may be withdrawn, quiet and sleepy and it is more difficult to recognise than hyperactive delirium when the person can be restless, agitated and aggressive.

Prevalence of delirium at admission is variable ranging from 10 to 31% whilst the incidence of new cases of delirium ranges from 3 to 29% and the occurrence rate per admission varies between 11 and 42% [77].

NICE suggests four risk factors for developing delirium when people first present to hospital: aged 65 years or older; with a history of cognitive impairment (past or present) or dementia; current hip fracture; and the presence of severe illness [49]. These recommendations were developed from studies of a wide range of clinical populations including from surgical and intensive care settings and the methodology used may have limitations [77]. Other predictive models for delirium in older people with general medical admission include a wider range of factors. A systematic review focusing on risk factors for incident delirium in older medical inpatients [77] identified a greater number of factors. The commonest were dementia, older age, co-morbid illness, severity of medical illness, infection, 'high-risk' medication use, diminished activities of daily living, immobility, sensory impairment, urinary catheterisation, urea and electrolyte imbalance and malnutrition. In pooled analyses, dementia, illness severity, visual impairment, urinary catheterisation, low albumin level and length of hospital stay were statistically significantly associated with delirium [77].

Older adults ≥65years with coronavirus 2019 (COVID-19) commonly present to the emergency department (ED) with delirium, and delirium should be considered as an important presenting symptom of COVID-19. Of 817 older ED patients with COVID-19 presenting at seven sites in the USA, 28% had delirium at presentation. Among delirious patients, 16% presented with delirium as a primary symptom and 37% had no typical COVID-19 symptoms such as cough or fever [78].

It can be very difficult to decide whether a person has delirium and/or dementia and some people will have both conditions; if there is diagnostic uncertainty, then it is wiser to manage the patient initially for delirium [49].

Diagnosis

At presentation, information should be gathered regarding changes or fluctuations in behaviour over the recent hours or days. Changes may include altered cognitive function and confusion, visual or auditory hallucinations, restlessness, agitation, sleep disturbance, lack of cooperation with reasonable requests or alterations in communication, mood and/or attitude. Features particularly suggestive of hypoactive delirium include worsened concentration, slow responses, reduced mobility, reduced movement, changes in appetite and being withdrawn [NICE 45].

A more formal assessment is useful, for example, based on the short Confusion Assessment Method (short CAM) as recommended by NICE or the 4 'A's Test (4AT, www.the4AT.com). A prospective diagnostic test accuracy study of 843 acute medical patients aged ≥70 seen in emergency departments or acute medical wards at three UK sites has compared the short CAM and the 4AT for detection of delirium [79]. Delirium was present in 12.1% of 785 evaluable subjects using DSM-IV as the reference standard assessment, 14.3% by the 4AT and 4.75% by CAM. The 4AT had a sensitivity of 76% and specificity of 94%, whilst the CAM had a sensitivity of 40% and specificity of 100%. The 4AT had a high area under the receiver operating curve of 0.90 (95% Confidence Interval 0.84–0.96) providing support for its use as a delirium assessment instrument in clinical practice with an acceptable overall diagnostic test accuracy.

In this study, the CAM showed a lower (40%) sensitivity than in many published studies although sensitivity does vary widely across studies. This may partly reflect studies where raters lacked full training in the CAM or specialist training in psychiatry [80].

The 4AT does not require specific training and takes less than 2 min to perform. The 4 'A's are Alertness, Abbreviated Mental Test-4, Attention (Months Backwards test) and Acute changes or fluctuating course. Its method of scoring means that it can be scored in the absence of history from an informant at the time of assessment and if cognitive testing is not possible. It is designed to give a score even in patients who are too unwell to be interviewed or tested for cognition and all patients can thus be assessed. This may be particularly useful in the general hospital setting and the 4AT essentially identifies that further assessment is required. The patient should therefore still be assessed by a suitably experienced clinician whenever possible to confirm the diagnosis. It is also important to continue checking patients at risk for delirium regularly noting any changes or fluctuations in behaviour but the 4AT is not designed for repeated use within the same day.

Interventions to Prevent or Reduce Delirium

There is evidence to suggest that delirium incidence can be reduced in older people admitted to medical services using multi-component interventions that target delirium risk factors. Examples of potential interventions are shown in Table 15.1.

Treating Delirium

It is important to try and treat any potential underlying cause. Re-evaluation is vital if the delirium fails to resolve and it is important to consider the presence of a possible underlying dementia, where such a diagnosis has not previously been made. It may be more appropriate for this possibility to be followed up after the patient has left hospital.

Effective communication should be maximised including reorientation as to where the patient is and who you are. This may be helped by the involvement of family and friends who can also provide reassurance to the individual.

When someone is distressed or considered to be a risk to themselves or to others, verbal and non-verbal techniques should be used to try and defuse the situation. If these fail or are not applicable, then it may be necessary to consider a short-term course of haloperidol using the lowest appropriate dose and increasing cautiously if necessary. The latest NICE guidance has removed its previous recommendation to also consider olanzapine as a possible treatment (NICE) and the use of antipsychotics should be avoided or used with extreme caution in people with dementia with Lewy bodies or Parkinson's disease and Parkinson's disease dementia. Such patients may experience serious adverse effects to antipsychotics but the Lewy Body Association's Scientific Advisory Committee (www.lbda.org/treatment-options/) does suggest quetiapine can be considered when other treatments have failed and

Table 15.1 Addressing issues that may prevent or reduce delirium [49]

Cognitive impairment and/or disorientation	Appropriate lighting and clear signage including a clock and a calendar Explain where they are, who they are, and who you are and your role Cognitively stimulating activities, e.g. reminiscence Visits from family and friends
Dehydration and/or constipation	Adequate fluid intake orally if possible but subcutaneously or intravenously if necessary (care if heart failure or chronic kidney disease)
Hypoxia	Optimise oxygen saturation
Infection	Investigate (and repeat) as necessary Avoid catheterisation
Immobility/limited mobility	Mobilise soon after surgery Encourage walking (with aids readily available) Range of motion exercises even if not mobile
Pain	Assess carefully including for non-verbal signs of pain (grimacing, moaning, etc.) Treat and review regularly
Medication	Review regularly and optimise
Nutrition	Encourage eating and assist if necessary Check dentures, swallowing
Sensory impairment	Treat reversible causes, e.g. ear wax Ensure availability of glasses and working hearing aids
Sleep problems	Minimise procedures during sleeping hours Reduce noise to a minimum

quality of life dictates the need for treatment with potential risks of morbidity or mortality. Specialist advice should be sought whenever possible and initiation of therapy should be with a low dose (12.5 or 25 mg nocte).

Whilst delirium is unpleasant it is also associated with poor outcomes. The adverse consequences of delirium developing in patients in hospital include an increased risk of hospital-acquired complications, new dementia, new admission to an institution, extended in-hospital stay and increased mortality [81]. The cost-effectiveness of multi-component interventions for delirium prevention has been demonstrated and is associated with an incremental net monetary benefit of £2200 using a cost-effectiveness threshold of £20,000 per quality-adjusted life year and was cost-effective in 96.8% of the simulations [81].

Case: Jill's Story

I was fit and active in my early 70s—playing tennis at the local club and generally enjoying retirement. I was still doing some odd jobs (I'd been an accountant for many years and helped some of the neighbours with their accounts). I was 77 when I started noticing some minor issues with forgetfulness. I realised that I'd made some silly mistakes with the neighbour's accounts which was rather embarrassing.

There were a few other incidents—for instance, I got lost going to my sister's house although she'd lived there for 30 years. I ended up being referred to the memory clinic. After some testing and a brain scan they gave me a diagnosis of Alzheimer's disease and started some medication for my memory...

Jill's husband Pete takes up the story... about two years after her diagnosis Jill fell in the garden when raking up leaves. It shook her confidence—her mother had fallen and broken her hip at a similar age and never really recovered. She wasn't keen to leave the house after that. We tried to muddle through, as you do, but Jill just got more and more unsteady. She fell several more times and broke her wrist. A physiotherapy programme was discussed but never started due to concerns that Jill's memory was too poor to complete the course. We had some help—carers twice a day, but about 6 months after she broke her wrist, she fell trying to get out of bed to go to the toilet. It was just as she feared—she had broken her hip.

Jill had a tricky time in hospital. She was very disorientated, the pain was difficult to manage and staff struggled to interpret when she was in pain. Jill wasn't able to consent to the operation but we had set up a Power of Attorney some years back with me as Jill's attorney for health and welfare so I was able to give consent on her behalf. She had an operation the day after arriving in hospital and the therapy team did their best to get her up and about again but it was difficult. The ward team encouraged me to come in and it clearly helped when I was there at lunch time. The dementia coordinator was brilliant and helped with planning how we would get Jill home from day one. After a week or so she reached something of a plateau and we took the plunge and went home with help from carers four times a day. It was tough but we have managed and things gradually improved, at least from a physical point of view but you know, we are managing...

There are several aspects to highlight from Jill's story. Some apply to the situation prior to hospital admission but still warrant consideration, while the remainder relate to her in-hospital care.

People with dementia (like Jill) or mild cognitive impairment have at least a two-fold risk of falling compared to their cognitively intact peers [82, 83]. In addition, having fallen, they are at higher risk of sustaining a fracture, particularly a hip fracture [84] and have a poorer recovery than the general population [56]. Evidenced-based interventions that reduce the risk of fracture are therefore welcomed.

NICE recommends that fracture risk assessment be considered in all women aged over 65, all men aged over 75 and younger people (>50 years) in the presence of risk factors [85]. The presence of cognitive impairment is a risk factor for falling and fracturing [86]. Therefore, a suspected or diagnosed cognitive impairment should ideally prompt a fracture risk assessment (using a recognised tool such as FRAX® [87]), which should then be acted upon. Ideally a fracture risk assessment should have been carried out at the point of Jill's diagnosis. Given the family history of hip fracture, Jill's fracture risk would be elevated, and a risk assessment would have potentially led to initiating medication that would have reduced her risk of a fracture. Certainly at the point when she sustained a fracture treatment should have been discussed. A comprehensive assessment and multifactorial falls intervention program may have reduced Jill's risk of falls sufficiently to have prevented the fractured hip in the first place.

Jill's experience of the inpatient management of her hip fracture is not untypical. Within the UK there is some variation in the precise model of care for older people with hip fractures. However, all receive input from a specialist orthogeriatrician and multidisciplinary team. The strongest evidence of benefit is from the use of a hip fracture programme where there is evidence of improved functional outcomes at 1 year and reduced mortality at discharge [88]. It is less clear whether more intense inpatient rehabilitation for people with dementia is more effective than standard care. The incidence of delirium may be lower with enhanced care [89]. Further work is in progress to examine whether an enhanced community based rehabilitation programme may have benefit [90].

Pain in people with dementia is often poorly recognised and undertreated [91]. As has been discussed people with dementia typically live with multiple chronic health complaints including painful conditions such as osteoarthritis. People with more advanced cognitive impairment than Jill may struggle to verbalise the existence of pain leading to the emergence of behavioural changes which healthcare staff may not realise are being driven by pain [92]. In Jill's case the hip fracture had been identified and could be expected to cause pain. However, even with an unambiguous painful condition such as a hip fracture people with dementia appear less likely to receive adequate analgesia than their cognitively intact peers [93]. Assessment of pain in people with dementia should include both verbal and observational components. Clinicians should use a tool developed to identify pain in someone with dementia such as the Abbey pain scale [94]. Pain should be treated using a stepwise protocol [95].

It is also worth highlighting the multidisciplinary working and discharge planning that occurred during Jill's admission. This started from day one and involved the dementia coordinator to help oversee the planning. It involved Jill and her husband working with the team to plan a successful discharge.

Summary

The dementia syndrome has many causes and work is underway across the world to elucidate disease pathways and develop disease modifying treatments. Perhaps one day effective intervention for this condition will be available. However, at present dementia remains incurable and the prevalence of this condition continues to increase. We have seen how people with dementia will typically also be living with multiple other health and social conditions and will be more likely therefore to require hospital services. People with dementia admitted to hospital are more likely to die, stay in hospital for longer and are less likely to be discharged to their own home than their cognitively intact peers.

The hospital at the beginning of the twenty-first century is not a safe place for people with dementia. Interventions that keep people with dementia independent and reduce the risk of major health events such as falls or fractured hips are vital.

However, people will still become unwell and will still benefit from admission to hospital in the same way that people without dementia do. There are ways and means of significantly improving the hospital experience for people with dementia and their carers. Developing a dementia-friendly environment and designing hospital facilities for the people who are very likely to be using them are clearly important but staff training and a move to a person-centred approach are also required.

Despite people with dementia being some of the most frequent users of healthcare services research underpinning good quality care in hospital is lacking. A robust evidence base is needed to drive investment and guidance for policy makers.

Changes to practice in the hospital environment are possible and could potentially benefit a large population of people who are currently being let down by the healthcare system. The question remains, however, is there the will to change?

References

1. Vincent C. Building improvement capacity in mental health services. BJPsych Int. 2020;17(4):75–6.
2. Parke B, Boltz M, Hunter KF, Chambers T, Wolf-Ostermann K, Adi MN, et al. A scoping literature review of dementia-friendly hospital design. Gerontologist. 2017;57(4):e62–74.
3. Reynish EL, Hapca SM, De Souza N, Cvoro V, Donnan PT, Guthrie B. Epidemiology and outcomes of people with dementia, delirium, and unspecified cognitive impairment in the general hospital: prospective cohort study of 10,014 admissions. BMC Med. 2017;15(1):140.
4. Burton JK, Guthrie B, Hapca SM, Cvoro V, Donnan PT, Reynish EL. Living at home after emergency hospital admission: prospective cohort study in older adults with and without cognitive spectrum disorder. BMC Med. 2018;16(1):231.
5. Krumholz HM. Post-hospital syndrome—an acquired, transient condition of generalized risk. N Engl J Med. 2013;368(2):100–2.
6. Keeble E, Roberts HC, Williams CD, Van Oppen J, Conroy SP. Outcomes of hospital admissions among frail older people: a 2-year cohort study. Br J Gen Pract. 2019;69(685):e555–e60.
7. Welsh TJ. Multimorbidity in people living with dementia. Case Rep Womens Health. 2019;23:e00125.
8. Jackson TA, MacLullich AM, Gladman JR, Lord JM, Sheehan B. Undiagnosed long-term cognitive impairment in acutely hospitalised older medical patients with delirium: a prospective cohort study. Age Ageing. 2016;45(4):493–9.
9. Kitwood T. Dementia reconsidered: the person comes first. New York: Open University Press; 1997.
10. Epp T. Person-centred dementia care: a vision to be refined. Can Alzheimer Dis Rev. 2003;5:14–8.
11. Godfrey M, Young J, Shannon R, Skingley A, Woolley R, Arrojo F, et al. The person, interactions and environment Programme to improve care of people with dementia in hospital: a multisite study. Southampton (UK): NIHR Journals Library; 2018 Jun.
12. Pan JL, Chochinov H, Thompson G, McClement S. The TIME Questionnaire: a tool for eliciting personhood and enhancing dignity in nursing homes. Geriatr Nurs. 2016;37(4):273–7.
13. Handley M, Bunn F, Goodman C. Dementia-friendly interventions to improve the care of people living with dementia admitted to hospitals: a realist review. BMJ Open. 2017;7(7):e015257.
14. Dewing J, Dijk S. What is the current state of care for older people with dementia in general hospitals? A literature review. Dementia (London). 2016;15(1):106–24.

15. Banks P, Waugh A, Henderson J, Sharp B, Brown M, Oliver J, et al. Enriching the care of patients with dementia in acute settings? The Dementia Champions Programme in Scotland. Dementia (London). 2014;13(6):717–36.
16. RUH. Dementia Care in Hospital. [cited 2020; Available from: https://www.ruh.nhs.uk/patients/your_care_inpatient/dementia_care.asp
17. Bateman C. Research into practice: volunteers improving person centred dementia care in a rural hospital: an intervention study. Master's thesis. University of Canberra. 2012.
18. Pritchard E, Soh SE, Morello R, Berkovic D, Blair A, Anderson K, et al. Volunteer programs supporting people with dementia/delirium in hospital: systematic review and meta-analysis. Gerontologist. 2020; https://doi.org/10.1093/geront/gnaa058.
19. Roots M. The Dementia Volunteer Project: a mixed methods investigation to study the effects of a volunteer programme for hospital in-patients with dementia. London: King's College; 2019.
20. England N. Achieving better access to 24/7 urgent and emergency mental health care—part 2: implementing the evidence-based treatment pathway for urgent and emergency liaison mental health services for adults and older adults—guidance. NHS England; 2016.
21. George T, Rafik S, Paul K, Nageen M, Eliza J, Rachel P, et al. Impact of an integrated rapid response psychiatric liaison team on quality improvement and cost savings: the Birmingham RAID model. Psychiatrist. 2013;37(1):4–10.
22. Bowen M, Edgar DF, Hancock B, Haque S, Shah R, Buchanan S, et al. The Prevalence of Visual Impairment in People with Dementia (the PrOVIDe study): a cross-sectional study of people aged 60–89 years with dementia and qualitative exploration of individual, carer and professional perspectives. Health Serv Deliv Res. 2016;4(21) https://doi.org/10.3310/hsdr04210.
23. Liu CM, Lee CT. Association of hearing loss with dementia. JAMA Netw Open. 2019;2(7):e198112.
24. Waller S, Masterson A. Designing dementia-friendly hospital environments. Future Hosp J. 2015;2(1):63–8.
25. The Centre for Excellence in Universal Design. [cited 2020 12/11/20]. Available from: http://universaldesign.ie/
26. Pinkert C, Faul E, Saxer S, Burgstaller M, Kamleitner D, Mayer H. Experiences of nurses with the care of patients with dementia in acute hospitals: a secondary analysis. J Clin Nurs. 2018;27(1–2):162–72.
27. Grey T, Xidous D, Kennelly S, Mahon S, Mannion V, de Freine P, et al. Dementia friendly hospitals from a universal design approach: design guidelines. TrinityHaus Research Centre, Tallaght University Hospital, O'Connell Mahon Architects; 2018.
28. McGuinness B, Todd S, Passmore P, Bullock R. Blood pressure lowering in patients without prior cerebrovascular disease for prevention of cognitive impairment and dementia. Cochrane Database Syst Rev. 2009;2009(4):CD004034.
29. Scerri A, Innes A, Scerri C. Dementia care in acute hospitals—a qualitative study on nurse managers' perceived challenges and solutions. J Nurs Manag. 2020;28(2):399–406.
30. Elvish R, Burrow S, Cawley R, Harney K, Graham P, Pilling M, et al. 'Getting to Know Me': the development and evaluation of a training programme for enhancing skills in the care of people with dementia in general hospital settings. Aging Ment Health. 2014;18(4):481–8.
31. Nichols JN, Heller KS. Windows to the heart: creating an acute care dementia unit. J Palliat Med. 2002;5(1):181–92.
32. Goldberg SE, Bradshaw LE, Kearney FC, Russell C, Whittamore KH, Foster PE, et al. Care in specialist medical and mental health unit compared with standard care for older people with cognitive impairment admitted to general hospital: randomised controlled trial (NIHR TEAM trial). BMJ. 2013;347:f4132.
33. Ellis G, Whitehead MA, Robinson D, O'Neill D, Langhorne P. Comprehensive geriatric assessment for older adults admitted to hospital: meta-analysis of randomised controlled trials. BMJ. 2011;343:d6553.
34. Welsh TJ, Gordon AL, Gladman JR. Comprehensive geriatric assessment—a guide for the non-specialist. Int J Clin Pract. 2014;68(3):290–3.

35. Stuck AE, Siu AL, Wieland GD, Adams J, Rubenstein LZ. Comprehensive geriatric assessment: a meta-analysis of controlled trials. Lancet. 1993;342(8878):1032–6.
36. Ellis G, Whitehead MA, O'Neill D, Langhorne P, Robinson D. Comprehensive geriatric assessment for older adults admitted to hospital. Cochrane Database Syst Rev. 2011;7:CD006211.
37. Tinetti ME, Fried T. The end of the disease era. Am J Med. 2004;116(3):179–85.
38. George J, Long S, Vincent C. How can we keep patients with dementia safe in our acute hospitals? A review of challenges and solutions. J R Soc Med. 2013;106(9):355–61.
39. Cook R, Lamont T, Martin R, Centre ND. Steps to better understanding resistant behaviours in hospitalised patients with dementia. BMJ. 2019;366:l4912.
40. Lin FR, Metter EJ, O'Brien RJ, Resnick SM, Zonderman AB, Ferrucci L. Hearing loss and incident dementia. Arch Neurol. 2011;68(2):214–20.
41. McCormack A, Fortnum H. Why do people fitted with hearing aids not wear them? Int J Audiol. 2013;52(5):360–8.
42. Bowker-Brady G. personal communication, 2020.
43. Vellas B, Villars H, Abellan G, Soto ME, Rolland Y, Guigoz Y, et al. Overview of the MNA—its history and challenges. J Nutr Health Aging. 2006;10(6):456–63. discussion 63-5
44. Food for life: nutrition for older people. 2020 [cited 27/12/20; Available from: https://foodforlife.org.uk/~/media/files/better%20care/resources/03_sa_bcr_resources_v3_aw_web.pd].
45. Healthcare improvement Scotland: standards for food, fluid and nutritional care. 2014 [cited 27/12/20; Available from: http://www.healthcareimprovementscotland.org/our_work/standards_and_guidelines/stnds/nutritional_care_standards.aspx].
46. Caccialanza R, Constans T, Cotogni P, Zaloga GP, Pontes-Arruda A. Subcutaneous infusion of fluids for hydration or nutrition: a review. JPEN J Parenter Enteral Nutr. 2018;42(2):296–307.
47. Mecocci P, von Strauss E, Cherubini A, Ercolani S, Mariani E, Senin U, et al. Cognitive impairment is the major risk factor for development of geriatric syndromes during hospitalization: results from the GIFA study. Dement Geriatr Cogn Disord. 2005;20(4):262–9.
48. Sampson EL, Blanchard MR, Jones L, Tookman A, King M. Dementia in the acute hospital: prospective cohort study of prevalence and mortality. Br J Psychiatry. 2009;195(1):61–6.
49. NICE. Delirium: prevention, diagnosis and management. https://www.guidelines.co.uk/mental-health/nice-delirium-guideline/455015.article; July 2010 (last updated March 2019).
50. Anderson D. Who cares wins: improving the outcome for older people admitted to the general hospital: guidelines for the development of liaison mental health services for older people. London: Royal College of Psychiatrists; 2005.
51. Graversen SB, Pedersen HS, Sandbaek A, Foss CH, Palmer VJ, Ribe AR. Dementia and the risk of short-term readmission and mortality after a pneumonia admission. PLoS One. 2021;16(1):e0246153.
52. Tonelli M, Wiebe N, Straus S, Fortin M, Guthrie B, James MT, et al. Multimorbidity, dementia and health care in older people:a population-based cohort study. CMAJ Open. 2017;5(3):E623–E31.
53. Welsh TJ, Gordon AL, Gladman JR. Treatment of hypertension in people with dementia: a multicenter prospective observational cohort study. J Am Med Dir Assoc. 2019;20(9):1111–5.
54. Klinge M, Aasbrenn M, Öztürk B, Christiansen CF, Suetta C, Pressel E, et al. Readmission of older acutely admitted medical patients after short-term admissions in Denmark: a nationwide cohort study. BMC Geriatr. 2020;20(1):203.
55. NICE. Multimorbidity: clinical assessment and management. NICE; 2016.
56. Givens JL, Sanft TB, Marcantonio ER. Functional recovery after hip fracture: the combined effects of depressive symptoms, cognitive impairment, and delirium. J Am Geriatr Soc. 2008;56(6):1075–9.
57. Stewart R, Xue QL, Masaki K, Petrovitch H, Ross GW, White LR, et al. Change in blood pressure and incident dementia: a 32-year prospective study. Hypertension. 2009;54(2):233–40.
58. Harrison JK, Van Der Wardt V, Conroy SP, Stott DJ, Dening T, Gordon AL, et al. New horizons: the management of hypertension in people with dementia. Age Ageing. 2016;45(6):740–6.
59. Clegg A, Young J, Iliffe S, Rikkert MO, Rockwood K. Frailty in elderly people. Lancet. 2013;381(9868):752–62.

60. Fried LP, Tangen CM, Walston J, Newman AB, Hirsch C, Gottdiener J, et al. Frailty in older adults: evidence for a phenotype. J Gerontol A Biol Sci Med Sci. 2001;56(3):M146–56.
61. Rolfson DB, Majumdar SR, Tsuyuki RT, Tahir A, Rockwood K. Validity and reliability of the Edmonton frail scale. Age Ageing. 2006;35(5):526–9.
62. Mhaoláin AM, Gallagher D, Crosby L, Ryan D, Lacey L, Coen RF, et al. Frailty and quality of life for people with Alzheimer's dementia and mild cognitive impairment. Am J Alzheimers Dis Other Dement. 2012;27(1):48–54.
63. Newnham W. Remarks on the present aspect of medicine. Prov Med Surg J. 1848;12(12):309–14.
64. Cherubini A, Eusebi P, Dell'Aquila G, Landi F, Gasperini B, Bacuccoli R, et al. Predictors of hospitalization in Italian nursing home residents: the U.L.I.S.S.E. project. J Am Med Dir Assoc. 2012;13(1):84.e5–10.
65. Nobili A, Garattini S, Mannucci PM. Multiple diseases and polypharmacy in the elderly: challenges for the internist of the third millennium. Journal of Comorbidity. 2011;1:28–44.
66. Welsh TJ, van der Wardt V, Ojo G, Gordon AL, Gladman JRF. Anticholinergic drug burden tools/scales and adverse outcomes in different clinical settings: a systematic review of reviews. Drugs Aging. 2018;35(6):523–38.
67. Fox C, Livingston G, Maidment ID, Coulton S, Smithard DG, Boustani M, et al. The impact of anticholinergic burden in Alzheimer's dementia-the LASER-AD study. Age Ageing. 2011;40(6):730–5.
68. Carriere I, Fourrier-Reglat A, Dartigues JF, Rouaud O, Pasquier F, Ritchie K, et al. Drugs with anticholinergic properties, cognitive decline, and dementia in an elderly general population: the 3-city study. Arch Intern Med. 2009;169(14):1317–24.
69. Anderson K, Stowasser D, Freeman C, Scott I. Prescriber barriers and enablers to minimising potentially inappropriate medications in adults: a systematic review and thematic synthesis. BMJ Open. 2014;4(12):e006544.
70. By the 2019 American Geriatrics Society Beers Criteria® Update Expert Panel. American Geriatrics Society 2019 Updated AGS Beers Criteria® for potentially inappropriate medication use in older adults. J Am Geriatr Soc. 2019;67(4):674–94.
71. O'Mahony D, O'Sullivan D, Byrne S, O'Connor MN, Ryan C, Gallagher P. STOPP/START criteria for potentially inappropriate prescribing in older people: version 2. Age Ageing. 2015;44(2):213–8.
72. Barnett NL, Oboh L, Smith K. Patient-centred management of polypharmacy: a process for practice. Eur J Hosp Pharm. 2016;23(2):113–7.
73. Reeve E, Shakib S, Hendrix I, Roberts MS, Wiese MD. Review of deprescribing processes and development of an evidence-based, patient-centred deprescribing process. Br J Clin Pharmacol. 2014;78(4):738–47.
74. Ailabouni NJ, Nishtala PS, Mangin D, Tordoff JM. Challenges and enablers of deprescribing: a general practitioner perspective. PLoS One. 2016;11(4):e0151066.
75. Farrell B, Pottie K, Thompson W, Boghossian T, Pizzola L, Rashid FJ, et al. Deprescribing proton pump inhibitors: evidence-based clinical practice guideline. Can Fam Physician. 2017;63(5):354–64.
76. Harrison J, Conroy S, Welsh T, Van der Wardt V, Gladman J. Proposed antihypertensive medication withdrawal protocol. East Midlands Research into Ageing Network (EMRAN) Discussion Paper Series. 2016(8).
77. Ahmed S, Leurent B, Sampson EL. Risk factors for incident delirium among older people in acute hospital medical units: a systematic review and meta-analysis. Age Ageing. 2014;43(3):326–33.
78. Kennedy M, Helfand BKI, Gou RY, Gartaganis SL, Webb M, Moccia JM, et al. Delirium in older patients with COVID-19 presenting to the emergency department. JAMA Netw Open. 2020;3(11):e2029540.
79. Shenkin SD, Fox C, Godfrey M, Siddiqi N, Goodacre S, Young J, et al. Delirium detection in older acute medical inpatients: a multicentre prospective comparative diagnostic test accuracy study of the 4AT and the confusion assessment method. BMC Med. 2019;17(1):138.

80. MacLullich AM, Shenkin SD, Goodacre S, Godfrey M, Hanley J, Stíobhairt A, et al. The 4 'A's test for detecting delirium in acute medical patients: a diagnostic accuracy study. Health Technol Assess. 2019;23(40):1–194.
81. Akunne A, Murthy L, Young J. Cost-effectiveness of multi-component interventions to prevent delirium in older people admitted to medical wards. Age Ageing. 2012;41(3):285–91.
82. Muir SW, Gopaul K, Montero Odasso MM. The role of cognitive impairment in fall risk among older adults: a systematic review and meta-analysis. Age Ageing. 2012;41(3):299–308.
83. Shaw F. Prevention of falls in older people with dementia. J Neural Transm. 2007;114(10):1259–64.
84. Hippisley-Cox J, Coupland C. Derivation and validation of updated QFracture algorithm to predict risk of osteoporotic fracture in primary care in the United Kingdom: prospective open cohort study. BMJ. 2012;344:e3427.
85. NICE. NICE Clinical Guideline 146. Osteoporosis: assessing the risk of fragility fracture. 2012.
86. Ambrose AF, Paul G, Hausdorff JM. Risk factors for falls among older adults: a review of the literature. Maturitas. 2013;75(1):51–61.
87. Kanis J. FRAX(R): fracture risk assessment tool. 2008 [cited 2018 1/11/18]; Available from: https://www.sheffield.ac.uk/FRAX/index.aspx.
88. NICE. Hip fracture: management. In: NICE, editor. NICE; 2011 (Last updated 2017).
89. Smith TO, Gilbert AW, Sreekanta A, Sahota O, Griffin XL, Cross JL, et al. Enhanced rehabilitation and care models for adults with dementia following hip fracture surgery. Cochrane Database Syst Rev. 2020;2:CD010569.
90. Williams N, Dodd S, Hardwick B, Clayton D, Edwards RT, Charles JM, et al. Protocol for a definitive randomised controlled trial and economic evaluation of a community-based rehabilitation programme following hip fracture: fracture in the elderly multidisciplinary rehabilitation-phase III (FEMuR III). BMJ Open. 2020;10(10):e039791.
91. Morrison RS, Siu AL. A comparison of pain and its treatment in advanced dementia and cognitively intact patients with hip fracture. J Pain Symptom Manag. 2000;19(4):240–8.
92. Husebo BS, Ballard C, Sandvik R, Nilsen OB, Aarsland D. Efficacy of treating pain to reduce behavioural disturbances in residents of nursing homes with dementia: cluster randomised clinical trial. BMJ. 2011;343:d4065.
93. Moschinski K, Kuske S, Andrich S, Stephan A, Gnass I, Sirsch E, et al. Drug-based pain management for people with dementia after hip or pelvic fractures: a systematic review. BMC Geriatr. 2017;17(1):54.
94. Lichtner V, Dowding D, Esterhuizen P, Closs SJ, Long AF, Corbett A, et al. Pain assessment for people with dementia: a systematic review of systematic reviews of pain assessment tools. BMC Geriatr. 2014;14:138.
95. NICE. Dementia: assessment, management and support for people living with dementia and their carers. NICE. 2018. www.nice.org.uk/guidance/ng97

Long-Term Care for Patients with Dementia

16

Kathryn Mullan, Anthony Peter Passmore, Bernadette McGuinness, and Joseph P. M. Kane

Introduction

When an individual takes up residency in a long-term care (LTC) facility, it is a watershed event in their lives. Irrespective of whether it is a long-anticipated result of insidious progression of illness, or a hastily arranged placement to facilitate discharge from acute care, it represents a significant transition for the patient, their family, and their healthcare. This transition may have come in the wake of other significant changes, such as the death or illness of a caregiver, or the emergence of a physical disability. Clinicians providing care to LTC residents must be cognisant of the significance of this transition and responsive to the difficulties brought by it.

This chapter discusses some of the clinical issues specific to the care of people with dementia in LTC. By its very nature, LTC is home to higher proportions of people with more severe disease and more complex needs than in other settings. Delirium and urinary incontinence are common, and seldom come with quick-fix solutions; interventions like behavioural management and non-pharmacological treatments may require consideration in a comprehensive care plan. The risk and care burden associated with problems like decreased oral intake and incontinence may have contributed to the decision to admit to LTC, whilst pain and infection can commonly manifest themselves in unconventional and deceptive ways in people with dementia. A case history illustrating some common issues, and how they might be addressed, is included.

Next, we consider how LTC can influence some of our approaches to the treatment of people with dementia, discussing aspects of the administration of both vaccines and antibiotic therapy, and the emergence of telemedicine. In the following section, we discuss the important issue of death and dying in LTC. Most people with

K. Mullan · A. P. Passmore · B. McGuinness · J. P. M. Kane (✉)
Centre for Public Health, Queen's University Belfast, Belfast, Northern Ireland
e-mail: kmullan13@qub.ac.uk; p.passmore@qub.ac.uk; b.mcguinness@qub.ac.uk; joseph.kane@qub.ac.uk

K. S. Frederiksen, G. Waldemar (eds.), *Management of Patients with Dementia*,
https://doi.org/10.1007/978-3-030-77904-7_16

dementia admitted to LTC will die there; around a third within a year of admission [1, 2]. We explore the importance of routine adoption of advance care planning in anticipating clinical challenges that can arise in LTC. One such significant challenge is the determination of thresholds for hospital transfer; another is ensuring that palliative care needs are met. Both of these are detailed in this section.

Finally, we conclude the chapter by considering the potential legacy of the COVID-19 pandemic on provision of LTC. In many countries, the virus itself has had a significant impact on the mortality of people with dementia, particularly in LTC, but it has also interfered with the care of many of the clinical issues discussed in this chapter. Moreover, COVID-19 has posed important questions as to how our LTC facilities, and healthcare systems, operate; we consider how the pandemic may affect the care of people with dementia for years to come.

Admission to Long-Term Care

Any transition can bring its own set of problems for a person with dementia. It is therefore important to ensure good communication between healthcare providers when such individuals are admitted to LTC. In one US study, hospital-to-LTC transitions were perceived as distressing for patients and their caregivers. These transitions were seen as being dominated by dementia-related behavioural symptoms, which were thought to be purposely under-communicated by hospital personnel in discharge documentation [3].

Adoption of nurse-led care coordination programmes such as the Transitional Care Model appear to reduce preventable hospital readmission by identifying individuals at risk of poor outcomes at the interface between acute care and LTC, facilitating regular communication and follow-up [4, 5]. The development of this model included identification of six overlapping categories of problems associated with negative outcomes amongst older adults, with and without cognitive impairment, transitioning between hospital and either LTC or community settings: lack of patient engagement; absent or inadequate communication; lack of collaboration amongst team members; limited follow-up and monitoring; poor continuity of care; and serious gaps in services as patients move between healthcare professionals (clinicians) and across care settings. The Transitional Care Model aims to remedy these issues by focusing on nine core components of effective transitionary care; screening, staffing, maintaining relationships, engaging patients and family caregivers, assessing and managing risks and symptoms, educating and promoting self-management, collaborating, promoting continuity, and fostering coordination. Each element is separately defined but interconnected with the others as part of a holistic care process.

Another study highlighting the importance of communication at the acute care-LTC interface identified nine geriatric syndromes; weight loss, decreased appetite, incontinence, pain, depression, delirium cognitive impairment, falls and pressure ulcers, present in more than 90% of hospitalised adults referred to nursing homes [6]. However, treating hospital physicians commonly did not recognise and document these syndromes in discharge summaries [6].

When a person with dementia is admitted to LTC, it is very important to carry out a detailed assessment which will inform staff about the personal details of the patient, their medical history and medications, the reasons for their admission, their location prior to admission, presence of any advance directives, and the views of their caregivers. This is often performed by nursing staff and should include medical input to this process as soon as possible after admission. In some countries, mechanisms for the systematic collection of such data exist; use of the Resident Assessment Instrument/Minimum Data Set (RAI/MDS) is a requirement for all US LTC facilities participating in Medicare and Medicaid national insurance programmes [7].

In the United Kingdom (UK) most of the decisions about community clinical management are taken by the general practitioner (GP) but it is unclear how often they participate in this type of admission assessment. Most LTC residents remain under the care of the GP who managed their care prior to admission so facilities may have numerous GPs from different organisations providing care to their residents. In some countries, where LTC facilities are managed by a core group of GPs, practitioners may be more experienced at managing presentations in people with dementia and able to tailor management accordingly [8].

A recurring theme in this chapter is the importance of establishing and maintaining accurate, timely and regular communication between the patient, their family, LTC staff, and healthcare staff. The transition between care settings is a critical juncture for this practice, and early effective communication can be instrumental in establishing therapeutic relationships and important components of ongoing care.

Common Clinical Issues in People with Dementia

Residents in LTC have higher levels of physical dependency, multimorbidity, and polypharmacy than those in the general population, some of which may disguise or complicate the detection of a number of common medical issues [9, 10]. Several of these issues, including dementia detection (Chap. 3) and pharmacological management (Chap. 5), behavioural and psychological symptoms and of dementia (Chap. 7), potentially inappropriate medication (Chap. 6) and pain (Chap. 9) are addressed elsewhere in this book.

Delirium

Delirium, although also discussed elsewhere in this book, is important to discuss specifically in the context of LTC. Risk factors for delirium, such as pain, sensory impairment, and dementia are more prevalent in LTC populations than in community settings. Research into delirium detection and management has largely been focused on the acute inpatient setting, but it is no less important an issue in the LTC population, where delirium predicts mortality and hospitalisation [11]. LTC facilities themselves, perhaps due to the many environmental features they share with hospitals, may increase the risk of delirium; those admitted to hospital from LTC facilities have higher rates of delirium than people admitted from their own home [11].

Delirium detection, however, is likely to be worse in the LTC population than in hospitals; older age and dementia, both more prevalent in LTC, are factors associated with delirium under recognition by acute care nurses [12]. Detection may be further complicated by differences between new-onset delirium residents and those in acute care [13]. The onset can be insidious, and patients can demonstrate prodromal symptoms of subclinical delirium in the 2 weeks preceding recognition by the clinician [14].

Estimating the scale of the problem that delirium poses to LTC is difficult; reported prevalence rates indicate that 1.4 and 70.3% of residents over the age of 65 experience delirium [15, 16]. These vary considerably on the basis of the methods used to determine the presence of delirium (e.g., expert assessment, assessment tool, clinical documentation), the setting, and the timescale employed [17]. Different diagnostic criteria (ICD-10, DSM-III, DSM-III-R, DSM-IV) applied as part of the same study, produce prevalence rates ranging from 10.1 to 24.9% [18].

Despite this observed variation, a consistent finding throughout epidemiological studies has been that those using structured assessment tools detect higher rates of prevalence than studies determining the presence of delirium through clinical documentation. Such tools may therefore have an important role in routine clinical practice. The Confusion Assessment Method (CAM) [19] is the most widely used assessment tool in delirium research, and has been adapted for use in nursing home populations (NH-CAM) [20]. NH-CAM uses information retrieved from the Minimum Data Set, the government mandated process for clinical assessment of residents in US LTC settings. Although CAM has been well validated, NH-CAM has not been validated against an external reference standard [20]. The 4 "A" s test (4AT) has emerged as a valid and feasible alternative to CAM in the acute setting [21]. 4AT has demonstrated a much higher sensitivity (76%) than CAM (40%) with comparable specificity (4AT 94%, CAM 100%) [22]. Although unvalidated in LTC cohorts, 4AT would appear to be an excellent alternative to specialist assessment and ideal for use by clinicians working in these areas; it is quick, structured, and accessible to non-specialists [23].

When compared with the data supporting hospital-based interventions for preventing delirium, the evidence relating to prevention in LTC is limited. A 2019 Cochrane review of prevention methods in LTC facilities included three cluster randomised controlled trials [24]. All three studies included in the review describe minimisation of risk factors, either through pharmacovigilance [25], adequate hydration [26] or educating staff to address risk factors [27]. It identified, in a computerised system to identify medications that may contribute to delirium risk, only moderate evidence for a reduction in delirium incidence (12-month HR 0.42), with little or no strong evidence to support a decrease in mortality, hospital admissions or falls. No pharmacological interventions were identified. In spite of the paucity of evidence for intervention in this population, the foundations of delirium care advocated in inpatient environments should be retained in its prevention in LTC facilities; vigilance for risk factors, systematic screening in at-risk populations and supportive, non-pharmacological basic therapeutic approaches, supported my interdisciplinary education and care [28].

The management of delirium in LTC should be no different to that in acute care and is discussed in greater detail elsewhere in this book and in clinical guidelines. Identification and management of the underlying cause are of paramount importance in delirium management, and non-pharmacological strategies should be adopted wherever possible. Interdisciplinary collaboration is critical and communication with the patient, their family and other professionals is encouraged. As a common harbinger of occult dementia, and a risk factor for dementia in and of itself, those diagnosed with delirium should be routinely followed up to monitor cognitive and functional recovery [29].

To conclude, LTC residents, particularly those with dementia, are at greater risk of delirium than their counterparts living at home. Like dementia, delirium is under detected in LTC, and in the absence of specialist assessment a structured assessment tool such as 4AT should be considered. There is a paucity of evidence specifically relating to both delirium prevention and management in this setting, but the core principles of delirium care in acute environments remain helpful in LTC settings.

Urinary Incontinence

Urinary incontinence is a burdensome and common condition facing people with dementia [30]. As a function dependent predominantly controlled by the medial prefrontal cortex and the brainstem, continence is vulnerable to neurodegenerative illness. The loss of cortical modulation of micturition and the development of global autonomic dysfunction can result in urinary incontinence in the early stages of frontotemporal dementia and Lewy body dementias respectively, but symptoms can occur in any subtype, particularly in advanced disease [31].

The factors influencing urinary incontinence go beyond the mechanistic, however; impairment in cognition, mobility, motivation, and communication, all commonly observed amongst in LTC residents, can contribute to urinary dysfunction. Thus, the terms "*functional incontinence*" or "*toileting difficulty*" have been adopted.

The prevalence of incontinence is higher in people with a dementia diagnosis (53%), than in those without (13%) [32–34]. The rate in females with dementia (38%) is reported to be twice that in males with dementia (19%) [35], reflecting the greater vulnerability of the female continence system and the underreporting of symptoms within the male population [36]. The prevalence of urinary incontinence also is higher amongst LTC residents than those in the community [37], with embarrassment and stigma often cited amongst the main reasons those affected avoided seeking help prior to institutionalisation [38]. Whilst a dementia diagnosis remains the strongest predictor of LTC placement [39], urinary incontinence also significantly increases that risk [40–43].

There are many negative effects of urinary incontinence on people with dementia, including an increased risk of local skin infections, pressure ulcers, urinary tract

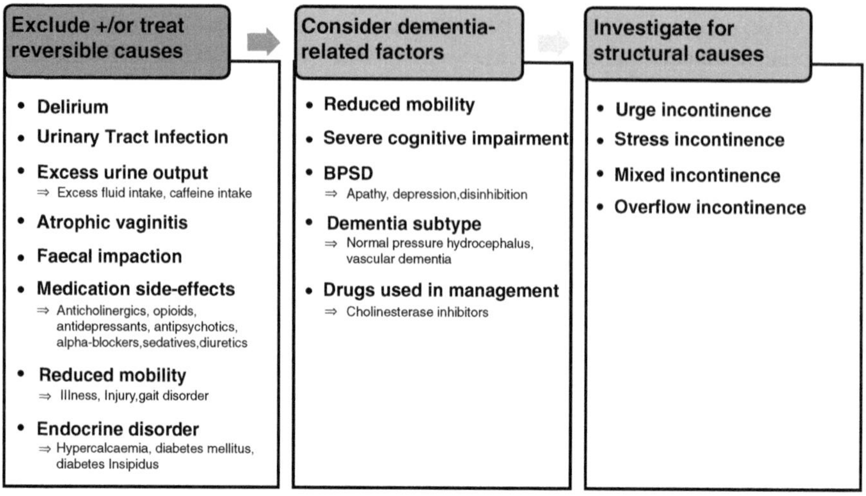

Fig. 16.1 Principles of a comprehensive continence assessment in people with dementia

infections, falls and fall-related injuries [44]. The aetiology of urinary incontinence in people with dementia is multifactorial and effective management therefore warrants consideration of the stage and type of dementia, comorbidities, and behavioural, social, pharmacological, and psychological factors. A comprehensive assessment is essential to an individualised care plan [45].

Three key considerations should be adopted in a structured continence assessment (Fig. 16.1). The first step in the evaluation is to identify "*reversible*" causes. These refer to medical factors that may be easily addressed, often in a primary care setting, where early detection and management allows for significant improvement in symptoms. These do not involve a primary problem within the genitourinary system but may co-exist with structural causes of urinary incontinence [46]. Notably, failure to address these reversible causes may result in poor treatment outcomes for those with established structural causes of urinary incontinence should they co-exist [47]. An important feature of reversible causes of urinary incontinence is the sudden onset of symptoms. For example, a short history of passive wetting in a previously continent individual with an acute on chronic disturbance in mental status is highly suggestive of an underlying delirium.

Several medications commonly prescribed in dementia populations represent reversible causes of urinary incontinence. Opioids and anticholinergic agents, such as tricyclic antidepressants and antipsychotics, cause constipation and inhibit detrusor muscle contractions, leading to urinary retention and subsequent overflow incontinence [48]. Similarly, sedatives, hypnotics, and narcotics may compromise the ability to recognise and respond appropriately to bladder filling [49]. Diuretics causing polyuria and increased contractions, can inhibit the ability to delay urgency, resulting in urge incontinence. Acetylcholinesterase inhibitors can cause urge incontinence through parasympathetic overstimulation [50], an effect which is dose-dependent and attenuated in those with advanced disease [51, 52]. The potential to worsen incontinence is therefore an important consideration when commencing acetylcholinesterase inhibitors [53].

After rectification of reversible causes, the second step in a comprehensive assessment should involve consideration of dementia-related factors contributing to incontinence. Although the degree of cognitive impairment is a significant predictor of urinary incontinence in people with dementia [54–56], immobility and the inability to transfer independently demonstrate a stronger correlation with incontinence than dementia severity itself [57]. Promotion of independence and maintenance of mobility are therefore crucial first-line strategies in preserving continence.

The loss of executive function and orientation skills often seen in dementia can interfere with patients' successful location and use of a toilet, whilst loss of insight, judgement, and inhibition can result in inappropriate toileting behaviours and incontinence. Behavioural and psychological symptoms of dementia (BPSD), including apathy and depression can manifest as lack of volition to maintain continence, and can give rise to the adoption of unhelpful caregiving strategies such as the use of restraints (which further impairs mobility) and inappropriate use of continence pads (which may result in loss of learned behaviours).

Dementia subtype can influence both the stage at which urinary incontinence presents and the mechanisms behind the symptom. Incontinence can appear much earlier in vascular dementia compared to AD and despite its recognition as a pathognomic feature of normal pressure hydrocephalus, incontinence is often not apparent until the later stages of disease [58]. Due to frontal cortex dysfunction and subsequent detrusor hyperactivity, urge incontinence is the mechanism most commonly reported in both AD and vascular dementia [59, 60].

If urinary incontinence persists after dealing with reversible causes and consideration of dementia-related factors, a third step in assessment is consideration of the four structural mechanisms of incontinence: urge, flow, stress, and functional incontinence. As with reversible causes, appropriate choice of investigations and management can improve symptoms and quality of life for people with dementia, but the feasibility of these investigations must be carefully considered. The measurement of postvoid residual urine with ultrasound imaging is a minimally invasive, acceptable means of differentiating between urge and overflow incontinence. Similarly, rectal examination may confirm prostate enlargement or constipation [61].

Like its aetiology, the approach to the management of urinary incontinence should be multifaceted. This is complicated by the relative paucity of research in populations with dementia, and guidelines in the management of incontinence have often excluded people with dementia [62–64]. The suitability of pharmacological and non-pharmacological strategies for urinary incontinence in people with dementia should therefore be assessed on an individual basis and reviewed regularly, taking into account the severity of cognitive impairment, degree of immobility and the caring environment. It is important to recognise that for many, especially those with severe cognitive and mobility impairment, the aim is to reduce symptom burden to contain the condition in a dignified manner.

Basic principles in the management of incontinence, including adequate hydration and environment alterations, should be considered in every case. Modification of fluid amount, type and timing of intake can help. Excessive intake in the evening, especially caffeinated drinks, can lead to nocturia and incontinence, but strict fluid restriction may increase the risk of dehydration, UTI, and acute kidney injury. Ideally, an individual assessment of voiding habits should be undertaken with a target intake of 1–1.5 l allocated throughout the day. Effective multidisciplinary input from occupational and physiotherapists can help identify areas of improvement within the caring environment. The addition of mobility aids, raised toilet seats, grab bars, commodes, and bed pans can help facilitate independent toileting in a person with reduced mobility and thus reduce frequency of incontinence. Introducing visual cues to help locate the toilet, decluttering the surrounding area and ensuring adequate lighting can increase chances of successful toileting. Finally, altering clothing to replace zips and button fastenings with elasticated waistbands and Velcro has shown to be beneficial in people with dementia [65].

Other non-pharmacological interventions include behavioural management with individualised toileting programmes to promote continence. Scheduled voiding involves toileting at predetermined times to reduce frequency of wetting but is reported to carry an intensive caregiver burden. Similarly, prompted voiding involves a regular schedule with the addition of regular prompts and offers of assistance with positive reinforcement to encourage the resident to initiate their own toileting. Success of the abovementioned strategies is only reported in early-stage dementia and is largely dependent on sustained caregiver motivation, which may prove challenging in LTC facilities with staffing shortages [66]. Despite this, it has been highlighted as one of the most successful strategies in dementia populations with a reported 32% reduction in episodes of incontinence [60]. There is little evidence to support the use of bladder training or pelvic muscle rehabilitation, for the treatment or urge and stress incontinence respectively, in people with dementia [67].

Effective management of urinary incontinence should not be dependent on disease severity, yet treatment options are often limited in those with advanced disease who are unable to modify behaviours [68]. The use of continence aids should be deemed a last resort and denotes a shift towards a palliative approach focusing on promoting perineal hygiene, preventing skin infections, pressure ulcers, falls, and reducing caregiver burden. Examples include absorbent pads and pants, as well as external and indwelling catheters, the latter of which should be discouraged until all options have been exhausted. Nonetheless, their use may be warranted in cases of acute urinary retention, fluid monitoring, sacral wound care, and end-of-life care. It has been proven that the use of incontinence pads and indwelling urinary catheters increase the risk of developing a UTI in LTC residents [69]. Often this can precipitate a delirium, with subsequent urethral trauma ensuing as a result of pulling on the catheter. Consequently, the International Continence Society discourages the use of indwelling urinary catheters in severe cognitive impairment due to "the danger of interference to the catheter" [70]. Despite this guidance, a study found that people with dementia were twice as likely to receive a urinary catheter, and to receive it sooner, than those without dementia [71]. In light of these adverse effects, it is imperative that clinicians and caregivers re-evaluate their rationale and avoid inappropriate usage whereby convenience and ease of care load is prioritised over risk avoidance.

Pharmacological management of urinary incontinence is limited to instances in which the underlying structural aetiology includes urge and overflow incontinence alone. There is little evidence to support the use of such agents in dementia populations, particularly when the cause of incontinence is often multifactorial, and side effects and polypharmacy are prevailing concerns. The key principles of prescribing in elderly populations apply; commence minimal agents are at the lowest possible dose, titrate upwards if necessary and discontinue if no therapeutic benefit is achieved. In cases of overflow incontinence secondary to benign prostatic hypertrophy, smooth muscle relaxants such as tamsulosin are often considered either as monotherapy or in combination with 5α-Reductase Inhibitors such as dutasteride and finasteride. Caution should be exercised when prescribing α-blockers in people with dementia due to the risk of postural hypotension increase falls risk [72].

Where urge incontinence has been identified as the predominant pathology, anticholinergic agents are often considered, but an increased anticholinergic load represents a major deterrent to their use in people with dementia. Commonly reported side effects of these medications also include constipation, visual disturbances, insomnia, which themselves increase risk of delirium [52, 73].

Encouragingly, one study in older populations reported reduced urinary leakage with newer, modified-release anticholinergic agents such as darifenacin and tolterodine [74]. These drugs target selective muscarinic receptors without crossing the blood–brain barrier, resulting in fewer central nervous system side effects. However, tolterodine can still precipitate delirium in people with dementia if combined with acetylcholinesterase inhibitors, so co-prescription should be avoided [75, 76].

In summary, urinary incontinence is common and burdensome in people with dementia. Aetiology is usually multifactorial, so a detailed and systematic assessment of contributing factors, including reversible causes and the effect of dementia itself, should be conducted.

Weight Loss, Decreased Appetite, and Feeding

Weight loss is very common in the latter stages of dementia. This can occur due to lack of appetite and insufficient intake but can also be a feature in the context of an adequate intake. One of the great clinical challenges is that weight loss can be a manifestation of other significant underlying health problems, including malignancy, and the clinical status of the patient means that there is often little or no possibility of useful investigation. Furthermore, when eating difficulties and weight loss occur, health care providers and families often feel they should continue oral feeding or opt for feeding tube placement; making such decisions in patients with advanced dementia can be challenging.

Cachexia is a complex metabolic process associated with advanced dementia, although the exact pathophysiological mechanisms remain unknown [77]. Loss of body weight in AD is typically associated with sarcopenia, which leads to further functional decline, greater disability, and increased clinical vulnerability. This perpetuates the cycle of altered food consumption and decreased energy intake. Whilst it is still suggested that the weight loss associated with AD may be entirely prevented by dealing with predisposing causes, there is also strong evidence that weight loss is probably a genuine manifestation of the disease [77]. However, in the advanced stages of dementia, the acceleration of weight loss seems to share similar features with cachexia.

Cachexia is a hypercatabolic state, and, theoretically, nutritional interventions containing 1.5 g per kilo of body weight per day of protein should be sufficient to counteract catabolism [78]. However, both European Society for Clinical Nutrition and Metabolism [79] and National Institute for Health and Care Excellence guidelines [80] indicate there is insufficient evidence to support the use of dietary supplements to maintain the nutritional status of people with dementia. Enteral nutrition may be useful in patients with mild to moderate dementia and reversible malnutrition, but neither guideline recommends the use of enteral nutrition in the terminal phase of dementia, although the physician's decision will be influenced by the individual general prognosis and preferences. The Japan Gastroenterological Endoscopy Society has recommended percutaneous endoscopic gastrostomy (PEG) tube placement in patients with malnutrition due to cerebrovascular disease or dementia, with the rationale that early PEG placement is associated with longer survival [81].

Nutritional interventions for patients with severe dementia are inconsistent, and comorbidity complicates the generalisation of existing studies. Thus, cachexia can be considered a refractory symptom in the clinical trajectory of dementia. Therefore, in late-stage dementia, therapy and care should be shifted towards end-of-life and palliative issues, in order to maximise dignity and quality of life [82]. Dysphagia secondary to advanced dementia is a progressive, irreversible, and incurable condition with a multifactorial aetiology that involves dyspraxia, cognitive fluctuation, impulsivity, reduced physical mobility, poor dentition, and dependence for feeding and medications. Tube feeding has been proposed as a means of protein and calorie supplementation for patients in the final stages of dementia to maintain skin integrity, prevent aspiration pneumonia and other infectious complications, improve functional status, and extend survival. Artificial nutrition and hydration have been made popular as a caring intervention, whilst forgoing such measures has been equated with neglect [77].

Studies investigating feeding tube placement in patients with severe dementia have been retrospective in nature, using mixed populations. They have concluded that feeding tubes confer little clinical benefit. PEG placement is relatively straightforward in comparison to the surgical interventions previously favoured. It can, however, be associated with high rates of tube-related complications, as well as mechanical complications, which are frequently overlooked. There can be other major complications and agitation and self-extubation can reduce quality of life. Direct mortality from the placement of a PEG tube is generally low (0–2%) but complication rates may range from 15 to 70%. It has been reported that weight loss and severe depletion of lean and fat body mass persisted in tube-fed patients with advanced dementia even after a standard enteral formula was provided daily for 1 year [83]. Other studies have shown that nutritional markers do not improve after feeding tube placement. It has also been shown that weight loss progressively worsened in parallel with the duration of the tube feeding. This evidence highlights the irreversible progression of cachexia alongside the limitations and potentially detrimental effects of artificial nutrition and hydration [77].

A 2009 Cochrane review of observational studies concluded that there was insufficient evidence to support the benefits of tube feeding in patients with advanced dementia in terms of survival, quality of life, nutrition, functional status, prevention of aspiration, or prevention and healing of pressure ulcers [84]. Feeding tubes do not appear therefore to be a useful palliative measure, and the use of artificial nutrition and hydration in end-stage dementia should be generally discouraged, as it can prolong the process of dying and may also increase discomfort and suffering. Therefore, it is not possible to define an internationally approved treatment or recommendation for reversing cachexia and advanced dementia at present.

The Choices, Attitudes, and Strategies for Care of Advanced Dementia at the End of Life (CASCADE) study prospectively enrolled LTC residents and followed them up until death (median survival 1.3 years). Eating problems were very common (86%) [85, 86]. Clinical observations have confirmed the benefit of minimal interventions including swabs, sips of water, ice chips, lubrication of the lips, and oral comfort feeding. Oral comfort feeding provides a number of advantages and mitigates artificial nutrition hydration and nutrition. However, this remains a very sensitive area, and the subject of debate as an international Delphi study with experts from 23 countries, full consensus was agreed on almost all aspects of palliative care in dementia but not on rehydration being inappropriate in the dying phase [87].

In conclusion, cachexia can be considered a refractory symptom in the clinical trajectory of dementia, with complex underlying pathology. Tube and enteral feeding are neither without complication nor are they associated with an improvement in outcomes, and in advanced dementia palliative approaches should be explored.

Lower Respiratory Tract Infections

The common problems seen with advancing dementia, such as dysphagia, weakness, and immobility, can combine to result in lower respiratory tract infections (LRTIs). LRTI is the cause of death in up to two thirds of patients with dementia and 6-month mortality is 74% [88]. Thus, there will be a considerable demand for LRTI treatment and use of antibiotics in this population. From a wider perspective, appropriate antibiotic use is important because of concerns regarding increased antimicrobial resistance. Consideration should also be paid to the possibility of Clostridium difficile infection and outbreaks.

Administration of antibiotics for LRTI in individuals with advanced dementia are aimed at extension of life and improvement of discomfort caused by the infection. In a study of male LTC residents with advanced dementia and LRTI, mortality was substantial despite antibiotic treatment; 48% died within 10 days and 74%

within 6 months. Antibiotics prolonged life, but in many cases only for several days. Benefit from antibiotics was less likely with inadequate fluid intake [89]. Treatment decisions regarding antibiotics must therefore take into account that although antibiotics improve short-term mortality, they may also prolong the dying process [89]. In the US LTC facility involved in the aforementioned study where there is a long tradition of hospice care and advance care planning. In Dutch LTC facilities approaches to antibiotic therapy are similar; therapy is withheld in about a quarter of residents with dementia and physician's diagnosis of pneumonia. This is especially the case in particularly vulnerable residents, almost all of whom die when not treated [90]. The authors refer to the fact that US treatment strategies are significantly driven by family wishes. They conclude that a more balanced decision-making process might be achieved by educating families and clinicians in the modest effectiveness of antibiotics in either prolonging life or diminishing suffering in those with advanced dementia.

LRTI can be anticipated to some degree, and the management will depend on the physical state of the patient as well as the stage of the dementia, the prognosis, the presence of any advanced directive, and patient's best interests. The medical practitioner is usually faced with a decision about the extent of treatment and extent of escalation of care which can mean the need for assessment in ED and possible hospitalisation. The notes should contain a care plan, so that even if the medical practitioner is not the usual medical attendant, it should be clear what management should entail. The care plan should include details of the ceiling of care that has been agreed with the family. After initial assessment of the severity of any LRTI the management decision will depend on the above considerations but usually involves decisions about use of antibiotics and need for adjunctive measures such as hydration and oxygen. Oral fluids are preferred where possible and safe to administer and, in some cases, subcutaneous fluids can be appropriate. If antibiotics are to be used, then they should be started as soon as possible.

In conclusion, LRTIs do not represent innocuous events in LTC residents, particularly in the presence of severe illness. Expectations of treatment should be reasonable in neither promising long-term survival nor alleviation of distress, and families of people with dementia should be informed of this both when advance care plans are discussed and when contributing to unplanned discussions of more immediate treatment. Advance care planning is discussed later in this chapter.

Pressure Ulcers

Pressure ulcers occur when an area of skin, or the tissues below, is damaged as a result of pressure or distortion (shearing forces). Consequently, blood supply is interrupted, and tissue death occurs.

Such shearing forces can occur when an individual is lifted or moved. Anyone, of any age, will develop such damage if the skin is subject to unrelieved pressure, but pressure sores are particularly common in those with severe illness, mobility impairment, poor posture, neurological impairment, compromised skin or malnourishment. Three major factors contribute to the development of pressure ulcers: pressure, shear, and friction. The areas of the body most at risk of damage are the sacrum, heels, buttocks, and greater trochanters. Almost half of all pressure sores develop on the sacrum and almost 20% develop on the heels [91].

The incidence and prevalence of pressure ulcers have reduced markedly in recent times. Previously they resulted in a steady stream of referrals to medical practitioners and were frequently responsible for hospital admissions. In a recent European study of 791 people with dementia in LTC, however, the overall prevalence of pressure ulcers was 6.7%; this ranged between 2.5 and 13.9% at different sites [92, 93]. This decrease is likely to be in no small part due to advances in the progression of pressure ulcer prevention.

Pressure at the interface between bony prominences and support surfaces, sufficient to occlude or reduce blood flow, is thought to cause pressure ulcers. The key measures for reducing pressures lie in the provision of support surfaces that redistribute pressure, and adoption of regular turning regimens. High-density foam mattresses distribute pressure more evenly and have largely replaced springform mattresses. A study by Li et al. [94] found a steady decrease in pressure ulcers in 2-year increments from 2002 to 2008. The authors attributed this to the use of high-density foam mattresses, providing a margin of error so great that, even when turning did not occur as recommended, the properties of the mattresses protected residents from excessive pressure [95].

Regular turning regimens are also important. In a 3-week prospective study of pressure ulcers in 942 LTC residents (71.3% OF whom had dementia) [96] the effects of 2-, 3-, and 4-h turning regimens were compared. The incidence (2%) of pressure ulcers in this moderate- and high-risk cohort was comparable with that observed in low risk LTC cohorts (2%) and was considerably lower than the 10% prevalence reported amongst high-risk, long-stay residents. They found that turning at 3- and 4-h intervals was no worse than turning every 2 h. The authors concluded that less frequent turning might increase sleep, improve quality of life, reduce staff injury, and save time for such other activities as feeding, walking, and toileting.

In assessment of risk, the most commonly used scales are the Waterlow scale [97] and the Braden scale [98], which allow the state of the skin and extent of pressure sore to be graded. Urinary or faecal incontinence can result in an incontinence-associated dermatitis, which can lead to skin breakdown and the development or worsening of pressure ulcers. Risk mitigation involves frequent positional changes at least every 6 h, increasing to every 4 h for those assessed as being at high risk of developing pressure ulcers. Tissue viability services can be very helpful in advising about prevention and if pressure ulcers develop early referral to tissue viability services can prevent deterioration.

Nutritional supplements are recommended in those with established deficiency, but they should not be offered specifically to prevent or treat a pressure ulcer in adults whose nutritional status is adequate [99]. A Cochrane review found no clear evidence of a benefit associated with nutritional interventions for either the prevention or treatment of pressure ulcers [100].

Table 16.1 Principles of prevention of pressure ulcers

Risk assessment
Skin assessment
Nutrition
Skin moisture
Repositioning for prevention of pressure ulcers
Support surfaces

In conclusion, people with dementia often have impaired mobility, prevention of pressure ulcers in LTC is a very important aspect of management (Table 16.1). Prevention involves the use of appropriate pressure relieving mattresses and regular turning, with evidence that a 3- or 4-h turning regimen is as effective as regular 2 hourly turning.

Vaccinations

Influenza and pneumococcal infections are the eighth leading cause of death in the USA [101]. Nearly half of these deaths occur amongst individuals who are 65 years of age and older and amongst frail older people residing in LTC. These infections also cause considerable morbidity. As a result, influenza vaccination is recommended annually in older persons, including LTC facility residents in most developed countries [102]. Given its low burden of risk and its beneficial effect in the short term and on the community, influenza vaccination is likewise recommended in older adults with poor prognosis or advanced dementia. Dementia has been shown to be an independent risk factor for influenza complications in older adults, so vaccination is particularly relevant in this high-risk population, particularly because early symptoms of influenza are difficult to recognise in individuals with dementia.

The Advisory Committee on Immunization Practices recommends that all adults 65 years or over receive both the recently introduced polysaccharide-protein conjugate vaccine against 13 pneumococcal serotypes (PCV13) as well as the polysaccharide vaccine against 23 pneumococcal serotypes (PPSV23) [103]. This was endorsed by The Society for Post-Acute and Long-Term Care Medicine (AMDA) [104].

In a recent study of 6275 residents from 175 French LTC facilities, influenza vaccination was achieved in 92% of residents with dementia and 88% of those without dementia. In the UK, influenza vaccine uptake was 83.3% in care home patients with dementia. In a fully adjusted model, compared with community patients without dementia, patients with dementia in the community were significantly less likely to receive vaccination (RR: 0.96). LTC residents with (RR: 1.06) and without (RR: 1.03) dementia were significantly more likely to receive vaccination. In LTC, people with dementia were marginally but significantly more likely to receive vaccination (RR: 1.03, 1.01–1.06) compared with patients without dementia.

Immunisation programmes appear to have an immediate effect on mortality. In a recent prospective European cohort study collecting information on residents admitted to 57 nursing homes in eight countries (Czech Republic, England, Finland, France, Germany, Italy, The Netherlands, and Israel) incident mortality was recorded during 1-year follow-up. A shared-frailty Cox regression model was used to assess the impact of vaccination status on mortality. In total, 81.7 and 27.0% received influenza and pneumococcal vaccination, respectively. Overall, 727 (20.7%) residents died during the follow-up period. After adjusting for potential confounders, which included age, sex, number of diseases, depression, cognitive and functional status, influenza, and the combination of influenza and pneumococcal vaccination, but not pneumococcal vaccination alone, were associated with a statistically significant reduction in mortality compared to no vaccinations [105]. Immunogenicity studies comparing the pneumococcal vaccines PCV13 and PPSV23 in frail elderly patients have been conducted in both LTC and hospital settings. Subjects recruited in these studies included very frail elderly individuals with significant levels of dependency and cognitive impairment. Regardless of setting, subjects were able to mount a significant antibody response.

There is some evidence of disparity in receipt of the immunisations. A US study reported that African American LTC residents were significantly less likely to receive influenza and pneumococcal vaccinations than their white counterparts. The likelihood of not being offered the influenza and vaccination pneumococcal vaccination was significantly greater for African American and Hispanic residents respectively when compared to white residents. The study also found that no racial/ethnic group met the US national vaccination targets (90% or more) between 2010 and 2013 [106].

Most developed countries have national policies and ambitious targets relating to influenza and pneumococcal immunisation. The World Health Organisation targets, incorporating recommendations for less developed countries, are slightly lower (75%). People with dementia in LTC appear to receive these immunisations in higher numbers than their community-based equivalents, but there is evidence supporting racial inequity in their availability. LTC residents with dementia should receive the influenza and pneumococcal immunisations.

Antibiotics

There is an increasing focus in healthcare systems on antibiotic stewardship. The frequent use of antibiotics contributes to the development of multidrug-resistant microorganisms and is associated with adverse events. The particular problem seen in LTC residents with dementia is Clostridium difficile. Respiratory and urinary tract infections (UTIs) are regularly diagnosed and treated in LTC populations, and it is therefore useful to have policies in place mitigating resistance and the development of Clostridium difficile.

Use of antimicrobial agents is very common in people with advanced dementia; 40% of patients are prescribed them during the last 2 weeks of life [107]. In one Italian study, investigators analysed 109 episodes of pneumonia amongst 77 nursing home patients with stage 7 on the Functional Assessment Staging Tool. Most decisions (90%) referred to treatment with antibiotics [88].

Antimicrobials were found to be unjustifiably used in one fifth of respiratory chest infections and over two-thirds of cases of acute bronchitis, suggesting a need for programmes to improve antibiotic prescribing at LTC facilities [108]. An estimated 60% of LTC residents are colonised with multidrug-resistant organisms [107] and colonisation rates amongst those with advanced dementia are reportedly three times higher than those of other residents [109].

In the Study of Pathogen Resistance and Exposure to Antimicrobials in Dementia (SPREAD), 362 LTC residents with advanced dementia were studied prospectively over 12 months. A total of 496 episodes were recorded, comprising respiratory tract (29.8%), urinary tract (39.5%), and skin (13.9%) infections as well as instances of fever of unclear source (16.7%). Only 44% of treated episodes met minimum clinical criteria for antimicrobial treatment initiation. Colonisation by multidrug-resistant organisms was extensive; over 12 months, 67% of residents were colonised, and the cumulative incidence rate of multidrug-resistant organism acquisition amongst residents not previously colonised at baseline was 48%. The authors suggested an approach that may improve the quality of these decisions. Firstly, as part of advance care planning, families of patients with dementia should be counselled to expect infections in the latter stages of the disease. Secondly, the risks and benefits involved in assessing and treating infections should be reviewed and aligned with the goals of care. If the decision is made to forego antimicrobial agents, suspected infections should not be investigated; symptoms should be treated solely with palliative measures. Finally, if the use of antimicrobials persists, treatment initiation should be guided by consensus criteria. A more judicious approach to infection management in advanced dementia may avoid unnecessary treatment burden in these terminally ill patients and reduce the rapidly growing public health threat of multidrug-resistant organism [107].

In another nested case-control study amongst 137 people with dementia in LTC who did not receive antimicrobials, 44 acquired a multidrug-resistant organism. Risk factors for acquisition included prescription of gastrointestinal medications affecting the gut microbiome, a higher number of visits from healthcare workers, pressure ulcers, and not residing in a specialist dementia unit [110].

In institutionalised older adults, UTI is common and difficult to differentiate from asymptomatic bacteriuria. Asymptomatic bacteriuria prevalence rates in LTC are high, ranging from 25 to 50% in women and from 15 to 40% in men [111]. In a recent study of LTC residents, 23% of whom had dementia, asymptomatic bacteriuria, mostly caused by Escherichia coli, occurred in approximately 40% of participants. Long-term asymptomatic bacteriuria (over 3 months) was found in 30% of the subjects and was most common in frail women with urinary incontinence and dementia. The authors concluded that women in LTC with incontinence have asymptomatic bacteriuria prevalence rates of about 80% and are often persistent carriers. These prevalence rates should be considered in clinical decision-making as they devalue the significance of a positive urine culture as a criterion to diagnose infection [112]. The decision about the need for antibiotics for urinary infections should therefore be carefully considered in those with chronic incontinence.

There should be a high level of vigilance regarding Clostridium difficile infection in people with dementia where antibiotics are prescribed, particularly in the case of recurrent prescription. Liaison with local microbiology departments about appropriate choice of antibiotics is very useful and any guidance should be reviewed regularly.

Telemedicine in People with Dementia

In the previous section, we discussed several clinical difficulties specific to the management of people with dementia in LTC. In the following section we highlight telemedicine as an opportunity that LTC homes may provide in optimising the care of their residents, helping facilitate contact with services that individuals might not have previously accessed.

Over the last 20 years, telecommunications technology has developed dramatically, and telemedicine, defined by the American Academy of Neurology as "*consultation at a distance, or not in person, using various technologies to achieve connectivity, including the telephone and the Internet* [113]" has evolved accordingly. The care of people with dementia, perhaps a more interview-driven process than that for other groups of disorders, has drawn considerable focus in this field. Although dementia practitioners largely have been slow to implement telemedicine into their routine, the restrictions imposed by COVID-19 may catalyse its adoption across routine clinical care [114–116].

The advantages offered by telemedicine, whilst not all adequately supported by published research, are too numerous and significant to readily dismiss. Telemedicine would appear to be particularly advantageous to residents of nursing homes, enhancing patients' access to specialist care whilst surrounded by a comfortable environment and familiar faces, avoiding the challenges often posed by outpatient facilities to those with visual impairment, poor mobility or continence issues. To providers, telemedicine could enhance access to services without the human resources and planning necessary to facilitate attendance at outpatient clinics. Finally, it provides clinicians with the opportunity to reduce the time spent on travel [117, 118] and in many cases provides workload flexibility; one study reports that 17 of 30 telemedicine clinics described would have otherwise been cancelled had travel to a rural clinic site been required [119].

Practical obstacles in the implementation of telemedicine in nursing homes might include the availability of appropriate equipment to conduct such examinations; only 13% of American physicians conducting work in nursing homes reported that they had access to telemedicine facilities, despite widespread support for the medium amongst those surveyed. The same survey reported geriatric psychiatrists and neurologists were amongst the most enthusiastic proponents for the use of telemedicine [120]. Provision of adequate facilities is crucial; the United States Centers for Medicare and Medicaid Services had previously only recognised telehealth that comprised both two-way audio and video components. These regulations were only amended to include telephone consultations shortly after the emergence of the COVID-19 pandemic [121], and only 20% of US states require reimbursement parity between telemedicine reviews and face-to-face consultations [116]. It is therefore crucial that clinicians considering practicing telemedicine consult local regulations and guidelines regarding its use.

Although discomfort and unfamiliarity with technology has been cited as a barrier to effective implementation of telemedicine [122], both patients and their families [117, 123, 124], as well as care providers [124–126] have reported high levels of satisfaction with programmes provided care via telemedicine. Patients experiencing assessment via both telemedicine and face-to-face consultation also report comparable levels of satisfaction between the two modalities [127].

Evidence supports the validity, as well as the acceptability, of telemedicine assessment in the assessment of people with dementia. A 2019 systematic review and meta-analysis exploring the use of telemedicine in the diagnosis of dementia and mild cognitive impairment [128] noted that four case-control accuracy studies, nine paired comparative accuracy studies, and two prospective single-arm accuracy studies reported high levels of agreement between assessments conducted in person and those performed using telemedicine. The review identified only one study reporting that telemedicine assessment led to an overestimation of cognitive ability in more severely impaired patients when compared with their traditional consultations [129]. In spite of the encouraging evidence base on this topic, however, there is a recognition that more randomised controlled trials are needed with respect to dementia assessment using telemedicine [113].

Nonetheless, a potential barrier to the successful implementation of telemedicine might include clinicians' access to, and familiarity with, modified appropriate structured neuropsychological tests long established in routine practice. Validated modifications to tools such as the MMSE allow cognitive assessment via telephone and demonstrate good sensitivity and specificity [130]. When video consultation is available, it may be more feasible to use the Montreal Cognitive examination (MoCA) or Addenbrooke's Cognitive Examination. The electronic version of MoCA (eMoCA) has been validated; scores produced paper and electronic versions were within 2 points in 76% of patients [131].

Cognitive examinations in telemedicine are not without their disadvantages; sensory impairment may artificially decrease cognitive scores, as might the environment, particularly if noisy or uncomfortable [132]. It may be more difficult to engage the patient using telemedicine facilities than in person, and again this should be taken into account where possible. Similarly, the savvy interviewee may use visual cues (such as calendars), enlist the assistance of companions, or write down items expected to be recalled, all without the examiner being aware. These underline the importance of recognition of neuropsychological tools as adjuncts to effective and comprehensive history-taking, rather than diagnostic tests themselves, irrespective of the medium. Where diagnostic uncertainty exists, consideration should be made to a face-to-face interview.

Another important caveat of the above is that cognitive assessment via telemedicine is a well circumscribed process that fails to integrate a valuable, more global, clinical appraisal, which cannot be reliably obtained through any other means than face-to-face examination. Appraisal of the patient with possible delirium, for example, benefits from observation of clinical signs ranging from skin turgor to abdominal tenderness and ketotic fetor. This, of course, is all the more important when assessing patients with multimorbidity, which is common in LTC residents.

Facets of physical examination via telemedicine have been evaluated; the Unified Parkinson's Disease Rating Scale, and the Abnormal Involuntary Movement Scale have been reported as noninferior when used via telemedicine over face-to-face evaluation [133, 134]. Similarly, observation of gait analysis via brief video clips allowed experienced geriatricians to reliably identify gait abnormalities [135]. Nevertheless, these represent small components of the comprehensive clinical assessment that is often necessary in the care of residents in LTC, and underline that telemedicine is an adjunct to, not a replacement for, face-to-face consultation.

The use of telemedicine in dementia care is not confined to diagnosis; studies have been conducted into its use in cognitive rehabilitation [136], post-diagnostic support for patients and caregivers [137], and in the management of neuropsychiatric symptoms [138, 139]. Although the evidence base relating to continuing care is much less developed than that relating to dementia diagnosis [128, 140], the importance of global clinical assessment highlighted above may suggest that telemedicine is best suited to routine follow-up of patients in LTC who have already undergone a robust initial assessment.

A combination of an emerging supportive evidence base and the clear practical benefits of delivery of telemedicine to individuals in nursing homes would suggest that its use will continue to grow in the coming years. Encouraging familiarity and comfort with telemedicine are likely to be important considerations in its implementation, but the foundations of traditional clinical care, particularly in the practice of dementia assessment, are as important and valid in virtual consultations.

Death and Dying in Long-Term Care

Planning for a comfortable and dignified death is an important, if sometimes overlooked, facet of the care of older people. The majority of people with dementia admitted to LTC will die there; a quarter within 6 months. In this section we discuss important issues facing the clinician regarding death, and how they can be anticipated and the preparations that can be made to best facilitate a good death.

Course of Care and Mortality in LTC

A recent study reported a significant increase in the number of residents who died within 6 months of being admitted into LTC facilities (2006–2012) [141]. A quarter (26%, adjusted for censoring) did not survive the first 6 months. The estimated survival rates for 1, 2, and 3 years after admission are 66%, 54%, and 47%, respectively. In a recent systematic review, mortality within the first 6 months after admission varied from 0 to 34% (median 20.2%) [142]. The authors concluded that there appears to be a difference in rates of mortality before and after a period of 6 months following admission; this period is therefore used as a benchmark of early mortality following admission. The causes of deaths were not reported, and increased mortality was not wholly explained by intrinsic resident factors such as dementia. Only two studies investigated the influence of factors relating to facilities themselves, reporting an increased risk in facilities with high rates of antipsychotic prescription [142]. Any transition from residence to another should be recognised as representing a risk to patient safety, not least due to fragmentation in care delivery and insufficient communication between health providers [143, 144]. The transition can result in new adverse health events or an acute deterioration of pre-existing conditions. These include delirium, worsening disability, malnutrition, falls, injury, and medication-related events [145].

If one survives the first 6 months of institutional life, then long-term survival is more likely than not. Amongst the LTC population, cognitive impairment, severe mental abnormality, urinary incontinence, need for intense nursing, functional impairment, physical dependence, and poor physical mobility are related to high mortality [146–150]. With regard to psychosocial factors, mortality is predicted by apathy, lack of social support, and social isolation [150–152]. Advanced age and being male sex are also associated with higher mortality in most studies, reflecting well established life expectancy patterns in the general population. Epidemiological studies help provide insight into patient management, particularly in those who survive longer in LTC. They inform and aid discussions with relatives and caregivers regarding immediate management and advance care planning.

Advance Care Planning

Advance care planning is a process of discussion, between a person and a care worker, taken in anticipation of a future deterioration in that patient's condition [153]. It aims to support patients in understanding and sharing their personal values, life goals and preferences regarding future medical care [154]. It puts in place plans to ensure that these preferences can be met when, as is may be the case in individuals with dementia, the person no longer has the capacity to express their wishes [155].

Advance care planning is of particular importance amongst LTC residents due to their older age and more complex care needs than the general population; the course of their care can be unpredictable and, in many cases, punctuated by emergency hospital admissions. Such admissions may not only be distressing and/or unnecessary, but may increase the risk of dying in hospital, against most patient's wishes [156]. Individuals with advance care plans, however, are associated with lower rates of crisis hospital admission and death in hospital and are associated with quality indicators such as adequate pain management, access to sufficient support and an overall satisfaction with care [157]. In contrast, the absence of advance care planning has been hypothesised to be at least partly responsible for inadequate end-of-life care in people with dementia [158] and limited access to palliative care services when compared with cognitively healthy individuals [159, 160].

Implementation of advance care planning in LTC facilities has proved challenging, with low levels (<12%) of engagement reported in residents in Germany, Belgium, and the UK [161–163]. Uptake amongst older people is historically higher in USA (75%) but lower rates are observed in both people with dementia and in non-white and lower income communities [164]. Countries like the UK are increasingly promoting advance care planning as part of national strategy and policy, recognising it as an indicator of quality care in and of itself [158].

Ideally, discussion around advance care plans should take place at or before the point of diagnosis, when support, information, and education about dementia itself should be combined with discussion of issues around palliative and end-of-life care [165]. In most cases this is long before their admission to LTC [166]. If advance care planning is not already in place upon admission, it should be addressed early in the patient's residency. Cognitive impairment will be present in a large proportion of individuals admitted to LTC, but residents' capacity to engage in the process of care planning should in all cases be presumed, unless a lack of capacity for such decisions has been previously established. Where capacity is in doubt, structured cognitive tests like MMSE are useful adjuncts to, but not replacements for, comprehensive capacity assessment.

Where no advance care plan is in place upon admission, every effort should be made to support residents and their relatives early in the process. This should be balanced with the need for the individual to be comfortable and familiar with the care worker engaging them in the pathway. No single professional is responsible for exercising this role; it is best done so by whomever the patient is most comfortable, ideally at a time when their health is relatively stable.

There is no single way to discuss advance care planning, with either people with dementia or those without. The need for contextualisation and adaptation of the discussion based on the patient themselves is demonstrated by the observations that studies from Western countries emphasise the reliance on autonomy as a driver for advance care plans, whilst those from Asian countries identify a more important role for family, community, and medical opinion in decision-making [167]. Many LTC facilities preface any discussion with a written introduction to the process; this can help put residents and their families at ease and can demonstrate assurance that such conversations are part of usual procedures within the facility [168]. A useful way to approach the discussion is through use of open questions that determine what the person values most (Table 16.2), and what concerns them the most. Acknowledging that emotional intensity of the conversation is helpful; it may be necessary to propose resumption of the conversation at another time if proving too difficult for a person with dementia. Ending the interaction in a conversational "safe space", perhaps discussing less taxing topics, is advisable [168].

Involving families as early as possible not only allows additional support to the individual but also provides an excellent opportunity to engage caregivers that may, then or a later point, be approached to act as a proxy informant. However, as

Table 16.2 Questions to consider when discussing advance care planning (Adapted from Stobbart-Rowlands and Thorn [168])

"At this time in your life, what is it that makes you happy?"
"What do you hope for? What do you enjoy doing?"
"What or who is important to you?"
"Is there anything you're particularly worried about?"
"What elements of care are important to you and what would you like to happen in the future?"
"Is there anything that you worry about or fear happening? What would you not want to happen?"
"What would help you cope? What is helping most right now?"

previously mentioned, a large proportion of people with dementia may already require a proxy to advise on their behalf at the point of LTC admission. Often family members feel unprepared for such decision-making responsibilities, particularly at the point of LTC; feelings of guilt and a sense of failure can add further burden [159, 169, 170].

An important point to reinforce to both professionals and relatives is that the role of the proxy is to advise on what the person with dementia would have wished for regarding their care, rather than the family member having decision-making power. As such, irrespective of capacity, the person with dementia should continue to be consulted and their hopes and concerns canvassed, even if the proxy is the one to communicate a clear conclusion. Education and support for families at this point is therefore crucial and are associated with improved outcomes; targeted end-of-life care education and a supportive advance care planning program for relatives can reduce unnecessary hospital admission and reduce mortality of LTC residents [171].

In conclusion, advance care planning works well in LTC, and should be systematically offered to every resident. When employed effectively it can improve a range of outcomes and is an important component of end-of-life care. Although people with dementia, by the time of LTC admission may not have the capacity to engage in such discussions, early involvement from families can produce similar beneficial outcomes when provided with adequate support and education.

Managing Transfers

Although a palliative approach to care is recommended for people with advanced dementia, approximately 25% of LTC residents with advanced dementia are hospitalised in the last 6 months of life [172]. In one study, around half of all hospitalisations fell into the major diagnostic categories of diseases or disorders of the respiratory system (22%), circulatory system (15%), and kidney or urinary tract (13%). It is important to examine the objective data to see how these patients are best managed. In another study, 47% of all LTC residents experienced at least one transfer to the emergency department (ED) over the course of a year. At their first

ED transfer, 36.4% of subjects were admitted to the hospital. The median time to first ED visit for subjects with advanced stage dementia was 258 days, whilst it was 250 days for subjects with early to moderate stage dementia and 202 days for subjects with no dementia. Multivariate proportional hazard modelling showed that age, race, number of comorbidities, number of hospitalisations in the year prior, and DNR status, but not dementia severity, all influenced subjects' time to first ED visit [173].

In a recent study which examined the processes involved in hospital transfers of people with dementia, the investigators found that decision-making regarding hospital transfer comprised two phases. "Phase One" took place shortly after admission and consisted of obtaining surrogates' preferences in response to hypothetical acute events. This process was influenced by the ability of the providers to effectively establish trust, foreshadow, and illuminate the hazards of hospitalisation. "Phase Two" began at the start of an acute event and ended when a decision was made to either treat the resident in LTC or transfer to the hospital. Responding to the acute event was influenced by the ability to care for residents in the LTC, the providers' comfort with end-of-life conversations, and surrogates' preferences [174].

Transfer of nursing home residents is frequently considered avoidable, although this judgement is often made based on analysis of diagnoses made in the hospital. Identified strategies for reducing hospital transfers of nursing home residents include improving communication during an acute change in status event, recognition of available resources to treat residents in-house, access to clinicians and rapid diagnostic testing, and timely access to advance care planning and palliative care [175].

A study in Italian LTCs examined the critical decisions made for patients with advanced dementia. The major critical decisions were in relation to LRTI and other infections (46.6%), nutritional and hydration problems (20.6%), and the worsening of a pre-existing disease (9.3%). The most frequent type of decision amongst LTC patients concerned the prescription of antibiotics (41.1%) and the most frequent purposes of the critical decisions were in reducing symptoms or suffering (81.1%) and prolonging survival (27.5%). In 3.8% of cases, the purpose was to ease death or not to prolong life. The overall conclusions were that decisions critical for the survival or quality of life of patients with advanced dementia were made for approximately one half of the patients during a 6-month period. LTC patients were more frequently hospitalised, and a sizeable minority of these patients were treated with the goal of prolonging survival. Italian patients with advanced dementia may benefit from the implementation of palliative care principles [176].

The decision to send to ED can be a very difficult one. The importance of initial assessment therefore cannot be underestimated. This will facilitate the "Phase One" intervention described above. Where that does not occur, dealing with an acute event can be problematic and the practices are very varied. Too often, people with advanced dementia are sent to hospital when the LTC facility, usually a comfortable and recognisable environment, can provide adequate care.

Palliative Care

Palliative care is a very important consideration as dementia progresses. It is very difficult to determine when patients enter the last few months of their illness. However, for those in LTC the focus on palliative care should be high on the patient management agenda. The topic is discussed in greater detail in Chap. 17.

Persons with advanced dementia usually have severe memory impairment, minimal verbal communication, poor mobility, are very dependent functionally and have urinary and faecal incontinence. LTC residents with advanced dementia survive a median of 1.3 years, yet they are commonly subjected to burdensome interventions toward the end of life. These interventions include a variety of transitions between health care facilities, invasive procedures, and in some cases, physical restraints. These interventions are often avoidable, may not improve comfort, and are frequently distressing to residents and their families.

There are global differences in the approach to palliative care in LTC. For example, a focus on palliative care for residents with dementia is much more common in Dutch facilities than in the USA. In one study investigators compared treatment and mortality in the USA and Dutch LTCs amongst residents with LRTIs, often the immediate cause of death in dementia. People with dementia were more often treated without antibiotics in the Netherlands (23%) than in Missouri (15%) [177].

In a large Canadian study of 27 243 LTC residents with advanced dementia (mean age 88 years), burdensome interventions were common in the last 30 days of life, especially amongst men. Of these, 21.8% residents were hospitalised and 0.8% received mechanical ventilation. Almost 30% were physically restrained, and more than one third (36%) of all residents in this study received an antibiotic. These findings reinforce the need for the expansion of palliative care and end-of-life antimicrobial stewardship in nursing homes [178]. As discussed in the section on hospital transfers, provision of palliative care in LTC should be more universally accepted. The use of restraint in particular seems extreme and it is very difficult to see why someone with advanced dementia should receive mechanical ventilation.

Covid-19 and Long-Term Care

It would be remiss to overlook COVID-19 in any discussion of the care for LTC residents. Variation has been noted in how different jurisdictions recorded COVID-19 mortality, but in most countries, LTC residents have comprised a large proportion of deaths due to the disease; over half of COVID-related deaths in Belgium (53%), France (51%), Ireland (60%), Norway (60%), and Canada (62%) were in LTC residents [179]. Several characteristics of LTC populations have been recognised as conferring risk of mortality, amongst them increased age, multiple comorbidities, and dementia diagnosis [180, 181].

An outbreak of COVID-19 in an LTC facility in Washington's King County highlighted the potential of the disease to spread rapidly. Within 3 weeks of identification of an index case, 167 residents, staff and visitors, linked to the same facility had tested positive for the virus [182]. Over a third of COVID-19-positive residents in this cohort died, and over half of infected staff and visitors required hospitalisation. The rapid spread of COVID-19 in some LTC facilities may have been compounded by limited recognition of its symptoms; residents may initially present with postural instability or diarrhoea, rather than with typical respiratory symptoms and fever [183]. Delirium, particularly in its hypoactive form, appears to have occurred in a high proportion of people with dementia [180] and is often severe and protracted [184]. Of the residents testing positive for COVID-19 in the King County cohort, approximately half were asymptomatic [185].

Once a case is suspected, staff should isolate that resident to their room and arrange for a swab test for SARS-CoV-2. They should be mindful of the distress that swab tests may cause to people with dementia and allow extra time to provide the necessary emotional support to such residents. Appropriate personal protective equipment should be worn at all times. The possibility of false negative tests should be borne in mind; where there is a strong suspicion of COVID-19 based on clinical findings, residents should stay in isolation for the full period of 14 days, irrespective of swab result. Step down from isolation should be considered on a case-by-case basis but erring on the side of caution is advisable [186].

When cases of COVID-19 are identified, LTC facilities may adopt zoning approaches, enabling residents with suspected or confirmed disease, to be managed in separate parts of the home from those without COVID-19. Plans for this should be developed and revised where necessary in advance of any outbreak. The routes by which people enter and exit the facility, and where they don, doff, and dispose of personal protective equipment, should also be standardised where possible to further decrease cross-contamination [186]. Heat maps have been identified as a helpful way of tracking and managing spread in LTC homes [187].

Some LTCs may request that residents remain in their room during outbreaks. Whilst this will undoubtedly reduce the risk of cross infection amongst residents, it presents challenges to safe staffing levels and, in many cases, residents' psychological wellbeing. These risks and benefits should again be appraised on a case-by-case basis. Residents with BPSD and those who walk with purpose may be particularly challenged by such measures. Nevertheless, pharmacological treatment remains a last resort in patients, and restraint is not justified. A behavioural approach should be used to understand and modify this behaviour, in collaboration with residents' families, and mental health services.

The commonly adopted practice of restricting visits from family and friends, in an effort to prevent movement of infection into LTC facilities, is advisable. In the case of some people with dementia, however, particularly those with severe disease, BPSD or those approaching the end of life, it may offer a more favourable risk-benefit ratio in reducing distress, and visits may be explored on a case-by-case basis. Where possible, visits should be held in areas with adequate space for social distancing, such as gardens, should be used. However, visiting will not always be possible, and LTC staff seeks to mitigate separation by facilitating use of video messaging through smartphones and tablets [186].

COVID-19 has illustrated many of the suggestions for routine care made elsewhere in this chapter. Guidelines for LTC published by the British Geriatric Society (BGS), note that "(COVID-19) *represents an important opportunity for care home staff to revisit, or visit for the first time, advance care planning, including plans about escalation to hospital, for all their residents*" [186]. The same document advocates the use of telemedicine should GPs or specialist staff be required to contribute to such discussions and underline the importance of communication with family and professionals involved in the patient's care. Where advanced care discussions regarding admission to hospital do occur, they should acknowledge that severity of frailty plays a significant role in assessment for, and prognosis in, critical care settings. It is suggested that individuals with a Clinical Frailty Scale [188] of five or more are therefore less likely to benefit from escalation to critical care [189].

COVID-19 may encourage a change in the way LTC facilities are run, and how prospective residents and their families choose the right facility for them. An analysis of COVID-19 infection mortality data in 215 nursing homes found that lower levels of registered nurse staffing were strongly associated with higher numbers of cases and deaths [190]. Previous studies have previously observed that higher nurse staffing levels increase hospitals' ability to respond to outbreaks of emerging infections [191]. For profit chains of nursing homes, those with larger resident populations, and those with lower quality of care ratings were more severely than affected by smaller, independently run facilities. The Connecticut study was also testament to the importance of transparency and availability of such data in determining, and responding to, outbreaks such as COVID-19; such data was published in only 36 of 50 US states at the time of writing.

LTC homes may consider adjusting work hours and shifts to decrease the risk of cross-contamination, cohorting staff so that they exclusively look after those with COVID-19 and those without. Promoting a positive organisation culture that supports staff well-being is crucial; one sixth of staff working in LTC facilities in New England had a second job where they worked over 20 h per week [192]. The majority of those surveyed described a culture of presenteeism within their workplace and a lack of provision of paid sick leave in some jurisdictions may compound this [193].

The pandemic may also encourage greater political focus on more longstanding inequalities affecting both LTC residents and wider society. The well-documented disparities in COVID-19-related outcomes for racial and ethnic minorities [194], and for groups with lower socioeconomic status [195] appear to extend to LTC residents. Li and colleagues' study of US facilities reported that LTC homes with higher concentrations of racial and ethnic minority residents, and those provided by Medicaid experienced more cases, and more deaths than other facilities [190].

COVID-19 has had a dramatic impact upon LTC residents with dementia, particularly with respect to mortality. Access to personal protective equipment, regular testing for staff and residents, and adoption of zoning measures are critical in both preventing and limiting the extent of outbreaks. Isolation from family and friends may prove particularly challenging to people with dementia and staff should explore mechanisms of mitigating this. As significant and unprecedented as the pandemic has been, COVID-19 has underlined the importance of several of the principles of quality LTC discussed throughout this chapter, such as advance care planning and close collaboration between the patient, their family and other professionals. It has also reinforced that the implementation of blanket measures, such as restricting visitors, may be helpful in some scenarios but that a case-by-case approach is likely necessary for many clinical decisions.

Case Study

Mrs A, an 84-year-old woman, was admitted to LTC from hospital in April. She had been diagnosed with AD 6 years previously and had just spent 32 days in hospital, where she had been admitted with a UTI and delirium. Previously, she had lived at home with her husband, aged 87, who had struggled to cope prior to her hospital admission, despite a care package comprising four care calls daily. She was quite dependent, requiring help from two people to walk, and needed help dressing and with personal hygiene. Her last Mini mental State Examination (MMSE) was 11/30 whilst in acute care, and MMSE 6 months previously was 13/30. During her acute admission, she had been aggressive at times and had experienced some visual hallucinations.

Her past medical history comprised ischaemic heart disease, atrial fibrillation, congestive cardiac failure, urinary frequency, osteoarthritis, osteoporosis, and chronic kidney failure. Her medications comprised bisoprolol 10 mg od, isosorbide mononitrate 50 mg od, nicorandil 10 mg bd, apixaban 2.5 mg bd, atorvastatin 40 mg od, donepezil 10 mg od, memantine 20 mg, fesoterodine 4 mg od, furosemide 40 mg od, perindopril 4 mg od, risperidone 0.5 mg bd, paracetamol 1 g 4–6 hourly PRN, risedronate 35 mg weekly, and calcium and vitamin D bd.

Mrs A was confused upon her admission to the LTC facility and was at times quite aggressive. She repeatedly stated that she wanted to go home. She had a urinary catheter in situ. She was admitted by nursing staff and her medications were continued unchanged. She was very dependent, needed help with all activities of daily living and needed two to transfer. She was unable to mobilise.

A comprehensive assessment was performed within 48 h. The only immediate information was that provided by the hospital and the details were as described above. Her husband was able to attend to speak to the staff, allowing collection of a full collateral history. The details about dementia and medical history were confirmed. There was no advanced directive in place. Her husband was asked specifically about whether she had ever expressed any specific wishes in relation to management of her condition and lifesaving interventions, but he knew of no such wishes. He stated that all of the family were in agreement that she should be kept comfortable and that they would prefer that hospital attendances or admission could be avoided. He stated that she had become very confused after admission to hospital and that this had settled a little in the week prior to discharge. She had no cardiovascular problems for a long time and had not been in pain. He felt that he was unable to manage her at home.

Examination revealed a thin older lady. She was not distressed and was not aggressive or agitated. She was disorientated and clearly confused. She was in atrial fibrillation with a heart rate of 52 bpm. Blood pressure was 118/78. Examination was otherwise unremarkable. There were no problems with her skin, and this was corroborated by the nursing staff. Urine was tested and was negative for infection. The electronic records were checked, and most recent bloods were satisfactory, apart from an eGFR of 45.

Mrs A's catheter was removed, and a care plan was drawn up. Her medications were changed; bisoprolol was reduced to 2.5 mg, furosemide was reduced to 20 mg, and isosorbide, nicorandil, and fesoterodine were discontinued. Risperidone was maintained at 0.5 mg bd. Discussion with her husband revealed that she had been taking treatment for osteoporosis for 8 years so risedronate was stopped. The new therapeutic regimen therefore bisoprolol 2.5 mg, apixaban 2.5 mg bd, donepezil 10 mg, memantine 20 mg, risperidone 0.5 mg bd, furosemide 20 mg, perindopril 4 mg, paracetamol as required and calcium and vitamin D.

Over the next 2 weeks Mrs A settled into the LTC facility. The degree of confusion was persistent but there was no suggestion of any delirium. There were some episodes of agitation which did not create any management problems. Appetite and sleep pattern were satisfactory. She was incontinent of urine. There were no concerns of a cardiovascular nature and no concerns about pain. Risperidone was reduced to 0.5 mg od.

There then followed a period of 7 months without major complications. Agitation continued but at a very low level, and risperidone was stopped 6 weeks after admission. Mrs A had one episode where she became distressed and seemed to have lower abdominal pain. Her urine tested positive for infection and she was treated with a course of antibiotics. The agitation returned to a degree but resolved quite quickly and medication was not deemed necessary. She did not have a great appetite and did lose some weight. Nursing staff had to encourage oral fluids on a regular basis. Her heart rate stabilised at 62 beats per minute. Systolic blood pressure was regularly recorded at 110 mmHg. Furosemide was stopped, as was perindopril, without any complications. Influenza vaccine was administered in September.

In December she then seemed to have some difficulty with swallowing. There was no evidence of any new neurological deficit. Speech and language therapy were consulted, and they assessed the situation. They suggested some positional changes during feeding and also recommended thickened fluids. There was one episode of likely chest infection which was treated with amoxicillin. At this time, Mrs A's her fluid intake was very poor, and after discussion with her family the agreement was to encourage oral fluids and avoid any artificial hydration. Her condition then settled. There was some deterioration in her overall condition, and she was more confined to bed, ate little and drank less fluid.

After a further 2 months she had another episode of LRTI, which was thought to be on the basis of aspiration. Discussion with the family took place and a management strategy was agreed upon. The nature of the aspiration pneumonia was discussed, and the possibility of regular episodes was explained. She was treated with a course of antibiotics and oral fluids were encouraged. There was general agreement that further episodes would be managed using a palliative approach. Donepezil, memantine, and calcium supplements were stopped, leaving her on bisoprolol, apixaban, and paracetamol as needed. Her condition settled somewhat, but she was much weaker and oral intake became very difficult. She was drowsy and slept for long periods. Over the next 3 weeks, her oral intake became negligible. All medication was discontinued. She was reviewed regularly to ensure she was comfortable and that there was no pain. She was turned regularly throughout her stay and at no stage was there any problem with pressure areas. She became less responsive and drifted into a coma from which she did not recover.

Commentary

This case illustrates the benefits of a comprehensive assessment soon after admission to LTC. It shows the importance of an initial discussion with family to understand the issues pertaining to the individual. At this time the likes and dislikes of the patient can be documented. It is also useful to document the nature of the physical health and how it has changed as the dementia has progressed. This enables the appropriate care plan to be established and facilitates rationalisation of medication. In this case, heart rate and blood pressure were low and there were no recent cardiovascular symptoms, allowing reduction/discontinuation of certain medication. It was likely that the lady had an unresolved delirium at time of discharge. Removal of her catheter was possible which contributed to maintenance of her dignity. It was also important to reduce and stop the risperidone. This is not always possible, but in this case the delirium resolved, so there was no need for long-term treatment. The relevant preventive medication was continued which was a reassurance to the family and the dementia medication was left unchanged. This lady remained stable for 7 months which does reflect a common situation. She had a proven urinary tract infection which was important to detect and helps sanction the proper use of antibiotics. She received the annual influenza vaccination according to the recommendations. She then developed problems with swallowing and resultant aspiration pneumonia which became recurrent. The liaison with family to explain the nature of the complications together with the formulation of an immediate and prospective management plan meant that a comprehensive approach was put in place with a clear plan for palliation at the right time. The initial discussion about preferences for management was important—there was no advance directive in place—and together with subsequent updated communication meant that there was no referral or attendance at Accident and Emergency and no hospital admission.

Summary

This chapter has discussed some clinical issues that characterise residency in LTC. We explored some of the clinical challenges brought by LTC in providing end-of-life care, and how facilities might change in the wake of the COVID-19 pandemic. Possible advantages brought by LTC were also discussed, in particular, the use of telemedicine and the opportunities to facilitate advance care planning.

One theme that has emerged throughout these topics has been the need for an early, assertive approach to determining the wishes and needs of the patient and their family with respect to ongoing treatment. It also necessitates frank and realistic discussion of the disadvantages associated with decisions such as hospital admission, and the limitations of approaches like antibiotic prescription. Once these wishes have been determined, these wishes are best enshrined in advance care planning documentation.

Almost all of the clinical issues discussed have been multifactorial and challenging to rectify, with quick and effective solutions few and far between. Understanding the problems from the perspective of the patient, particularly equipped with information from initial assessment, can transform our approach to management. In many cases we observed a paucity of research specific to management in LTC when compared with that of acute care, but frequently the core principles remained the same; non-pharmacological, low risk management that focused on the comfort of the patient.

Finally, the theme of communication and collaboration has run throughout this chapter. Communication between hospital and LTC, between staff and patient, staff and families, and between professionals of all backgrounds is the foundation of maintaining the safety of LTC residents. As previously discussed, transition to LTC is significant for all involved, and is not without inherent risk; accurate and timely communication is the most effective way to navigate this transition.

References

1. Shah SM, Carey IM, Harris T, DeWilde S, Cook DG. Mortality in older care home residents in England and Wales. Age Ageing. 2013;42:209–15.
2. Van Dijk PTM, Mehr DR, Ooms ME, Madsen R, Petroski G, Frijters DH, Margriet Pot A, Ribbe MW. Comorbidity and 1-Year Mortality Risks in Nursing Home Residents. J Am Geriatr Soc. 2005;53:660–5.
3. Gilmore-Bykovskyi AL, Roberts TJ, King BJ, Kennelty KA, Kind AJH. Transitions from hospitals to skilled nursing facilities for persons with dementia: a challenging convergence of patient and system-level needs. Gerontologist. 2017;57(5):867–79.
4. Naylor MD, Hirschman KB, Hanlon AL, Bowles KH, Bradway C, McCauley KM, Pauly MV. Comparison of evidence-based interventions on outcomes of hospitalized, cognitively impaired older adults. J Comp Eff Res. 2014;3:245–57.
5. Hirschman KB, Shaid E, McCauley K, Pauly MV, Naylor MD. Continuity of care: the transitional care model. Online J Issues Nurs. 2015;20(3):1.
6. Bell SP, Vasilevskis EE, Saraf AA, Jacobsen JML, Kripalani S, Mixon AS, Schnelle JF, Simmons SF. Geriatric syndromes in hospitalized older adults discharged to skilled nursing facilities. J Am Geriatr Soc. 2016;64:715–22.
7. Hutchinson AM, Milke DL, Maisey S, et al. The resident assessment instrument-minimum data set 2.0 quality indicators: a systematic review. BMC Health Serv Res. 2010;10:166.
8. Pain T, Stainkey L, Chapman S. AgedCare+GP: description and evaluation of an in-house model of general practice in a residential aged-care facility. Aust J Prim Health. 2014;20(3):224–7.

9. Gordon AL, Franklin M, Bradshaw L, Logan P, Elliott R, Gladman JR. Health status of UK care home residents: a cohort study. Age Ageing. 2014;43(1):97–103.
10. Moore KL, Boscardin WJ, Steinman MA, Schwartz JB. Patterns of chronic co-morbid medical conditions in older residents of U.S. nursing homes: differences between the sexes and across the agespan. J Nutr Health Aging. 2014;18(4):429–36.
11. Dosa D, Intrator O, McNicoll L, Cang Y, Teno J. Preliminary derivation of a Nursing Home Confusion Assessment Method based on data from the Minimum Data Set. J Am Geriatr Soc. 2007;55(7):1099–105.
12. Inouye SK, Foreman MD, Mion LC, Katz KH, Cooney LM Jr. Nurses' recognition of delirium and its symptoms: comparison of nurse and researcher ratings. Arch Intern Med. 2001;161(20):2467–73.
13. Tune LE. How acute is delirium in nursing homes: an observational study from Wesley Woods at Emory. Am J Geriatr Psychiatry. 2008;16(9):786.
14. Voyer P, McCusker J, Cole MG, et al. Prodrome of delirium among long-term care residents: what clinical changes can be observed in the two weeks preceding a full-blown episode of delirium? Int Psychogeriatr. 2012;24(11):1855–64.
15. Shega JW, Ellner L, Lau DT, Maxwell TL. Cholinesterase inhibitor and N-methyl-D-aspartic acid receptor antagonist use in older adults with end-stage dementia: a survey of hospice medical directors. J Palliat Med. 2009;12(9):779–83.
16. Voyer P, Richard S, Doucet L, Carmichael PH. Detecting delirium and subsyndromal delirium using different diagnostic criteria among demented long-term care residents. J Am Med Dir Assoc. 2009;10(3):181–8.
17. de Lange E, Verhaak PF, van der Meer K. Prevalence, presentation and prognosis of delirium in older people in the population, at home and in long term care: a review. Int J Geriatr Psychiatry. 2013;28(2):127–34.
18. Laurila JV, Pitkala KH, Strandberg TE, Tilvis RS. The impact of different diagnostic criteria on prevalence rates for delirium. Dement Geriatr Cogn Disord. 2003;16(3):156–62.
19. Inouye SK, van Dyck CH, Alessi CA, Balkin S, Siegal AP, Horwitz RI. Clarifying confusion: the confusion assessment method. A new method for detection of delirium. Ann Intern Med. 1990;113(12):941–8.
20. Wei LA, Fearing MA, Sternberg EJ, Inouye SK. The confusion assessment method: a systematic review of current usage. J Am Geriatr Soc. 2008;56(5):823–30.
21. Bellelli G, Morandi A, Davis DH, et al. Validation of the 4AT, a new instrument for rapid delirium screening: a study in 234 hospitalised older people. Age Ageing. 2014;43(4):496–502.
22. Shenkin SD, Fox C, Godfrey M, et al. Delirium detection in older acute medical inpatients: a multicentre prospective comparative diagnostic test accuracy study of the 4AT and the confusion assessment method. BMC Med. 2019;17(1):138.
23. MacLullich AM, Shenkin SD, Goodacre S, et al. The 4 'A's test for detecting delirium in acute medical patients: a diagnostic accuracy study. Health Technol Assess. 2019;23(40):1–194.
24. Woodhouse R, Burton JK, Rana N, Pang YL, Lister JE, Siddiqi N. Interventions for preventing delirium in older people in institutional long-term care. Cochrane Database Syst Rev. 2019;4(4):CD009537.
25. Lapane KL, Hughes CM, Daiello LA, Cameron KA, Feinberg J. Effect of a pharmacist-led multicomponent intervention focusing on the medication monitoring phase to prevent potential adverse drug events in nursing homes. J Am Geriatr Soc. 2011;59(7):1238–45.
26. Culp K, Mentes J, Wakefield B. Hydration and acute confusion in long-term care residents. West J Nurs Res. 2003;25(3):251–73.
27. Siddiqi N, Cheater F, Collinson M, et al. The PiTSTOP study: a feasibility cluster randomized trial of delirium prevention in care homes for older people. Age Ageing. 2016;45(5):652–61.
28. American Geriatrics Society Expert Panel on Postoperative Delirium in Older Adults. Postoperative delirium in older adults: best practice statement from the American Geriatrics Society. J Am Coll Surg. 2015;220(2):136–48.e1.

29. National Institute for Health and Care Excellence. Delirium: prevention, diagnosis and management. [London]: NICE; 2010 [updated 2019 Mar; cited 2020 July 02]. Clinical guideline [CG103].
30. Offermans MP, Du Moulin MF, Hamers JP, Dassen T, Halfens RJ. Prevalence of urinary incontinence and associated risk factors in nursing home residents: a systematic review. Neurourol Urodyn. 2009;28(4):288–94.
31. Allan LM. Diagnosis of autonomic dysfunction in dementia syndromes. Curr Treat Options Neurol. 2019;21(8):38.
32. Campbell AJ, Reinken J, McCosh L. Incontinence in the elderly: prevalence and prognosis. Age Ageing. 1985;14(2):65–70.
33. Byles J, Millar CJ, Sibbritt DW, Chiarelli P. Living with urinary incontinence: a longitudinal study of older women. Age Ageing. 2009;38(3):333–251.
34. Miu DK, Lau S, Szeto SS. Etiology and predictors of urinary incontinence and its effect on quality of life. Geriatr Gerontol Int. 2010;10(2):177–82.
35. Maggi S, Minicuci N, Langlois J, Pavan M, Enzi G, Crepaldi G. Prevalence rate of urinary incontinence in community-dwelling elderly individuals: the Veneto study. J Gerontol A Biol Sci Med Sci. 2001;56(1):M14–8.
36. Milsom I, Kaplan SA, Coyne KS, Sexton CC, Kopp ZS. Effect of bothersome overactive bladder symptoms on health-related quality of life, anxiety, depression, and treatment seeking in the United States: results from EpiLUTS. Urology. 2012;80(1):90–6.
37. Rose A, Thimme A, Halfar C, Nehen HG, Rübben H. Severity of urinary incontinence of nursing home residents correlates with malnutrition, dementia and loss of mobility. Urol Int. 2013;91(2):165–9.
38. Drennan VM, Cole L, Iliffe S. A taboo within a stigma? A qualitative study of managing incontinence with people with dementia living at home. BMC Geriatr. 2011;11:75.
39. Luppa M, Luck T, Weyerer S, König HH, Brähler E, Riedel-Heller SG. Prediction of institutionalization in the elderly. A systematic review. Age Ageing. 2010;39(1):31–8.
40. Tilvis RS, Hakala SM, Valvanne J, Erkinjuntti T. Urinary incontinence as a predictor of death and institutionalization in a general aged population. Arch Gerontol Geriatr. 1995;21(3):307–15.
41. O'Donnell BF, Drachman DA, Barnes HJ, Peterson KE, Swearer JM, Lew RA. Incontinence and troublesome behaviors predict institutionalization in dementia. J Geriatr Psychiatry Neurol. 1992;5(1):45–52.
42. Eaker ED, Vierkant RA, Mickel SF. Predictors of nursing home admission and/or death in incident Alzheimer's disease and other dementia cases compared to controls: a population-based study. J Clin Epidemiol. 2002;55(5):462–8.
43. Schluter PJ, Ward C, Arnold EP, Scrase R, Jamieson HA. Urinary incontinence, but not fecal incontinence, is a risk factor for admission to aged residential care of older persons in New Zealand. Neurourol Urodyn. 2017;36(6):1588–95.
44. Farage MA, Miller KW, Berardesca E, Maibach HI. Incontinence in the aged: contact dermatitis and other cutaneous consequences. Contact Dermatitis. 2007;57(4):211–7.
45. Bravo CV. Urinary and faecal incontinence and dementia. Rev Clin Gerontol. 2004;14:129–36.
46. Fonda D, Benvenuti F, Cottenden A, DuBeau CE, Kirshner-Hermann R, Miller K, et al. Urinary incontinence and bladder dysfunction in older persons. Incontinence 2nd consultation on incontinence. United Kingdom: Health Publication; 2002. p. 629–700.
47. Casey G. Incontinence and retention—how the bladder misfunctions. Nurs N Z. 2011;17(7):26–3.
48. Gormley EA, Griffiths DJ, McCracken PN, Harrison GM. Polypharmacy and its effect on urinary incontinence in a geriatric population. Br J Urol. 1993;71(3):265–9.
49. Hashimoto M, Imamura T, Tanimukai S, Kazui H, Mori E. Urinary incontinence: an unrecognised adverse effect with donepezil. Lancet. 2000;356(9229):568.
50. Starr JM. Cholinesterase inhibitor treatment and urinary incontinence in Alzheimer's disease. J Am Geriatr Soc. 2007;55(5):800–1.

51. Gill SS, Mamdani M, Naglie G, et al. A prescribing cascade involving cholinesterase inhibitors and anticholinergic drugs. Arch Intern Med. 2005;165(7):808–13.
52. Kay G, Crook T, Rekeda L, et al. Differential effects of the antimuscarinic agents darifenacin and oxybutynin ER on memory in older subjects. Eur Urol. 2006;50(2):317–26.
53. Sink KM, Thomas J 3rd, Xu H, Craig B, Kritchevsky S, Sands LP. Dual use of bladder anticholinergics and cholinesterase inhibitors: long-term functional and cognitive outcomes. J Am Geriatr Soc. 2008;56(5):847–53.
54. Ouslander JG, Zarit SH, Orr NK, Muira SA. Incontinence among elderly community-dwelling dementia patients. Characteristics, management, and impact on caregivers. J Am Geriatr Soc. 1990;38(4):440–5.
55. Jirovec MM, Wells TJ. Urinary incontinence in nursing home residents with dementia: the mobility-cognition paradigm. Appl Nurs Res. 1990;3(3):112–7.
56. Jerez-Roig J, Santos MM, Souza DL, Amaral FL, Lima KC. Prevalence of urinary incontinence and associated factors in nursing home residents. Neurourol Urodyn. 2016;35(1):102–7.
57. Resnick NM, Yalla SV. Detrusor hyperactivity with impaired contractile function. An unrecognized but common cause of incontinence in elderly patients. JAMA. 1987;257(22):3076–81.
58. Sakakibara R, Panicker J, Fowler CJ, et al. Is overactive bladder a brain disease? The pathophysiological role of cerebral white matter in the elderly. Int J Urol. 2014;21(1):33–8.
59. Lee SH, Cho ST, Na HR, Ko SB, Park MH. Urinary incontinence in patients with Alzheimer's disease: relationship between symptom status and urodynamic diagnoses. Int J Urol. 2014;21(7):683–7.
60. Skelly J, Flint AJ. Urinary incontinence associated with dementia. J Am Geriatr Soc. 1995;43(3):286–94.
61. Yu LC, Rohner TJ, Kaltreider DL, Hu TW, Igou JF, Dennis PJ. Profile of urinary incontinent elderly in long-term care institutions. J Am Geriatr Soc. 1990;38(4):433–9.
62. Hägglund D. A systematic literature review of incontinence care for persons with dementia: the research evidence. J Clin Nurs. 2010;19(3–4):303–12.
63. National Institute for Health and Care Excellence. Urinary incontinence in neurological disease: assessment and management. [London]: NICE; 2012 [cited 2020 July 02]. Clinical guideline [CG148].
64. DuBeau CE, Kuchel GA, Johnson T 2nd, Palmer MH, Wagg A, Fourth International Consultation on Incontinence. Incontinence in the frail elderly: report from the 4th International Consultation on Incontinence. Neurourol Urodyn. 2010;29(1):165–78.
65. Brink CA. Absorbent pads, garments, and management strategies. J Am Geriatr Soc. 1990;38(3):368–73.
66. Engberg S, Sereika SM, McDowell BJ, Weber E, Brodak I. Effectiveness of prompted voiding in treating urinary incontinence in cognitively impaired homebound older adults. J Wound Ostomy Continence Nurs. 2002;29(5):252–65.
67. Yap P, Tan D. Urinary incontinence in dementia—a practical approach. Aust Fam Physician. 2006;35(4):237–41.
68. Orme S, Morris V, Gibson W, Wagg A. Managing urinary incontinence in patients with dementia: pharmacological treatment options and considerations. Drugs Aging. 2015;32(7):559–67.
69. Omli R, Skotnes LH, Romild U, Bakke A, Mykletun A, Kuhry E. Pad per day usage, urinary incontinence and urinary tract infections in nursing home residents. Age Ageing. 2010;39(5):549–54.
70. Cottenden A, Bliss DZ, Buckley B, Fader M, Getliffe K, Paterson J, et al. Management using continence products. In: Abrams P, Cardozo L, Khoury S, Wein A, editors. Incontinence. 4th ed. Paris: Health Publication; 2009. p. 1519–642.
71. Grant RL, Drennan VM, Rait G, Petersen I, Iliffe S. First diagnosis and management of incontinence in older people with and without dementia in primary care: a cohort study using The Health Improvement Network primary care database. PLoS Med. 2013;10(8):e1001505.
72. Testa G, Ceccofiglio A, Mussi C, et al. Hypotensive drugs and syncope due to orthostatic hypotension in older adults with dementia (syncope and dementia study). J Am Geriatr Soc. 2018;66(8):1532–7.

73. Bell JS, Mezrani C, Blacker N, et al. Anticholinergic and sedative medicines—prescribing considerations for people with dementia. Aust Fam Physician. 2012;41(1-2):45–9.
74. Samuelsson E, Odeberg J, Stenzelius K, et al. Effect of pharmacological treatment for urinary incontinence in the elderly and frail elderly: a systematic review. Geriatr Gerontol Int. 2015;15(5):521–34.
75. Edwards KR, O'Connor JT. Risk of delirium with concomitant use of tolterodine and acetylcholinesterase inhibitors. J Am Geriatr Soc. 2002;50(6):1165–6.
76. Triantafylidis LK, Clemons JS, Peron EP, Roefaro J, Zimmerman KM. Brain over bladder: a systematic review of dual cholinesterase inhibitor and urinary anticholinergic use. Drugs Aging. 2018;35(1):27–41.
77. Morris JC, Rubin EH, Morris EJ, Mandel SA. Senile dementia of the Alzheimer's type: an important risk factor for serious falls. J Gerontol. 1987;42(4):412–7.
78. Minaglia C, Giannotti C, Boccardi V, et al. Cachexia and advanced dementia. J Cachexia Sarcopenia Muscle. 2019;10(2):263–77.
79. Op den Kamp CM, Langen RC, Haegens A, Schols AM. Muscle atrophy in cachexia: can dietary protein tip the balance? Curr Opin Clin Nutr Metab care. 2009;12(6):611–6.
80. National Institute for Health and Care Excellence. Dementia: assessment, management and support for people living with dementia and their carers. [London]: NICE; 2018 [updated 2018 Jun; cited 2020 July 02]. (NICE guideline [NG97]).
81. Kumagai R, Kubokura M, Sano A, Shinomiya M, Ohta S, Ishibiki Y, et al. Clinical evaluation of percutaneous endoscopic gastrostomy tube feeding in Japanese patients with dementia. Psychiatry Clin Neurosci. 2012;66(5):418–22.
82. Stewart JT, Schultz SK. Palliative care for dementia. Psychiatr Clin North Am. 2018;41(1):141–51.
83. Henderson CT, Trumbore LS, Mobarhan S, Benya R, Miles TP. Prolonged tube feeding in long-term care: nutritional status and clinical outcomes. J Am Coll Nutr. 1992;11(3):309–25.
84. Candy B, Sampson EL, Jones L. Enteral tube feeding in older people with advanced dementia: findings from a Cochrane systematic review. Int J Palliat Nurs. 2009;15(8):396–404.
85. Mitchell SL, Kiely DK, Jones RN, Prigerson H, Volicer L, Teno JM. Advanced dementia research in the nursing home: the cascade study. Alzheimer Dis Assoc Discord. 2006;20(3):166–75.
86. Mitchell SL, Teno JM, Kiely DK, Shaffer ML, Jones RN, Prigerson HG, et al. The clinical course of advanced dementia. New Engl J Med. 2009;361(16):1529–38.
87. van der Steen JT, Radbruch L, Hertogh CMPM, de Boer ME, Hughes JC, Larkin P, et al. White paper defining optimal palliative care in older people with dementia: a Delphi study and recommendations from the European Association for Palliative Care. Palliat Med. 2014;28(3):197–209.
88. van der Steen JT, Di Giulio P, Giunco F, Monti M, Gentile S, Villani D, et al. Pneumonia in nursing home patients with advanced dementia: decisions, intravenous rehydration therapy, and discomfort. Am J Hosp Palliat Care. 2018;35(3):423–30.
89. van der Steen JT, Lane P, Kowall NW, Knol DL, Volicer L. Antibiotics and mortality in patients with lower respiratory infection and advanced dementia. J Am Med Dir Assoc. 2012;13(2):156–61.
90. Helton MR, van der Steen JT, Daaleman TP, Gamble GR, Ribbe MW. A cross-cultural study of physician treatment decisions for demented nursing home patients who develop pneumonia. Ann Fam Med. 2006;4(3):221–7.
91. Bhattacharya S, Mishra RK. Pressure ulcers: current understanding and newer modalities of treatment. Indian J Plast Surg. 2015;48(1):4–16.
92. Joyce NR, McGuire TG, Bartels SJ, Mitchell SL, Grabowski DC. The impact of dementia special care units on quality of care: an instrumental variables analysis. Health Serv Res. 2018;53(5):3657–79.

93. Beerens HC, Sutcliffe C, Renom-Guiteras A, Soto ME, Suhonen R, Zabalegui A, et al. Quality of life and quality of care for people with dementia receiving long term institutional care or professional home care: the European RightTimePlaceCare study. J Am Med Dir Assoc. 2014;15(1):54–61.
94. Li Y, Yin J, Cai X, Temkin-Greener J, Mukamel DB. Association of race and sites of care with pressure ulcers in high-risk nursing home residents. JAMA. 2011;306(2):179–86.
95. Bergstrom N, Horn SD. Racial disparities in rates of pressure ulcers in nursing homes and site of care. JAMA. 2011;306(2):211–2.
96. Bergstrom N, Horn SD, Rapp M, Stern A, Barrett R, Watkiss M, et al. Preventing pressure ulcers: a multisite randomized controlled trial in nursing homes. Ont Health Technol Assess Ser. 2014;14(11):1–32.
97. Waterlow J. Practical use of the Waterlow tool in the community. Br J Community Health Nurs. 1997;2(2):83–6.
98. Bergstrom N, Braden B. A prospective study of pressure sore risk among institutionalized elderly. J Am Geriatr Soc. 1992;40(8):747–58.
99. National Institute for Health and Care Excellence. Pressure ulcers: prevention and management. [London]: NICE; 2014 [cited 2020 Jul 26]. (Clinical guideline [CG179]). Available from: https://www.nice.org.uk/guidance/cg179
100. Langer G, Fink A. Nutritional interventions for preventing and treating pressure ulcers. Cochrane Database Syst Rev. 2014;6:CD003216.
101. Murphy SL, Xu J, Kochanek KD, Arias E. Mortality in the United States, 2017. NCHS Data Brief. 2018;328:1–8.
102. van Essen GA, Palache AM, Forleo E, Fedson DS. Influenza vaccination in 2000: recommendations and vaccine use in 50 developed and rapidly developing countries. Vaccine. 2003;21(16):1780–5.
103. Tomczyk S, Bennett NM, Stoecker C, Gierke R, Moore MR, Whitney CG, et al. Use of 13-valent pneumococcal conjugate vaccine and 23-valent pneumococcal polysaccharide vaccine among adults aged ≥65 years: recommendations of the Advisory Committee on Immunization Practices (ACIP). MMWR Morb Mortal Wkly Rep. 2014;63(37):822–5.
104. Nace DA, Archbald-Pannone LR, Ashraf MS, Drinka PJ, Frentzel E, Gaur S, et al. Pneumococcal vaccination guidance for post-acute and long-term care settings: recommendations from AMDA's Infection Advisory Committee. J Am Med Dir Assoc. 2017;18(2):99–104.
105. Poscia A, Collamati A, Carfì A, Topinkova E, Richter T, Denkinger M, et al. Influenza and pneumococcal vaccination in older adults living in nursing home: a survival analysis on the shelter study. Eur J Pub Health. 2017;27(6):1016–20.
106. Travers JL, Dick AW, Stone PW. Racial/ethnic differences in receipt of influenza and pneumococcal vaccination among long-stay nursing home residents. Health Serv Res. 2018;53(4):2203–26.
107. Mitchell SL, Shaffer ML, Loeb MB, Givens JL, Habtemariam D, Kiely DK, et al. Infection management and multidrug-resistant organisms in nursing home residents with advanced dementia. JAMA Intern Med. 2014;174(10):1660–7.
108. Vergidis P, Hamer DH, Meydani SN, Dallal GE, Barlam TF. Patterns of antimicrobial use for respiratory tract infections in older residents of long-term care facilities. J Am Geriatr Soc. 2011;59(6):1093–8.
109. Pop-Vicas A, Mitchell SL, Kandel R, Schreiber R, D'Agata EMC. Multidrug-resistant gram-negative bacteria in a long-term care facility: prevalence and risk factors. J Am Geriatr Soc. 2008;56(7):1276–80.
110. D'Agata EMC, Varu A, Geffert SF, Araos R, Mitchell S, Situ A, et al. Acquisition of multidrug-resistant organisms in the absence of antimicrobials. Clin Infect Dis. 2018;67(9):1437–40.
111. Nicolle LE. Asymptomatic bacteriuria and bacterial interference. Microbiol Spectr. 2015;3(5) https://doi.org/10.1128/microbiolspec.

112. Biggel M, Heytens S, Latour K, Bruyndonckx R, Goossens H, Moons P. Asymptomatic bacteriuria in older adults: the most fragile women are prone to long-term colonization. BMC Geriatr. 2019;19(1):170.
113. Hatcher-Martin JM, Adams JL, Anderson ER, Bove R, Burrus TM, Chehrenama M, et al. Telemedicine in neurology: telemedicine work group of the American Academy of Neurology update. Neurology. 2020;94(1):30–8.
114. Greenhalgh T, Wherton J, Shaw S, Morrison C. Video consultations for covid-19. BMJ. 2020;368:m998.
115. Smith AC, Thomas E, Snoswell CL, Haydon H, Mehrotra A, Clemensen J, et al. Telehealth for global emergencies: implications for coronavirus disease 2019 (COVID-19). J Telemed Telecare. 2020;26(5):309–13.
116. Hollander JE, Carr BG. Virtually perfect? Telemedicine for covid-19. New Engl J Med. 2020;382(18):1679–81.
117. Powers BB, Homer MC, Morone N, Edmonds N, Rossi MI. Creation of an interprofessional teledementia clinic for rural veterans: preliminary data. J Am Geriatr Soc. 2017;65(5):1092–9.
118. Morgan DG, Crossley M, Kirk A, McBain L, Stewart NJ, D'Arcy C, et al. Evaluation of telehealth for preclinic assessment and follow-up in an interprofessional rural and remote memory clinic. J Appl Gerontol. 2011;30(3):304–31.
119. Azad N, Amos S, Milne K, Power B. Telemedicine in a rural memory disorder clinic-remote management of patients with dementia. Can Geriatr J. 2012;15(4):96–100.
120. Driessen J, Chang W, Patel P, Wright RM, Ernst K, Handler SM. Nursing home provider perceptions of telemedicine for providing specialty consults. Telemed J E Health. 2018;24(7):510–6.
121. Pachana NA, Beattie E, Byrne GJ, Brodaty H. COVID-19 and psychogeriatrics: the view from Australia. Int Psychogeriatr. 2020;12:1–7.
122. Almathami HKY, Win KT, Vlahu-Gjorgievska E. Barriers and facilitators that influence telemedicine-based, real-time, online consultation at patients' homes: systematic literature review. J Med Internet Res. 2020;22(2):e16407.
123. Lindauer A, Seelye A, Lyons B, Dodge HH, Mattek N, Mincks K, et al. Dementia care comes home: patient and caregiver assessment via telemedicine. Gerontologist. 2017;57(5):e85–93.
124. Tso JV, Farinpour R, Chui HC, Liu CY. A multidisciplinary model of dementia care in an underserved retirement community, made possible by telemedicine. Front Neurol. 2016;7:225.
125. Barton C, Morris R, Rothlind J, Yaffe K. Video-telemedicine in a memory disorders clinic: evaluation and management of rural elders with cognitive impairment. Telemed J E Health. 2010;17:789–93.
126. McGee M, Potter C, Kane JPM. Are UK care homes ready for the telemedicine revolution? BJPsych Bull. 2020;44(5):222.
127. Morgan DG, Crossley M, Kirk A, McBain L, Stewart NJ, D'Arcy C, et al. Evaluation of telehealth for preclinic assessment and follow-up in an interprofessional rural and remote memory clinic. J Appl Gerontol. 2010;30(3):304–31.
128. Costanzo MC, Arcidiacono C, Rodolico A, Panebianco M, Aguglia E, Signorelli MS. Diagnostic and interventional implications of telemedicine in Alzheimer's disease and mild cognitive impairment: a literature review. Int J Geriatr Psychiatry. 2020;35(1):12–28.
129. Allain P, Foloppe DA, Besnard J, Yamaguchi T, Etcharry-Bouyx F, Le Gall D, et al. Detecting everyday action deficits in Alzheimer's disease using a nonimmersive virtual reality kitchen. J Int Neuropsychol Soc. 2014;20(5):468–77.
130. Roccaforte WH, Burke WJ, Bayer BL, Wengel SP. Validation of a telephone version of the mini-mental state examination. J Am Geriatr Soc. 1992;40(7):697–702.
131. Berg JL, Durant J, Léger GC, Cummings JL, Nasreddine Z, Miller JB. Comparing the electronic and standard versions of the Montreal cognitive assessment in an outpatient memory disorders clinic: a validation study. J Alzheimers Dis. 2018;62(1):93–7.

132. Castanho TC, Amorim L, Zihl J, Palha JA, Sousa N, Santos NC. Telephone-based screening tools for mild cognitive impairment and dementia in aging studies: a review of validated instruments. Front Aging Neurosci. 2014;6:16.
133. Hubble JP, Pahwa R, Michalek DK, Thomas C, Koller WC. Interactive video conferencing: a means of providing interim care to Parkinson's disease patients. Mov Disord. 1993;8(3):380–2.
134. Amarendran V, George A, Gersappe V, Krishnaswamy S, Warren C. The reliability of telepsychiatry for a neuropsychiatric assessment. Telemed J E Health. 2011;17(3):223–5.
135. Russell TG, Jull GA, Wootton R. The diagnostic reliability of Internet-based observational kinematic gait analysis. J Telemed Telecare. 2003;9(Suppl 2):S48–51.
136. Burton RL, O'Connell ME. Telehealth rehabilitation for cognitive impairment: randomized controlled feasibility trial. JMIR Res Protoc. 2018;7(2):e43.
137. Wisniewski SR, Belle SH, Coon DW, Marcus SM, Ory MG, Burgio LD, et al. The resources for enhancing Alzheimer's Caregiver Health (REACH): project design and baseline characteristics. Psychol Aging. 2003;18(3):375–84.
138. Williams K, Arthur A, Niedens M, Moushey L, Hutfles L. In-home monitoring support for dementia caregivers: a feasibility study. Clin Nurs Res. 2013;22(2):139–50.
139. Piau A, Nourhashemi F, De Mauléon A, Tchalla A, Vautier C, Vellas B, et al. Telemedicine for the management of neuropsychiatric symptoms in long-term care facilities: the DETECT study, methods of a cluster randomised controlled trial to assess feasibility. BMJ Open. 2018;8(6):e020982.
140. Bateman DR, Srinivas B, Emmett TW, Schleyer TK, Holden RJ, Hendrie HC, et al. Categorizing health outcomes and efficacy of mHealth apps for persons with cognitive impairment: a systematic review. J Med Internet Res. 2017;19(8):e301.
141. Schön P, Lagergren M, Kåreholt I. Rapid decrease in length of stay in institutional care for older people in Sweden between 2006 and 2012: results from a population-based study. Health Soc Care Community. 2016;24(5):631–8.
142. Ferrah N, Ibrahim JE, Kipsaina C, Bugeja L. Death following recent admission into nursing home from community living: a systematic review into the transition process. J Aging Health. 2018;30(4):584–604.
143. Boling PA. Care transitions and home health care. Clin Geriatr Med. 2009;25(1):135–48, viii.
144. Naylor M, Keating SA. Transitional care. Am J Nurs. 2008;108(9 Suppl):58–63.
145. LaMantia MA, Scheunemann LP, Viera AJ, Busby-Whitehead J, Hanson LC. Interventions to improve transitional care between nursing homes and hospitals: a systematic review. J Am Geriatr Soc. 2010;58(4):777–82.
146. Goldfarb AI. Predicting mortality in the institutionalized aged. A seven-year follow-up. Arch Gen Psychiatry. 1969;21(2):172–6.
147. Engle VF, Graney MJ. Predicting outcomes of nursing home residents: death and discharge home. J Gerontol. 1993;48(5):S269–75.
148. Shapiro E, Tate R. Who is really at risk of institutionalization? Gerontologist. 1988;28(2):237–45.
149. Brauer E, Mackeprang B, Bentzon MW. Prognosis of survival in a geriatric population. Scand J Soc Med. 1978;6(1):17–24.
150. Kelman HR, Thomas C. Transitions between community and nursing home residence in an urban elderly population. J Community Health. 1990;15(2):105–22.
151. Wolinsky FD, Johnson RJ. Perceived health status and mortality among older men and women. J Gerontol. 1992;47(6):S304–12.
152. Diesfeldt HF, van Houte LR, Moerkens RM. Duration of survival in senile dementia. Acta Psychiatr Scand. 1986;73(4):366–71.
153. NHS End of Life Care. Advance care planning: a guide for health and social care staff. [Nottingham]: NHS End of Life Care; 2007 [cited 2020 Jul 26]. Available from: http://www.

stlukes-hospice.org.uk/wp-content/uploads/2017/06/ACP-Guide-for-Health-and-Social-Care-Staff-.pdf
154. Rietjens JAC, Sudore RL, Connolly M, van Delden JJ, Drickamer MA, Droger M, et al. Definition and recommendations for advance care planning: an international consensus supported by the European Association for Palliative Care. Lancet Oncol. 2017;18(9):e543–51.
155. Teno JM. Advance directives for nursing home residents: achieving compassionate, competent, cost-effective care. JAMA. 2000;283(11):1481–2.
156. Higginson IJ, Gomes B, Calanzani N, Gao W, Bausewein C, Daveson BA, et al. Priorities for treatment, care and information if faced with serious illness: a comparative population-based survey in seven European countries. Palliat Med. 2014;28(2):101–10.
157. Dixon J, King D, Knapp M. Advance care planning in England: is there an association with place of death? Secondary analysis of data from the National Survey of Bereaved People. BMJ Support Palliat Care. 2019;9(3):316–25.
158. Sampson EL, Gould V, Lee D, Blanchard MR. Differences in care received by patients with and without dementia who died during acute hospital admission: a retrospective case note study. Age Ageing. 2006;35(2):187–9.
159. Dening KH, Jones L, Sampson EL. Advance care planning for people with dementia: a review. Int Psychogeriatr. 2011;23(10):1535–51.
160. Hanrahan P, Luchins DJ. Access to hospice programs in end-stage dementia: a national survey of hospice programs. J Am Geriatr Soc. 1995;43(1):56–9.
161. Sommer S, Marckmann G, Pentzek M, Wegscheider K, Abholz HH, in der Schmitten J. Advance directives in nursing homes: prevalence, validity, significance, and nursing staff adherence. Dtsch Arztebl Int. 2012;109(37):577–83.
162. Vandervoort A, Houttekier D, Van den Block L, van der Steen JT, Vander Stichele R, Deliens L. Advance care planning and physician orders in nursing home residents with dementia: a nationwide retrospective study among professional caregivers and relatives. J Pain Symptom Manag. 2014;47(2):245–56.
163. Knight T, Malyon A, Fritz Z, Subbe C, Cooksley T, Holland M, et al. Advance care planning in patients referred to hospital for acute medical care: results of a national day of care survey. EClinicalMedicine. 2020;19:100235.
164. Harrison KL, Adrion ER, Ritchie CS, Sudore RL, Smith AK. Low completion and disparities in advance care planning activities among older Medicare beneficiaries. JAMA Intern Med. 2016;176(12):1872–5.
165. Kirchhoff KT, Hammes BJ, Kehl KA, Briggs LA, Brown RL. Effect of a disease-specific planning intervention on surrogate understanding of patient goals for future medical treatment. J Am Geriatr Soc. 2010;58(7):1233–40.
166. Banerjee S, Willis R, Matthews D, Contell F, Chan J, Murray J. Improving the quality of care for mild to moderate dementia: an evaluation of the Croydon Memory Service Model. Int J Geriatr Psychiatry. 2007;22(8):782–8.
167. Jimenez G, Tan WS, Virk AK, Low CK, Car J, Ho AHY. Overview of systematic reviews of advance care planning: summary of evidence and global lessons. J Pain Symptom Manag. 2018;56(3):436–459.e25.
168. Stobbart-Rowlands M, Thorn M. Experience of the use of advance care planning in care homes. In: Thomas K, Lobo B, Detering K, editors. Advance care planning in end of life care. New York: Oxford Universtity Press; 2018.
169. Davies S, Nolan M. "Making the move": relatives' experiences of the transition to a care home. Health Soc Care Community. 2004;12(6):517–26.
170. Ryan AA, Scullion HF. Nursing home placement: an exploration of the experiences of family carers. J Adv Nurs. 2000;32(5):1187–95.
171. Caplan GA, Meller A, Squires B, Chan S, Willett W. Advance care planning and hospital in the nursing home. Age Ageing. 2006;35(6):581–5.

172. Lamberg JL, Person CJ, Kiely DK, Mitchell SL. Decisions to hospitalize nursing home residents dying with advanced dementia. J Am Geriatr Soc. 2005;53(8):1396–401.
173. LaMantia MA, Stump TE, Messina FC, Miller DK, Callahan CM. Emergency department use among older adults with dementia. Alzheimer Dis Assoc Disord. 2016;30(1):35–40.
174. Palan Lopez R, Mitchell SL, Givens JL. Preventing burdensome transitions of nursing home residents with advanced dementia: it's more than advance directives. J Palliat Med. 2017;20(11):1205–9.
175. Unroe KT, Carnahan JL, Hickman SE, Sachs GA, Hass Z, Arling G. The complexity of determining whether a nursing home transfer is avoidable at time of transfer. J Am Geriatr Soc. 2018;66(5):895–901.
176. Toscani F, van der Steen JT, Finetti S, Giunco F, Pettenati F, Villani D, et al. Critical decisions for older people with advanced dementia: a prospective study in long-term institutions and district home care. J Am Med Dir Assoc. 2015;16(6):535.e13–20.
177. Mehr DR, van der Steen JT, Kruse RL, Ooms ME, Rantz M, Ribbe MW. Lower respiratory infections in nursing home residents with dementia: a tale of two countries. Gerontologist. 2003;43(Spec No 2):85–93.
178. Stall NM, Fischer HD, Fung K, Giannakeas V, Bronskill SE, Austin PC, et al. Sex-specific differences in end-of-life burdensome interventions and antibiotic therapy in nursing home residents with advanced dementia. JAMA Netw Open. 2019;2(8):e199557.
179. Comas-Herrera A, Zalakaín J, Litwin C, Hsu AT, Lemmon E, Henderson D et al. Mortality associated with COVID-19 outbreaks in care homes: early international evidence. International Long-term Care Policy Network. 2020. https://ltccovid.org/2020/04/12/mortality-associated-with-covid-19-outbreaks-in-care-homes-early-international-evidence/. Accessed Jul 26 2020.
180. Bianchetti A, Rozzini R, Guerini F, Boffelli F, Ranieri P, Minelli G, et al. Clinical presentation of COVID19 in dementia patients. J Nutr Health Aging. 2020;24:1–3.
181. Atkins JL, Masoli JAH, Delgado J, Pilling LC, Kuo CLC, Kuchel G, et al. Preexisting comorbidities predicting severe COVID-19 in older adults in the UK Biobank community cohort. Biorxiv. 2020;75(11):2224–30. https://doi.org/10.1101/2020.05.06.20092700.
182. McMichael TM, Currie DW, Clark S, Pogosjans S, Kay M, Schwartz NG, et al. Epidemiology of covid-19 in a long-term care facility in king county, Washington. New Engl J Med. 2020;382(21):2005–11.
183. Lithander FE, Neumann S, Tenison E, Lloyd K, Welsh TJ, Rodrigues JCL, et al. COVID-19 in older people: a rapid clinical review. Age Ageing. 2020;49(4):501–15.
184. De Biase S, Cook L, Skelton DA, Witham M, ten Hove R. The COVID-19 rehabilitation pandemic. Age Ageing. 2020;49(5):696–700. https://doi.org/10.1093/ageing/afaa118.
185. Arons MM, Hatfield KM, Reddy SC, Kimball A, James A, Jacobs JR, et al. Presymptomatic SARS-CoV-2 infections and transmission in a skilled nursing facility. New Engl J Med. 2020;382(22):2081–90.
186. British Geriatrics Society. COVID-19: managing the COVID-19 pandemic in care homes for older people. British Geriatrics Society. 2020. https://www.bgs.org.uk/resources/covid-19-managing-the-covid-19-pandemic-in-care-homes. Accessed Jul 26 2020.
187. Blackman C, Farber S, Feifer RA, Mor V, White EM. An illustration of SARS-CoV-2 dissemination within a skilled nursing facility using heat maps. J Am Geriatr Soc. 2020;68(10):2174–8. https://doi.org/10.1111/jgs.16642.
188. Rockwood K, Song X, MacKnight C, Bergman H, Hogan DB, McDowell I, et al. A global clinical measure of fitness and frailty in elderly people. CMAJ. 2005;173(5):489–95.
189. National Institute for Health and Care Excellence. COVID-19 rapid guideline: critical care in adults. [London]: NICE; 2020 [cited 2020 Jul 26]. (NICE guideline [NG159]). Available from: https://www.nice.org.uk/guidance/ng159

190. Li Y, Temkin-Greener H, Gao S, Cai X. COVID-19 infections and deaths among Connecticut nursing home residents: facility correlates. J Am Geriatr Soc. 2020;68(9):1899–906. https://doi.org/10.1111/jgs.16689.
191. Stone PW, Clarke SP, Cimiotti J, Correa-de-Araujo R. Nurses' working conditions: implications for infectious disease. Emerg Infect Dis. 2004;10(11):1984–9.
192. Van Houtven CH, DePasquale N, Coe NB. Essential long-term care workers commonly hold second jobs and double- or triple-duty caregiving roles. J Am Geriatr Soc. 2020;68(8):1657–60. https://doi.org/10.1111/jgs.16509.
193. Barnett ML, Grabowski DC. Nursing homes are ground zero for COVID-19 pandemic. JAMA Health Forum. 2020;1(3):e200369.
194. Hooper MW, Nápoles AM, Pérez-Stable EJ. COVID-19 and racial/ethnic disparities. JAMA. 2020;323(24):2466–7.
195. van Dorn A, Cooney RE, Sabin ML. COVID-19 exacerbating inequalities in the US. Lancet. 2020;395(10232):1243–4.

17 End-of-Life Care in Patients with Advanced Dementia

Marie-José H. E. Gijsberts and Wilco Achterberg

List of Abbreviations

ACP	Advance care planning
BPSD	Behavioural and psychological symptoms of dementia
EOLD-CAD	End-of-Life in Dementia-Comfort Assessment in Dying
EOLD-SWC	End-of-Life in Dementia-Satisfaction with Care
FPCS	Family Perceptions of Care Scale
FPPFC	Family Perception of Physician-Family caregiver Communication
MSSE	Mini-Suffering State Examination
PAIC15	Pain Assessment in Cognitive Impairment

Introduction

Determining when an individual with dementia has entered the end-of-life stage is often difficult as a gradual decline in health and frailty are generally part of the disease trajectory. It is not uncommon for the advanced stage of dementia to last several years. A recently developed model using indicators of survival probability: higher age, male, increased comorbidity burden, lower cognitive function at diagnosis and non-Alzheimer dementia (e.g. frontotemporal dementia or Lewy body

M.-J. H. E. Gijsberts (✉)
Faculty of Medicine, Vrije Universiteit Brussel, Brussels, Belgium
e-mail: Marie-Jose.Gijsberts@vub.be

W. Achterberg
Department of Public Health and Primary Care, Leiden University Medical Center, Leiden, The Netherlands
e-mail: W.P.Achterberg@lumc.nl

K. S. Frederiksen, G. Waldemar (eds.), *Management of Patients with Dementia*,
https://doi.org/10.1007/978-3-030-77904-7_17

dementia) can provide physicians and others with an estimation of life expectancy [1].

Good quality care for patients with dementia is chiefly defined as person-centred care designed to relieve biomedical and physical symptoms, but that also takes psychological, social and spiritual issues in to consideration:

> Person-centred care should not only be directed at compensating for what people with dementia cannot do, but also at facilitating their interests, pleasure and use of their capacities. Thus, as research progresses beyond caregiving to embrace the wider concepts outlined by Kitwood, person-centred care may become a facilitator for people with dementia to live life as fully as possible, whether they are supported in the own home or in a care home. [2]

The relative importance of these aspects of care will vary across time as well as between patients, changing in keeping with the individual's experience of dementia. Although physical concerns and treatments may be given more attention at the time of diagnosis and in the terminal phase, it is important to focus on them in all phases of the disease, keeping in mind that expressing discomfort in stages that are not end of life can be equally challenging. Thc inclination is to view challenging behaviour as a medical problem to address with medication. Behavioural and psychosocial symptoms of dementia (BPSD), including challenging behaviour, however, require a person-centred diagnostic approach that incorporates the biomedical domain. Conclusions on the underlying causes should only be made based if the evidence supports them or if arguments can be made that the behaviour is caused by a specific underlying cause. This type of approach may limit the risk of medicalisation and of overlooking serious but treatable medical causes [3]. The social aspects of dementia care primarily concern the people with dementia themselves and involve their capacity to meet their potential and fulfil their obligations; their ability to manage life with some degree of independence; and participation in social activities [4]. Social aspects also comprise supporting family caregivers, keeping them informed, ensuring their participation in advance care planning (ACP) and offering support as they gradually lose their loved, an aspect that remains important throughout the disease trajectory. Studies show that a good match between care providers and families in need of support leads to better quality of care [5]. At the time of diagnosis spiritual concerns may arise as an existential crisis, while at the end of life the need for reconciliation and being at peace with the life they lived may develop, making spiritual and religious support increasingly important as death becomes imminent [3].

Where people die when they have dementia differs greatly between countries. A study of five European countries showed that a majority of people with dementia died in long-term care facilities, ranging from 50.2% in Wales to 92.3% in the Netherlands, 89.4% of whom died in a specialised nursing home and 10.6% in a general care home for older adults. More people with dementia died in hospital in the United Kingdom (England 36.0%; Wales 46.3%; Scotland 33.9%) and Belgium (22.7%) than in the Netherlands (2.8%). In Belgium 11.4% died at home, while 5% or less did so in the other countries. Less than 1% died in a hospice [6]. A 2014 study performed in 14 European and non-European countries reported that death in long-term care facilities was highest in the Netherlands (93.1%) and lowest in Korea (5.5%). There were no deaths in long-term care reported in Hungary and Mexico. Death in hospital was highest in Korea (73.0%) and lowest in the Netherlands (3.8%). Dying at home with dementia was highest in Mexico (69.3%), and lowest in Canada (3.4%), while death with dementia in a hospice setting was highest in the USA (2.9%) [7]. The disease trajectory varies depending on comorbidities, type of dementia and other factors [8]. Often, dementia follows a pattern of decline, leading to frailty and severe disabilities in the last years of life, with a substantial deterioration in function (e.g. increased ADL dependency) in the last months of life. Concurrent illnesses may accelerate the decline but generally patients suffer a steady "prolonged dwindling" [9]. Some patients, however, will not live to advanced stages and may die with mild dementia.

As the disease progresses, the prioritisation of care goals may change. Three care goals stand out when health declines, also in dementia: prolonging life, maintaining function and maximising comfort [10]. At the end of life, when the first two goals are no longer relevant, comfort care is the best option. Figure 17.1, which depicts how care goals and priorities change during the various stages of dementia, illustrates how some care goals may apply simultaneously but are of varying relevance depending on the stage of dementia. For example, with moderate dementia the three goals may apply simultaneously, though maintenance of function and maximisation of comfort can be prioritised over prolongation of life. In end-of-life care,

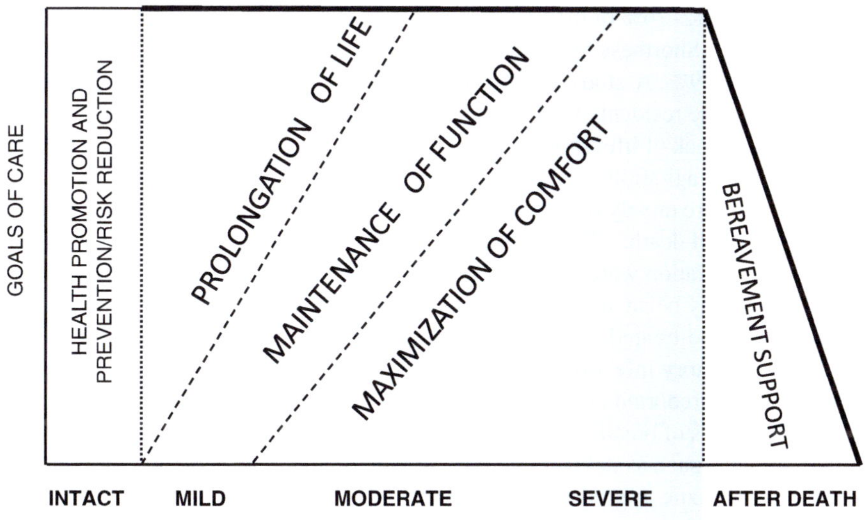

Fig. 17.1 Dementia progression and suggested prioritisation of care goals (Source: van der Steen et al. [9]). An evaluation of palliative care contents in national dementia strategies in reference to the European Association for Palliative Care white paper; First published online 13 February 2015. Miharu Nakanishi, Taeko Nakashima, Yumi Shindo, Yuki Miyamoto, Dianne Gove, Lukas Radbruch, and Jenny T. van der Steen. International Psychogeriatrics (2015), 27:9, 1551–1561 C [1] International Psychogeriatric Association 2015. doi:10.1017/S1041610215000150

maximisation of comfort is the most appropriate care goal. Comfort care does not aim to hasten death or to prolong life, which means it does not preclude treating health issue such as infections with antibiotics, as this may be the best way to resolve burdensome symptoms. This type of goal-oriented approach may simplify ACP discussions and the process of shared decision making for professionals, family caregivers and patients [9].

Domains of Good End-of-Life Care in Dementia

Concordant with major studies and publications, the following domains of end of-life care in dementia are currently being promoted: (1) optimal treatment of physical symptoms, providing comfort, avoiding burdensome or futile treatment, (2) optimal treatment of challenging behaviour BPSD, (3) social support, family support and involvement in care, (4) spiritual support and (5) ACP and shared decision making [3, 9].

1. *Optimal treatment of physical symptoms, providing comfort and avoiding burdensome or futile treatment*
   Pain and shortness of breath frequently occur in patients with dementia at the end of life [8], with a prevalence that is about as frequent as in other diseases, such as cancer, acquired immunodeficiency syndrome, chronic obstructive pulmonary disease, heart disease and renal disease [11]. For instance, two studies show that pain occurs 12–76% of the time in people with dementia, and in 35–96% in cancer patients. Shortness of breath is reported in dementia in 8–80% of the time, in cancer 12–79%. A study on symptom prevalence and prescribed treatment in nursing home residents with dementia, and their association with quality of life in the last week of life, showed that pain was the most common symptom (52%), followed by agitation (35%) and shortness of breath (35%). Pain and shortness of breath were mostly treated with opioids and agitation mainly with anxiolytics. On the day of death, 77% received opioids and 21% received palliative sedation. Pain and agitation were associated with lower quality of life [1]. Since shortness of breath may be an alarming symptom, it may attract more attention from caregivers and be treated early, contributing to better quality of dying [12]. Death from respiratory infection was associated with the largest symptom burden, and studies have reported undertreatment of symptoms, specifically treatment of pain and shortness of breath with opioids, possibly due to concerns about undesirable side effects, such as delirium [1, 9].

   Symptomatic treatment trends, such as symptom relief in patients with dementia with pneumonia, for example, with antipyretics are becoming more common, providing more comfort for the patient [9]. Other reported conditions are aspiration and pressure ulcers, especially in nursing home residents. Although undertreatment of symptoms is reported to be a concern, overtreatment with burdensome interventions is also a concern, and a supportive or palliative approach may be more applicable than hospital admission in older people with dementia

[13]. Tube feeding and antibiotics are an example of areas where under- or over-treatment occur. Using antibiotics in severe dementia at end of life is a complex choice, as they may prolong life but often only for days, which is why complex treatment decisions should take into account that death may be delayed death but the dying process prolonged [14]. A prognostic model that includes gender, respiratory rate, respiratory difficulty, pulse rate, decreased alertness, fluid intake, eating dependency and pressure sores as variables has been developed and tested to support physicians in predicting the mortality risk in nursing home residents. The model allows physicians to substantiate the initiation of palliative care when applicable [15]. In several countries, patients with dementia are sent to the emergency department or hospitalised shortly before death, and sometimes even admitted to an intensive care unit [16]. In this prospective study, within 1.5 years, more than half of the residents had infectious episodes, and 86% had eating problems. Survival was poor after the onset of these complications. Families and caregivers must be told that the underlying cause of death will be a major illness, in this case dementia, and that using potentially burdensome interventions of unclear benefit, such as tube feeding and hospitalisation, in nursing home residents with advanced dementia nearing the end of life is not recommended. In Israel, a quarter of all resources in medical wards are used on patients with dementia in the last stage of disease, and shared decision making and ACP may prevent burdensome interventions and hospitalisations [17]. Shared decision making and ACP may also prevent the use of medication that is no longer useful, which is unfortunately still a widespread practice in many countries [18].

2. *Optimal treatment of challenging behaviour and BPSD*
   Agitation, which also frequently occurs in patients with dementia at the end of life, is less often assessed in studies on the last phase of life but may be as common as pain and shortness of breath [8]. Agitation may be related to other problems, such as cognitive impairment, depression or pain. A study showed that comprehensive training in behavioural management, where pain medication is the first consideration, resulted in less observed pain [19], improved behaviour and reduced use of psychotropic medication [20]. Other BPSD, including behaviour that may be problematic for the patient, such as apathy, are another important aspect of dementia [9]. A multidisciplinary palliative approach may be helpful in anticipating, assessing and managing problems. With challenging behaviour, integrating specific expertise from geriatrics and dementia care specialists is recommended, just as (clinical) psychology can play a significant role. Evidence shows that a stepwise approach with a combination of medical and psychosocial interventions is most useful [19, 21].
3. *Social support, family support and involvement in care*
   An example of family support is providing social support when relatives suffer from caregiver burden and perhaps struggle to combine caring with their other obligations. They may also need support with the institutionalisation of the patient, when a major decline in health occurs and death is near. Families may need education regarding the progressive course of the dementia and (palliative

care) treatment options. This should be a continuous process addressing specific needs in different stages that is based on an assessment of how receptive the family is to learn more. Families need support in their new role as (future) proxy decision maker. They may also need education and support in dealing with patient's challenging behaviours [9].

Family involvement should be encouraged as many families wish to be involved in care, even when the patient is admitted to a long-term care home. Professional caregivers should have an understanding of family needs related to suffering from chronic or prolonged grief through the various stages, and with evident decline. In addition, bereavement support should be offered. Following the death of the patient, family members should be allowed adequate time to adjust after often a prolonged period of caring for the patient. Taking care of the body of their deceased loved one may be a first step in this process [9]. Some interesting and promising interventions have been developed, such as Reclaiming Yourself, a structured writing tool for bereaved spouses of people with dementia that captures the overall bereavement experience, describing the need for both continuity and growth as the spouses renegotiate life and their identity after the end of caregiving and the death of their loved one. The tool guides and encourages reflection on these themes: experiences as a caregiver, navigating regrets, changes in oneself, personal strength and support networks [22].

4. *Spiritual support*

   A consensus definition of spirituality is: "the dynamic dimension of human life that relates to the way persons (individual and community) experience, express and/or seek meaning, purpose and transcendence, and the way they connect to the moment, to self, to others, to nature, to the significant and/or the sacred" [23]. Although this appears to be a rather abstract concept in the context of patients with severe dementia at the end of their lives, it may still be particularly important for their well-being.

   A variety of interventions can support patients with dementia in terms of their spiritual well-being. For example, spiritual caregiving in dementia should as a minimum include an assessment of religious affiliation and involvement, sources of support and spiritual well-being. Patients and their families can provide this information upon admittance to a nursing home, e.g. in the form of a biography (life story) that includes meaningful events and encounters, positive and negative, and sources of support (e.g. people, but also religious or spiritual support). A concrete example is life story work, which is intended to underpin person-centred care in dementia [24]. If the patient is in spiritual distress, referral to experienced spiritual counsellors, psychologists or social workers working in nursing homes may be appropriate when available [9, 25]. Conversations and possibly rituals with such professionals may be beneficial not only to the patient and their loved ones but provide essential information that may also be supportive to families and professionals.

   Paying attention to familiar religious rituals, artefacts and symbols may give people a deep sense of connection with the significance of their religion. Singing hymns or religious songs, praying, reading the *Bible*, *Koran*, *Tora* or other religious books, holding a rosary or other holy artefact, looking at a statue of Buddha or the Virgin Mary, may provide a meaningful connection not based on overt cognition [9].

Our connectedness to and knowing of ourselves is expressed and constituted through the narrative of our lives. Our selves are held within a web of narratives, which is why it is important to facilitate people with dementia in sharing their life narratives, to co-construct their life stories with their loved ones [26]. By inviting nursing home residents with dementia to tell their life stories, or even early memories, they are invited to make sense of themselves and of their place in the world. This may support their self-worth, reduce anxiety, improve their mood and boost the way they feel. Through spiritual reminiscence, the personal narrative and the importance of spirituality may be explored, even in severe dementia. Mackinlay and Trevitt developed a practical guide that teaches caregivers how to facilitate engaging and stimulating spiritual reminiscence sessions with older people, particularly people with dementia. The guide provides a set of questions and discussion topics for a 6-week group programme that contains step-by-step strategies to prompt discussions on grief, guilt, fears, regrets, joys and issues concerning death and dying, giving meaning, hope and perspective to the experiences and feelings of people living with dementia [27].

5. *ACP and shared decision making*

ACP and shared decision making may help in providing person-centred care that maximises comfort for patient and families at the end of life [28]. ACP may be defined as: "a continuous, dynamic process of reflection and dialogue between an individual, those close to them and their healthcare professionals, concerning the individual's preferences and values concerning future treatment and care, including end-of-life care" [29]. Despite recognition of the importance of ACP, it still happens infrequently. Within the ACP process, a three-step systematic approach to shared decision making may be helpful in supporting decisions on treatment choices. In step one, all relevant information can be shared with patients and their families; second, treatment options can be described to aid them in the process of deliberating treatment choices; and in the last step, patients and their families can be given help to explore their preferences and make decisions [30]. The literature identifies these key triggers for ACP conversations: admission to a nursing home, initiation of palliative care, deterioration of the condition or upon request. Specifically, for dementia, key moments might be the period around diagnosis, while discussing the overall general care plan and/or when changes occur in health status, place of residence or financial situation [29]. As dementia progresses, cognitive activity and abstract thinking may become more and more difficult. This does not preclude ACP but does make discussing it more difficult, especially at the end of life. Consequently, it is important to adjust the communication style and content to suit the individual's current level, just as it is best to hold ACP conversations on several occasions over a period of time. In addition, healthcare professionals should include significant people in the patient's life in ACP and people with the ability to be involved in ACP conversations and to become surrogate decision makers [29]. In nursing homes, ACP was found to positively influence the quality of care and provide greater harmony between residents at the end of lives, their loved ones and continuity of care. Similar interventions in the outside community improved the quality of life for patients but did not influence the level of compliance between patient wishes and the care provided [31].

The Use of Measurement Instruments in End-of-Life Dementia Care

People with end-stage dementia often have difficulty expressing their level of comfort verbally, and since comfort care is the primary care goal, validated measurement instruments can aid in monitoring and providing optimal care. The End-of-Life in Dementia-Satisfaction with Care and the Family Perceptions of Care Scale, which are the most valid and reliable for measuring quality of care, are administered by family members in the last month of life and validated in nursing home/long-term care populations. The End-of-Life in Dementia-Comfort Assessment in Dying and Mini-Suffering State Examination are valuable for measuring quality of dying [32, 33].

Developed internationally, validated in a population of people with dementia and administered by nurses, the Pain Assessment in Cognitive Impairment scale [34, 35] specifically assesses pain in dementia, and its use in practice is promising [36]. A short training in using the instrument's facial descriptor items is required.

As physician communication with family caregivers is essential at the end of life, the Family Perception of Physician-Family caregiver Communication instrument can be of importance in assessing family perceptions of communication between physicians and family caregivers [37]. To evaluate the knowledge of the staff on palliative care, the Palliative Care Survey is also a useful tool [38]. Finally, the functional assessment of chronic illness therapy—spiritual well-being scale, which is self-administered by patients and validated in nursing home residents with and without dementia, is valuable for assessing spiritual aspects in patients with dementia [39].

In summary, an increasing amount of scientific evidence supports the use of measuring instruments in end-of-life care in dementia (Table 17.1).

Conclusion

In end-of-life care for patients with advanced dementia, person-centred care is preferred that focuses on biomedical, psychological, social and spiritual concerns. Comfort care is the most appropriate care goal. Important domains in good end-of-life care in dementia are: physical symptoms (most frequently pain and shortness of breath). Psychological concerns may be overlooked or medicalised. Agitation, a neuro-psychiatric symptom that often occurs at the end of life in dementia, may be related to other issues. A stepwise approach that contains a combination of medical

Table 17.1 Overview of relevant instruments in end-of-life dementia care

Measurement instrument	Measuring	Validated in population	Respondent
EOLD-SWC	Quality of care	Nursing home residents with advanced dementia	Family
FPCS	Quality of care	Long-term care facility residents	Family
EOLD-CAD	Quality of dying	NH residents with advanced dementia	Family/ professionals
MSSE	Quality of dying	Patients with dementia	Family/ professionals
PAIC15	Pain	Persons with dementia	Nurses
FACIT-Sp	Spirituality	Nursing home residents with/without dementia	Patients
FPPFC	Physician communication with family	Long-term care facility residents who passed away	Family

EOLD-CAD End-of-Life in Dementia-Comfort Assessment in Dying, *FPPFC* Family Perception of Physician-Family caregiver Communication, *MSSE* Mini-Suffering State Examination, *EOLD-SWC* End-of-Life in Dementia-Satisfaction with Care, *FPCS* Family Perceptions of Care Scale, *PAIC15* Pain Assessment in Cognitive Impairment, *EOLD-SWC* End-of-Life in Dementia-Satisfaction with Care

and psychological interventions appears to be the most useful for these symptoms. In the social domain, family support, family education, family involvement in caregiving and bereavement support are cornerstones of good patient-centred care. Spiritual support should at least involve an assessment of religious affiliation and involvement, but also focus on familiar religious rituals, artefacts and symbols, in addition to the life narrative of the patient, using spiritual reminiscence to explore this, also in severe dementia. ACP and the three-step systematic approach of shared decision making may be supportive in providing person-centred care that makes the patient at the end of life and their families as comfortable as possible. The use of measurement instruments is helpful in end-of-life care for patients with dementia who often have difficulty verbally expressing their level of comfort for in the end stage of the disease. Validated and reliable instruments are available to assess quality of care and dying, pain and spirituality, physician communication with family caregivers and staff knowledge on palliative care to help achieve the aim of good comfort care that is person-centred.

References

1. Haaksma ML, Eriksdotter M, Rizzuto D, Leoutsakos J-MS, Olde Rikkert MGM, Melis RJF, Garcia-Ptacek S. Survival time tool to guide care planning in people with dementia. Neurology. 2020;94:e538–48. https://doi.org/10.1212/WNL.0000000000008745.
2. Vernooij-Dassen M, Moniz-Cook E. Person-centred dementia care: moving beyond caregiving. Aging Ment Health. 2016;20(7):667–8. https://doi.org/10.1080/13607863.2016.1154017.

3. Houttekier D, Cohen J, Bilsen J, Addington-Hall J, Onwuteaka-Philipsen BD, Deliens J. Place of death of older persons with dementia. A study in five European countries. JAGS. 2010;58(4):751–6. https://doi.org/10.1111/j.1532-5415.2010.02771.x.
4. Dröes RM, Chattat R, Diaz A, Gove D, Graff M, Murphy K, Verbeek H, Vernooij-Dassen M, Clare L, Johannessen A, Roes M, Verhey F, Charras K. Social health and dementia: a European consensus on the operationalization of the concept and directions for research and practice. Aging Ment Health. 2017;21(1):4–17. https://doi.org/10.1080/13607863.2016.1254596.
5. Dam AEH, Boots LMM, Boxtel MPJ, Verhey FRJ, de Vugt ME. A mismatch between supply and demand of social support in dementia care: a qualitative study on the perspectives of spousal caregivers and their social network members. Int Psychogeriatr. 2018;30(6):881–92. https://doi.org/10.1017/S1041610217000898.
6. Hendriks SA, Smalbrugge M, Hertogh CM, van der Steen JT. Dying with dementia: symptoms, treatment, and quality of life in the last week of life. J Pain Symptom Manag. 2014;47(4):710–20. https://doi.org/10.1016/j.jpainsymman.2013.05.015.
7. Reyniers T, Deliens L, Pasman LH, Morin L, Addington-Hall J, Frova L, Cardenas-Turanzas M, Onwuteaka-Philipsen B, Naylor W, Ruiz-Ramos M, Wilson DM, Loucka M, Csikos A, Joo Rhee Y, Teno J, Cohen J, Houttekier D. International variation in place of death of older people who died from dementia in 14 European and non-European countries. J Am Med Dir Assoc. 2015;16(2):165–71. https://doi.org/10.1016/j.jamda.2014.11.003.
8. van der Steen JT. Dying with dementia: what we know after more than a decade of research. J Alzheimers Dis. 2010;22(1):37–55. https://doi.org/10.3233/JAD-2010-100744.
9. van der Steen JT, Radbruch L, Hertogh CM, de Boer ME, Hughes JC, Larkin P, Francke AL, Jünger S, Gove D, Firth P, Koopmans RT, Volicer L. White paper defining optimal palliative care in older people with dementia: a Delphi study and recommendations from the European Association for Palliative Care. European Association for Palliative Care (EAPC). Palliat Med. 2014;28(3):197–209. https://doi.org/10.1177/0269216313493685. Epub 2013 Jul 4.PMID: 23828874.
10. Gillick MR. Adapting advance medical planning for the nursing home. J Palliat Med. 2004;7(2):357–61. https://doi.org/10.1089/109662104773709521.
11. Solano JP, Gomes B, Higginson IJ. A comparison of symptom prevalence in far advanced cancer, AIDS, heart disease, chronic obstructive pulmonary disease and renal disease. J Pain Symptom Manag. 2006;31(1):58–69. https://doi.org/10.1016/j.jpainsymman.2005.06.007.
12. Caprio AJ, Hanson LC, Munn JC, et al. Pain, dyspnea, and the quality of dying in long-term care. J Am Geriatr Soc. 2008;56:683e688.
13. Sampson EL, Leurent B, Blanchard MR, Jones L, King M. Survival of people with dementia after unplanned acute hospital admission: a prospective cohort study. Int J Geriatr Psychiatry. 2013;28(10):1015–22. https://doi.org/10.1002/gps.3919.
14. van der Steen JT, Lane P, Kowall NW, Knol DL, Volicer L. Antibiotics and mortality in patients with lower respiratory infection and advanced dementia. J Am Med Dir Assoc. 2012;13(2):156–61. https://doi.org/10.1016/j.jamda.2010.07.001.
15. Rauh SP, Heymans MW, van der Maaden T, Mehr DR, Kruse RL, de Vet HCW, van der Steen JT. Predicting mortality in nursing home residents with dementia and pneumonia treated with antibiotics: validation of a prediction model in a more recent population. J Gerontol A Biol Sci Med Sci. 2019;74(12):1922–8. https://doi.org/10.1093/gerona/gly260.
16. Mitchell SL, Teno JM, Kiely DK, et al. The clinical course of advanced dementia. N Engl J Med. 2009;361(16):1529–38. https://doi.org/10.1056/NEJMoa0902234.
17. Salz IW, Carmeli Y, Levin A, Fallach N, Braun T, Amit S. Elderly bedridden patients with dementia use over one quarter of resources in internal medicine wards in an Israeli hospital. Isr J Health Policy Res. 2020;9(1):21. https://doi.org/10.1186/s13584-020-00379-0.
18. Rausch C, Hoffmann F. Prescribing medications of questionable benefit prior to death: a retrospective study on older nursing home residents with and without dementia in Germany. Eur J Clin Pharmacol. 2020;76(6):877–85. https://doi.org/10.1007/s00228-020-02859-3.
19. Pieper MJC, van der Steen JT, Francke AL, Scherder EJA, Twisk JWR, Achterberg WP. Effects on pain of a stepwise multidisciplinary intervention (STA OP!) that targets pain and behavior

in advanced dementia: a cluster randomized controlled trial. Palliat Med. 2018;32(3):682–92. https://doi.org/10.1177/0269216316689237.
20. Pieper MJC, Francke AL, van der Steen JT, Scherder EJA, Twisk JWR, Kovach CR, Achterberg WP. Effects of a stepwise multidisciplinary intervention for challenging behavior in advanced dementia: a cluster randomized controlled trial. J Am Geriatr Soc. 2016;64(2):261–9. https://doi.org/10.1111/jgs.13868.
21. Zwijsen SA, Gerritsen DL, Eefsting JA, Smalbrugge M, Hertogh CMPM, Pot AM. Coming to grips with challenging behaviour: a cluster randomised controlled trial on the effects of a new care programme for challenging behaviour on burnout, job satisfaction and job demands of care staff on dementia special care units. Int J Nurs Stud. 2015;52(1):68–74. https://doi.org/10.1016/j.ijnurstu.2014.10.003.
22. Peacock S, Bayly M, Gibson K, Holtslander L, Thompson G, O'Connell M. Development of a bereavement intervention for spousal carers of persons with dementia: the Reclaiming Yourself tool. Dementia (London). 2020;20(2):653–71. https://doi.org/10.1177/1471301220909604.
23. Nolan S, Saltmarsh P, Leget C. Spiritual care in palliative care: working towards an EAPC Task Force. Eur J Palliat Care. 2011;18(2):86–9.
24. McKinney A. The value of life story work for staff, people with dementia and family members. Nurs Older People. 2017;29(5):25–9. https://doi.org/10.7748/nop.2017.e899.
25. Gijsberts MJHE, van der Steen JT, Hertogh CMPM, Deliens L. Spiritual care provided by nursing home physicians: a nationwide survey. BMJ Support Palliat Care. 2019; https://doi.org/10.1136/bmjspcare-2018-001756.
26. Baldwin C. Narrative, supportive care, and dementia: a preliminary exploration. In: Hughes JC, Lloyd-Williams M, Sachs GA, editors. Supportive care for the person with dementia. Oxford: Oxford University Press. isbn:978019955413.
27. Mackinlay E, Trevitt C. Finding meaning in the experience of dementia: the place of spiritual reminiscence work. London: Jessica Kingsley; 2012. isbn:9781849052481
28. Dening KH, Sampson EL, De Vries K. Advance care planning in dementia: recommendations for healthcare professionals. Palliat Care Soc Pract. 2019; https://doi.org/10.1177/1178224219826579.
29. Piers R, Albers G, Gilissen J, De Lepeleire J, Steyaert J, Van Mechelen W, Steeman E, Dillen L, Vanden Berghe P, Van den Block L. Advance care planning in dementia: recommendations for healthcare professionals. BMC Palliat Care. 2018;17:88. https://doi.org/10.1186/s12904-018-0332-2.
30. Elwyn G, Frosch D, Thomson R, Joseph-Williams D, Lloyd A, Kinnersley P, Cording E, Tomson D, Dodd C, Rollnick S, Edwards A, Barry M. Shared decision making: a model for clinical practice. J Gen Intern Med. 2012;27(10):1361–7. https://doi.org/10.1007/s11606-012-2077-6.
31. Kelly AJ, Luckett T, Clayton JM, Gabb L, Kochovska S, Agar M. Advance care planning in different settings for people with dementia: a systematic review and narrative synthesis. Palliat Support Care. 2019;17(6):707–19. https://doi.org/10.1017/S1478951519000257.
32. Pivodic L, Smets T, Van den Noortgate N, et al. Quality of dying and quality of end-of-life care of nursing home residents in six countries: an epidemiological study. Palliat Med. 2018;32(10):1584–95. https://doi.org/10.1177/0269216318800610.
33. van Soest-Poortvliet MC, van der Steen JT, Zimmerman S, et al. Psychometric properties of instruments to measure the quality of end-of-life care and dying for long-term care residents with dementia. Qual Life Res. 2012;21(4):671–84. https://doi.org/10.1007/s11136-011-9978-4.
34. Corbett A, Achterberg W, Husebo B, Lobbezoo F, de Vet H, Kunz M, Strand I, Constantinou M, Tudose C, Kappesser J, de Waal M, Lautenbacher S. An international road map to improve pain assessment in people with impaired cognition: the development of the Pain Assessment in Impaired Cognition (PAIC) meta-tool. BMC Neurol. 2014;14(1):229. https://doi.org/10.1186/s12883-014-0229-5.
35. Kunz M, de Waal MWM, Achterberg WP, Gimenez-Llort L, Lobbezoo F, Sampson EL, van Dalen-Kok AH, Defrin R, Invitto S, Konstantinovic L, Oosterman J, Petrini L, van der Steen JT, Strand L-I, de Tommaso M, Zwakhalen S, Husebo BS, Lautenbacher S. The Pain Assessment in Impaired Cognition scale (PAIC15): a multidisciplinary and international

approach to develop and test a meta-tool for pain assessment in impaired cognition, especially dementia. Eur J Pain. 2020;24(1):192–208. https://doi.org/10.1002/ejp.1477.
36. Lautenbacher S, Walz AL, Kunz M. Using observational facial descriptors to infer pain in persons with and without dementia. BMC Geriatr. 2018;18(1):88. https://doi.org/10.1186/s12877-018-0773-8.
37. Biola H, Sloane PD, Williams CS, Daaleman TP, Williams SW, Zimmerman S. Physician communication with family caregivers of long-term care residents at the end of life. JAGS. 2007;55(6):846–56. https://doi.org/10.1111/j.1532-5415.2007.01179.x.
38. Van den Block L, Honinx E, Pivodic L, et al. Evaluation of a palliative care program for nursing homes in 7 countries: the PACE cluster-randomized clinical trial. JAMA Intern Med. 2019;180(2):1–10. https://doi.org/10.1001/jamainternmed.2019.5349.
39. Santana-Berlanga NDR, Porcel-Gálvez AM, Botello-Hermosa A, Barrientos-Trigo S. Instruments to measure quality of life in institutionalised older adults: systematic review. Geriatr Nurs. 2020;S0197-4572(20):30054–9. https://doi.org/10.1016/j.gerinurse.2020.01.018.

Systematic Medical Follow-Up of Patients with Dementia

18

Kristian Steen Frederiksen and Gunhild Waldemar

Introduction

Dementia is defined as a syndrome of acquired cognitive decline which causes loss of the ability to carry out activities of daily living independently. However, this definition fails to capture the many ways in which dementia affects the patient with dementia including many aspects of health, and medical issues.

Dementia may be caused by many different underlying conditions, and a majority of these are neurodegenerative disorders. These conditions carry a high likelihood of progression compounding the difficulties in maintaining adequate everyday function and quality of life. In many regions and countries, patients with a dementia disorder, including neurodegenerative dementia disorders, are not followed up regularly by medical specialists, which is in contrast to patients with other comparable disorders such as Parkinson's disease, or cancer. This may be related to the fact that these disorders are considered, to some extent curable, or at least manageable, whereas dementia disorders are not. However, although neurodegenerative dementia disorders are not curable, they are also manageable. For example, symptomatic treatment for Alzheimer's disease or Lewy body dementia, and treatment of cerebrovascular risk factors may slow progression and diagnosing and treating epilepsy may also improve functioning and quality of life. For these and other reasons, a European Academy of Neurology guideline on dementia recently recommended regular medical follow-up for patients with dementia [1].

K. S. Frederiksen (✉) · G. Waldemar
Danish Dementia Research Centre, Department of Neurology, Rigshospitalet, University of Copenhagen, Copenhagen, Denmark
e-mail: Kristian.steen.frederiksen@regionh.dk

K. S. Frederiksen, G. Waldemar (eds.), *Management of Patients with Dementia*,
https://doi.org/10.1007/978-3-030-77904-7_18

Why Is Follow-Up in Patients with Dementia Important

As already mentioned, follow-up in patients may be motivated by a number of reasons which are listed below and further expanded on. See also Fig. 18.1.

Lack of Insight and Cognitive Impairment Many patients with dementia have some degree of lack of insight. It may be partial, or it may be almost complete meaning that patients denies the presence of the disease and the existence of symptoms. This has several adverse effects such as failure to report symptoms or seeking out medical attention when needed. This may be further compounded by cognitive impairment such as memory problems affecting, e.g., compliance. A proactive approach in terms of preplanned follow-up may be necessary and eliciting complaints by enquiring about specific symptoms. As with many other aspects, the caregiver plays a key role in order to safeguard appropriate follow-up.

Co-morbidities Patients with dementia are more likely to suffer from a variety of other disorders compared to age-matched persons. These include epilepsy, diabetes, stroke, atrial fibrillation, falls, thyroid disorders, vision problems, hearing loss, anemia, coronary disease, and infections [2, 3]. Furthermore, dementia patients are more likely to suffer from more than one of these disorders [4]. Adequate management is as important in patients with dementia as in cognitively unimpaired, but for the reasons mentioned in the preceding paragraphs, a number of barriers exist to accomplish this. This may be one of the driving factors behind an increased short-term and long-term mortality following infections in patients with dementia [5]. Management of these and other co-morbidities may help to slow progression and improve functional status and quality of life.

Other Symptoms of Dementia Cognitive impairment in patients with dementia may be accompanied by other symptoms associated with the neurodegenerative disease such as motor symptoms, changes in behavior, and psychiatric symptoms.

Progression Patients with a neurodegenerative disease are likely to progress and develop new or worsening of symptoms which should be monitored in order to be able to institute new treatments or activate stage-appropriate support. Follow-up in a multiprofessional setting will be necessary for some patients.

Information and Patient Education Patients and caregivers need access to continuous information and counseling and may have questions about the disease or emerging, new symptoms.

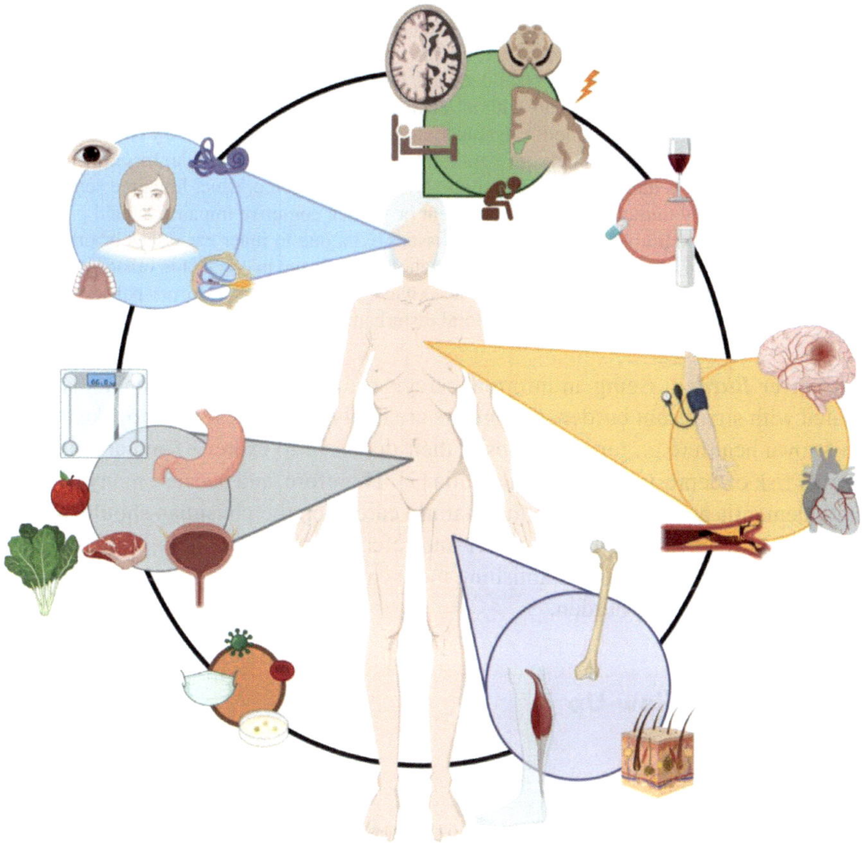

Fig. 18.1 Key elements in the medical follow-up of patients with dementia. Legend: The figure presents an overview of important issues to keep in mind when following up patients with dementia. Green: Assessment of cognitive function is important to assess disease trajectory, including progression from the MCI to dementia stage (together with functional assessment) and dementia staging. Not only the general cognitive functional level must be assessed but also specific domains if there is evidence of impairment (e.g., visuocognitive functions). This may have bearing on the ability of the patient to drive a car. Sleep, mood, other psychiatric and behavioral changes, other neurological signs and symptoms (e.g., hemiparesis, Parkinsonian features) should be evaluated and may elicit initiation of treatment or reconsideration of the initial diagnosis. The clinician should also be vigilant of possible presence of epileptic seizures. Red: Review of medication should be done at each visit. Further, assessing compliance as well as ensuring that the patient is getting help to administer medication in a safe manner is important. Enquiring about alcohol habits and substance abuse should also be considered. Yellow: Vascular risk factors such as hypertension should be screened for and proper pharmacological treatment should be ensured to reduce the risk of cerebro- and cardiovascular disease. Purple: Bone health and disuse atrophy associated with inactivity should be addressed and referral to physiotherapy where appropriate. Skin problems such as bed sores or due to reduced hygiene may be other issues. Orange: Dementia is associated with an increased risk of infections which may have long-lasting negative health consequences. Therefore, it is important to reduce the risk of infections by adequate hygiene, adherence to hygiene guidelines (e.g., hand wash and use of masks), etc. Diagnosing ongoing or recurrent infec-

(continued)

tions is also important. Gray: Weighing patients will help to uncover unintended weight loss, which is a common occurrence in patients with dementia as they may forget to eat or have reduced appetite (e.g., due to side effects of cholinesterase inhibitors). Weight loss may also be due to another underlying disease and this should always be considered. Healthy eating is as important for patients with dementia as patients without dementia. Constipation may be a very bothersome symptom and may be due to autonomic dysfunction such as in patients with Lewy body disease but also due to inappropriate food intake, low fluid intake, or a sedentary lifestyle. Incontinence may be a consequence of dementia, but other causes should be considered. Blue: Impaired senses (i.e., hearing, vision) may mimic cognitive impairment or worsen cognitive impairment and providing aids may improve cognitive function. Balance issues, e.g., due to inner ear issues or orthostatic hypotension (e.g., in Lewy body disease) may be another issue and may result in falls. Teeth decay or ill-fitting dentures (e.g., following weight loss) may give rise to discomfort or pain which may lead to avoidance of food or drink or behavioral disturbances

Caregiver Burden Being an informal caregiver to a patient with dementia is associated with significant burden. Caregivers are likely to have less time to take care of their own health (e.g., for check-ups at their doctor or to exercise) and are also at a higher risk of depression [6] and dementia [7]. Therefore, and because many patients with dementia are dependent on their family caregiver, the physician should also be attentive to the health of the caregiver and refer to appropriate help such as a doctor's appointment. Further, establishing more care in the home or days in a day care center may reduce the burden.

Contents of Follow-Up

Role of Caregivers

The patient should be the focal point of the consultation and it is important always to start by enquiring about how he or she is feeling and experiencing the disease and any complaints the patient may have. The wishes and opinions of the patient should, to the extent possible, be incorporated into any decisions made, and respect for the patients' autonomy and consent is important. Nevertheless, competency and capacity for decisions and the ability to convey an accurate assessment is frequently impaired in patients with dementia. Moreover, any interventions which may be instituted are likely to involve the caregiver, and reliant on the participation of the caregiver. This underlines the importance of involving the caregiver when possible and accepted by the patient. Although some patients with dementia may be able to give an accurate account of their situation, it is important to have the information verified by a caregiver with regular contact to the patient.

Monitoring Disease Progression and Emergence of New Symptoms

Many patients with dementia will have an underlying neurodegenerative disorder with subsequent worsening of symptoms as the disease progresses. Monitoring the progression will help to stage the disease and safeguard the appropriate care in terms of declining activities of daily functions. In patients with MCI, progression to dementia is a significant transitional phase both in medical terms and in everyday life. In patients with Alzheimer's disease, cholinesterase inhibitors may be started, and with progression from mild to moderate stages, memantine may be prescribed. Very rapid decline should give rise to suspicions of a co-morbid condition (e.g., chronic subdural hemorrhage, infection, cardiac disease) or new medication. Affection of specific cognitive functions may also occur and may need to be addressed specifically. For example, language impairment may develop, giving rise to the need for communications aids, difficulties in topographic orientation may be helped by a Global Positioning System device, and visuocognitive impairments may be a concern in terms of, e.g., driving. Non-cognitive symptoms such as motor symptoms (e.g., Parkinsonian symptoms, dyskinesias, gait impairment), autonomic dysfunction (e.g., obstipation, orthostatic hypotension, erectile dysfunction), sleep disorders (e.g., insomnia or Rapid Eye Movement-sleep behavior disorders), epilepsy, delirium, urinary incontinence, etc., are commonly occurring in patients with dementia and should be enquired about when relevant. In some instances, the emergence of new symptoms may lead to the initial diagnosis be reconsidered. Weight loss is common in patients with dementia. This may be due to forgetfulness, reduced appetite, or another underlying disease. Behavioral and psychological symptoms are common also in the initial phases of the dementia disorder and should thus be considered throughout the disease.

Co-morbidities

As already discussed, co-morbidities are common in patients with dementia. Therefore, assessing for these and when discovered, instituting appropriate treatment should be a part of follow-up. Measurement of blood pressure and weighing the patient, and physical and neurological examination are bedside approaches that are important. Moreover, asking the patient and caregiver about specific symptoms is also important such as pain, symptoms of (recurrent) infection, sensory impairment, dental and gum disease, etc., should also be done. Ordering ancillary investigations should be considered (e.g., analysis of blood). In many instances, co-morbidities such as vascular risk factors and pain may be treated according to guidelines for patients without cognitive impairment, but due consideration with regard to compliance and anticholinergic effects are important.

Review of Pharmacological Treatment

Review of pharmacological treatment should also be done at each follow-up as potentially inappropriate prescriptions, polypharmacy, and lower threshold for developing unwanted side effects are common in patients with dementia. We refer to Chap. 6 for further information on the matter.

Alcohol and Other Substance Abuse

A substantial number of patients with dementia will have an ongoing alcohol or other substance abuse at the time of diagnosis. It may be that lifelong alcohol abuse is the main cause of the dementia [8], sometimes as a consequence of Wernicke's encephalopathy. Treatment of the addiction may be complicated by the dementia but should be encouraged as patients with cognitive impairment are likely to be more adversely affected by alcohol than others resulting in cognitive worsening, falls, etc. Starting treatment with disulfiram in patients with dementia will in many instances be inappropriate due to the risk of forgetting, and accidentally ingesting alcohol. Another concern in patients with alcohol abuse is malnourishment leading to vitamin deficiency. Therefore, starting vitamin supplements such as thiamine and B12 vitamin should be considered. It should be highlighted that it is not alcohol that causes the vitamin deficiency, but rather that is takes the place of other sources of nutrients. Therefore, conditions such as Wernicke's encephalopathy may also arise in patients with dementia and no alcohol abuse where the malnutrition results due to other causes. Patients with dementia may also receive medications with a potential for abuse such as benzodiazepines and morphine, and it may be relevant to try and wean off patients if treatment with the medications is not indicated.

Assessment of Competency, Driving, and Other Legal Issues

Assessment of competency is an important aspect of dementia care but may sometimes be neglected by physicians as it is often not straight forward. Competency may be viewed as a process with four core features [9]: (1) understanding (i.e., the ability to comprehend information relevant to a decision), (2) appreciation (i.e., the ability to apply that information to one's own situation); (3) reasoning (i.e., the ability to evaluate the potential consequences of one's own decisions); and (4) expression of choice (i.e., the ability to communicate one's own choices). Clinical competency may be evaluated by specific interviews, vignette methods, neuropsychological tests, but also by general clinical judgement. It is important to keep in mind that competency is not necessarily compromised in patients with dementia, but as the disease progresses, it becomes more likely that it will become compromised. Competency is also dependent on the situation and may be compromised in some situations and not in others depending on, e.g., the complexity of the situation.

An important part of preparing for the future for patients with dementia and their caregivers will include legal matters. Legal issues and possibilities will differ across countries but may include legal wills, and advance directories which may govern how the patient's future life should be organized when the patient will not be able to express his or her wishes. The physician may stimulate the patient to consider these issues and may also be involved in some legal procedures, e.g. to judge whether the patient has preserved capacity. The regulations governing driving in dementia will also differ across countries but may involve the physician. The physician may be tasked with evaluating whether patients with dementia may have retained abilities for driving. In patients with advanced dementia with severe cognitive impairment and impairment of activities of daily living it will often be straight forward to make an accurate assessment. However, in mild cognitive impairment and mild dementia, it becomes more difficult. There are several reasons for this. Firstly, mapping cognitive abilities to driving abilities is complex. Secondly, impairments of specific cognitive domains may have disproportionate impact on driving ability thereby short-circuiting the relationship between the level of cognitive impairment and driving abilities. For example, although most patients with mild cognitive impairment are likely to be able to drive safely, impairment in, e.g., visuospatial abilities or mental speed may severely impact driving abilities but not lead to impairment in activities of daily living. Thirdly, other factors such as behavioral changes or other disabilities may also play a role in the ability to drive. A number of off-road approaches have been tested for the assessment of driving abilities in patients with cognitive impairment such as virtual reality, measurement of reaction time, and neuropsychological assessment and may be a part of the assessment of driving abilities [10–12].

The reason for assessing driving abilities in patients with dementia is to avoid traffic accidents caused by the cognitive impairment of patients with dementia. Given this aspect, it may seem most reasonable to "err on the side of safety" and have a very low threshold for imposing a driving ban. However, a number of countering factors should be kept in mind. For example, for some patients driving is an important part of their identity, enables a higher degree of independence and mobility, and may be a prerequisite for living in rural areas where public transportation is limited or non-existent. Further, estimates of the risk of patients with dementia causing traffic accidents vary between studies and remain uncertain [13, 14]. While the aforementioned should not override a genuine concern for the driving abilities in a patient with dementia, it also constitutes arguments against a blanket driving ban for all patients with dementia.

Ensuring Adequate Support, Information, and Counseling

This section of the chapter deals with important aspects of the care of patients with dementia. However, it is usually not aspects in which the physician will play a major role. Rather, it will often be supplied by primary care teams or similar services. Nevertheless, the physician should be knowledgeable about these aspects.

By definition, all patients with dementia will require some form of support in their life to maintain activities of daily living. In the early stages, the need for practical help and care may be minimal such as helpful reminders or help with medication. However, the need for information and counseling of the patient may be equally higher as the patient may be more capable to comprehend and has a larger need for information about the disease, prognosis, treatment, and legal decisions. This should be readily available optimally both in terms of information delivered at consultations but also as written information. As the dementia progresses, the need for care will usually increase and most patients will need 24-h care at some stage which may be in a care home or similar facility. For patients with family or other networks, care may be delivered by a family member or friend, but often in the advanced stages, formal care becomes inevitable. The transitional phase when the patient moves out of their old home to a new one is, as with the delivery of the diagnosis, often a difficult one which may evoke feelings of sorrow, sadness, anger, feelings of uncertainty and hopelessness for both caregivers and patients. Caregivers which may have been instrumental in the move, may also feel doubt, guilt (e.g., at feeling relieved) and uncertainty in the decision. Patients may feel betrayed by their loved ones. It is important to counsel the patient and caregiver that these emotions are common and that as written above, most patients with dementia will at some point require 24-h care which cannot be delivered at home. Explaining that the new living arrangements may also give opportunities to spend time on those activities that give pleasure and joy, may help to give hope. The need for counseling does not decline, but focus may shift from the patient to informing the caregiver.

Organization of Medical Follow-Up in Patients with Dementia

How medical follow-up is organized is likely to vary greatly across regions and countries [15], due to differences in availability of resources and organization of the general health care system as well as other factors. Optimally, follow-up should be preplanned as patients with dementia may not seek out medical attention. Follow-up in a multiprofessional setting such as a memory clinic would be ideal but is not realistic in most countries (if any). Indeed, for some patients being followed by their general practitioner with easy access to dementia experts may safeguard a fully acceptable level of medical management.

Conclusion

A cure for the underlying disease which causes dementia, is not available for most patient, but managing symptoms and co-morbidities is, and should be ensured by regular and preplanned follow-up with a physician. This will help to overcome some of the barriers for patients with dementia in receiving the adequate diagnostic and treatment opportunities which may present itself. In this chapter we have outlined which elements the physician should consider when seeing patients with dementia for follow-up. This includes addressing comorbidities such as vascular risk factors and epilepsy, information to the patient and caregiver, and legal matters. The caregiver will in most instances play an important role in this process as the informant, coordinator, and ambassador for the patient. Lastly, the physician should be mindful of caregiver burden and stress.

References

1. Frederiksen KS, Cooper C, Frisoni GB, Frölich L, Georges J, Kramberger MG, et al. A European Academy of Neurology guideline on medical management issues in dementia. Eur J Neurol. 2020:1–16. Available from: http://doi.wiley.com/10.1111/ene.14412
2. Clague F, Mercer SW, Mclean G, Reynish E, Guthrie B. Comorbidity and polypharmacy in people with dementia: insights from a large, population-based cross-sectional analysis of primary care data. Age Ageing. 2017;46(1):33–9.
3. Bauer K, Schwarzkopf L, Graessel E, Holle R. A claims data-based comparison of comorbidity in individuals with and without dementia. BMC Geriatr. 2014;14(1):10.
4. Barnett K, Mercer SW, Norbury M, Watt G, Wyke S, Guthrie B. Epidemiology of multimorbidity and implications for health care, research, and medical education: a cross-sectional study. Lancet. 2012;380(9836):37–43. Available from: https://doi.org/10.1016/S0140-6736(12)60240-2
5. Janbek J, Taudorf L, Musaeus CS, Frimodt-Møller N, Laursen TM, Waldemar G. Increased short- and long-term mortality following infections in dementia: a nationwide registry-based cohort study. Eur J Neurol. 2020:ene.14595. Available from: https://onlinelibrary.wiley.com/doi/10.1111/ene.14595
6. Alfakhri AS, Alshudukhi AW, Alqahtani AA, Alhumaid AM, Alhathlol OA, Almojali AI, et al. Depression among caregivers of patients with dementia. Inq J Heal Care Organ Provision Financ. 2018;55:004695801775043. Available from: http://journals.sagepub.com/doi/10.1177/0046958017750432
7. Norton MC, Smith KR, Østbye T, Tschanz JT, Corcoran C, Schwartz S, et al. Greater risk of dementia when spouse has dementia? The Cache County Study. J Am Geriatr Soc. 2010;58(5):895–900. Available from: http://doi.wiley.com/10.1111/j.1532-5415.2010.02806.x
8. Ridley NJ, Draper B, Withall A. Alcohol-related dementia: an update of the evidence. Alzheimers Res Ther. 2013;5(1):3. Available from: http://alzres.biomedcentral.com/articles/10.1186/alzrt157
9. Appelbaum PS. Assessment of patients' competence to consent to treatment. N Engl J Med. 2007;357(18):1834–40. Available from: http://www.nejm.org/doi/abs/10.1056/NEJMcp074045
10. Piersma D, Fuermaier ABM, de Waard D, Davidse RJ, de Groot J, Doumen MJA, et al. Prediction of fitness to drive in patients with Alzheimer's dementia. Ginsberg SD, editor. PLoS One. 2016;11(2):e0149566. Available from: https://dx.plos.org/10.1371/journal.pone.0149566
11. Piersma D, Fuermaier ABM, De Waard D, Davidse RJ, De Groot J, Doumen MJA, et al. Assessing fitness to drive in patients with different types of dementia. Alzheimer Dis Assoc Disord. 2018;32(1):70–5. Available from: https://journals.lww.com/00002093-201801000-00010
12. Fuermaier ABM, Piersma D, de Waard D, Davidse RJ, de Groot J, Doumen MJA, et al. Assessing fitness to drive—a validation study on patients with mild cognitive impairment. Traffic Inj Prev. 2017;18(2):145–9. Available from: https://www.tandfonline.com/doi/full/10.1080/15389588.2016.1232809
13. Fraade-Blanar LA, Ebel BE, Larson EB, Sears JM, Thompson HJ, Chan KCG, et al. Cognitive decline and older driver crash risk. J Am Geriatr Soc. 2018;66(6):1075–1081. Available from: http://doi.wiley.com/10.1111/jgs.15378
14. Petersen JD, Siersma V, Nielsen CT, Vass M, Waldorff FB. Dementia and traffic accidents: a Danish register-based cohort study. JMIR Res Protoc. 2016;5(3):e191. Available from: http://www.researchprotocols.org/2016/3/e191/
15. Frederiksen KS, Nielsen TR, Appollonio I, Andersen BB, Riverol M, Boada M, et al. Biomarker counseling, disclosure of diagnosis and follow-up in patients with mild cognitive impairment: a European Alzheimer's disease consortium survey. Int J Geriatr Psychiatry. 2020;36(2):324–33.

Index

K. S. Frederiksen, G. Waldemar (eds.), *Management of Patients with Dementia*,
https://doi.org/10.1007/978-3-030-77904-7

E

GPSR Compliance

The European Union's (EU) General Product Safety Regulation (GPSR) is a set of rules that requires consumer products to be safe and our obligations to ensure this.

If you have any concerns about our products, you can contact us on ProductSafety@springernature.com

In case Publisher is established outside the EU, the EU authorized representative is:

Springer Nature Customer Service Center GmbH
Europaplatz 3
69115 Heidelberg, Germany

Batch number: 10732076

Printed by Printforce, the Netherlands